MANAGEMENT AND CARE OF
THE CATARACT PATIENT

Management and Care of the Cataract Patient

EDITED BY

FRANK J. WEINSTOCK
MD, FACS
Professor of Ophthalmology,
Northeastern Ohio Universities College of Medicine,
Canton, Ohio; and
Clinical Assistant Professor of Ophthalmology,
The Ohio State University College of Medicine,
Columbus, Ohio

FOREWORD BY

NORMAN S. JAFFE
MD

BOSTON

BLACKWELL SCIENTIFIC PUBLICATIONS

OXFORD LONDON EDINBURGH

MELBOURNE PARIS BERLIN VIENNA

© 1992 by
Blackwell Scientific Publications, Inc.
Editorial offices:
3 Cambridge Center, Cambridge
    Massachusetts 02142, USA
Osney Mead, Oxford OX2 0EL, England
25 John Street, London WC1N 2BL, England
23 Ainslie Place, Edinburgh EH3 6AJ, Scotland
54 University Street, Carlton
    Victoria 3053, Australia

Other editorial offices:
Librairie Arnette SA
2, rue Casimir-Delavigne
75006 Paris
France

Blackwell Wissenschafts-Verlag
Meinekestrasse 4
D-1000 Berlin 15
Germany

Blackwell MZV
Feldgasse 13
A-1238 Wien
Austria

First published 1992

Set by Excel Typesetters Company, Hong Kong
Printed and bound in the United States of America by
Maple-Vail, New York

92 93 94 95   5 4 3 2 1

DISTRIBUTORS

USA
  Blackwell Scientific Publications, Inc.
  3 Cambridge Center
  Cambridge, MA 02142
  (*Orders*: Tel: 800 759-6102
              617 225-0401)

Canada
  Times Mirror Professional Publishing, Ltd
  5240 Finch Avenue East
  Scarborough, Ontario M1S 5A2
  (*Orders*: Tel: 416 298-1588
              800 268-4178)

Australia
  Blackwell Scientific Publications
  (Australia) Pty Ltd
  54 University Street
  Carlton, Victoria 3053
  (*Orders*: Tel: 03 347-0300)

Outside North America and Australia
  Marston Book Services Ltd
  PO Box 87
  Oxford OX2 0DT
  (*Orders*: Tel: 0865 791155
              Fax: 0865 791927
              Telex: 837515)

Library of Congress
Cataloguing-in-Publication Data

Management and care of the cataract patient/
    edited by Frank J. Weinstock.
        p.   cm.
    Includes bibliographical references
    and index.
    ISBN 0-86542-185-4
    1. Cataract—Surgery.   2. Cataract—
Surgery—Patients—Mental health.
    3. Physician and Patient.
    I. Weinstock, Frank J., 1933–
    [DNLM: 1. Cataract—psychology.
    2. Cataract Extraction—adverse effects.
    3. Cataract Extraction—methods.
    4. Cataract Extraction—rehabilitation.
    WW 260 M2657]
    RE451.M345   1992
    617.7'42—dc20
    DNLM/DLC

To my supportive family—wife, Saragale,
and children, Michael, Jill, and Jeffrey—
and to two exemplary surgeons,
my late father, Michael B. Weinstock MD,
and my late father-in-law, Samuel S. Reinglass MD,
both of whom always respected patients
and cared for them as people
demonstrating the ultimate care of
and concern for patients

Contents

List of Contributors

DAVID J. APPLE MD, *Departments of Ophthalmology and Pathology, Center for Intraocular Lens Research, Storm Eye Institute, 171 Ashley Avenue, Medical University of South Carolina, Charleston, SC 29425-2236*

ROBERT C. ARFFA MD, *Department of Ophthalmology, Medical College of Pennsylvania, 320 East North Avenue, Pittsburgh, PA 15212*

FREDERICK C. BLODI MD, *Department of Ophthalmology, University of Iowa Hospitals, Iowa City, IA 52242*

WILLIAM A. BOROVER, *Ophthalmic Practice Improvement, PO Box 506, Chula Vista, CA 92012*

DEBBIE BRANDEL MS, *Preferred Health Strategies, 50 Main Street, Suite 1000, White Plains, NY 10606*

JAMES B. BYRNE JR MD, *Retina and Vitreous Associates of Alabama–Birmingham, 700 18th Street South, Suite 601, Birmingham, AL 35233*

ROBERT J. CIONNI MD, *Cincinnati Eye Institute and Outpatient Eye Surgery Center, 10494 Montgomery Road, Cincinnati, OH 45242*

MICHAEL COBO MD, *Duke Eye Center, PO Box 3802-200, Durham, NC 27710*

AUGUST COLENBRANDER MD, *2340 Clay Street, PPMC Annex, Room 636, San Francisco, CA 94115; Department of Ophthalmology, California Pacific Medical Center*

DAVID B. DAVIS II MD, *Medical–Surgical Eye Center, 1237 B Street, Hayward, CA 94541-2977*

PETER C. DONSHIK MD, FACS, *Division of Ophthalmology, University of Connecticut School of Medicine, Farmington, CT 06032*

WILLIAM H. EHLERS MD, *Division of Ophthalmology, University of Connecticut School of Medicine, Farmington, CT 06032*

MARIANNE E. FEITL MD, *Department of Ophthalmology, Geisinger Medical Center, Danville, PA 17821*

DONALD C. FLETCHER MD, *Department of Ophthalmology, University of Missouri at Kansas City, 2300 Holmes, Kansas City, Missouri 64108*

BARBARA GRENELL PhD, *Preferred Health Strategies, 50 Main Street, Suite 1000, White Plains, NY 10606*

WILLIAM H. HAVENER MD *(deceased), Department of Ophthalmology, Ohio State University College of Medicine, 456 W 10th Avenue, Columbus, OH 43210*

LEE HOFFER PhD, MD, *Rt. #1, Box 368, Bolivar, Ohio 44612; Northeastern Ohio Universities College of Medicine; Barberton Citizens Hospital, Barberton, OH*

WILLIAM L. HOPPES MD, FACP, *Infectious Diseases, Northeastern Ohio Universities, College of Medicine, Affiliated Hospitals of Canton, Medical Center Professionals Building, Suite 322, 1330 Timken Mercy Drive NW, Canton, OH 44708*

NORMAN S. JAFFE MD, *16400 NW 2nd Avenue, North Miami Beach, FL 33169*

MILTON KAHN MD, *Department of Ophthalmology, Lenox Hill Hospital, 100 E 77th Street, New York, NY 10021*

JAMES A. KIMBLE MD, *Retina and Vitreous Associates of Alabama–Birmingham, 700 18th Street South, Suite 601, Birmingham, AL 35233*

MANUS C. KRAFF MD, *Northwestern University, 5600 W. Addison St., Chicago, IL 60634*

RICHARD P. KRATZ MD, *Suite 3011441, Avocado Ave., Newport Beach, CA 92206*

THEODORE KRUPIN MD, *Department of Ophthalmology, Ward Building 2–186, Northwestern University Medical School, Chicago, IL 60611*

SIDNEY LERMAN MD, *New York Medical College, Eye Research Lab, 100 Grasslands Road, Room 41, Valhalla, NY 10595*

EDWARD S. LIM MD, *Department of Ophthalmology, Center for Intraocular Lens Research, Storm Eye Institute, 171 Ashley Avenue, Medical University of South Carolina, Charleston, SC 29425-2236*

NICK MAMALIS MD, *University of Utah, Department of Ophthalmology, Intermountain Ocular Research Center, 50 N Medical Drive, Salt Lake City, UT 84132*

MARK R. MANDEL MD, *Medical–Surgical Eye Center, 1237 B Street, Hayward, CA 94541–2977*

DAVID D. MICHAELS MD, *1441 W. 7th St, San Pedro, CA 90732*

ROBIN C. MORGAN MD, *Department of Ophthalmology, Center for Intraocular Lens Research, Storm Eye Institute, 171 Ashley Avenue, Medical University of South Carolina, Charleston, SC 29425-2236*

MICHAEL A. NOVAK MD, *Retina Associates of Cleveland, Inc., 26900 Cedar Road #303, Beechwood, OH 44122*

STEPHEN A. OBSTBAUM MD, *115 East 39th Street, New York, NY 10016*

ROBERT H. OSHER MD, *Cincinnati Eye Institute and Outpatient Surgery Center, 10494 Montgomery Road, Cincinnati, OH 45242*

SANDER MARC RABIN MD, JD, FCLM, *151 Upton Lake Toad, Clinton Corners, New York 12514*

JAMES G. RAVIN MD, *The Eye Center of Toledo, Suite 100, 3000 Regency Court, Toledo, OH 43623*

JOHN A. RETZLAFF MD, *Medical Eye Centre PC, 2900 Barnett Road, Suite 2, Medford, OR 97504–8331*

THOMAS A. RICE MD, *Retina Associates of Beechwood, Inc., 26900 Cedar Road #303, Cleveland, OH 44122*

GARY S. RUBIN PhD, *Lions Vision Research Center, Johns Hopkins University School of Medicine, 550 North Broadway, Baltimore, MD 21205*

DAVID D. SAGGAU MD, *Wolfe Clinic, 309 E Church Street, Marshalltown, IA 50153*

DONALD R. SANDERS MD, PhD, *University of Illinois at Chicago, 815 W Van Buren, Chicago, IL 60607*

H. JOHN SHAMMAS MD, *3510 Martin Luther King Boulevard, Lynwood, CA 90602*

LAWRENCE J. SINGERMAN MD, *Retina Associates of Cleveland, Inc., 26900 Cedar Road #303, Cleveland, OH 44122*

JAN D. SMITH MB, MRCP, FACP, *University of Pittsburgh School of Medicine, Pittsburgh, PA 15261*

KEVIN G. SMITH MD, *408 South Main Street, Greenville, PA 161125*

THOMAS STANK MD, *804 S Washington, Moscow, Idaho 83843*

WALTER J. STARK MD, *Wilmer Eye Institute, Johns Hopkins University School of Medicine, 600 North Wolfe Street, Baltimore, MD 21205*

RICHARD A. THOFT MD, *203 Lothrop Street, Pittsburgh, PA 15213–2592*

SPENCER P. THORNTON MD, *Mid-State Medical Center, 2010 Church Street, Nashville, TN 37203*

ROBERT L. TOMSAK MD, PhD, *Division of Neuro-Ophthalmology, Department of Neurology, University Hospitals of Cleveland and Case Western Reserve University School of Medicine, 2074 Abington Road, Cleveland, OH 44106*

JULIE C. TSAI MD, *Department of Ophthalmology, Center for Intraocular Lens Research, Storm Eye Institute, 171 Ashley Avenue, Medical University of South Carolina, Charleston, SC 29425-2236*

FRANK J. WEINSTOCK MD, FACS, *Canton Ophthalmology Associates, Inc., 2912 West Tuscarawas, Canton, OH 44708*

Foreword

The technology of cataract surgery has progressed at a blinding pace during the past 4 decades. Surgeons of the 1960s would not recognize the cataract operation as it is presently performed. The intracapsular procedure reigned supreme until 1967 when Kelman introduced phacoemulsification and Binkhorst taught us the advantages of the extracapsular method. In addition, 1967 marked the year that Galin, Hirschman, Byron, and I introduced intracapsular lens implantation to the American ophthalmologist. Since then, the ophthalmic literature and several texts have documented the dynamic changes that have placed modern cataract surgery in its current exalted position. It is now the most frequently performed surgical procedure on patients over 65 years of age. There are now more than 1300 000 cataract/lens implantation operations performed annually in the USA alone and more abroad. A surgical procedure that was initially met with academic scorn has become the standard operation for patients afflicted with cataracts. The indications for the surgery itself have been liberalized because of its high rate of success. The seemingly endless number of complications that may confront the cataract surgeon have been either eliminated or minimized as a result of ophthalmologists' rational approach to their management.

The beginning ophthalmologist and his or her more experienced colleagues have at their disposal a variety of resource materials to assist them in learning the techniques of cataract surgery and managing their complications. The emphasis has clearly been on the technical aspects of the surgery itself while consideration of the patient as a whole probably received insufficient attention. Dr Weinstock has recognized this. He has made an effort to present material that is not easily available in reference to the older cataract patient. Thus this is not simply another book on cataract surgery, but a volume on where the others have left off.

Mainstream ophthalmologists fully appreciate the importance of mastering the techniques of contemporary cataract surgery and its complications but recognize that they serve only to improve the quality of life of their patients.

NORMAN S. JAFFE MD

Introduction

Most books and discussions in reference to cataracts emphasize the lens and its manipulation. It is essential not to forget that the lens is situated in the eye of an individual—the patient.

In this book we are trying to concentrate on the cataract patient and his or her needs—in addition to the cataract surgery. The eye and its abnormalities evoke a flood of emotions in patients. It is necessary to deal with these emotions and concerns from the time of the diagnosis until after surgery, regardless of whether the result of the surgery is successful or unsuccessful.

Cataract surgery is a technical skill, but we must remember the art of practicing medicine and dealing with patients. In reference to the science of ophthalmology, technical state-of-the-art information is presented by leading experts. We have also concentrated heavily on the art of dealing with patients and some of the management considerations which are so necessary to incorporate in modern ophthalmology practices.

There are some "fun" chapters dealing with cataract surgery in history and art which serves to emphasize the high level of achievement that we have attained in reference to management of cataracts and patients. Fortunately we do not have to deal with the intense anxiety, depression and reactions that occurred in Monet. The rapidity and ease of cataract surgery can lull us into a false sense of security and may tend to cause ophthalmologists to forget that a patient lurks behind that cataract with many of the same feelings of Monet, but muted due to the speed at which diagnosis is made, surgery scheduled and then carried out.

FRANK J. WEINSTOCK MD, FACS

MANAGEMENT AND CARE OF
THE CATARACT PATIENT

1: The History of the Cataract Operation

FREDERICK C. BLODI

For thousands of years the cataract operation has been surrounded by a certain mystique because this procedure removes an obstacle which may cause blindness, rendering the patient unable to work, and may even from the beginning cause a marked deterioration of vision and a severe change in the patient's lifestyle. The frequency with which cataracts occur and the startling success with which the operation restores vision have made the cataract operation the fulcrum of surgical ophthalmic endeavors.

Cataract operations have been performed for more than 2000 years. Our approach to this operation has changed over time and especially during the last 240 years since we are capable of extracting a cataract, thereby raising the success rate dramatically over the previous palliative couching of the opaque lens.

The ancient Sanskrit manuscripts already mention and describe the cataract operation. The first known description is found in the Susruta in which couching is performed with two instruments. A lancet perforates the eyeball and another such instrument or a needle opens the cataract. The couching itself is attributed more to the patient who by breathing heavily dislocates the cataract. The couching instrument is only of secondary importance. The second lancet is wrapped in hemp or wool and only the point is left bare, thereby protecting the iris. These manuscripts were probably written around the birth of Christ or in the first century AD. It is quite likely, however, that the cataract operations were performed in India much earlier though we cannot determine who actually invented this procedure.

To Hippocrates and his pupils the cataract was unknown, at least they did not describe it. It took several centuries and contact with the Eastern civilizations before the Greeks accepted the concept of a cataract and its operation.

The ancient physicians thought that *glaucósis* and *hypochýma* were identical conditions; later authors declared glaucoma a disease of the crystalline lens (a light blue discoloration of the pupil) and hypochyma an outpouring of fluid which then gels and lies between the iris and the crystalline body. Glaucomas were considered incurable, but most hypochymas were thought to be amenable to treatment.

This dogma was based on the assumption that the crystalline lens is the main organ of vision, as stated in the canon presented by Aristotle and adhered to for 15 hundred years. It was therefore concluded that if a disease leading to discoloration of the pupil is curable, e.g. hypochyma, it cannot be an affection of the lens.

The Romans translated hypochyma to *suffusio*; the Arabs called it a "downpour of water" which was again translated back into Latin as *gutta opacta* or *cataracta*.

In Roman times a great number of myths surrounded the cataract and its operation. It was seriously suggested that couching of a cataract (a procedure which the Romans had accepted from the East) had been copied from animals. The fairy tale claims that when a goat notices that its vision becomes cloudy it will go to a special bush and then pierce its eyes with a thorn. Fluid will escape, but the pupil remains intact and the goat will immediately see again. This myth was told by Claudius Aelianus (around AD 222) and is also mentioned in one of the non-authentic manuscripts of the Galen collection.

The first description of a cataract operation which has been preserved into our time comes from Cornelius Celsus, who lived at the time of Emperor Nero. This Roman physician presented exact guidelines on not only how to operate, but also when to perform the operation.

Celsus describes the procedure thusly (Fig. 1.1). The patient should be seated on a chair facing the sun. The room should be bright and the physician should sit opposite the patient on a somewhat higher stool. The assistant stands behind the patient and should immobilize the patient's head by holding it tightly. The eye should be immobilized by putting a wool compress over the other eye. The operation should be performed with the right hand for the left eye and with the left hand for the right eye. The needle should be applied perpendicular to the ocular surface exactly at the middle between the black of the eye (corneal limbus) and the external canthus, opposite the center of the cataract (i.e. in the horizontal meridian of the eye); when the needle has entered the eye it is turned toward the cataract and the cataract is pushed toward the lower pupillary margin (Fig. 1.1).

If the cataract remains dislocated downward, the operation is terminated. If the cataract rises again, it has to be cut with the needle which has remained in the eye.

This then presented an enormous progress against the Hippocratic canon which recognized only four operations, all on the external eye and lids.

The Greek concepts on the cataract operation were summarized by Antyllus in the second century AD representing the Hellenistic period of civilization and by Paullus of Aegina, a physician who lived during the seventh century AD representing the Byzantine period of civilization.

During the Middle Ages, the Arabian physicians described two methods of couching a cataract: (a) the Greek method using a pointed needle to press the lens downward. This is the procedure also described by Celsus; and (b)

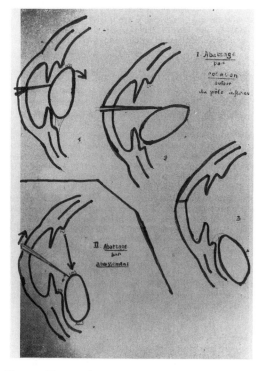

Fig. 1.1 The couching maneuver illustrated in schematic drawings.

an incision was made into the sclera with a small knife and through that wound a blunt needle was introduced to dislocate the lens downward.

In addition, the Arabian surgeon Ammar introduced the suction method whereby a hollow needle was placed into the eye and the surgeon aspirated lens material directly.

The Arabian surgeons used two different cataract needles: (a) one with a rounded end (*Mihatt*); and (b) another one with a triangular point (*Miqdah*). The entrance point of the needle should be the same as described by Celsus or it should lie at a distance from the limbus which equals the width of the needle's handle, i.e. approximately the size of a grain of barley or about 4 mm (Fig. 1.2).

In Europe during the Middle Ages and up to the middle of the eighteenth century couching of cataracts remained the only cataract operation known. Some refinements evolved, e.g. cutting a loose conjunctiva over the sclera with a lancet and then introducing the needle. The needle was frequently wrapped in fresh cot-

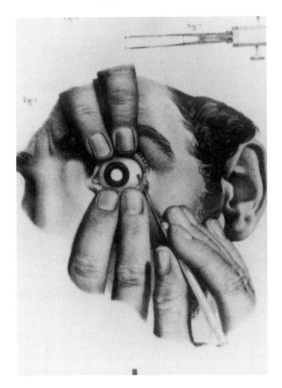

Fig. 1.2 The couching needle approaches the left eye. The Scarpa needle is used here. It is held like a pencil, perforates the sclera, and then pushes the cataract downward.

ton so that only the tip remained uncovered. During this time the surgeons left the cataract operation more and more to itinerant barbers. This applied to all of Europe and, as a matter of fact, the surgeons themselves disdained to perform a cataract operation because, like lithotomy and setting bones, the cataract operation was below the dignity of a well-educated surgeon.

Slowly it became evident that the cataract was indeed an opacification of the lens itself and not a membrane on it. The great German astronomist and mathematician Johannes Kepler early in the seventeenth century had already determined on the basis of simple experiments and calculations that the retina was the organ of visual perception and the lens was only a refracting body. His revolutionizing concept was published in 1610, but practically no physician or surgeon paid heed to this discovery. It took another hundred years before this concept was appreciated by the medical community.

The first one who clearly recognized the lens as the site of a cataract was the French physician, Pierre Brisseau, who in a brief monograph in 1705 reported his results of dissecting autopsy eyes. His finding was completely corroborated by Antoine Maître Jean, who in 1707 made important experiments proving that an animal can see without the lens. These findings were extensively discussed at various meetings of the French Academy of Sciences and officially accepted in 1708.

It remained for a genial French surgeon, Jacque Daviel, to change the situation suddenly and dramatically. This brave man, who valiantly fought a cholera epidemic in the Provence, became an excellent ophthalmologist who knew how to couch a cataract. When one of his patients, a one-eyed eremite, became blind in his second eye after Daviel had dislocated the lens, this conscientious surgeon realized that another surgical approach had to be found. Accepting the new concept that the lens is the site of the cataract, Daviel began to experiment on autopsy eyes and on animals. As soon as he was convinced that the lens could be extracted, he performed this operation in 1750 on the living human eye. Daviel used a corneal incision to cut into the cataract and extract it. The incision was usually semicircular, often close to the limbus forming a "corneal flap." The incision was made near the lower limbus, because of the patient's tendency to roll the eye upward. He made a keratome incision and enlarged it with scissors (Fig. 1.3).

It would have been impossible to predict the strange events which followed the memorable session of the French Academy of Surgery on November 15, 1752 when Daviel reported for the first time on his new procedure. From there the method embarked on a victorious course all over the civilized world and yet several decades later there was still considerable controversy about the best way to operate on a cataract. The dispute between those favoring extraction and those favoring couching lasted another century.

Several circumstances contributed to this delayed dispute: a considerable percentage of

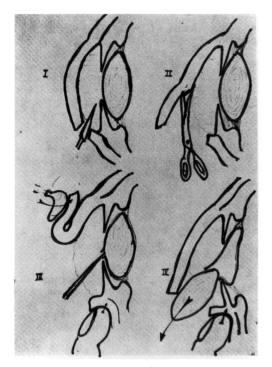

Fig. 1.3 Daviel's extraction procedure illustrated in schematic drawings.

the operations were failures, either because of a purulent infection, or an iris prolapse led to a staphyloma, or the procedure was too difficult for the less skillful. Daviel had already stated that "the extraction is only for skillful and experienced hands." C.F. Graefe, the father of Albrecht von Graefe, stated in 1823 "a certain preference by some physicians for the couching operation is due to the fact that the corneal incision requires a high degree of skill which not every surgeon can muster."

In addition there was during the early decades this unfortunate tendency to change and modify constantly the procedure, especially the incision. This is always quite popular among ambitious surgeons, but may impede progress by attempting to repair something which has not broken down. One step forward was, however, to replace the lancet by a knife (Fig. 1.4).

The couching procedure had never been completely abandoned and during the last decades of the eighteenth century, a vivid dispute which reached a crescendo of acrimony and vehemence during the beginning of the nineteenth century was carried on.

At first England attacked France, then the controversy raged in Germany and in Italy. One of the most ardent opponents of the extraction method was the great surgeon of St Bartholomew's Hospital in London, Percival Pott (1713–1783). He declared the cataract extraction a "kind of fashion" and stated "it may possibly be supposed, that I have conceived a prejudice against the operation of extraction. Of this I am not conscious . . . the preference will be found justly due to the needle."

Pott does not present any convincing evidence. It is quite possible that soft cataracts can be couched, but Pott relied too heavily on absorption of the lens material after the capsule had been opened; he even wanted to leave untouched a hard lens dislodged into the anterior chamber until it had dissolved.

It is curious that in his short monograph Pott repeatedly defends himself against prejudice and partiality; we know how he was angered by the success of the itinerant ophthalmologist Wenzel, who had performed cataract extractions in London. However, Pott found followers in England. Joseph Beer gives the following evaluation: "Some of the English ophthalmologists rejected the extraction method in order to please Mr Pott, others in order to stand out among the crowd. A third group did it out of national pride and out of hate of all French. And a fourth group did it because they had bad results due to prejudice or clumsiness."

The able surgeon Jonathan Wathen defended with the power of his conviction the cataract extraction in London in 1785, but the great B. Bell of Edinburgh expressed himself in the first edition of his *System of Surgery* (1783–1787) again in favor of the couching procedure. Wathen's previous partner, James Ware, published an excellent monograph about the extraction method (1795). It was not as eagerly accepted by his compatriots as it was by August Gottlieb Richter and Beer, who already were convinced that this was the better operation. Richter published his experiences in book form (1773) dealing exclusively with the cataract extraction, while Beer incorporated his concept in a textbook (1792).

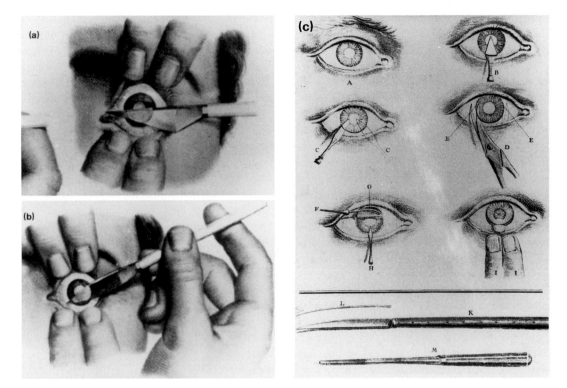

Fig. 1.4 (a) Preparing a corneal flap with a triangular knife. The inferior keratotomy is performed with a Richter knife. The upper lid is retracted by the assistant's index and middle finger. The lower lid is retracted by the surgeon using the same fingers. (b) Preparing a corneal flap with the cataract knife of Wenzel using an oblique keratotomy. (c) Extraction method of Daviel. Inferior keratotomy at 6 o'clock with a lancet (B), enlarging the wound (C), also with correct scissors (D), incising the capsule with a needle (H), and expressing the cataract.

The dispute had only one good result which must be acknowledged by the impartial observer. It led to the development of the discission operation (the term was first used in 1824). This procedure developed into an independent operation and became the method of choice for soft cataracts.

Celsus already mentions in antiquity the fragmentation of cataracts as a complementary procedure to couching, if the latter does not achieve the desired result. The Arabian surgeons used fragmentation only exceptionally in cases when couching was impossible.

Thomas Woolhouse was the first who in 1726 declared on the basis of his experience that fragmentation should always be performed when possible. Discission became an important operation when the dispute between extraction and couching raged in Europe. Pott was the first to push this procedure, though he considerably overestimated its importance.

Dislocation of the cataract became again more popular when in 1785 Willburg advised replacing the usual couching by the reclination method, i.e. dislodging the lens backward. The advantages of this procedure were recognized by Beer, who admitted that this was the best method of couching a cataract. The Italian Scarpa became the champion of this method and in 1801 he wrote quite precisely: "Experience speaks for the reclination." Under his influence, the countries of romance languages accepted reclination as the method of choice. In France the main proponents were Dupuytren and Luzardi, who in 1827 boasted to have performed 5034 cataract operations, most of them by reclination. Up to the middle of the nineteenth century, reclination was the accepted method of operating a cataract in France.

In Germany in the meantime Buchhorn published a thesis in which he recommended a corneal incision to couch a cataract. He called this "keratonyxis." A special rounded needle is used to perforate the cornea and incise the lens capsule. This approach could also be used to fragment the cataract. The procedure was enthusiastically accepted by the famous Langenbeck, professor of surgery in Göttingen. In 1819, Langenbeck declared that keratonyxis and depression of the cataract had replaced extraction to such an extent that one could read nothing but reports about the depression and keratonyxis procedures.

His colleague, Karl Himly, professor of medicine and director of the Academic Hospital in Göttingen, declared in 1816 that it is much more reasonable to recline the cataract than to extract it. He reported among 50 reclinations only two failures, whereas the statistics on extractions were less favorable.

The condition was different in Berlin. C.F. Graefe, the great father of a greater son, performed the extraction and left the needle operation to less skillful surgeons; on the other hand, his pupil and successor, Jüngken, relapsed in his old days and performed reclinations.

It remained to the Austrian school to carry the cataract extraction to its final victory over couching. This was achieved by Joseph Beer and his son-in-law, Friedrich Jaeger, his grandson, Eduard Jaeger, and his direct and indirect pupils, Rosas, Fischer, Arlt, and Hasner. Their teaching and their example disseminated the concept of the cataract extraction not only over Germany, but brought it back to France. The method reached England and all other European countries, and the other side of the Atlantic.

Friedrich Jaeger also introduced the incision at the upper limbus as the procedure of choice. This approach had originally been performed by Richter. Covering the wound with the upper lid protected the eye against an infection.

Beer established firmly that couching of a partly or totally solid cataract is only an apparent cure, a palliative relief. A cataract will never dissolve in the vitreous. He found on anatomic examinations a small lens in the eye even 20 years after couching. In one eye he saw the lens rise again 30 years after couching.

Around the middle of the nineteenth century it was generally accepted (only a few outsiders disagreed) that the extraction of a cataract with a classical semicircular ("corneal flap") incision was the method of choice for the mature cataract, whereas for the immature soft cataract fragmentation was recommended. The final victory of the extraction method could only be achieved when better postoperative care and anesthetics became available.

Postoperatively vision with a cataract lens can be superb so that the patient is able to perform almost any task (including a cataract operation!). Unfortunately, this ideal, perfect result was obtained in only 50% of the patients. In many patients there was iris prolapse or incarceration of the iris into the wound with corresponding pupillary distortion; the scar was frequently broad and ectatic; vision was therefore often mediocre only.

The worst complication, however, and the saddest results were due to purulent endophthalmitis. In the hands of most surgeons this complication occurred in about 10% of all operations. Only a few ophthalmologists who operated under especially favorable conditions in private institutions and who were extremely skillful and exerted greatest caution could reduce this complication rate to 6–7%.

Nevertheless, nobody dared to suggest a substantial modification of the "sacred" corneal flap incision. Some of the surgeons placed the incision at the upper limbus. This had occasionally been done by Wenzel, was often performed by Parmard (1784), and became the routine procedure for Friedrich Jaeger in 1825, and for Rosas in 1830. The idea was that this could improve wound healing by covering the incision with the upper lid.

Nobody dared to make the incision smaller. It had been previously well known that this would lead to most unpleasant complications, including massive vitreous loss. A hard lens could only be extracted when the incision was large enough.

Two modifications were proposed in the

following years. The first one was by Mooren of Düsseldorf. Based on the success of Graefe's iridectomy, Mooren introduced the preparatory iridectomy thereby reducing his failure rate from 11 to 3.5%. J. Jacobson of Königsberg recommended in 1863 an incision which extended into the scleral lip. He combined the extraction with an iridectomy and operated under deep chloroform anesthesia.

A brand new approach was suggested and performed by A. von Graefe in 1864. He devised a peripheral linear incision. This new procedure seemed to avoid unnecessary gaping of the semicircular corneal incision. The question was what kind of an incision on the spherical surface of the eyeball would correspond to a linear incision on a plane surface anywhere else in the body? Graefe recognized that the shortest distance between two points on a sphere is represented by the smaller part of the major circle encompassing these two points. He therefore performed the incision with a thin pointed knife (which he devised himself) a nearly linear incision through the upper limbus at 12 o'clock extending for 412 lines. This incision could be covered by a small conjunctival flap which would remain on the corneal wound edge and could be cut with the same knife as used for the incision. Graefe then performed an iridectomy in the same area and opened the lens capsule with a small curved lancet, extracting the opaque lens material by mild external pressure while applying a rubber spoon at the lower limbus.

This new peripheral linear incision soon spread all over the world and was performed by nearly every ophthalmic surgeon. The new procedure was unanimously praised at the International Ophthalmological Congress in Paris in 1867 and similarly at the Heidelberg Congress in 1868.

For the majority of ophthalmologists, the Graefe method reduced the failure rate from 10% down to 5% and the incidence of purulent endophthalmitis down to 2–3%. After Graefe's death, numerous doubts were expressed about this new procedure. However, it was clear that because of less gaping, it reduced the chances of infection. In time, most ophthalmic surgeons returned to the semicircular limbal incision and

performed a peripheral iridectomy. Hasner in Prague was a proponent of the latter procedure and he never switched to the linear extraction. The French ophthalmologists returned to the corneal incision and called it the "method of Daviel."

Looking back, it is clear that both methods had their advantages and disadvantages. However, with better asepsis, suturing, and improved instruments, the semicircular limbal incision was probably the method of choice, but it was not suitable for all types of cataracts. Just as Beer had a hundred years earlier still preferred couching for special cases, it was then decided to perform under unusual circumstances, a linear incision with segmental iridectomy, e.g. for eyes with posterior synechiae, shallow anterior chamber, or on patients with severe cardiac or pulmonary complications. In these cases the safety of a good procedure was preferred over the hazards of a better one.

The intracapsular cataract extraction was actually performed as long as the extracapsular one. Daviel reported that in one case he performed an intracapsular procedure unintentionally on a patient with a long-standing liquefied cataract with thickening and adhesions of the anterior capsule. Daviel grasped the capsule with a small forceps and while severing the adhesions, extracted the entire lens.

During the second half of the eighteenth century, the intracapsular extraction was performed occasionally by a few surgeons. A.G. Richter says in his treatise on cataract extraction (1773) that occasionally the lens can be mobilized and extracted within the capsule. In these patients this method is not a complication, but a desired event which certainly prevents the formation of an aftercataract. Richter himself reported (1776) a new method for an intracapsular extraction by mobilizing the lens with a small tubule.

It remained for Beer to make this procedure a standard operation. He published a monograph (1799) on the intracapsular extraction listing as its advantages quicker healing, better postoperative vision, and the avoidance of aftercataract.

This publication involved Beer in a bitter

argument with his competitor, Johann Adam Schmidt. Schmidt, who was then professor at the Surgical Academy Josephinum in Vienna, declared after numerous spiteful and slanderous remarks—accusing Beer of lack of skill, calling him a dilettante and regarding the procedure as crude—that he had no success with Beer's procedure on autopsy eyes, in animals, and in three attempts on a living human eye. Schmidt then asked the rhetorical question: Does the moral law have to be quiet when the police laws do not speak? Beer answered in a dignified way. He pointed out some mistakes committed by Schmidt, but the feud continued. For a time Beer performed the intracapsular procedure nearly exclusively.

Another champion of the intracapsular operation was Justus Arnemann, who in his book which appeared around the turn of the century (1800–1810) described a corkscrew-like instrument to dislodge the lens. Schmidt thereupon commented sarcastically "the eye is not a wine bottle."

However, during the next decades the intracapsular cataract extraction lost in favor. Only in 1866 a monograph appeared by Alexander Pagenstecher of Wiesbaden in which he again recommends the intracapsular extraction as the method of choice. Pagenstecher admits freely that this technique presents unusual difficulties and that deep chloroform anesthesia is absolutely necessary.

During the early twentieth century, English physicians performed this procedure in India. The most prominent was Henry Smith, who practiced in the Punjab. He expressed the entire lens by pressure only. The surgeon places with his left hand a Daviel spoon on the lower half of the cornea, corresponding to the lower third of the lens. The surgeon's right hand holds a blunt squint hook which is applied to the upper limbus. The squint hook is moved laterally and slight pressure is exerted. As soon as the lens equator appears in the wound, the spoon follows it upward.

Two great advances in cataract operations developed in the second half of the nineteenth century. The first was the introduction of anesthesia. General anesthesia had been introduced early in the century, but it remained

to the great American ophthalmologist, Henry Willard Williams (1821–1895), to use ether routinely for all cataract extractions. This certainly made it easier for the patients to tolerate the operation and it facilitated maneuvering for the surgeon.

In addition, Karl Koller discovered in 1884 the local anesthetic effect of cocaine. He proved this on the cornea and conjunctiva of a frog and within a few weeks this method of anesthesia was applied to the human eye. Local anesthesia for ophthalmology was then reported at the Heidelberg Congress of the same year and, of course, it was accepted practically immediately all over the world. Within 2 weeks Hermann Knapp used this method in New York.

The second advance was the introduction of sutures to close the wound. This was again initiated by Henry Willard Williams, who reported in 1865 that he had placed a suture at 12 o'clock at the limbus. Williams used a pointed sewing needle and as a thread he took a strand of fine glover's silk. Suturing the wound was then nearly forgotten for 30 years, but it was reintroduced by Kalt in France (1894) who used corneoscleral sutures. Conjunctivoscleral sutures were first used by Verhoeff in 1916 and Suarez de Mendoza recommended in 1891 for the first time preplacing the limbal sutures.

The first part of the twentieth century provided additional advances in the form of akinesia and anesthesia. Elschnig advised in 1928, for the first time, the retrobulbar injection of an anesthetic to improve anesthesia and immobilize the globe. Van Lint of Brussels was the first to immobilize the orbicularis oculi muscle in 1914. He injected the anesthetic directly into the muscle fibers.

In the twentieth century the intracapsular extraction slowly gained the upper hand. This procedure was championed especially by Hermann Knapp of Heidelberg and New York, who used the tumbling procedure in which the lower equator of the lens is grasped and by rotating the lens this portion exits first through the wound. Verhoeff of Boston, on the other hand, preferred the sliding method in which the lens equator is grasped at 12 o'clock and by rotating motions the zonule fibers are broken.

The extraction of the cataract had up to then

been effected by mechanical means, e.g. pressure, pulling with a forceps, depression with a spoon, or other devices. Ignacio Barraquer of Barcelona constructed in 1917 the first erysophake by which the cataract could be extracted using suction.

During World War II and shortly thereafter, the intracapsular cataract extraction with peripheral iridectomy had become perfected to such an extent that many physicians thought that this method of operating a cataract was so ideal and complete that no improvement or change could be expected.

Enormous advances developed during the second half of the twentieth century after World War II. The first was the introduction of microsurgical methods for ophthalmology. Devices for magnification, especially loupes, had been used for several decades, but it remained for Harms in Tübingen and Barraquer in Barcelona to modify, in the 1950s, the Zeiss surgical microscope for ophthalmic purposes. This method was soon accepted and ocular surgery without it is nowadays practically unimaginable.

During these decades two methods were advised to improve the extraction of the cataract. The first was published by Joaquin Barraquer in 1958 in Barcelona. He used α-chymotrypsin for enzymatic zonulolysis. This certainly facilitates an intracapsular cataract extraction. A fresh solution of the enzyme in a 1:5000 or 1:10000 dilution has to be injected into the chambers to obtain this effect.

The second improvement was the use of a cold probe to extract the cataract. T. Krwawicz of Lublin, Poland pioneered in 1961 the cryoextraction. This allowed an easier and better grasp on the lens than any forceps or suction method. Kelman improved on this in 1962 and 1963 by developing the first hand-held cryostylet for cataract removal.

The development of new methods accelerated during this and the next decade. In 1967, Charles D. Kelman devised the first ingenious apparatus for phakoemulsification. In this method soft lens material is fragmented by ultrasound energy, irrigated, and aspirated. In the early stages this device required a complicated and sophisticated computer system to control the various functions. In the meantime this has been considerably streamlined. This method allows a cataract operation through an extremely small wound which makes postoperative care and rehabilitation of the patient much easier. Use of the aspirating aspect of the Kelman/Cavitron phakoemulsification unit allowed it to be used for either phakoemulsification or planned extracapsular cataract surgery. In conjunction with the development of viscoelastics, cataract surgery has evolved to a unprecedented high degree of sophistication.

Although early ambulation of cataract patients began with Galin and Williamson in the 1960s, the modern cataract operation has made ambulatory surgery the rule, rather than the exception. In addition to a significant decrease in morbidity, this has resulted in a major reduction in the expense of surgery.

The second giant step forward was initiated by Harold Ridley of London, who performed in 1949 the first intraocular lens implant after observing that certain plastics could be tolerated by the ocular tissues. The first lenses were heavy and clumsy and therefore caused a good number of complications. It took another 10 years before Binkhorst in The Netherlands modified the intraocular lens. In 1972, the same author switched to an extracapsular cataract extraction with implanting the lens into the posterior chamber. Kelman was a main force in the evolution of small implants (foldable and non-foldable) which could be used in small incision surgery. Intraocular lenses followed the use of contact lenses for the improvement of vision to mimic normal vision and eliminated the need for the distortion-producing thick spectacles of the past.

In summary, we can say that couching was performed for about 2000 years and came to the Western World from India. The suction method was accepted for a short time only and was practiced by Arabian physicians during the early Middle Ages. It remained to the great French surgeon, Jacques Daviel, to devise around 1750 the first planned cataract extraction. This was not an act of serendipity, but based on careful experimental work. The procedure was initially not favorably received and it remained for the Austrian school (Beer,

Jäger, and Arlt) to elevate the extraction method to the procedure of choice. The genial A. von Graefe introduced the linear extraction which gaped less and therefore became less often infected. The fragmentation method, introduced by Arabian physicians, was perfected to the discission procedure by English surgeons. The intracapsular extraction was practiced by Beer around 1800, but became the standard method only between the two World Wars. Since 1950 microsurgery, phakoemulsification, extracapsular cataract surgery, and intraocular lenses have established a new era of cataract surgery which is continuing to evolve at a dazzling pace.

Further reading

Duke-Elder. *System of Ophthalmology*, vol. XI. St Louis: CV Mosby, 1969: 248–64.

Hirsch A. Geschichte der Augenheilkunde. In: *Graefe-Saemisch Handbuch der Gesammten Augenheilkunde*, vol. VII. Leipzig: Wilhelm Engelmann, 1877: 235.

Hirschberg J. *The History of Ophthalmology*, volumes I–XI. (Translated by Frederick C. Blodi.) Bonn: Wayenborgh, 1982–1988.

Kirby D. *Surgery of Cataract*. Philadelphia: JB Lippincott, 1950: 3–35.

Magnus H. *Die Geschichte des Grauen Staares*. Leipzig: Veit, 1876.

Münchow W. *Geschichte der Augenheilkunde*. Stuttgart: F Enke, 1984.

Shastid Th. H. History of ophthalmology. In: Wood CA, ed. *The American Encyclopedia and Dictionary of Ophthalmology*, vol. XI. Chicago: Cleveland Press, 1917: 8524–904.

2: The Effects of Cataracts on Three Famous Artists

JAMES G. RAVIN

Cataracts have caused serious disability to several artists of major importance. The best example is Claude Monet, the famous French Impressionist. Poor vision due to cataracts interrupted work on his famous *Waterlilies* project. Following surgery he was able to resume painting a series of waterlily paintings for which he is well known.

Honoré Daumier, another nineteenth century French artist, underwent cataract surgery late in his life. His eye problems coincided with other medical problems and this combination put an end to his career. Mary Cassatt, the famous American Impressionist, suffered from cataracts and diabetes. Visual troubles caused her great distress, and forced her to end her artistic work many years before her death.

These three artists are excellent examples of the effect of cataracts on artists. For each of them health data is available that can be correlated with their oeuvre.

Monet

Claude Monet (1840–1926) was a leader of the French Impressionist group. He was fortunate to live 86 years, but developed cataracts. The cataracts became a severe problem late in his life.

Monet first attracted critical attention at the Salon of 1866, where he exhibited a portrait of the woman who was to become his first wife. Zola, the famous novelist and journalist who defended Dreyfus vociferously, found Monet's art compelling:

> His painting speaks whole volumes to me about energy and truth. Oh, yes, here is someone with a temperament, here is a man among all these eunuchs. Look at the paintings nearby and see how crestfallen they look next to this open window on nature! Here we have more than a realist, someone who knows how to interpret each detail with delicacy and power, yet without lapsing into tediousness. [1]

The term Impressionism originated from Monet's painting *Impression: Sunrise* of 1872. Until recently this painting was on exhibition at the Marmottan Museum in Paris. In a spectacular daylight robbery, it was stolen in 1985 and has yet to be recovered.

An astute critic noted that the Impressionist group of artists attempted to depict the general appearance of a landscape rather than an exact rendition [2]. But another French satirical writer drew attention to Monet's canvas in a humorous review that linked forever the names of Monet and his colleagues with the term Impressionism:

> The poor man was peacefully raving in his fashion and nothing led me to see the misfortune that was to ensue from his visit to this revolutionary exhibition . . . "Ha, ha" he laughed diabolically, "this one's pretty good! . . . Here's an impression if I don't say so myself . . . Only, tell me what these countless little black licking marks at the bottom of the painting?"
>
> "Those, they are people strolling."
>
> "Is that what I look like when I stroll down the Boulevard des Capucines? . . . Hell and damnation! Are you trying to make a fool of me?" . . .
>
> "Ah! This is it, this is it!" He cried in front

of number 98, "This one is Papa Vincent's favorite! What is this a painting of? Look in the catalogue."

"Impression: Sunrise."

"Impression—I knew it. I was just saying to myself, if I am impressed, there must be an impression in there." [3]

Some critics disliked Monet's work, while others went beyond themselves to extol his virtues. J.K. Huysmans, the decadent novelist and critic, described Monet in the following terms:

> M. Monet has been spattering for some time, dropping little improvisations, botching bits of landscapes, bitter salads of orange peels, green onions, and blue ribbons that simulated the flowing waters of a river. One thing was certain: this artist's vision was high strung. [4]

Another critic, writing in the prestigious *Gazette des Beaux-Arts*, described Monet in superhuman terms:

> M. Monet's eyesight is highly unusual; he sees in a way that most human beings do not, and, because he is sincere, he attempts to produce what he sees. We know that the solar spectrum includes a range of rays that the cornea intercepts, and that, therefore, the retina does not receive. This range is called ultraviolet, because it extends beyond the violet range that everyone sees. It does play a significant part in nature but its effects are not optical. Recent experiments by M. Chardonnet, however, have proven positively that some people respond strongly to this invisible part of the spectrum. Without a doubt, M. Monet belongs to this number; he and his friends see ultraviolet: the masses see something different . . . The brilliance of the yellow rays stimulates the painter's nervous sensibility, then blinds him; at that point he undergoes a well known physiological phenomenon: the complimentary color is evoked; he sees violet. Those that are fond of this color will be pleased: M. Monet executes for them an exquisite symphony in violet. [5]

Monet's failing eyesight

As an Impressionist, Monet employed a method of painting that is based on an intended lack of fine detail. This deliberate lack of precision caused the visually related blurriness of his work to become apparent much later in his career than would have been the case if he had painted in greater detail. His loss of vision was first evident in his works created on a visit to Venice in 1908 [6]. Works painted during that Italian sojourn (Plate 2.1, facing p. 110) show an imprecision of detail and are less convincing in their depiction of space than are his earlier paintings. His use of color still appeared to be unaffected. During the decade from 1908 to 1918, his cataracts became an increasing problem. A country physician advised him that he had cataracts, and in 1912 an ophthalmologist in Paris confirmed the diagnosis. Being afraid of the consequences, he sought the opinions of many other doctors. When a writer came to his home at Giverny to interview him, he described his problems:

> It is extremely difficult work and very seductive. To catch the fleeing moment, or at least its sensation, is terribly difficult when the play of light and color is concentrated on one fixed point, a cityscape or a motionless landscape in the country. But water, which moves constantly and is always changing, is a real and appealing problem, for with each passing moment, there is something new and unforeseen.

> One could spend his life at his work. I did for eight or nine years, then I suddenly stopped in a severe sense of anguish.

> I did not perceive colors with the same intensity. I was not painting light with the same accuracy. Reds appeared muddy, pink tones were dull, and the intermediate or deeper colors escaped me. As for forms, they always appeared clear, and I was able to paint them with the same result.

> At first I tried to be stubborn. Time after time, near the little footbridge where we are now, I remained for hours under the most severe sunlight, seated on my little

chair, in the shade of my parasol, forcing myself to resume the interrupted task of painting and regain the freshness that had disappeared from my palette. All the efforts were in vain. I painted more and more in dark tones. The paintings looked like very old works, and when my effort was over, I would compare it with previous works. I would be overcome with a wild rage and would slash all my canvases with my penknife.

It is not necessary to tell you that, in the meantime, I consulted all of the well known ophthalmologists. The contradictory diversity of their responses scared me. Some told me it was old age and progressive weakness of the visual organ. Others, and I believe that these were the correct ones, led me to understand, with a thousand precautions, that I had the beginning of a cataract and that an operation at the appropriate time would cure me. They did not let me ignore that the slow progression of symptoms showed a slow development of the problem, and that it would be years before an operation would be possible. Both groups were in accord only on one point, the necessity of absolute rest.

I had spent many cruel hours in my life, but never had I lived with as much torture as the five or six months which followed. One day however, a blessed day, I felt that the problem was temporarily stopped. I attempted a series of experiments destined to give me an idea of the limits and possibilities of my vision, and I joyfully noticed that although I remained unaware of the delicacy and gradations of color at near, my eyes did not fool me when I took a step back and looked at the canvas—this was the starting point for the compositions that you are going to see in my studio.

To tell the truth, this was a very modest point of departure. I mistrusted myself and did not want to leave anything to chance. Slowly I tested my strength in innumerable rough sketches that convinced me at first that work in bright light was not possible, but reassured me by revealing that if small variations of tone and variations of color were not possible, I could still see as clearly as ever when it was a question of vivid colors isolated within a mass of dark tones.

What was I going to make out of this?

Little by little I clarified my intentions. I had had the idea, since reaching sixty years of age, of engaging myself in several categories of work that had taken my attention in the past, a kind of synthesis in which I could condense in one or perhaps two canvases all my impressions and sensations from previous times. I gave up that thought, since it would have been necessary to travel considerably, and it would take much time to visit each of the places where I had painted, to feel the same emotions again. Travel now fatigues me. Trips of two or three days in an automobile exhaust me. What would happen if several months of travel were required? And, besides, I am pleased here. The flowers of my garden in the springtime, the waterlilies of my pond on the Epte River in summer are part of my daily habits, the daily salt of my life. Therefore, I gave up the project. The cataract made me return to it. I had always loved the sky and the water, the verdure and the flowers. All these elements were plentiful in my little pond. Occasionally in the morning or the evening—I had stopped working in extremely bright daylight and in the afternoon I only come here to rest. I told myself that a series of impressions of the whole scene, created at the time of day when my vision had the best chance of being accurate, would not lack interest. I waited for the idea to take shape, until the arrangement and composition of the motifs inscribed themselves little by little on my brain, and when the day came that I felt I had sufficient trump cards in my hand to try my luck with some real hope of success I resolved to act and I did. [7]

This journalist was overcome by the sumptuousness, richness and intensity of Monet's paintings. At first he felt that Monet was trying to fool him in describing visual problems. Soon he found evidence that Monet was correct. He visited Monet's studio and examined many paintings that were done when cataracts began to be a severe problem for him. The colors appeared false and distorted. Although the artist was still evident in the design, the composition and overall impression showed that his sense of color was gone. Monet, the marvelous painter, no longer was a success. Monet told him:

> If I have rediscovered the sense of color in the canvases which I will show you, it is because I have adapted my method of work to my vision. Most of the time I have laid down colors at random, relying only on the labels of the tubes, and by maintaining an unvaried order for the paints on my palette. I soon got used to this method and have never made an error. I should add that my visual problem has had remissions. Several times my color vision has returned, and I have profited by making the required changes. [7]

We can understand by Monet's admission, that he was no longer able to distinguish colors, that he found it necessary to maintain an unchanging order of paints on his palette in order to avoid confusing colors. We do not know, however, what effect may have resulted from other individuals looking at his works and telling him he was having difficulty. After his cataract surgery, Monet reportedly noted with surprise how peculiar the colors were that he had chosen prior to the operation. He scolded some members of his family for having let him continue to paint in this manner without telling him. But later he changed his mind, having decided that they had been right not to say anything, since he could not have done anything about it. The situation would have merely upset him without helping him in the least [8]. The changes in his vision were not something that he could control.

Slowly Monet's vision worsened. The weeping willows and waterlilies of the 1920s reveal increasingly poor depiction of form (Plates 2.2 and 2.3). Colors lacked variety, as one observer has noted: "The symphony in color became more and more monochrome in the blues and yellows" [9].

In a letter to a critic who was preparing an article about him, Monet wrote the following:

> I shut my door to everyone all winter. I felt that otherwise, each day would be diminished and I wished to profit from what little [remained of] my vision in order to bring certain of my *Decorations* to completion. And I was gravely mistaken. For in the end, I had to admit that I was ruining them, that I was no longer capable of making anything of beauty. And I destroyed several of my panels. Today I am almost blind and I have to renounce work completely. It's hard, but that's how it is: a sad ending despite my good health! [10]

On arriving at Monet's home, the critic saw the frames in the studio:

> Shreds and shreds of slashed canvas hang from the stretchers. The knife's trace is still vivid, and the painting bleeds like a wound. The nails are in place; the border of the painting is stretched. An enraged, powerful, deeply moved hand has lacerated the panel without troubling to remove the canvas patiently like a precious carpet which one rolls up. Suffering commanded the gesture, a vexed overexcitement accomplished it. Look at these hands, these supple hands which have massacred their work. [10]

Clemenceau

The French physician and statesman, Georges Clemenceau (1841–1929), was a close friend of Monet and a very strong influence on him. Clemenceau was a dominant figure in French politics, premier of France (1870–1920), a major contributor to the allied victory in World War I, and a framer of the Treaty of Versailles. With his knowledge of medicine, he was able to exert a strong influence on Monet. Due to Clemenceau's persistence, Monet consented to have cataract surgery, and to create the series of waterlily paintings that he gave to France. This was Monet's contribution to the country during its struggle for survival. Clemenceau had great respect for Monet, saying:

> Amongst all the men I have known, Monet is perhaps the one who most gave me an insight into all sorts of things. This describes him doesn't it? He stands before a light, he takes that light, breaks it into its component parts, puts it together again. From the point of view of science there is nothing more interesting. Once I said to him, Monet, the rest of us, seeing a field or a sky, think, "this is a field and that's a sky"; but for you that is not so. The words "field" and "sky" have no meaning for you . . .
>
> He was a fellow with a knack, never satisfied with his work, yet appreciating its worth—he found the means to reconcile both those characteristics. I have known him in bad times as well as good . . .
>
> Despite his cataract (he was in a terrific funk of physical pain) . . . I did all I could to make him have it [surgery]. He was afraid of it—despite his cataract he could see well enough to paint and even to improve his canvases. [11]

Clemenceau was an astute man, but all his psychologic ability and cunning were needed to manage Monet.

Coutela, Monet's surgeon

At the urging of Clemenceau, Monet consulted a distinguished Parisian ophthalmologist, Charles Coutela MD, in September 1922. Coutela (1876–1969) was 46 years of age. He had trained in ophthalmology at the Hotel-Dieu under Professor de Lapersonne, and later at Saint-Antoine Hospital under Dr Dupuy-Detemps. He served as an ophthalmologist in military service during World War I. Although his military obligation had been completed, he served with the Ministère de la Defense Nationale in World War II. He received the prestigious award of Chevalier de la Legion d'Honneur in 1917, later becoming an officer and commander of the Legion. Coutela served in many administrative positions and was a medicolegal expert. He was secretary general of the Syndicat National des Oculistes in 1920,

and later was honorary president of that group. He was the author of a great number of scientific works including studies on eye movements and visual problems following cranial trauma [12].

Coutela diagnosed bilateral senile cataracts. He found that Monet could discern only light and the direction from which it was projected with his right eye, while his visual acuity with the left eye was 20/200 [13]. On September 13, 1922, Monet wrote to Coutela:

> My dear Doctor,
> I have to tell you, today, of the effect produced by the drops [eucatropine, a mydriatic] that you have ordered for my left eye. It is all simply marvelous. I see as I have not seen for a very long time, so well that I regret having not seen you sooner! The drops have permitted me to paint good things instead of the bad paintings which I had persisted in making when seeing nothing but fog.
>
> I see everything in my garden. I revel in all the colors. One singular point: the right eye is still purple in color. Can I continue this treatment so that I can do more pressing things? A word of response would oblige me. [14]

Monet wrote Clemenceau as well, looking for encouragement. Clemenceau did his best:

> September 19, 1922
> Dear Friend,
> Thank you for your letter which must have taken so much effort. It will be necessary to agree with the decisions of the doctor. Once operated, I will not be surprised if in closing the good eye, which is only half opened, you will be able to paint as before. There are great resources in the impossible. [15]

Monet wrote Coutela again on October 20, 1922:

> My dear Doctor,
> I believe that the time is approaching when I ought to come to you in full confidence, but not without anxiety, I confess. The first operation can be done during the first week of November at Giverny, as you promised me, and the second fifteen days later at Paris. I am doing very well thanks

to your drops which make my vision much better, not to say good. But I have lost your prescription and the address of the supplier. I would be very obliged if you would send me a second ampule, and as soon as possible, for I will be sad to miss it for only a day.

Claude Monet. [16]

But Monet's good feelings soon changed, as may be seen in a letter he wrote to Clemenceau on November 9, 1922:

Dear Doctor and Friend,

I cannot decide to make up my mind. I have too great a fear of the result. I am going to beg you to say no to the clinic and to inform Dr Coutela of this. If I change my mind and decide otherwise, it will be a little later.

I am not going out of fear. In brief I am in too troubled a state to let myself be operated.

Kindly,

Claude Monet. [17]

Clemenceau reminded Monet of his promise to finish a series of paintings for France. He convinced Monet to undergo surgery. This was done on December 22, 1922, at the Clinic of Neuilly.

In Coutela's words, "I proceeded directly to extract the cataract, extracapsularly, washing out as much of the lens as was possible. That evening the anterior chamber was reformed, which was a great encouragement for me" [18]. Coutela may have used one silk suture to close the incision. At the time topical cocaine was the only anesthesia available. Rapid surgery was necessary because of the patient's tendency to move during the operation.

Jean-Pierre Hoschedé, one of Monet's six stepchildren, described certain aspects of Monet's cataract problems. With his one brother and four sisters, Hoschedé was raised by Monet and his mother, who became Monet's second wife. He had also been a model for Monet since infancy. In his book entitled, *Claude Monet Ce Mal Connu*, Hoschedé has a chapter entitled "The Truth About the Cataract of Claude Monet." Hoschedé says at first Monet did not want to hear any talk about the cataract. This was 1922. He was afraid, not of the operation

itself, but of what would occur to his vision afterward. Fortunately, Clemenceau intervened to convince Monet what should be done. Hoschedé had an excellent understanding of the effect of cataract, since he himself developed cataracts and underwent surgery. Hoschedé describes what happened to Monet: "His vision became foggy, at first for distant objects, which appeared invisible, then near objects no longer appeared clear to him." In his own case, during surgery Hoschedé noted "an amazing spectacle of light with the most beautiful rainbow that one can imagine." He wrote:

I remember perfectly that Monet had told us about the marvelous colors which lasted only a few seconds. After the surgery came the suffering. Complete darkness with both eyes patched, the operated eye covered with a metal shield and the other bandaged. Placed in a bed completely flat without a pillow, totally immobilized, both arms placed alongside his body, the head not being allowed to move in any circumstance, neither to the right nor the left, nor lifted up. Nourishment consisted simply of vegetable bouillon or lime tea which a nurse placed in the mouth of the convalescent to be certain that there was no movement. All of this lasted for ten days. In the beginning drops were instilled in the operated eye every hour and later every two hours. There were injections for pain. Gradually came the possibility to move the arms, then the legs, but never the head. Later a pillow was allowed. Finally, the unoperated eye was opened. Twelve to fifteen days later, a pair of temporary glasses was given, replaced after three weeks by a pair of glasses with an individualized prescription to aid vision for near and for writing. For the first few days following surgery, the patient had a guardian with him, a watchman, since under the influence of cocaine, the patient could be delirious and pull off his dressing, destroying the effect of the surgery. [19]

Hoschedé did mention the possible complication of delirium induced by bilateral patching and lack of visual stimulation. Since the patient had a guardian with him, who could converse with him at all times, delirium was not a problem. Hoschedé confirms that Monet was not an easy patient, and, in particular, adapted poorly to his glasses. He credits Dr Jacques Mawas with allowing Monet to finish successfully his gigantic task of creating the waterlily canvases he was to present to France. Hoschedé says Monet's perception of colors returned postoperatively. It was Hoschedé's sister Blanche, who was both Monet's step-daughter and daughter-in-law, who cared continually for Monet during his convalescence and who wrote most of Monet's correspondence during this period.

Clemenceau wrote to Coutela on February 26, 1923:

> My dear Colleague,
> I thank you cordially for your concise words. With you, I estimate that the morale of our friend ought to be managed above all, for he can be totally inflexible against a second operation later on.
>
> It is with the greatest pleasure that I will make the trip to Giverny with you. We can go have lunch there. The trip takes about two hours. Tell me when it will be convenient for you. Which day does not matter to me. What would you say to Wednesday? [20]

Monet wrote Coutela about these arrangements and advised him that his country doctor (Rebiere) had visited him that very morning and noted that healing was advancing normally, but slowly [21].

Monet dictated a letter which was transcribed by his daughter-in-law, Blanche, on April 9, 1923:

> My dear Doctor,
> Sadly I cannot give you as good news as I would like. You understand that I am counting the days until your visit of the sixteenth and I was greatly disappointed when Dr Rebiere told me that your visit was delayed until the twentieth. I have spent some bad days due to pains from neuralgia or some other cause, fortunately improved by pain pills. Besides I see less and less with or without tinted eye glasses. The excessive light that we have tires me so

much that I confine myself to the semi-darkness of my room. Today I had severe pains in the center of the eye and in addition, I continually have the feeling of water in the eye.
>
> Naturally I follow your advice of compresses and atropine drops twice a week. I am as patient as possible, but although you are satisfied with my condition, I find that it won't last long. This is to say that I look forward to your visit, which this time will not be put off. [22]

Monet was developing an opacity of his posterior lens capsule which rapidly decreased his vision. Coutela saw him some time between April 9 and June 15, 1923, Monet wrote Coutela again on June 15:

> I am doing well. I certainly read better, 15 to 20 pages a day, but out of doors and for distance the glasses do not help me any more than at the beginning and without glasses it is totally foggy. Beside that I am in perfect health, but I need to see you so that you will see what is occurring. [23]

On June 18, 1923, Monet wrote Coutela:

> I can read certainly, not badly, but the reduction of vision out of doors troubles me. Remember that in several days it will be six months since the first operation. This is hardly encouraging and I ought to admit to you that I regret having had this operation.
>
> In spite of that, my compliments. [24]

On June 22, 1923, Monet wrote Coutela this despairing letter:

> All my apologies for not having come to meet you. I am absolutely discouraged and as much as I read, not without effort from 15 to 20 pages per day, out of doors and at a distance, I cannot see any longer with or without glasses. And for two days black floaters have been troubling me.
>
> Remember that it has been six months since the first operation, five since I left the clinic, and four since I have been wearing glasses, which is far from four or five weeks to get used to my new vision. Six months that I would have been able to work, if you had told me the truth. I would

have been able to finish the *Decorations* which I was supposed to deliver in April and I am now certain not to be able to do them as I wanted.

It is to my great chagrin that I regret having had this terrible operation. Pardon me for speaking so frankly and let me tell you that it is criminal to have placed me in this situation.

Writing sadly to you,

Claude Monet. [25]

On June 28, 1923, he wrote a more apologetic letter to Coutela:

Since I understand the truth, I look forward to the day which will take me away from the sandbags and I regret that it wasn't sooner. Also I count on you for the seventeenth, beg you to correspond in advance with Dr Rebiere, to have everything you will need for that day and avoid any delay. All of that understood, I ought to tell you that since my return, having stopped all fatigue with glasses, I see absolutely better; but we have forgotten to ask you if it is necessary to continue or not hot compresses, although they don't help me, but I am asking you. [26]

An incision of his posterior lens capsule was done on July 17, 1923. Coutela described the effect:

Afterwards, as had been predicted, the inevitable thickening of the capsule occurred; this did not trouble me, but it caused some particularly troublesome moments for Monet. He was devastated. The period which followed at Giverny was a period of profound discouragement and despair. He saw himself blind forever and completely demoralized. He refused to leave his bed. When the eye calmed down, I proceeded with the extraction of this contrary membrane. The operation was done at Giverny, in his home, and allowed him to achieve 20/30 with the correction of $+10.00 + 4.00 \times 90$. I was reassured by the final result. [27]

On August 21, 1923, Coutela wrote Clemenceau:

The vision at near can be considered nearly perfect with correction . . . For distant vision, the result is less extraordinary: Monet has 20/50 to 20/70, which is not bad . . . But a little training is needed, for distant vision, he will be more or less restricted. In short, I am very satisfied. [28]

Difficulties with eyeglasses

On August, 27, 1923, Monet dictated a letter via his daughter-in-law, Blanche, to Coutela:

You have been wondering if I am anxiously awaiting the glasses. I have just received them today but I am absolutely brokenhearted, for in spite of all my good will, I feel that if I take a step it will be to fall down. To look at near, or far, everything is deformed, everything is doubled and it has become intolerable to see. To persist seems dangerous. What should I do? I await your response with impatience. And sadly. [29]

Again troubled by his glasses he wrote Coutela on August 29, 1923:

My dear Doctor,

Be reassured on the receipt of your note I resumed the glasses and I can read a little, but poorly with a little fatigue naturally. Things are deformed as before but I am trying courageously. It is very difficult for me to get about with the glasses. Today I began to paint a little longer . . . I am using the euphthalmine drops at six in the morning, and occupy myself with things I have to do until ten, when I begin painting again. I ought to tell you that to see, I have placed a piece of paper over the left lens. [30]

Quite naturally, Monet found that an occluder for one eye would cure the confusion of two images caused by his aphakic correction. The same day, Clemenceau wrote Coutela to thank him for sending a long, detailed report of Monet's progress [31]. Clemenceau hoped that with time Monet would get used to his new glasses and hoped to chat about operating the other eye in a few months.

Monet wrote Coutela, asking him to come to Giverny to see him at work and judge the effect of the new eye glasses. He had separate pairs of glasses for near and distant vision since he wrote:

> I suppose [they are] a little too strong, especially those for distance, which I absolutely cannot use.
>
> At near things are marvelous but this is not enough. I read fluently without drops for the left eye, yet it is impossible for me to get around. I am asking you to come see me for lunch if that is possible, or whenever may be better. [32]

On September 8, 1923, Clemenceau wrote Coutela:

> Dear Colleague,
>
> I cannot thank you too much for your kind correspondence. Monet writes reasonable things. It seems to me that it is time for the two of us to chat. His projects are to be done this winter, with several changes to two of his canvases, and that will have its advantages. It will be necessary for him to have good feet and good eyes in April for his inauguration. Therefore, I am permitting myself to ask you the following questions.
>
> First, with the reestablishment sought for his one eye can Monet paint properly? That is the most pressing problem.
>
> Second, if possible, the operation for the second eye ought to be put off. What do you think of this?
>
> Third, if this is not possible, when should it be? And if it is time to proceed with the new operation—suppose he should consent to it?
>
> Fourth, from the psychologic point of view, he has acquired an enthusiasm which will dispose him to give his assent.
>
> Fifth, for this reason, I incline to proceed as soon as possible, in a month for example. But the first rule is to conform to your advice. Thus you have the word. I ask of you only that this be between us, as though Monet's psychological state is not to be considered.
>
> Sixth, in any case it will be necessary to make corrections to the paintings in the month of March, which will be all right. [33]

Monet wrote to Coutela on September 14, 1923, describing his vision with his glasses:

> They are more and more perfect from the point of view of reading and writing. Black and white are perfect, but things are not the same for colors and forms, although I wear my glasses all the time . . . I continue to see green as yellow and the rest more or less blue. It isn't funny. I await your response. [34]

During an examination in September 1923, Dr Coutela found that Monet's vision was good, but a bit distorted. Coutela noted: "Monet is most upset by the colors: he sees everything too yellow"[35]. Soon he was to see everything too blue. Monet's yellow vision was due to the difference in the manner his two eyes perceived colors after having only one cataract removed. His cataracts had grown slowly for years, indicating that nuclear sclerosis of the lens was a major factor in causing his yellowish vision. After one of these yellow–brown filters (cataracts) was removed, he became able to see colors he had not seen for years, particularly violets and blues. Many individuals who have cataract surgery suddenly become aware of color changes, and an artist would be expected to be especially cognizant of this. After surgery to the right eye, when Monet compared colors seen with each eye independently, objects seen with his left eye would have appeared more yellow–brown than when looking with the right eye. Objects seen with his right eye would have appeared more violet or blue than those with the left eye. Since his cataract glasses only had power in the right lens, and since he could not have used both eyes simultaneously, he must have been particularly aware of the differences in colors.

I have examined the pair of Monet's glasses which are in the collection of the Marmottan Museum in Paris [36]. The lenses are held in a wire frame and are lightly yellow–green tinted. The prescription is right eye, +14.00 + 7.00 × 90; left eye, plano. The base curve on the front surface of the right lens is +14.00 and on the back surface plano vertically by +7.00 in the 180° meridian. A photograph of Monet in his garden taken about 1926 shows him wearing a pair of glasses that is probably this pair. Spectacles of this type were commonly prescribed in the 1920s and created some visual problems. First, the high power plus lens for his right eye was combined with a lens of no power for the left eye, which resulted in differences in image size for the two eyes. This prevented Monet from using both eyes together. Monet wrote Coutela saying that he blocked off the vision of his left eye with a piece of paper, which was a logical act to avoid confusion. Second, the field of view for this pair of glasses was very limited. Third, Monet had different pairs of glasses for near and for far vision. His distant glasses had no bifocal lens. This limited his ability to focus at various distances, a problem he mentioned in his letters. Fourth, the lenses of this type induce spherical and chromatic aberration. Fifth, the large amount of astigmatic correction for his right eye must have increased his problems. Sixth, the lenses lacked the corrected curves that are available today. Seventh, the high power of his right lens caused extreme magnification. Today we would use an intraocular lens or a contact lens to avoid the problems of magnification, any size difference, and restricted field of vision.

On October 13, 1923, he wrote Coutela to say:

Finally I am very happy to inform you that I am surprised with the progress of my vision from the point of view of colors, not daylight, but in the evening under artificial light. I am seeing as I formerly did, which makes me hope for better things in daylight. I hope that the new glasses which will come soon will be helpful. One thing astonishes me a little. For several days, I have sudden little sharp pains in the operated eye. [37]

On October 21, 1923, he wrote Coutela:

First—I have received the glasses from Germany, and to my great astonishment the result is very good. Again I can see green, red, and toned down blue. It would be perfect if the frame were better, for the lenses of the two eyes are too close together. [38]

On January 18, 1924, Monet wrote Coutela to ask him to send a summary of his fees for the first eye [39]. On January 29, 1924, Monet sent Coutela a check in the amount of 10 000 francs drawn on an account at the Societe Generale. He thanked Coutela for his

good care, for having endured my attacks of anxiety. I hope that for the other eye it will not be the same on my part at least, in case an operation becomes necessary. I ask you only not to forget the way to Giverny, and to come to have lunch one of these beautiful days. [40]

Clemenceau did his best to keep Monet encouraged. In a letter dated March 1, 1924, he wrote:

My poor old crazy one,
I believe truly that I like you better when you are stupid. In spite of the pleasure of loving you, I would prefer that this not happen too often.

You developed cataracts in each eye. These things happen to everyone. You resented this because you are an artist without equal, and when your vision failed you tried to make more beautiful things than when you had both eyes working. The most admirable thing is that you have succeeded. This is the cause of your present sadness.

You have spent your lifetime between crises of success and reactions of defiance against yourself. This is the same condition of your triumph. This continues with the aggravation of an overtired retina. You have decided that your work which was interrupted when you were at the end of the road, should be begun again with your half-vision. And you have found the means of producing a finished masterpiece. [41]

Monet was touching up some of his previous works, and was in danger of ruining them. Clemenceau wrote him on October 8, 1924, trying to dissuade him from this:

Now you have conceived the absurd idea of fixing up other works. Who knows better than you, that the impressions of a painter change each moment? If one were to take you back with your canvases before the Cathedral of Rouen what wouldn't you find to change? You have made new works, most of which were and still are masterpieces if you have not ruined them.

Then you have wanted to make super-masterpieces, with an instrument of vision that you have told me is imperfect.

And you are irritated at the idea that you cannot please yourself. That is a pure aberration. A true artist is never content with himself. [42]

Monet wrote Coutela on April 9, 1924, of further discouragement:

For months I have been working with obstinacy, without arriving with anything good. I destroy everything that is so-so. Is this due to my age? Is it defective vision? Both certainly, but especially my vision. You have given me the sight of black on white for reading and writing, and for that I cannot be too grateful, but the vision of a painter, when lost, I am certain, cannot return!

I am saying this to you confidentially. I hide it as much as possible, but I am terribly sad and discouraged. Life is a torture for me. I don't know what to tell you. You understand I am lavished with care and affection. Except for my near vision, I certainly see less and less. Only the first glasses helped me in artificial light, and one unique thing, I accidentally wore them out of doors, and I cannot verify my ability to see blue and yellow which you found with the tinted glasses. [43]

Three days later Monet again wrote Coutela, thanking him for his most recent letter:

Thank you for troubling yourself on my part with Clemenceau, who has completely reassured you on my part. But let me tell you that if I am creating masterpieces, it is he that says so. In that we are not in accord. That said, I am telling you that I have definitely stopped the tinted glasses. To paint and get about, I use the first glasses that you prescribed for me, and with which I see so badly. I ask you not to forget to send me the prescription for the first glasses, if you have a record of them, and send me also the prescription for the tinted glasses. [44]

On May 9, 1924, he wrote Coutela complaining about all his glasses:

Each time that I change glasses it seems to me that I see better, but sadly this doesn't last, and nothing is any good. There is always too much blue and yellow. Clemenceau has said that my last paintings were masterpieces. He is mistaken or else I am. Things are terrible and I need to see you . . . One thing seems possible. That would be to try glasses tinted more lightly than those that I have . . .

His daughter-in-law added to the end of the letter: "Monsieur Monet has forgotten to say that our euphthalmine is almost gone. He finds that the new formula worked more slowly. He asked me to ask you to send it to him if you can" [45].

On July 7, 1924, Monet wrote Coutela:

My dear Doctor and Friend,

You have had the kind idea to write my daughter-in-law and ask her of news about me, how I have been doing. In my last letter I told you that I have gone back to work outdoors and I continue with ardor but not without difficulty. The last untinted glasses that you have given me have not provided good results and I have stopped using them.

In the meantime I ought to tell you, my friend Barbier has made the acquaintance of Dr Mawas, who it appears is a specialist in optics, and is the only one who can order lenses from Zeiss. This doctor (who is your friend) has offered to come to take the measurements required for these marvelous glasses. I wanted to write you sooner but work absorbed me.

As this is vacation time, I would hope that you would not go away without coming to see me. I would like to know what you think of Dr Mawas. A word to announce you are coming before lunch.

All my friendship,

Claude Monet [46]

And so we introduce a new character into the continuing drama of Monet's changeable vision.

Jacques Mawas MD

Jacques Mawas (1885–1976) was a great figure in the history of French ophthalmology. He was just 38 years old when called upon to care for the grand old man of Impressionism. Born in Egypt, he studied medicine in Beirut, then came to France where he studied histology and astronomy. He worked at the Pasteur Institute in Paris until World War I. He served in the war and was gassed. He later returned to the Pasteur Institute. He became chief of the laboratory at the Clinique Nationale des Quinze-Vingts, later moving his laboratory to the Rothschild Hospital. He became chief of service of the Rothschild Foundation, then scientific director of the Foundation. He became so identified with this institution that when Baron Maurice Rothschild asked for information about the hospital founded by his Uncle Adolphe, he was answered, "Rothschild Foundation? I don't know it. You must be speaking of the Mawas Foundation?" Mawas was proud also to be director of the eye laboratory at the Ecole Practique des Hautes Etudes of the Sorbonne, where he followed in the footsteps of Javal and Tschernig. Mawas was an energetic researcher and a kind, generous, lovable man. He was a member of countless medical societies. Enthusiastic and vivacious, he was a pioneer in research but also aimed to be practical, concerned with clinical applications. Early, he worked on questions of anatomy and physiology. His late work was on the function of the pigment epithelium and the structure and development of the vitreous. He was well known for his classification of ocular tumors, his work on chorioretinal degeneration, histology of the angle, physiology of the eye, and did pioneer work in retinal photography. His bibliography of about 250 items includes several books [47–49].

Dr Mawas enjoyed retelling the story of his first meeting with Monet and the care that he provided the artist. When approached by Monet's friend Barbier, to take care of the aged artist, Mawas said that he took care of Maurice Denis, another artist, and that he was very interested in the vision of painters. The same day he wrote Monet to make arrangements to visit the artist at his home along with Clemenceau. Mawas told what happened at Giverny. He met Clemenceau and they discussed the situation. Later Monet joined them. After lunch Monet took Mawas to his studio and pointed out several of his most recent

canvases saying: "It is filthy, it is disgusting, I see nothing but blue." He spoke of destroying many of his paintings and said:

I see blue; I no longer see red or yellow. This annoys me terribly because I know that these colors exist, because I know that on my palette there is some red, some yellow, a special green and a certain violet. I no longer see them and I saw them previously, and I recall very well the colors that they gave me. [50]

Several very blue paintings date from this period including a view of his house at Giverny (Plate 2.4). This contrasts with a yellow–red view of the same scene which is signed and dated 1922, just before his cataract surgery (Plate 2.5). Mawas prescribed glasses with a yellow–green tint, which pleased Monet and brought him out of his despair. The overwhelming blue cast to his paintings disappeared and he began working on his waterlily canvases with more enthusiasm. He adapted well to his new glasses and wore them to paint. He preferred to use his right eye with glasses for painting. Before surgery he had relied on the left eye. In a photograph of Monet in his studio, his glasses are on a table only because this was a posed photograph (Fig. 2.1). Without the glasses he could not have used both eyes, and must have relied on the left eye alone. Careful observation of photographs of his glasses (Fig. 2.2) reveal that some of those he used after cataract surgery have a left lens that is much darker than the right one, an occlusive lens, blackened to blot out the input from the left eye.

Trying to keep both Coutela and Mawas happy, Monet wrote Coutela on August 11, 1924, asking that he and Mawas come together to visit him at Giverny [51]. He wrote Coutela again on October 6, 1924:

I do not hide from you that I am troubled that you have not given me any sign of life. I cannot believe that you are unhappy with me for having been obliged to receive Monsieur [sic] Mawas. I owe you too much to believe that.

If I have not written you since my last letter it is because I am waiting for a sign from Dr Mawas, but I have been

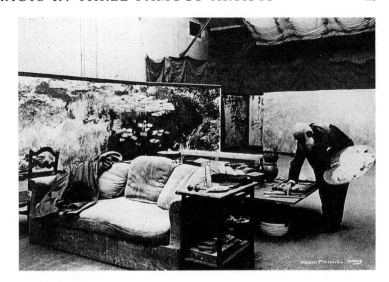

Fig. 2.1 Photograph of Monet in his third studio, 1924 or 1925 by Henri Manuel. Marmottan Museum, Paris.

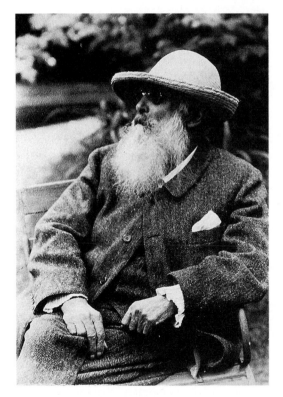

Fig. 2.2 Photograph of Monet in his garden, 1926 by Nicholas Muray. Museum of Modern Art, New York.

but it hasn't lasted and I am completely discouraged. [52]

Eight days later he wrote to Coutela:

Thank you for the kind letter which gave me great pleasure . . . Dr Mawas ought to come again to take more measurements for the excellent glasses but I don't know when. Excuse this scrawl and believe my best wishes. [53]

Clemenceau was not particularly pleased that Monet had consulted another doctor without asking him. Trying to keep on good terms with everyone, Monet wrote Coutela on January 16, 1925:

Dear Doctor and Friend,

I am late in thanking you for your good wishes. Intense work obsesses me, without the results that I would like. This is the only reason.

I am still in good health. My vision will give you the greatest pleasure.

My best wishes and my fond remembrances,

Your Claude Monet [54]

abandoned by you and by him! And don't speak of my friend Barbier.

You write that I am doing better. This is wrong. There has been little amelioration,

Monet's final years

During 1924 and 1925, Mawas obtained several more pairs of glasses in various tints for Monet. Like Clemenceau, Mawas was psychologically astute and understood what troubled Monet. Monet had outlived two wives and one of his two sons. He was no longer young and was frequently depressed. Monet's depression is evident in this quotation:

> At night I'm constantly haunted by what I'm trying to achieve. I get up exhausted every morning. The dawning day gives me back my courage. But my anxiety comes back as soon as I set foot in my studio . . . Painting is so difficult. And a torture. Last fall I burned six canvases along with the dead leaves from my garden. It's hopeless. Still I wouldn't want to die before saying all that I have to say, or at least having tried to say it. And my days are numbered. [55]

Monet's comments reveal his alternating moods. On December 8, 1924, he wrote Mawas of his pleasure with a new pair of untinted lenses, saying: "I see colors more clearly and I am able to work with greater assurance . . . I am very pleased, very happy to tell you this and thank you heartily" [56]. Nonetheless, his mood again became grim a few months later. On March 25, 1925, he wrote Dr Mawas:

> Dear Doctor,
>
> I am quite late in giving you news concerning the outcome of my new glasses, but they arrived at such a bad period. I was very discouraged and I no longer hoped for better, so that I discontinued using these glasses which I probably might have accustomed myself to had they not completely disturbed me— eyesight trouble, the slightest color tones broken and exaggerated.
>
> As soon as I am in a better frame of mind I will try to get used to them, though I am more than ever certain that a painter's eyesight can never be recovered. When a singer loses his voice he retires; the painter who has undergone an operation of the cataract must renounce painting; and this is what I have been incapable of. [57]

Monet's mood improved 4 months later. Here is an excerpt from a letter to his friend Andre Barbier, dated July 17, 1925: "Since your last visit my vision is totally ameliorated. I am working harder than ever, am pleased with what I do, and if the new glasses are better still I would like to live to be one hundred" [58].

Ten days later he was still content, as this quotation from a letter to Dr Coutela attests:

> I am very happy to inform you that finally I have recovered my proper vision and that nearly at a single stroke. In brief, I am happily seeing everything again and I am working with ardor. [59]

Monet continued to paint nearly to the time of his death from lung disease associated with smoking in December 1926. A group of his waterlily canvases was installed in the Orangerie des Tuileries, in May 1927, where they may be seen today.

Monet painted for more than 60 years. The paintings created during his long career span the period from early Impressionism to the vague scenes of his old age. For many years his late works were considered inferior to his earlier ones, but more recent critical opinion has changed. The late works are now generally considered to be a link to the abstract art of the twentieth century.

Honoré Daumier

Daumier (1808–1879) was a Frenchman who is remembered for his satirization of human frailties. A prolific artist, Daumier created some 4000 prints and a much smaller number of paintings and sculpture characterized by a graceful style. A man of the people, Daumier joined the typical citizen in his daily battle with the establishment. Pompous physicians were one of his targets. Daumier poked fun at patients as well, in a good natured manner. But doctors and their patients were more gently lambasted than were bureaucrats, politicians, policemen, and lawyers. Most of his prints were created for publication in newspapers and many were political cartoons. They served to make the reader laugh or to prod the public to correct injustice.

The record Daumier left behind is mainly his art. This major nineteenth-century artist left behind relatively few details of his life. Until old age, he enjoyed good health, but by age 64 his vision began to deteriorate. The following year he acquired a ptosis of one upper lid and frequent blinking. His physician advised him to stop work due to his poor eyesight. Daumier underwent cataract surgery during his last year or two of life but the surgery did him little good. The recovery period coincided with his first solo exhibition of his paintings and drawings. Daumier died a few months after suffering a stroke, just prior to his 71st birthday.

Mary Cassatt

Cassatt (1844–1926) is often considered the finest female artist that America has produced. Late in her career she developed cataracts and diabetes. Although she underwent several operations for cataracts, her vision never improved. As her sight decreased, a progressive looseness of artistic style occurred. Blindness followed, so that she stopped work totally for the last dozen years of her life.

She was born into a wealthy, sophisticated family in what is now Pittsburgh. When Cassatt decided to become an artist, her father objected strongly saying: "I would almost rather see you dead" [60]. Other family members never understood her devotion to art and considered her eccentric. Recognition of her merit as a significant artist came earlier in Europe than in the USA. She achieved official recognition when her works were accepted for exhibition at the Salon in Paris in 1868; she was only 24. Cassatt was particularly friendly with Degas and some of the other Impressionists. She accepted an invitation to exhibit with them, and showed her works at four of the eight Impressionist shows. She was the only American artist to exhibit with the Impressionists.

Cassatt is usually classified as an Impressionist artist, but her art differs from Impressionists such as Monet and Pissarro in several ways. Her themes are generally indoor scenes of mothers and children (Plate 2.6) rather than landscapes. Until visual problems troubled her, her paintings were carefully composed, without the broken brush strokes typical of Impressionism. Her close friend Degas said of her: "I am not willing to admit that a woman can draw that well" [61].

Recognition of her ability came earlier in France than in America, where she remained essentially unknown. When she returned home to Pennsylvania in 1898, after spending many years in France, a newspaper had this to say about her:

> Mary Cassatt, sister of Mr Cassatt, president of the Pennsylvania Railroad, returned from Europe today. She has been studying painting in France, and owns the smallest Pekinese dog in the world. [62]

With advanced age her medical problems became serious. She developed diabetes mellitus and was placed on a program of strict medical treatment. Part of the program was radiation therapy, radium by inhalation. On December 14, 1911, she wrote the following:

> I am at the doctor's, taking inhalations of radium. This is the eighth day, and I am suffering very much, which it seems, would prove that it is doing me good, that it will be a success, providing I can stand it. [63]

Radiation as a treatment for cataracts was tried by some well-known individuals at this time. Frederick C. Cordes MD (former chairman, Department of Ophthalmology, University of California at San Francisco) coauthored an article which appeared in the *American Journal of Ophthalmology* in 1920 entitled "Radium for cataract." The authors concluded: "Radium is of proven value in the treatment of incipient cataracts" [64]. The same year an article appeared in the *American Journal of Roentgenology* entitled "The technic of radium application in cataracts." The author concluded: "The application of radium is harmless to the normal tissues of the eye" [65]. Obviously things have changed since 1920.

Although this form of therapy seems misguided if not totally bizarre today, it should be viewed in the context of the time. The history of the treatment of diabetes reveals that a multitude of various forms of therapy were tried, many of which are strange, even harmful, by today's standards. In Cassatt's era Marie Curie won the Nobel Prize for her work with radium, and radiation was used then for a far greater range of diseases than today. The diabetes and radiation therapy may have caused her greatest medical problem—cataracts.

By 1911 Cassatt realized that her vision

was failing. She was examined in 1913 by the famous French ophthalmologist, Edmond Landolt, who told her that nothing could be done. Unfortunately, Landolt's records no longer exist. Although the conflict of World War I meant that most doctors were serving with the military and were unable to treat civilians, Cassatt found an American ophthalmologist in Paris to treat her, Dr Louis Borsch. He operated each of her eyes for cataracts but the results were poor.

On September 8, 1915, she sent a telegram to a friend describing some of her difficulties. It said: "Sick eyes. Iritis with adhesion under treatment . . . Ophthalmologist will be famous if he succeeds. Operation to be avoided" [66].

In 1917 the cataract in her right eye was removed but she was not pleased with the results. She wrote on December 12, 1917: "The operated right eye will not help my sight much even tho' the secondary cataract is absorbed altogether" [67]. Her mood had not improved by December 28, 1917, when she wrote:

I am nearer despair than I ever was. Operating on my right eye before the cataract was ripe is the last drop. I asked Borsch if it was ripe and he assured me that it was! The sight of that eye is inferior but I still saw a great deal in spite of the cataract. Now I see scarcely at all. [68]

Her situation had not improved by the summer of 1918. On July 13, 1918, she wrote:

The secondary cataract is covering the right eye which was operated in October, and no doubt that it can be removed in the fall. The operation which was made in October and was followed by so long a treatment was a complete failure and ought not to have been attempted if only it has not injured what there was of sight in that eye! The cataract over the left eye which is the eye in which depends my hope of future sight is not nearly ripe or I could not write you this. [69]

On August 24, 1918, she wrote: "My sight is getting dimmer every day. I find writing tires my eyes. I look forward with horror to utter darkness and then an operation which may end in as great a failure as the last one" [70].

Her cataract in the left eye was operated in October 1919. She described this in a letter dated November 14, 1919: "The operation was a very daring one as the cataract was not ripe, but he staked his reputation on the result. He is the only man in Paris capable of doing such an operation and I am told few anywhere in the US" [71]. She continued to do poorly as she remarked in a letter dated March 28, 1920:

I am old and so blind that I don't feel up to much . . . I see less with the eye that was operated in October than I did with the one with a secondary cataract in it! Borsch knew that would be so and spoke of a film that sometimes formed after an operation for cataract even when the operation was ripe and that it was nothing to make a slit and then one saw! Which means of course another operation which equally I must submit to. I think that state of my eyes, will I hope shorten my life. [72]

Apparently she had a discussion of the posterior capsule in the left eye for she wrote on May 18, 1920: "A secondary cataract is to be opened tomorrow" [73].

Even by 1921 her vision had not shown significant improvement. She wrote the following that year:

Last May I had an operation upon my best eye. The operation was very successful and the oculist promised me I should paint again, but a hidden abscess in an apparently sound tooth caused a violent inflammation and I have not yet recovered from it. Nor has the sight of the eye returned.

I have had a very serious operation for cataract several weeks ago and have my eye still bandaged and can only see very indifferently with the other eye which is my poor eye. I shall not be able to use my eyes, nor be allowed glasses for several months to come, after that my oculist promises great results. I do not allow myself such sanguine hopes. [74]

With the advancement of her lens opacities, she became unable to paint in her previous manner. Details were lost from her paintings. She found working with pastel crayons easier than painting with oils. The loose, sketchy nature of pastel did not require the sharp acuity of oil painting. It is curious that Cassatt's close friend, Degas, also switched from oil to pastel as his vision diminished from what was probably macular degeneration. He suffered from extreme loss of vision in one eye and had a central scotoma in the other eye. For both Cassatt and Degas, vision loss resulted in similar artistic results. Their late pastels were with broad strokes on large pieces of paper. Colors became limited in range and were harsh, even strident. Details became much less present in the later works. For each artist the delicacy of early creations was lost in the late works.

Cassatt was depressed, even embittered by her visual problems. After 1914 she stopped her artwork altogether. By 1918 she could not read. The vision loss shortened her artistic career by about 12 years. She died aged 81 in 1926, the same year that Monet died.

Mary Cassatt was a remarkable individual. In an era in which women tended to stay close to home, she ventured across the Atlantic and earned fame in Europe. Today her artistic reputation continues to increase as do prices for her works. In 1980 the San Francisco Museum of Art purchased a color print by Cassatt for about $80 000 at auction, which set a record for any American print. In 1988 another Cassatt print sold for $198 000. This is even more remarkable when we consider that prints are not one-of-a-kind items.

She took the old theme of mother and child and refashioned it with her own charm giving it a new vigor. She produced many emotionally touching works that were able to avoid a false sense of sentimentality or lack of genuine feeling. Today her art is appealing for its combination of careful modeling, simplified forms, influenced by Eastern art and the bright colors of Impressionism.

Acknowledgments

Several individuals provided valuable assistance with this article: Mlle Monique Delacour, Adolphe de Rothschild Ophthalmologic Foundation, Paris, who was a laboratory technician for Jacques Mawas MD; Edouard Mawas MD, Paris, nephew of Jacques Mawas; Pierre Amalric MD, Albi, France, an ophthalmologist who was instrumental in acquiring the Monet correspondence for the French Ophthalmologic Society in Paris; George Heard Hamilton PhD, director emeritus of the Clark Art Institute, Williamstown, Massachusetts; and Leslie Balkany MA, and Marc Gerstein PhD, Toledo Museum of Art.

References

1 Zola E. The Realists at the Salon. *Evenement*, 1866. In: Stuckey CF, ed. *Monet: a Retrospective*. New York: Levin, 1985: 34.

2 Castagnary J. The Exhibition on the Boulevard des Capucines. *Siecle*, April 29, 1874. In: Stuckey CF, ed. *Monet: a Retrospective*. New York: Levin, 1985: 58.

3 Leroy L. The Impressionist Exhibition. *Charivari*. April 25, 1874. In: Stuckey CF, ed. *Monet: a Retrospective*. New York: Levin, 1985: 57.

4 Huysmans JK. The Exhibition of the Independents of 1881. *Art Moderne Certains*, 1883. In: Stuckey CF, ed. *Monet: a Retrospective*. New York: Levin, 1985: 94.

5 de Lostalot A. Exhibition of the Works of M. Claude Monet. *Gazette Beaux-Arts*, April, 1883. In: Stuckey CF, ed. *Monet: a Retrospective*. New York: Levin, 1985: 103–4.

6 Moreau PG. La cataracte de Claude Monet. *L'Ophthalmologie des Origines a Nos Jours* 1981; **3**: 141.

7 Thiebault-Sisson F. *Les Nympheas* de Claude Monet a l'Orangerie des Tuileries. *Revue Art Ancien Moderne* 1927; **52**: 45–6.

8 Rouart D, Rey JD. *Monet Water-Lilies*. New York: Amiel, 1974: 67.

9 Moreau PG. La cataracte de Claude Monet. *L'Ophthalmologie des Origines a Nos Jours* 1981; **3**: 141.

10 Stuckey CF. Blossoms and blunders: Monet and the State, II. *Art Am* 1979; **68**: 116.

11 Martet J. *Georges Clemenceau*. New York: Langmans, Green, 1930: 203–5.

12 Offret G. Charles Coutela. Notices necrologiques. *Bull Soc Ophthalmol Fr* 1969; **81**: 120–1.

13 Dittiere M. Comment Monet recouvra la vue apres l'operation de la cataracte. *Sandorama* 1973; **32**: 30.

14 Monet to Coutela, September 13, 1922. French Ophthalmologic Society. (Translation of this and other letters by Ravin JG.)

15 Clemenceau to Monet, September 19, 1922. In: Suarez G. *La Vie Orgueilleuse de Clemenceau*. Paris: Editions de France, 1930: 622.

16 Monet to Coutela, October 20, 1922. French Ophthalmologic Society.

17 Monet to Coutela, November 9, 1922. French Ophthalmologic Society.

18 Dittiere M. Comment Monet recouvra la vue apres l'operation de la cataracte. *Sandorama* 1973; **32**: 30.

19 Hoschedé JP. *Claude Monet Ce Mal Connu*. Geneva: Cailler, 1960: 142–3.

20 Clemenceau to Coutela, February 26, 1923. French Ophthalmologic Society.

21 Monet to Coutela, March 11, 1923. French Ophthalmologic Society.

22 Monet to Coutela, April 9, 1923. French Ophthalmologic Society.

23 Monet to Coutela, June 15, 1923, French Ophthalmologic Society.

24 Monet to Coutela, June 18, 1923. French Ophthalmologic Society.

25 Monet to Coutela, June 22, 1923. French Ophthalmologic Society.

26 Monet to Coutela, June 28, 1923. French Ophthalmologic Society.

27 Coutela C. Comment Monet recouvra la vue apres l'operation de la cataracte. *Sandorma* 1973; **32**: 30.

28 Coutela to Clemenceau, August 21, 1923, *Ophthalmol* 1981; **3**: 142.

29 Monet to Coutela, August 27, 1923. French Ophthalmologic Society.

30 Monet to Coutela, August 29, 1923. French Ophthalmologic Society.

31 Clemenceau to Coutela, August 29, 1923. French Ophthalmologic Society.

32 Monet to Coutela, September 27, 1923. French Ophthalmologic Society.

33 Clemenceau to Coutela, September 8, 1923. French Ophthalmologic Society.

34 Monet to Coutela, September 14, 1923. French Ophthalmologic Society.

35 Coutela C. Monet's Giverny. In: Wildenstein D, ed. *Monet's Years at Giverny: Beyond Impressionism*. New York: Metropolitan Museum of Art, 1978: 40.

36 Ravin JG. Monet's cataracts. *JAMA* 1985; **254**: 394–9.

37 Monet to Coutela, October 13, 1923, French Ophthalmologic Society.

38 Monet to Coutela, October 21, 1923. French Ophthalmologic Society.

39 Monet to Coutela, January 18, 1924. French Ophthalmologic Society.

40 Monet to Coutela, January 29, 1924. French Ophthalmologic Society.

41 Clemenceau to Monet, March 1, 1924. In: Suarez G, ed. *La Vie Orgueilleuse de Clemenceau*. Paris: Editions of France, 1930: 622–3.

42 Clemenceau to Monet, October 8, 1924. In: Suarez G, ed. *La Vie Orgueilleuse de Clemenceau*. Paris: Editions of France, 1930: 625.

43 Monet to Coutela, April 9, 1924. French Ophthalmologic Society.

44 Monet to Coutela, April 12, 1924. French Ophthalmologic Society.

45 Monet to Coutela, May 9, 1924. French Ophthalmologic Society.

46 Monet to Coutela, July 7, 1924. French Ophthalmologic Society.

47 Hervouet F. Necrologie. Jacques Mawas. *Arch Ophthalmol* 1976; **36**: 273–6.

48 Baillart JP. Rapport moral du Secretaire General. *Bull Soc Ophthalmol Fr* 1977; **77**: 2–8.

49 Dollfus MA. *In memoriam*, Jacques Mawas. *Bull Cancer* 1976; **63**: 259–60.

50 Dittiere PG. La cataracte de Claude Monet. Comment Monet recouvra la vue apres l'operation de la cataracte. *Sandorama* 1973; **32**: 31; Moreau PG. La cataracte de Claude Monet. *L'Ophthalmologie des Origenes a Nos Jours*, 1981; **3**: 142–3.

51 Monet to Coutela, August 11, 1924. French Ophthalmologic Society.

52 Monet to Coutela, October 6, 1924. French Ophthalmologic Society.

53 Monet to Coutela, October 14, 1924. French Ophthalmologic Society.

54 Monet to Coutela, January 16, 1925. French Ophthalmologic Society.

55 Delange R. Interview with Monet. In: Gordon R, Forge A, eds. *Monet*. New York: Abrams, 1983: 247.

56 Monet to Mawas, December 8, 1924. In: Rouart D, Rey JD. *Monet Water Lillies*. New York: Amiel, 1974.

57 Monet to Mawas, March 25, 1925. French Ophthalmologic Society.

58 Monet to Barbier, July 17, 1925. In: Hoschede JP, ed. *Claude Monet ce Mal Connu*. Geneva: Cailler, 1960: 150–1.

59 Monet to Coutela, July 27, 1925. French Ophthalmologic Society.

60 Hale N. *Mary Cassatt*. New York: Doubleday, 1975: 31.

61 Hale N. *Mary Cassatt*. New York: Doubleday, 1975: 193.

62 Sweet FA. *Miss Mary Cassatt, Impressionist from Pennsylvania*. Oklahoma: Oklahoma University Press, 1966: 150.

63 Hale N. *Mary Cassatt*. New York: Doubleday, 1975: 244.

64 Franklin WS, Cordes FC. Radium for cataract. *Am J Ophthalmol* 1920; **3**: 643.

65 Levin I. Technic of radium application in cataracts. *Am J Roentgenol* 1920; **7**: 107.

66 Cassatt, Telegram to Louisine Havemeyer, September 8, 1915. Cassatt papers, Collection of National Gallery, Washington. DC.

67 Cassatt to Havemeyer, December 12, 1917. National Gallery.

68 Cassatt to Havemeyer, December 28, 1917. National Gallery.

69 Cassatt to Havemeyer, July 13, 1918. National Gallery.

70 Cassatt to Havemeyer, August 24, 1918. National

Gallery.

71 Cassatt to Havemeyer, November 14, 1919. National Gallery.

72 Cassatt to Havemeyer, March 28, 1920. National Gallery.

73 Cassatt to Havemeyer, May 18, 1920. National Gallery.

74 Sweet FA. *Miss Mary Cassatt, Impressionist from Pennsylvania*. Oklahoma: Oklahoma University Press, 1966: 198.

3: Cataractogenesis: Etiology, Risk Factors, and Therapy

SIDNEY LERMAN

Introduction

There is a considerable amount of variation relating to cataract incidence in the literature and this can be attributed to differences in determining what constitutes a cataract. Some investigators consider that any inhomogeneity in the lens is a cataract, irrespective of its size and location. However, most middle-aged and older people have some lens changes but do not suffer from any visual impairment. If we consider a cataract to be a disease state, then it should be defined as a change in lens transparency (opacity) which affects visual acuity, glare, and contrast sensitivity.

Studies by the World Health Organization demonstrate that at least 20 million people are blind because of cataracts [1,2]. While the incidence of cataracts in people older than 50 years is 15% in the West, in the developing countries it is much higher, reaching 40% in India [3]. A recent conference on the epidemiology of cataracts identifies several risk factors in the pathogenesis of senile (aging) cataracts [4]. Aside from aging itself, genetic factors, nutrition, and diabetes mellitus, ultraviolet (UV) radiation has been implicated as a significant risk factor in the generation of brunescent (brown) nuclear cataracts and it also plays a role in the pathogenesis of cortical and mixed (brown nuclear and cortical) cataracts [4–14]. The most frequent initial sites of senile cortical and mixed cataracts are the subcapsular and supranuclear zones [15,16]. While the brown cataract is probably a photo-induced nuclear change which represents a form of accelerated lens aging.

Cataract risk factors

While heredity plays a role in the genesis of the aging cataracts, it does not appear to exert a dominant genetic effect and we are as yet unable to manipulate human chromosomes; thus, this risk factor can only be acknowledged but not treated. Malnutrition is also a significant risk factor particularly in the underdeveloped countries which have the highest incidence of cataracts; the lack of which specific nutrient or nutrients play a role has yet to be determined. In addition to a lack of certain nutrients, there is the possibility that certain diets could contain cataractogenic or cocataractogenic factors which could play a role in the development of lenticular opacities. For example, in certain parts of the world the diet may consist of a large amount of vegetation which contains photosensitizing agents such as psoralen derivatives, thereby enhancing the role of UV radiation as a risk factor. Ocular phototoxicity and photosensitization as cataractogenic factors will be considered in a subsequent section.

A recent study has demonstrated that a group of presumptive risk factors previously considered to be of some significance, do not appear to have a cataractogenic influence. These include smoking, allergies, diseases of the pancreas, thyroid, respiratory and circulatory systems, with the latter showing more of an eye-related behavior rather than exerting a clear-cut cataractogenic effect [17].

Diabetes mellitus and experimental sugar cataracts

The lens derives most, if not all, of its metabolic energy from the oxidation of glucose. Almost all the enzyme systems required for the operation of anaerobic glycolysis, the Krebs' cycle, and the hexose monophosphate pathway of glucose oxidation, are present in this organ. The lens also contains a rather unusual pathway for the metabolism of glucose and other monosaccharides, known as the polyol or sorbitol pathway. This pathway involves the direct utilization of non-phosphorylated sugars, with the formation of sugar alcohols as an intermediate step. Alterations in the activity of the polyol pathway appear to be of major importance in initiating the chain of metabolic events leading to the development of the experimental sugar cataracts and the human juvenile diabetic and galactosemic cataracts. Transient refractive errors in the uncontrolled diabetic patient may also be related to the elevated aqueous glucose levels leading to an osmotic imbalance between the lens and aqueous. A sudden elevation of aqueous glucose concentration (e.g. above 250 mg%) could result in aqueous hyperosmolarity leading to a transient withdrawal of water from within the lens. The consequence of such a reaction would be a slight relative increase in density, and therefore refractive index, of this organ. Prolonged elevation of aqueous glucose levels will saturate the hexokinase (phosphorylating) enzyme system through which glucose enters the usual metabolic pathways (anaerobic glycolysis and the shunt pathway). This leads to increased activity of the polyol pathway where glucose need not be phosphorylated. The end result is an accumulation of sorbitol within lens fibers. Since cell membranes are relatively impermeable to polyols, there is an accompanying increase in osmolarity within the cortical fibers. Water is imbibed, the cells rupture, and hydropic degeneration develops. The snowflake peripheral cortical opacities seen in experimental sugar cataracts and in the juvenile

diabetic lens (poorly controlled patient) have been attributed to this process of hydropic degeneration initiated by the polyol pathway. This type of opacity is reversible if the blood and aqueous sugar levels are decreased by insulin therapy. However, if this process persists, a severe metabolic breakdown occurs with changes in transport, water balance, protein aggregation, etc., and the lens becomes irreversibly and completely opaque. It should be noted that the polyol pathway only plays a significant role in the pathogenesis of juvenile diabetic cataracts. Its role in cataracts developing in mature onset diabetes is questionable.

A similar correlation exists between the ease of induction of experimental sugar cataracts (galactose, diabetic, and xylose) and the age of the animal. The xylose cataract can only be induced in the young rat; the induction of the galactose cataract requires a short latent period in the young animal (6–10 days) and progressively longer periods of galactose feeding as the animal ages. The osmotic changes that initially accompany the accumulation of sugar alcohols (in the experimental sugar cataracts) do not seriously alter their viability since this process is reversible in the early stages (cortical snowflake opacities or vacuoles) if the blood glucose level is lowered below 250 mg% (by insulin therapy) or if galactose or xylose are removed from the diet. However, if the lens hydration is allowed to persist, other changes occur in such lenses, such as cation redistribution, loss of free amino acids and the relatively sudden development of a dense nuclear opacity [18]. On the enzymic level, the enzymes aldose reductase and polyol dehydrogenase (which constitute the sorbitol pathway) are present in sufficient concentration in the young animal lenses (employed in studying experimental sugar cataract), to rapidly generate levels of sugar alcohol at concentrations capable of exerting a severe osmotic effect. These studies have established that the sorbitol pathway is a major initiating factor in the genesis of sugar cataracts in young animals. In the young human lens, this pathway probably plays a similar role in the genesis of the juvenile diabetic cataract. The young human lens also contains sufficient levels of these enzymes and the

snowflake opacities which can suddenly appear
in an uncontrolled juvenile diabetic patient are
probably associated with the accumulation of
sorbitol resulting in an osmotic imbibition of
water into the lens cells followed by swelling
and hydropic degeneration (vacuolization).

However, the activity of the aldose reductase
enzyme (required to initiate the first step in the
sorbitol pathway) is much lower in the adult
human lens compared with the young lens and
its capacity to generate significant levels of
sugar alcohol is thereby limited [19]. Furthermore, the activity of this enzyme is not increased in the diabetic individual [19]. Thus the
role of the sorbitol pathway in the pathogenesis
of cataracts in mature onset diabetics is still
obscure as is the potential of the aldose reductase inhibitors which have been advocated in
the medical therapy (inhibition or prevention)
of cataracts [20,21]. A variety of aldose reductase inhibitors have recently been developed
[21] and several of them are undergoing clinical
testing. Most of these drugs are effective in
preventing or slowing the onset of experimental sugar cataracts in young animals but
their efficacy in mature onset diabetics remains
to be determined. One would anticipate that
these compounds will prove quite effective in
preventing the acute juvenile diabetic cataract.
Their efficacy as anticataract agents for the vast
majority of the so-called diabetic cataracts
(which are simply senile cataracts occuring at a
somewhat younger age than in non-diabetic
individuals) will require prolonged clinical
trials and evaluation utilizing newer biophysical techniques. One must also bear in
mind that these drugs are not entirely without
risk. For example, Sorbinil which is a potent
aldose reductase inhibitor carries with it a significant risk of skin rash and hepatic cellular
dysfunction. Furthermore, one can predict that
most of the aldose reductase inhibitors would
be potent photosensitizers, based on their
chemical structure (comprising a tricyclic
ring). A recent study on quercetrin, quercitin,
AY22-284, and Sorbinil has demonstrated that
intralenticular photobinding of these compounds can occur both *in vivo* as well as *in vitro*
[22]. The potential that such photobinding
might generate new intralenticular photo-

sensitizers with the consequent enhancement
of UV-induced photodamage to this organ,
must be further investigated.

Direct and photosensitized UV radiation

During the past decade, a considerable amount
of evidence has accumulated implicating UV
radiation (between 300 and 400 nm) as an important factor in the *in vitro* generation of
fluorescent compounds and in protein cross-
linking associated with lens aging and cataractogenesis in mouse, rat, and human lenses
[8,10,11]. The human ocular lens is constantly
exposed to ambient UV radiation (300–400 nm)
throughout life. The consequence of cumulative photochemical damage is an increasing
absorption of UV radiation and some visible
light as a result of the presence of photo-
chemically generated lens chromophores
(pigments). As these compounds increase
in concentration in the aging lens, the lens
nucleus becomes yellower and there is a progressive decrease in the transmission of visible
as well as UV radiation with age (Plate 3.1 and
Fig. 3.1).

It is now generally accepted that chronic
exposure to UV radiation (300–400 nm) over an
individual's lifetime leads to the generation and
increased accumulation of various fluorescent
chromophores in the lens that are, to some
extent, responsible for the increased yellow
color of the lens nucleus as it ages. In about
10% of the population in the USA, this process
progresses at a more rapid pace, resulting
in the development of the brown (nuclear)
cataract. This discoloration, in moderation, is
actually beneficial since it enables the lens to
become a very effective filter for UV and short
wavelength visible radiation (by the second to
the third decade), thus protecting the older
and metabolically less efficient retina from
cumulative photochemical damage that could
occur during our lifetime. Laboratory studies
have shown that $5 \, mW/cm^2$ (for 1000 s) of UVA
(320–400 nm) radiation exposure can cause
irreversible retinal photodamage in the aphakic
rhesus monkey.

These radiation levels approach the amount
of UV radiation in sunlight (which in the tem-

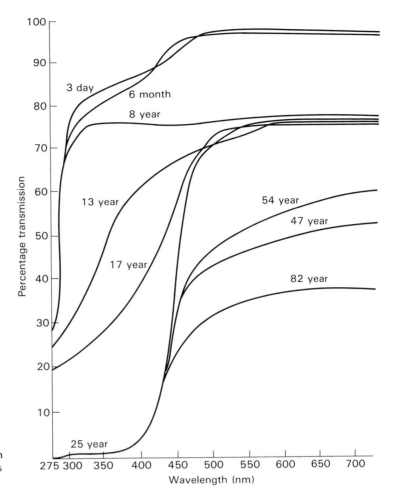

Fig. 3.1 Age-related changes in the transmission characteristics of the human lens.

perate zone has been measured at 2–4 mW/cm^2). These data are of particular importance for pseudophakes (as well as older aphakic patients) because clear artificial intraocular lenses are excellent transmitters of UVB (295–320 nm) as well as UVA (320–400 nm) radiation, which can penetrate the cornea. Aside from the effects of chronic exposure to ambient UV radiation, acute exposure to higher radiation levels can produce cortical opacities in human, rat, and rabbit lenses *in vitro* and *in vivo* [8]. Thus, more intense and acute UV can play a significant role in the generation of cortical cataracts while chronic (low level) exposure is more likely to be involved in the formation of the brown nuclear cataracts.

While UV radiation does play a role as a risk factor in cataractogenesis, one should also bear in mind that nature has enabled us to develop a natural UV-filtering capacity in our lenses by the third decade of life. This can be ascribed to the photochemical generation of the chromophores (pigments) caused by the eye's continuous exposure to ambient UV radiation. The beneficial effect of such exposure must be considered in deciding how to counsel patients regarding UV radiation exposure. In general, for most phakic patients living in the USA, UV-protective glasses are generally not necessary and could be counterproductive in youngsters who have not as yet had the time to develop proper UV-filtering capabilities in their lenses. Only those patients who by virtue of their life-style in sun-belt regions or who indulge in snow skiing (snow reflects 80% of UV radiation and can thus be much more damaging than the overhead sun) should consider proper UV-filtering glasses (or contact lenses when they become available). Of course, people who by virtue of their occupation are exposed to excessive UV radiation, should also be advised to wear such glasses. In addition, all patients (irrespective of age) who are undergoing phototherapy, must be protected with proper UV-filtering glasses, as well as all aphakes and pseudophakes with clear (non-UV filtering) intraocular lenses.

In addition to the demonstrated direct photochemical action of UV radiation on ocular tissues, particularly the cornea, lens, and retina, there is the possibility of photobiologic damage by means of photosensitized reactions due to the accumulation and retention of certain drugs within these tissues. For example, after the 13 mm stage of development, the ocular lens is completely encapsulated and never sheds its cells throughout life. Thus, photobinding a drug to the lens proteins and nucleic acids ensures its lifelong retention within the lens with the potential for enhanced photodamage if these compounds are capable of acting as photosensitizing agents. A similar situation exists in the neural retina which does not regenerate.

Two groups of compounds, the psoralens and the phenothiazines, have been clearly identified as intraocular photosensitizing agents that are capable of causing photochemical damage to the choroid, the retina, and the lens, in man as well as in experimental animals. The blood–aqueous and the blood–retinal barriers prevent intraocular penetration of many drugs. It is well known, for example, that it is difficult if not impossible to obtain an effective concentration of certain antibacterial, antimycotic, or antibiotic drugs in the interior of the normal eye, and this has been attributed to the relative impermeability of the blood–aqueous and the blood–retinal barriers [8]. Furthermore, the cornea and particularly the lens as it ages, provide effective filters for UV radiation and the shorter wavelengths of the visible spectrum, thereby nullifying any potential photosensitizing action of the drugs that are activated at these wavelengths which might accumulate in the posterior half of the globe. However, any photosensitizing agent that accumulates in the ocular lens or the retina might be a potential hazard if it becomes photobound to macromolecules within these tissues, since it would now be permanently retained there.

PSORALENS

The psoralen compounds are well known photosensitizing agents and have been used (under controlled conditions) in many dermatology clinics to treat psoriasis and vitiligo [23,24]. This form of phototherapy, commonly referred to as PUVA therapy, involves the ingestion of 8-methoxypsoralen (8-MOP) or related compounds, followed by exposure to UVA radiation (320–400 nm) for short periods of time. 8-MOP can be found in a variety of ocular tissues within 2 h after the patient is given a single dose (equivalent to a therapeutic level) and can become photobound to DNA and lens proteins if there is concurrent exposure to ambient levels of UVA radiation [25–31]. Since the mature ocular lens is a very effective filter for UVA radiation in most mammals (including humans) there can be no photobinding of 8-MOP in the retina. However, UVA radiation can penetrate to the retina in aphakic and pseudophakic experimental animals and in young eyes (where the ocular lens still permits significant penetration of UVA radiation) and 8-MOP photobinding can occur in their retinas.

PUVA therapy and cataract formation have now been documented in humans as well as in experimental animals [32–38]. These data provide objective proof that the drug can generate specific photoproducts in human lenses, which have been shown to be associated with the formation of PUVA cataracts in experimental animals. However, this observation should not deter anyone from prescribing such therapy, since simple and effective preventive measures are available. It should be noted that free 8-MOP can be found in the lens for only 24 h provided that the eye is protected from UVA radiation during this period, thus preventing permanent photobinding of this drug. Many dermatologists are now providing proper UV-filtering glasses to all their PUVA patients with instructions to put them on as soon as they ingest the drug and continue to wear them for at least 24 h. They must be worn indoors as well as outdoors, since there is sufficient UVA radiation in ordinary fluorescent lighting to photobind the 8-MOP [25,28]. A 2-year follow-up study utilizing UV slit-lamp densitography has proven the efficacy of this approach. All the patients wore proper UV-filtering glasses for at least 24 h following drug ingestion, and none developed enhanced or abnormal lens fluorescence levels. In contrast, patients whose eyes had not been properly protected (those treated prior to 1978) had anomalous and enhanced lens fluorescence and some developed PUVA cataracts. It should be noted that PUVA therapy could pose a potential hazard not only to the ocular lens but to the retina in young people whose lenses are not effective UV absorbers and/or in aphakic or pseudophakic individuals, particularly if they are exposed to repeated PUVA treatments [28,36–38]. The clear intraocular lenses are excellent transmitters of UV radiation and thus provide less protection from UV radiation than the natural lens or even ordinary glass, which can absorb UV radiation up to 320 nm. UV-absorbing intraocular lenses are now available and should provide a simple solution for preventing potential UV photodamage to the pseudophakic retina.

PHENOTHIAZINES

The phenothiazines, especially chlorpromazine, have long been recognized as having adverse ocular side effects [39]. Chlorpromazine is reported to be cataractogenic, with pigment deposits appearing in the lens as well as in the cornea and conjunctiva.

ALLOPURINOL

Allopurinol is a commonly used antihyperuricemic agent in treating gout. Scattered reports have appeared regarding the possible relationship between the development of lens opacities in relatively young patients (second to fourth decade) and chronic ingestion of this drug [40–42]. Studies suggest that allopurinol can act as a catactogenic-enhancing agent in some patients when it is permanently photobound within their lenses (probably as an additional extrinsically derived photosensitizer). Thus, chronic allopurinol therapy by itself does not necessarily result in the retention of allopurinol unless it becomes photobound. The relationship between levels of UVA exposure, circulating allopurinol levels and renal function in the genesis of photosensitized allopurinol cataracts will require further evaluation.

PORPHYRIN DERIVATIVES

The increasing interest in using hematoporphyrin derivatives (HPD) for phototherapy (and photodiagnostic procedures) merits careful evaluation regarding their phototoxic (or sensitizing) potential. The porphyrin derivatives absorb over a wide range in the UV and visible region of the electromagnetic spectrum and the fact that they appear to be slowly metabolized (HPD can be retained for 3 months after ingestion [43]) necessitates that adequate precautions be taken when such therapy is employed. These compounds can exert a photosensitizing action via the type I and II reactions. The photodynamic action is mediated via singlet oxygen and has been shown to polymerize lens proteins *in vitro* [44]. Patients undergoing HPD therapy must be monitored for ocular side effects, and they should also be informed about the potential for severe sunburn, particularly within the first 3 months following therapy.

RETINOIDS

There has been a resurgence of interest in the therapeutic uses of topical vitamin A acid (retinoic acid) and closely related compounds [45–47] particularly for skin conditions such as acne and related disorders, and psoriasis. In addition, such compounds have been tested as a method for treating corneal xerophthalmia, an ocular condition caused by a severe vitamin A deficiency. Considerable success has been claimed with such a therapeutic regime; however, the oral administration of isotretinoin has

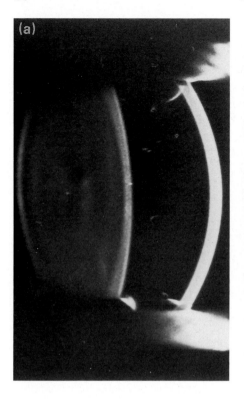
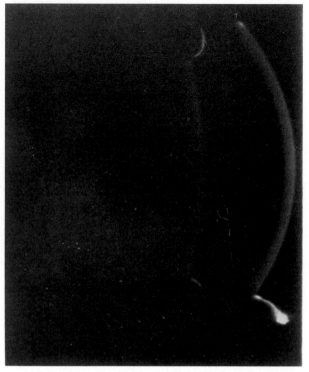

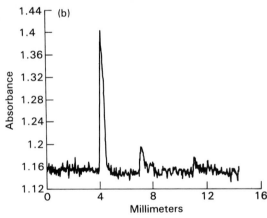

Fig. 3.2 (a) Visible (left) and ultraviolet (right) photographs of a 5-year-old normal eye. (b) Ultraviolet (fluorescence) densitogram.

resulted in some side effects; these include blepharoconjunctivitis or meibomianitis (33%), dry eyes (20%), contact lens intolerance (8%), and corneal opacities (5%). In addition, cataracts have now been reported in some patients, and the potential cataractogenic action of such drugs and the possibility of phototoxicity (and/ or photosensitization) should be considered, particularly with respect to the eye. Also, such drugs (which are analogs of retinoic acid)

could be incorporated into the rod photoreceptor elements during the continuous process of outer disc shedding and renewal. This might explain the complaint of impaired night vision, which can occur in some patients receiving these drugs. This side effect clears up rapidly, provided the drug is immediately discontinued. Patients undergoing clinical trials with these drugs should have careful ocular examinations prior to instituting therapy and be reevaluated at specific intervals to assess their ocular status.

Clinical studies

Since laboratory studies have demonstrated enhanced fluorescence in the ocular lens associated with aging and PUVA therapy and PUVA cataracts have recently been reported, a method to monitor lens fluorescence *in vivo* has been developed. A new slit-lamp densitographic apparatus (based on the Scheimpflug principle) capable of accurately and reproducibly recording visible changes in lens density as it ages was recently introduced [48]. This apparatus has been modified to utilize UV radiation (300–400 nm) to measure and quantitate age-related fluorescence levels in the normal lens *in vivo* and to correlate them with previously reported *in vitro* data [49–51]. Representative UV slit-lamp photographs (taken with the Scheimpflug Topcon SL45 camera) of normal eyes and corresponding densitograms show increased lens fluorescence with age. A series of UV and visible slit-lamp photographs of normal patients ranging in age from 5 to 65 years are shown in Figs 3.2 to 3.4. Note particularly the lack of fluorescence in the young lens and the progressive increase in fluorescence with age. These data can be expressed in graphic form showing the normal age-related increase in lens fluorescence (*in vivo*), which corresponds well with the *in vitro* data previously reported [52].

Aside from demonstrating the normal age-related increase in lens fluorescence, one can also detect abnormally enhanced fluorescence caused by occupational (or accidental) exposure to higher levels of UV radiation. This is shown in Fig. 3.5, which is a Scheimpflug photograph of a 40-year-old patient who was exposed to excessive UV in his workplace. The increased fluorescence can easily be appreciated by comparing this lens with a photograph of a normal 40-year-old eye (Fig. 3.6). Enhanced fluorescence and/or abnormal fluorescence emission can also occur in patients on PUVA therapy, and failure to properly protect such patients from all UV radiation (for at least 24 h following ingestion of the drug) can result in cataract

formation as shown in Fig. 3.7. This 52-year-old patient with psoriasis received 4 years of intermittent PUVA treatment (without proper eye protection). Although dermatology clinics now provide all PUVA patients with proper UV-absorbing or reflecting spectacles, data on a series of such patients who were treated prior to 1977 (when the potential for photosensitized lens damage from psoralen therapy was first demonstrated) and their densitograms, demonstrate a significant elevation of one of the lens fluorescence peaks (Fig. 3.8). Patients who have been on D-penicillamine therapy (for a variety of diseases) tend to have lower lens fluorescence intensities. This finding was anticipated since we had previously demonstrated that D-penicillamine (which is an excellent free radical scavenger as well as a chelating agent) is capable of entering the lens, as shown by *in vivo* as well as *in vitro* experiments. As a free radical scavenger, D-penicillamine aborts the UV-induced free radical reaction, thereby preventing photodamage.

These studies demonstrate the feasibility of obtaining *in vivo* lens fluorescence data that are objective, reproducible, and can be quantified. Thus, UV slit-lamp densitography can be used to objectively monitor one parameter of lens aging (fluorescence), as well as photosensitized lens damage, at a molecular level years before opacities become manifest by conventional slit-lamp examination, and measures can be instituted to retard or prevent UV-induced (direct or photosensitized) lens opacities. This approach actually measures total lens fluorescence *in vivo* (in the living eye) and aside from demonstrating abnormal and/or enhanced lens fluorescence resulting from phototoxicity or photosensitization, it has also demonstrated a normal age-related increase in lens fluorescence [51,53–57]. Aside from the marked increase in lens fluorescence in patients with brown cataracts, a more moderate elevation (Fig. 3.9) has also been noted in patients developing cortical cataracts [58]. Since UV radiation exposure plays a significant role in the generation of lens fluorescence, it is necessary to determine a "lens fluorescence aging index" for specific geographic locations (Fig. 3.10) because of variations in ambient solar UV radiation [59].

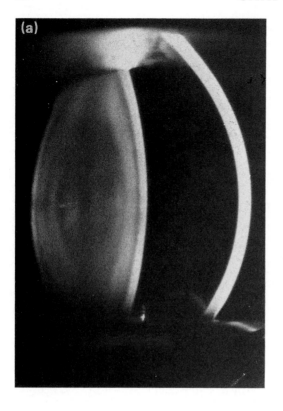

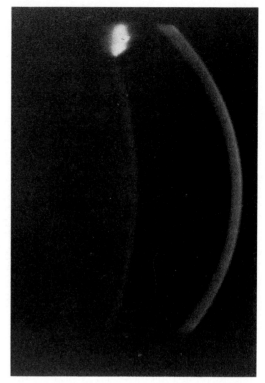

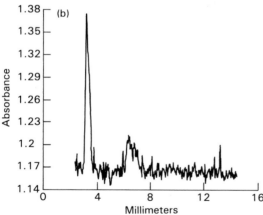

Fig. 3.3 (a) Visible (left) and ultraviolet (right) photographs of a 28-year-old normal eye. (b) Ultraviolet (fluorescence) densitogram.

While glare testing has been advocated as a means to monitor the precataractous state, studies performed on patients showed that this technique was incapable of detecting such changes, while lens fluorescence and certain nuclear magnetic resonance (NMR) techniques (to be considered later) were clearly able to detect precataractous molecular changes [60–62].

Cataracts caused by ocular medications

Although many ocular drugs have been implicated as potential cataractogenic agents, only steroids and strong miotics have been clearly demonstrated to be of significant clinical importance [63].

Prolonged local steroid therapy (as well as systemic steriods) can cause posterior

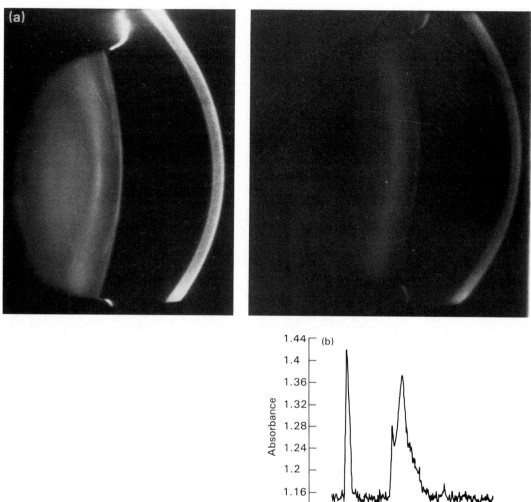

Fig. 3.4 (a) Visible (left) and ultraviolet (right) photographs of a 65-year-old normal eye. (b) Ultraviolet (fluorescence) densitogram.

subcapsular opacities (and glaucoma). Strong miotics such as echothiophate iodide can induce a variety of lens opacities and even pilocarpine has been implicated as a potential cataractogenic agent [64].

In vivo methods to evaluate ocular drug efficacy and side effects

Aside from a variety of ocular side effects which can occur with the use of ophthalmic medications, there is always the danger of unexpected eye problems with drugs used to treat a variety

of systemic conditions. This is well exemplified by the significant number of cataracts which were reported when the anticholesterol drug Triparanol was introduced several decades ago [65]. The ever-increasing proliferation of new drugs designed to affect an enzyme system or systems, or a specific metabolic pathway, could result in unexpected ocular side effects, particularly with respect to enhancing one or more of the multifactorial risk factors in human cataractogenesis. In addition, the recent development and increasing popularity of the phototherapeutic approach has already resulted in

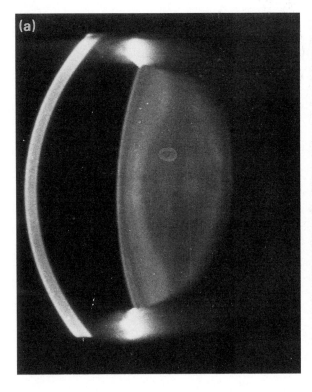

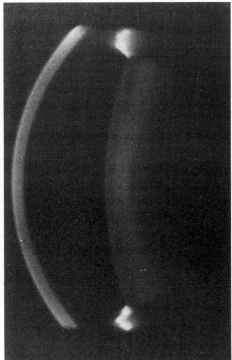

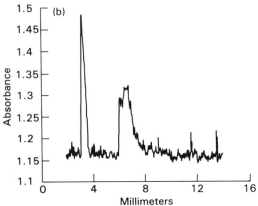

Fig. 3.5 (a) Visible (left) and ultraviolet (right) photos of a 40-year-old eye showing abnormal fluorescence due to excessive occupational ultraviolet exposure. (b) Ultraviolet (fluorescence) densitogram. Note enhanced fluorescence compared with normal 40-year-old lens (Fig. 3.6b).

the generation of "phototoxic" cataracts in man as well as in experimental animals as exemplified by the PUVA cataract [11].

Evaluation of anticataract drug therapy

Proof of efficacy has been a significant problem in the past since we had to rely on non-objective observations and variable subjective responses. It is generally recognized that simple visual acuity measurements are not a good parameter for a scientific evaluation of an anticataract agent. Simple variations in illumination, the patient's health and well-being, mental condition, etc., can significantly affect visual acuity measurements. Furthermore, many early cortical opacities vary in their appearance (size and density) in the same patient and can actually appear to regress at one time compared with their previous slit-

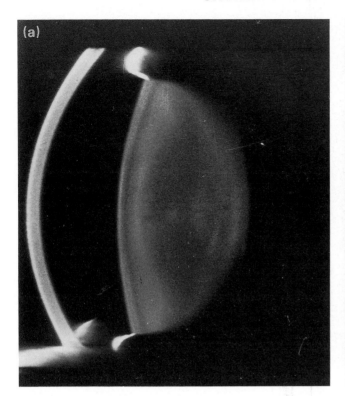
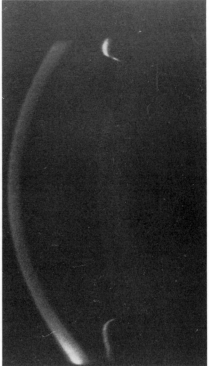

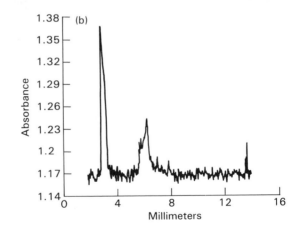

Fig. 3.6 (a) Visible (left) and ultraviolet (right) photographs of a normal 40-year-old eye. (b) Ultraviolet (fluorescence) densitogram.

lamp appearance, without any therapy. A proper scientific evaluation of any anticataract agent requires the methodology to objectively monitor the patient at periodic intervals utilizing parameters which are not subject to these variables. Recent technology now enables us to perform such evaluations utilizing techniques such as laser light scattering, *in vivo* lens fluorescence densitography, and magnetic resonance imaging (MRI). The Scheimpflug slit-lamp densitography approach has been employed by Hockwin *et al*. [66] to evaluate the efficacy of a drug containing glutathione, as well as several other amino acids. This drug, Phakon, appears to have a slight effect on some cortical lens opacities (when given locally or parenterally). The densitographic data reported by Hockwin *et al*. [66] indicate that there is a slowing in the

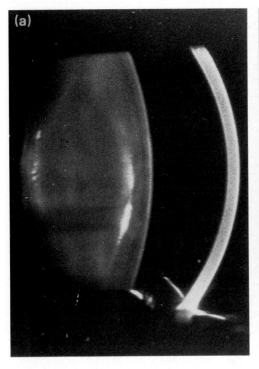
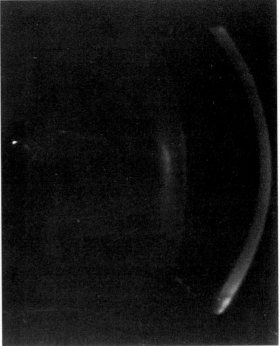

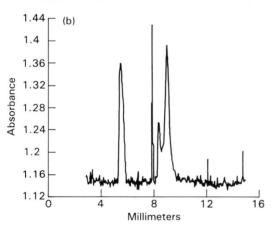

Fig. 3.7 (a) Visible (left) and ultraviolet (right) photographs of a psoralens and ultraviolet A induced cataract with abnormal fluorescence in a 52-year-old patient on psoralens and ultraviolet A therapy for 4 years. (b) Ultraviolet (fluorescence) densitogram.

progression of cortical lens opacities, but there is no effect on subcapsular or nuclear cataractogenesis [66]. Many more studies of this nature are required before one can determine whether this drug is truly effective in retarding one form of opacification. However, this study does provide us with the type of route one must undertake in attempting to evaluate drug efficacy as well as safety.

Visible densitography

Visible densitograms utilizing the Scheimpflug (Topcon SL45) slit-lamp camera and laser scanning apparatus to objectively evaluate the negatives [67] has enabled us to institute a protocol whereby we have been able to predict potential lenticular problems in patients undergoing clinical testing with new drugs. In

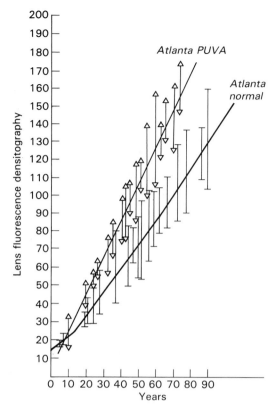

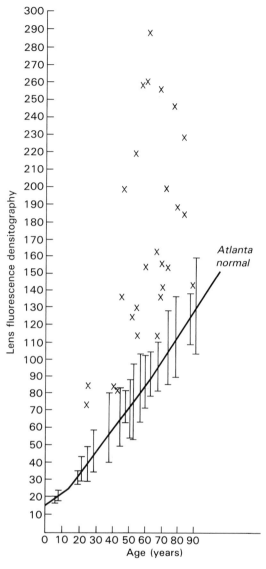

Fig. 3.8 Elevation of lens fluorescence densitograms in psoralens and ultraviolet A patients (◁——▷) compared with normal controls (├———┤).

Fig. 3.9 Lens fluorescence densitograms in patients with early cortical changes (×) compared with normal controls (├———┤).

essence, this approach involves an initial complete ocular examination in which Scheimpflug visible light slit-lamp photographs are obtained prior to instituting the drug regimen. The biometric data as well as the visible densitograms are compared with the data we have accumulated on over 1000 normal control patients. These data have been grouped by decade, from the first through to the ninth decade. Thus, any significant variation in the lens densitogram and lens thickness based on the patient's age (per decade) is immediately apparent. It should be noted that there is a variation in normal lens densitograms and lens thickness within each decade, and the ensuing repeat Scheimpflug studies for each specific patient are of greater importance than a simple comparison of the data with the corresponding values for this specific decade. This has been clearly demonstrated by Hockwin [68].

Utilizing this approach one can delineate a possible hazard in such patients, as shown in Figs 3.11 and 3.12. These patients were first seen after they had already been started on a new drug (as part of a clinical testing program) for several months. Their visible densitograms already demonstrated a significant enhancement of the supranuclear peaks compared with the normal densitography range in their age group (by decade), although their visual acuity

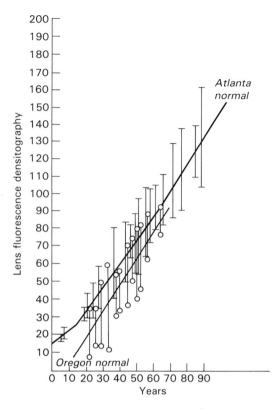

Fig. 3.10 Lens fluorescence "aging index" on patients in Atlanta, Georgia (⊢━━━━⊣) and patients in Portland, Oregon (○━━━━○).

tive data regarding a possible hazard to the ocular lens in patients undergoing clinical testing programs with new drugs.

A second observation derived from the biometric data obtained on such patients relates to an apparent cessation in the age-related increase in lens thickness (AP diameter) in some individuals developing manifest lens opacities. Such a trend was noted by O. Hockwin (personal communication) and biometric analysis appear to bear out this observation. Obviously, the foregoing must still be catagorized as preliminary conclusions and will require a large data base for further substantiation.

In addition to performing Scheimpflug densitography, the same photographs can also be utilized (with proper software) to obtain biometric measurements on these eyes including: (a) radius of curvature of the anterior and posterior cornea and corneal thickness; (b) depth of the anterior chamber; and (c) radius of curvature of the anterior and posterior lens surfaces and lens thickness [67]. Thus, the clinician can now obtain reproducible biometric data on the anterior segment ocular tissues and structures by simply utilizing the Scheimpflug slit-lamp photographic method. These data provide an accurate method for monitoring age-related changes in the normal eye (e.g. AC diameter, lens thickness, lens density, growth of lens nucleus, as well as abnormal or increased lens fluorescence). The progress of lenticular opacification can also be followed utilizing visible light slit-lamp densitography and lenticular and corneal fluorescence data can be obtained concurrently by substituting broadband UV radiation for the visible exciting light with appropriate filters.

These studies demonstrate the feasibility of obtaining *in vivo* lens fluorescence data which are objective, reproducible, and can be quantified. Thus, UV slit-lamp densitography can be used to objectively monitor one parameter of lens aging (fluorescence), as well as lenticular photodamage, at a molecular level, months to years before visible opacities become manifest by conventional slit-lamp examination, and measures can be instituted to at least retard if not prevent such lens opacities.

was not affected. Their lens fluorescence levels (as manifested by the UV densitograms) were within normal limits. Repeat studies 6 months later demonstrated a further enhancement of the supranuclear peaks although their visual acuity and lens fluorescence values remained unchanged.

Concurrent studies on control patients receiving placebos, as well as previous studies on normal individuals who had repeat densitography evaluations at 6-month intervals, did not show similar lens densitography changes within a 6-month period. Furthermore, such changes were not seen in another study involving a group of patients undergoing clinical testing with an entirely different drug. This type of evaluation suggests that precataractous drug-induced changes, as evidenced by visible Scheimpflug slit-lamp densitography, can provide significant objec-

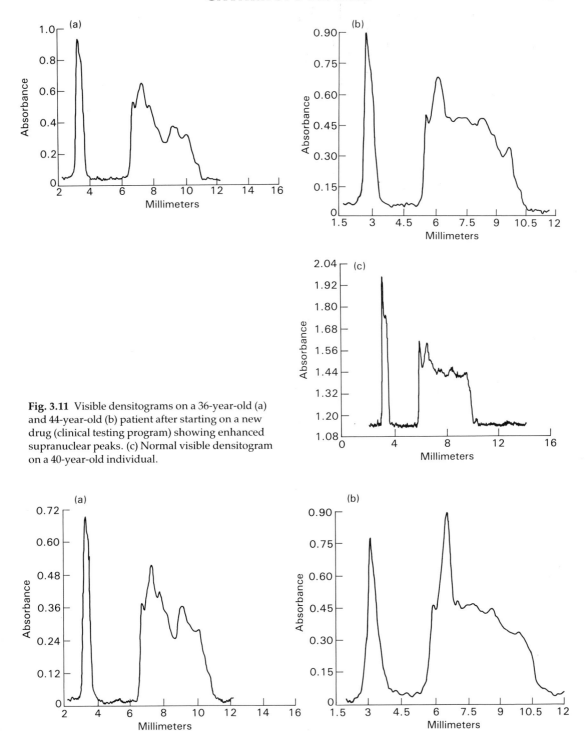

Fig. 3.11 Visible densitograms on a 36-year-old (a) and 44-year-old (b) patient after starting on a new drug (clinical testing program) showing enhanced supranuclear peaks. (c) Normal visible densitogram on a 40-year-old individual.

Fig. 3.12 Repeat visible densitograms on the 36- and 44-year-old patients (Fig. 3.11a) 6 months later.

Lens fluorescence densitography

In vivo lens fluorescence analyses are another objective way of evaluating drug efficacy. UV slit-lamp densitography has already demonstrated its ability to measure lens fluorescence *in vivo* as a reflection of ocular photodamage (hence degree of UV radiation exposure and/ or photosensitized damage) and can thus be utilized to monitor drugs which claim to be effective in preventing or aborting such changes.

Laser light scattering

Laser light scattering can also be employed as an *in vivo* method to monitor the development and progression of light-scattering elements within the lens at a level before they become manifest with our conventional slit-lamp examination [69–71]. Aside from the foregoing biophysical techniques already available, Raman and NMR spectroscopy are now becoming available for detecting and measuring molecular changes in the living lens at an early state in their development.

NMR

In NMR examinations, patients are subjected to long-wavelength radiation in a large chamber that exerts a magnetic field around them. Unlike radiation from a computerized tomographic (CT) scan, NMR radiation is non-ionizing and, thus, relatively harmless as it energizes atomic nuclei in the patient's body. The nuclei do not remain energized but tend to "relax" back to their normal, less energetic "ground state." In doing this they give off energy, or "resonate"—thus the term NMR. Current studies utilizing ^{31}P-NMR spectroscopy enable the investigator to monitor organophosphate metabolism in the lens *in vitro*. Such data provide dynamic rather than static information about the general metabolic state of this organ and quickly reflect changes in high energy phosphates (adenosine triphosphate, adenosine diphosphate, etc.) in sugar phosphates, inorganic phosphate and so forth. In experimental sugar cataracts (glucose,

galactose, or xylose) one can measure the accumulation of the sugar alcohols and the concomitant alterations in organophosphate levels as soon as these metabolic changes develop and well before any opacities become manifest.

MRI

In vivo NMR spectroscopy utilizing proton MRI permits us to visualize the ocular lens (as well as the entire globe and its related structures) within minutes [72–78]. In addition, it has recently been demonstrated that this technique enables us to obtain T1 and T2 values in the living lens which show an age-related correlation, thus confirming previously reported *in vitro* pulse relaxation studies [79].

In vitro pulse relaxation studies have shown an age-related increase in the T1 and T2 values in the normal human lenses derived from eye bank specimens (Fig. 3.13). These data demonstrate that the free water component (T1) in the human lens as well as the moderately bound water phase (T2a) show a normal aging change while the tightly bound water phase (T2b) remains unchanged as the lens ages. These experiments demonstrate a potential non-invasive parameter to evaluate "molecular changes" related to the aging process and cataractogenesis.

In order to perform such an *in vivo* evaluation, we developed a high resolution imaging method on human eyes with very small surface coils (Fig. 3.14) using the GE Signa imager (at 1.5 T). Figure 3.15 demonstrates representative images employing this technique. The higher resolution makes it possible to perform T2 relaxation measurements *in vivo* with less partial volume interference from adjacent tissues. We have measured relaxation times (T2 values) in a series of normal volunteers ranging in age from 22 to 62 years. There is an age-related change in the T2 value of the normal lens nucleus, from 16.4 msec in a 22-year-old individual to 30.3 msec in a 55-year-old person. A similar trend can be seen in the lens cortex where the T2 values range from 20.2 to 30.9 msec according to age. Our previous *in vitro* studies have shown that of the two

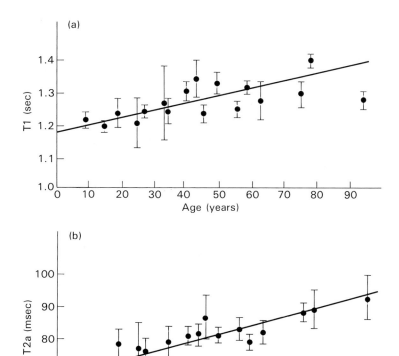

Fig. 3.13 (a) Normal age-related increase in free water component (T1) of the human lens. (b) Normal age-related increase in the moderately bound (T2a) water phase of the human lens.

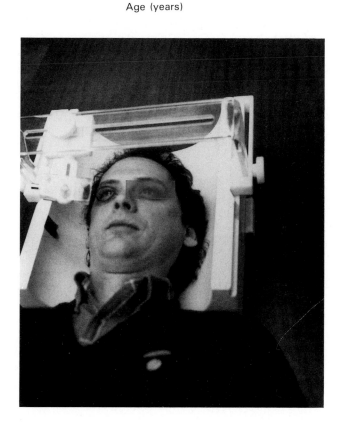

Fig. 3.14 Surface coil over right eye in patient undergoing magnetic resonance imaging study.

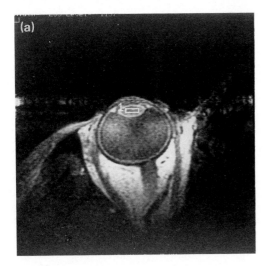
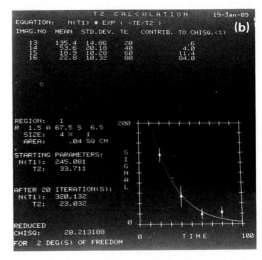

Fig. 3.15 (a) Representative magnetic resonance image. (b) T2 values obtained with the magnetic resonance imaging technique.

components constituting the T2 value, the tightly bound water phase (T2b) remains unchanged with aging and only the moderately bound water phase (T2a) shows an age-related increase, thus our current *in vivo* data demonstrate that there is a significant change in the moderately bound water phase in the human lens as it ages. Since the lens is a highly concentrated bag of proteins (over 30% v/v) it is not surprising that the moderately bound water phase reflecting protein water interaction changes with age. It is well known that there is a significant age-related change in the relative concentration of the α-, β-, and γ-crystallins and in the water insoluble protein fraction as aging progresses, and one would anticipate that such changes must be reflected by alterations in the degree of solvation of certain crystallins. For example, our previous studies have clearly demonstrated the apparent loss of at least one of the γ-crystallin fractions with age, and this has been corroborated by other laboratories. This γ fraction appears to be one of the most hydrophobic proteins in the lens and its apparent loss, probably by aggregation with other fractions, would result in altered H_2O solvation and this is reflected by the T2 values we have obtained.

These data clearly demonstrate that one can obtain reproducible T2 values using this approach, and that it is important to know the age of the patient in order to be able to monitor for abnormal T2 values in the precataractous lens, i.e. in the lens undergoing molecular changes on the road to manifest opacification. *In vivo* lens fluorescence data obtained with the Scheimpflug UV densitographic approach demonstrate our ability to monitor for abnormal and/or enhanced age-related lens fluorescence as a sign of eventual cataract formation due to ocular photodamage and the MRI data correlate well with these findings. We have shown that such lens fluorescence values are also significantly changed in patients with early senile cortical cataracts as well as in the mixed and/or brunescent cataracts and we have obtained similar findings with our MRI approach.

We are thus able to utilize these two noninvasive techniques to monitor for precataractous molecular changes in the living, clear lens months to years before any type of opacity becomes manifest with the conventional slit-lamp examination. These two techniques permit one to evaluate the anticataract drugs currently being studied by several pharmaceutical houses. Since such drugs are supposed to act by inhibiting and/or preventing the development of manifest opacification and not by reversing a cataract already present, it is important to utilize techniques which are capable of monitoring molecular changes in patients with clear lenses and normal visual acuity. The lens fluorescence technique can be performed in 4–6 min, and the MRI technique in 10–20 min, and thus they provide a rapid objective measure of the status of a lens as well as a truly objective monitor of anticataract drug efficacy.

References

1 WHO Chronicle. Data on blindness throughout the world. *Bull WHO* 1979; **33**: 275–83.

2 Dawson RJ, Schwab J. Epidemiology of cataract. A major cause of preventable blindness. *Bull WHO* 1981; **59**: 493.

3 Ohrloff C. Edpidemiology of "senile cataract." In: Hockwin O, Sasaki K, Leske MC, eds. *Risk Factors for Cataract Development. Proceedings of the Second International Symposium on Cataract Epidemiology.* Basel: Karger, 1989: 1–5.

4 Hockwin O, Sasaki K, Leske MC, eds. *Risk Factors for Cataract Development. Proceedings of the Second International Symposium on Cataract Epidemiology.* Basel: Karger 1989.

5 Lerman S, Kuck JF, Borkman R, Saker E. Introduction, acceleration and prevention (*in vitro*) of an aging parameter in the ocular lens. *Ophthalmol Res* 1976; **8**: 213–26.

6 Lerman S, Borkman RF. Spectroscopic evaluation and classification of the normal, aging and cataractous lens. *Ophthalmol Res* 1976; **8**: 335–53.

7 Lerman S, Borkman RF. Photochemistry and lens aging. In: Von Hahn HP, ed. *Interdisciplinary Topics in Gerontology* 1978; **13**: 154–82.

8 Lerman S. *Radiant Energy and The Eye.* New York: Macmillan, 1980.

9 Lerman S. An experimental and clinical evaluation of lens transparency and aging. *J Gerontol* 1983; **38**: 293–301.

10 Lerman S. Ocular phototoxicity. In: Fraunfelder F, Davidson SI, eds. *Recent Advances in Ophthalmology.* Edinburgh: Churchill-Livingstone, 1985: 109–36.

11 Lerman S. Photosensitizing drugs and their possible role in enhancing ocular toxicity. *Ophthalmology* 1986; **93**: 304–18.

12 Lerman S. Effects of sunlight on the eye. Ben-Hur E, Rosenthal J, eds. *Photomedicine.* Boca Raton: CRC Press, 1987: 79–122.

13 Pitts DG, Cameron LL, Jose JG, Lerman S, Moss E, Varma S *et al.* Optical radiation and cataracts. In: Waxler M, Hutchins VM, eds. *Optical Radiation and Visual Health.* Boca Raton: CRC Press, 1987: 5–41.

14 Lerman S. *In vivo* lens fluorescence as a cataract marker. In: Hockwin O, Sasaki K, Leske MC, eds. *Cataract Epidemiology. Proceedings of the Second International Symposium on Cataract Epidemiology.* Basel: Karger, 1989: 60–5.

15 Pau H. Clinical and biochemical aspects of the different types of senile cataract. *Lens Res* 1986; **3**: 265–70.

16 Goder G, Hubscher HJ, Luther K, Meinel U, Kraft H, Simon K. Results of an epidemiological study of lens opacifications. In: Hockwin O, Sasaki K, Leske MC, eds. *Risk Factors for Cataract Development.* Basel: Karger, 1989: 21–5.

17 Laser H, Ludtke R, Eckerskorn U, Hockwin O. Epidemiologic investigations into the determination of cataractogenic risk factors for cataract development. In: Hockwin O, Sasaki K, Leske MC, eds. *Risk Factors for Cataract Development.* Basel: Karger, 1989: 152–57.

18 Kinoshita JH. Mechanisms initiating cataract formation. *Invest Ophthalmol* 1974; **13**: 713.

19 Lerman S, Moran M. Sorbitol generation and its inhibition by sorbinil in the aging normal human and rabbit lens and human diabetic cataracts. *Ophthalmol Res* 1989; **20**: 348–52.

20 Varma SD. Aldose reductase and the etiology of diabetic cataracts. *Curr Topics Eye Res* 1980; **9**: 91.

21 Kador PF. Overview of the current attempt toward the medical treatment of cataract. *Ophthalmology* 1983; **90**: 352.

22 Lerman S, Megaw J, Gardner K. Optical spectroscopy as a method to monitor aldose reductase inhibitors in the lens. *Invest Ophthalmol Vis Sci* 1983; **24**: 1505–10.

23 Parrish JA, Fitzpatrick TB, Tannenbaum L, Pathak MA. Photochemotherapy of psoriasis with oral methoxsalen and longwave ultraviolet light. *N Engl J Med* 1974; **291**: 1207–11.

24 Parrish JA, Fitzpatrick TB, Shea C, Pathak MA. Photochemotherapy of vitiligo; use of orally administered psoralens and a high-intensity longwave ultraviolet light system. *Arch Dermatol* 1976; **112**: 1541–4.

25 Lerman S, Jocoy M, Borkman RF. Photosensitization of the lens by 8-methoxypsoralen. *Invest Ophthalmol Vis Sci* 1977; **16**: 1065–8.

26 Jose JG, Yielding KL. Photosensitive cataractogens, chlorpromazine and methoxypsoralen, cause DNA repair synthesis in lens epithelial cells. *Invest Ophthalmol Vis Sci* 1978; **17**: 687–91.

27 Lerman S, Megaw J, Willis I. Potential ocular complications from PUVA therapy and their prevention. *J Invest Dermatol* 1980; **74**: 197–9.

28 Lerman S, Megaw JM, Gardner K, Takei Y, Willis I. Localization of 8-methoxypsoralen in ocular tissues. *Ophthalmol Res* 1981; **13**: 106–16.

29 Wulf HC, Andreasen MP. Distribution of ^{3}H-8-MOP and its metabolites in rat organs after a single oral administration. *J Invest Dermatol* 1981; **76**: 252–8.

30 Wulf HC, Andreasen MP. Concentration of ^{3}H-8-

methoxypsoralen and its metabolites in the rat lens and eye after a single oral administration. *Invest Ophthalmol Vis Sci* 1982; **22**: 32–6.

31 Lerman S, Megaw J, Gardner K, Takei Y, Franks Y, Gammon A. Photobinding of ^{3}H-8-methoxypsoralen to monkey intraocular tissues. *Invest Ophthalmol Vis Sci* 1984; **25**: 1267–74.

32 Cloud TM, Hakim R, Griffin AC. Photosensitization of the eye with methoxsalen. I. Acute effects. *Arch Ophthalmol* 1960; **64**: 346–51.

33 Cloud TM, Hakim R, Griffin AC. Photosensitization of the eye with methoxsalen. II. Chronic effects. *Arch Ophthalmol* 1961; **66**: 689–94.

34 Freeman RG, Troll D. Photosensitization of the eye by 8-methoxypsoralen. *J. Invest Dermatol* 1969; **53**: 449–53.

35 Cyrlin MN, Pedvis-Leftick A, Sugar J. Cataract formation in association with ultraviolet photosensitivity. *Ann Ophthalmol* 1980; **12**: 786–90.

36 Lerman S. Psoralens and ocular effects in man and animals: *in vivo* monitoring of human ocular and cutaneous manifestations. *Natl Cancer Inst Monogr* 1984; **66**: 227–33.

37 Lerman S, Kuck JF Jr, Borkman RF, Saker E. Induction, acceleration and prevention (*in vitro*) of an aging parameter in the ocular lens. *Ophthalmol Res* 1976; **8**: 213–26.

38 Lerman S, Megaw J, Gardner K. PUVA therapy and human cataractogenesis. *Invest Ophthalmol Vis Sci* 1982; **23**: 801–4.

39 Potts AM, Gonasun LM. Toxicology of the eye. In: Casarett LJ, Doull J, eds. *Toxicology; The Basic Science of Poisons*. New York: Macmillan, 1975: 275–309.

40 Fraunfelder FT, Hanna C, Dreis MW, Cosgrove KW Jr. Cataracts associated with allopurinol therapy. *Am J Ophthalmol* 1982; **94**: 137–40.

41 Lerman S, Megaw JM, Gardner K. Allopurinol therapy and catactogenesis in humans. *Am J Ophthalmol* 1982; **994**: 141–6.

42 Lerman S, Megaw J, Fraunfelder FT. Further studies on allopurinol therapy and human cataractogenesis. *Am J Ophthalmol* 1984; **97**: 205–9.

43 Dayhaw-Barker P, Forbes D, Fox D *et al*. Drug phototoxicity and visual health. In: *FDA Symposium on the Long Term Visual Health Risks of Optical Radiation*. Bethesda, Maryland, September 1983: 24–27.

44 Roberts JE. The photodynamic effect of chlorpromazine, promazine, and hematoporphyrin on lens protein. *Invest Ophthalmol Vis Sci* 1984; **25**: 746–50.

45 Thomas JR III, Doyle JA. The therapeutic uses of topical vitamin A acid. *J Am Acad Dermatol* 1981; **4**: 505–13.

46 Ward A, Brogden RN, Heel RC *et al*. Etreinate: a review of its pharmacological properties and therapeutic efficacy in psoriasis and other skin disorders. *Drugs* 1983; **26**: 9–43.

47 Shalita AR, Cunningham WJ, Leyden JJ *et al*. Isotretinoin treatment of acne and related disorders: an update. *J Am Acad Dermatol* 1983; **9**: 629–38.

48 Dragomirescu V, Hockwin O, Koch HR, Sasaki K. Development of new equipment for rotating slit image photography according to Scheimpflug's principle. In: Hockwin O, ed. *Gerontological Aspects of Eye Research. Interdisciplinary Topics in Gerontology*, vol. 13. Basel: Karger, 1978: 118–30.

49 Lerman S, Hockwin O. Ultraviolet-visible slit lamp densitography of the human eye. *Exp Eye Res* 1981; **33**: 587–96.

50 Lerman S, Dragomirescu V, Hockwin O. *In vivo* monitoring of direct and photosensitized ultraviolet radiating damage to the lens. In: Henkind P, ed. *Acta XXIV International Congress of Ophthalmology*, San Francisco, October 31 to November 5, 1982. Philadelphia: JB Lippincott, 1983: 354–8.

51 Hockwin O, Sasaki K, Lerman S. Evaluating cataract development with the Scheimpflug camera. In: Masters B, ed. *New Developments in Non-Invasive Studies to Evaluate Ocular Function*. New York: Springer-Verlag, 1989.

52 Lerman S, Borkman R. Spectroscopic evaluation and classification of the normal, aging, and cataractous lens. *Ophthalmol Res* 1976; **8**: 335–53.

53 Lerman S. UV slit lamp densitography of the human lens. An additional tool for prospective studies of changes in lens transparency. In: Von Hahn HP, ed. *Aging of the Lens Symposium*, Strasburg. Munich: Integra, 1982: 139–54.

54 Lerman S, Dragomirescu V, Hockwin O. *In vivo* monitoring of direct and photosensitized UV radiation damage to the lens. *Acta XXIV International Congress of Ophthalmology* 1983; **1**: 354–8.

55 Klang G. Measurements and studies of the fluorescence of the human lens *in vivo*. *Acta Ophthalmol* 1984; **31** (suppl): 1.

56 Zeimer RC, North JM. A new method of measuring *in vivo* the lens transmission, the study of lens scatter, fluorescence and transmittance. *Ophthalmol Res*, 1984; **16**: 246.

57 Bleeker J, Van Best J, Vrij L, van der Veide E, Oosterhuis J. Autofluorescence of the lens in diabetic and healthy subjects by fluorophotometry. *Invest Ophthalmol Vis Sci* 1986; **27**: 791–4.

58 Lerman S. *In vivo* lens fluorescence as a cataract marker. *In*: Hockwin O, Leske MC, Sasaki K, eds. *Cataract Epidemiology. Proceedings of the Second International Symposium on Cataract Epidemiology*. Basel: Karger, 1989: 60–5.

59 Lerman S. Human lens fluorescence aging index. *Lens Res* 1988; **5**: 23–31.

60 Mandal K, Lerman S. *In vivo* NMR studies on the ocular lens. *Invest Ophthalmol Vis Sci* 1989; (suppl): 328.

61 Wandel T, Matthews N, Lerman S. *In vivo* lens

fluorescence and glare testing to monitor anti-cataract drug efficacy. *Invest Ophthalmol Vis Sci* 1989; (suppl): 498.

62 Lerman S. *In vivo* monitoring of pre-cataractous changes in the human lens: a fluorescence and MRI approach. *Proceedings of the Fifth Congress of the US–Japan Cooperative Cataract Research Group.* Uchinada, Japan, October, 1989.

63 Bonomi L. Cataracts induced by topical ocular medication in risk factors for cataract development. Hockwin O, Sasaki K, Leske MC, eds. *Developments in Ophthalmology Series*, vol. 17. Basel: Karger, 1989; 196–7.

64 Leopold JH. Cholinergic agents in management of intraocular pressure in glaucoma. In: Drance SM, Neufeld AH, eds. *Applied Pharmacology in Medical Treatment.* Grune & Stratton, 1984.

65 Kirby TJ Jr, Achor RWP, Perry HE, Winkelmann RK. Cataract formation after triparanol therapy. *AMA Arch Ophthalmol* 1962; **68**: 486.

66 Hockwin O, Weigelin E, Baur M. Erganzungen zur klinischen Studie uber die Wirksamkeit eines Antikatarakt-Preparates. *Fortschr Ophthal* 1985; **82**: 237–9.

67 Lerman S, Hockwin O. Automated biometry and densitography of anterior segment of the eye. *Greafes Arch Klin Exp Ophthal* 1985; **223**: 121–9.

68 Hockwin O. The causes and prevention of cataract blindness. *Endeavor* 1985; **9**: 132–8.

69 Ben-Sira I, Weinberger D, Bodenheimer J, Yassur Y. Clinical method for measurement of light backscattering from the *in vivo* human lens. *Invest Ophthalmol Vis Sci* 1980; **19**: 435.

70 Bettelheim FA, Siew EL, Shyne S, Farnsworth P, Burke P. A comparative study of human lens by light scattering and scanning electron microscopy. *Exp Eye Res* 1981; **32**: 125.

71 Nishio I, Weiss JN, Tanaka T et al. *In vivo* observation of lens protein diffusivity in normal and X-irradiated rabbit lenses. *Exp Eye Res* 1984; **39**: 61–8.

72 Moseley I, Brant-Zawadski M, Mills C. Nuclear magnetic resonance imaging of the orbit. *Br J Ophthalmol* 1983; **67**: 333–42.

73 Racz P, Tompa K, Pocsik I, Bank P. Water fractions in normal and senile cataractous eye lenses studied by NMR. *Exp Eye Res* 1983; **36**: 663–71.

74 Cheng HM, Lung Y, Barnett P et al. Proton magnetic resonance imaging of the ocular lens. *Exp Eye Res* 1987; **45**: 875–82.

75 Kolodny NH, Gragoudas S, D'Amico DJ et al. Proton and sodium magnetic resonance imaging of ocular tissues. *Arch Ophthalmol* 1987; **105**: 1532–6.

76 Aguayo JB, Blackband SB, Wehrle JP, Glickson JD, Mattingly MA. NMR microscopic studies of eyes and tumors with histological correlation. *Ann NY Acad Sci* 1988; **508**: 399–413.

77 Lerman S, Mandal K, Misrai B, Schechter A and Schenk J. Phototoxicity involving the ocular lens. *Photochem Photobiol* 1991; **53**: 243–247.

78 Lerman S, Wandel T, Schechter A, Schneck J, Souza SP. In vivo non-invasive studies on the human lens. *J Mag Res Imag* 1991; **9**: 525–32.

79 Lerman S, Moran M. NMR pulse relaxation studies on the normal aging and cataractous lens. *Exp Eye Res* 1989; **48**: 451–9.

4: Psychologic Aspects of Cataract Care

WILLIAM H. HAVENER

To understand and help your patients, you must be conscious that their perspective of a cataract is in all respects directly opposite from your perspective. To them, it is a disaster. You consider the dreadful alternatives and regard the patient as fortunate. You are comfortable in familiar territory while performing customary routine activity. The patient is insecure in a strange place and among unfamiliar persons. You are not being perforated, folded, stapled, and manipulated; the patient is. You slept last night, the patient tossed and turned with insomnia. No wonder misunderstandings and differences of opinion can arise!

As just described, the perspectives of patient and physicians are so totally different that they often fail to understand each other. The application of medicine to cataract patients requires the physician to approach the patient–physician relationship from the perspective of the patient. It has been said that a physician should personally have the patient's disease in order to fully understand the patient. Probably this is true, because emotional understanding is different from intellectual contemplation. However, human responses to adversity are subject to classification in only a relatively few categories, for instance, fear, denial, rising to a challenge, etc. The perceptive physician can identify, or shrewdly guess at, the type of response exhibited by a given patient. The next step is to select an appropriate management for that type of response.

Actually, when we comment about the psychologic management of cataract (or of any other patient status), we are really dealing with the *art of medicine*. This "art" is generally per-ceived as being a nebulous, perhaps even imaginary, sort of hocus pocus chicanery. The practitioners of modern scientific medicine tend to scoff at it and place their confidence in antibiotics, β-blockers, and microsurgery. However, the primary message of this chapter is to make clear that it is not only real, but is one of the most powerful strategies a physician can use. Further, the art of medicine is an essential part of every ideal patient–physician encounter which should be practiced with all patients.

I must therefore define precisely what it is and how it is done. Let us rename this strategy "Reassurance Therapy." The effective delivery of reassurance therapy requires an orderly sequence of steps which are: (a) history; (b) evaluation of affect; (c) physical examination; (d) diagnosis; (e) explanation; and (f) reassurance. These are simply the routine steps of medical practice. Delivery of reassurance therapy does not consume any more time than ordinary practice. It does, however, require the physician's conscious emphasis upon the need for reassurance.

Step 1: History

Physicians consider the history to exist as an effective means of learning information about the patient. From the physician's perspective, the history is solely for his or her benefit. From the different standpoint of the patient, the history is viewed as a very large proportion of the patient–doctor verbal communication. Since the success of the communication may determine whether the doctor makes the right diagnosis and provide the proper treatment, the patient is anxious to ensure total communication. This is the reason patients are so insistent on talking about minor and irrelevant details and are distressed if the doctor doesn't listen to them.

Be aware that the history is not merely a physician-informing procedure, but also serves an important patient-reassuring function. Do allow the patient to talk enough so that he or she is secure in the belief that adequate and necessary detail has been transmitted to you.

Step 2: Evaluation of affect

This is a primarily non-verbal, body-language evaluation which occurs throughout your contact with the patient. Your assessment of the emotional significance of the problem to the patient will determine the amount of reassurance therapy necessary in the given instance. Surprisingly, the greatest amount of reassurance is often necessary for the most minor problems. For example, migraine equivalents, posterior vitreous separation, and subconjunctival hemorrhages often terrify the patient but are dismissed by the physician as being of no significance. This discrepancy in perspective leads to patient insecurity.

With respect to cataract, you can assume that progressive and inexorable loss of sight with the prospect of surgery is terrifying. Cataract patients desperately need and deserve proper reassurance therapy.

Step 3: Physical examination

Again, physicians assume physical examination to be an activity designed solely for their discovery of information. To the patient, this part of the encounter is another way of assessing the physician. Communication with the patient is as effectively made by the physician's touch and manner as by voice, perhaps even more so. Touch gently and carefully and confidence is transmitted. Handle the patient roughly and he will not let you operate.

To the physician, a physical examination is a routine activity of no emotional significance. To the patient, it is an aggressive violation of personal privacy and a threat to physical integrity.

Do think of the emotional body-language message inevitably delivered, for good or bad, during your physical examination.

Step 4: Medical diagnosis

This is the only step of reassurance therapy that is reserved uniquely for the physician. Adroit quacks and charlatans perform the other five steps better than do most physicians—they have to be better at reassurance because they have nothing else to offer.

Be aware that the patient cannot know when or how the diagnosis is reached, nor can he or she judge your accuracy. The patient does not know that 90% of diagnoses are considered within the first 5 minutes of a new patient–physician encounter, and is unaware of your hypothesis-driven comparisons of diagnoses and of your use of probability considerations. The patient would be distressed to learn that the physician is never absolutely sure of anything, including the patient's response to therapy, and presumes that the great physician is deep in orderly thought after the completion of the examination. You know better. Your process of differential diagnosis is one of uncertainty, in which possible diagnosis is considered, then tentatively rejected or compared with yet another possibility.

Do not think out loud about your struggles with differential diagnosis, for this uncertain process will shatter the patient's confidence! A new young physician is especially vulnerable to self-destruction in this manner. If the patient learns that you doubt yourself, how can he or she trust you? *Do not think out loud about your uncertainties.*

Step 5: Explanation

Reassurance explanation is not a didactic mini-medical school course about the patient's disorder. It is not a transmission of scientific knowledge. Neither is it a legal presentation designed to meet the criteria of informed consent. An anesthesiologist once told me that there is no such thing as an informed consent to anesthesia. If everything were to be explained to the patient and despite this he consented to undergo anesthesia, then his consent would be invalid on the basis of insanity!

Although your cataract explanation should include some medical facts and meet an increasing number of legal obligations, none of these is reassuring. Reassurance therapy explanation is designed to transmit three beliefs to the patient who should believe that:

1 you are certain as to the process of arriving at the proper diagnosis;
2 you are certain as to the process of arriving at the proper therapy; and
3 you are sympathetic with the patient's needs.

Note carefully my wording. The physician cannot lie to the patient about knowing the diagnosis precisely or the response to treatment. But, the physician does know the steps whereby these decision thresholds critical to management of the individual case are reached.

And you cannot simply tell the patient: "Trust me, I know all the answers." That won't work very often. You must indirectly convey these three attitudes of faith to the patient by means of a combination of your words or actions. Remember that your reassurance transmission has already started with the very first time the patient hears your name, even before he or she arrives at the office. Your secretary's actions also contribute to your image.

Avoid being aloof and pretentious. The best way to convey sympathy is by being truly sympathetic to the patient's problems of declining eyesight and increasing hardships.

Step 6: Reassurance

The patient cannot be reassured until the first five preparatory steps have been attended to completely. Do not try. The effort will be counterproductive. It won't work. For example, attempted reassurance of a scared patient at the beginning of the history can convey only one of two adverse messages: (a) "I am willing to advise you before I know enough to understand your problem," or (b) "I'm not even bothering myself to listen to you whine about your problem."

Reassurance is defined as a *credible and accept-able prediction of the patient's future*. You cannot offer the patient this message until the details are known and the patient is prepared to receive the message. And you can't just say: "Don't worry, everything will be OK." The patient knows better.

The two critical words are *credible* and *acceptable*. The prediction must be believable to the patient. Credibility is achieved by presenting a series of steps into the future that can appear as being reasonably true. For example, you can describe the various steps involved in the preparations for surgery or in the postoperative care. "Acceptability" is also essential. If the patient has only minimal glare that does not interfere with lifetime activities, then the risks of cataract surgery are unacceptable. Six months later, however, a rapidly progressing posterior subcapsular cataract may change the risks of surgery to being not merely acceptable, but highly desirable.

I, myself, cannot process a cataract patient through the steps of reassurance therapy in less than a half hour, often considerably longer. This time is fully justified, because:

1 I am sure I have advised the patient properly;
2 if indicated, the patient will select me as his surgeon; and
3 the patient will be comfortable with a local anesthetic, which is far better for the health of an elderly patient than is a general anesthetic.

Each physician will do it differently, but the six step principles remain constant.

Negative placebo effect

A negative placebo effect is literally the result of a poison pill. It can harm the physician and the patient by causing patient non-wellbeing, physician misdiagnosis, active non-compliance, and malpractice litigation. Unavoidably, every patient–physician effect will result in a placebo effect of some sort. It is most assuredly worth your while to resolve that your effect will be positive.

Patient non-wellbeing refers to the attitude of your patient. Consciously or unconsciously, you modify your patient's attitudes. You can convey pessimism or optimism. You could even consider the patient to be a mirror, reflecting your attitudes. The patient is constantly interpreting your body language, often wrongly. Your frown or moment of hesitation can easily translate into: "He thinks my cataract is bad—maybe even inoperable."

Physician misdiagnosis results when a discrepancy is sensed between the patient's complaints and the physical findings. We are aware of the incompleteness of our knowledge of every patient and have adopted the fail-safe mechanism of seeking a correlation between history and physical evaluations. Whenever patient non-wellbeing distorts this correlation, we automatically search further, perhaps ordering a visual field for our cataract patient. Naturally, the result will be the finding of a non-specific field constriction. Explanation of this finding to the patient will, of course, result in additional non-wellbeing, thereby perpetuating the vicious cycle of more diagnostic uncertainty, more patient insecurity, etc.

Active non-compliance refers to the deliberate choice by the patient to disobey our recommendations. This is far worse than passive non-compliance, which is simply the absent-minded elderly patient forgetting the need to instill an eye drop. Before you scoff at the negative placebo effect, reflect upon whether it matters if the patient decides to have someone else operate on the cataract. Your negative placebo effect can and does cancel your effectiveness in the care of your patient. What matters your 4 years of medical school and Alpha Omega Alpha academic performance and 4 years of subsequent specialization in ophthalmology if the patient won't accept and act upon your advice?

Malpractice litigation is supposed to be inevitable in current medical practice. That is true, if you do not know about and avoid the negative placebo effect. I have consulted in very many malpractice cases. In almost every instance, the physician had earned the patient's enmity. Conversely, in 35 years of active practice, I have inevitably produced very many unfortunate visual results. Retinal detachments and cataracts do not always yield 20/20 vision, especially when associated with macular degeneration, glaucoma, and all the other eye disorders. Nevertheless, I have yet to be sued for malpractice, thanks to the tolerance of my very nice patients.

Malpractice litigation is not due to conniving lawyers or bad results, but is clearly a negative placebo effect. Ignore this at your own peril.

Positive placebo effect

The path of a patient is rocky, thorny, and generally difficult and unpleasant. The perspective of a hospital bed is different when you are in it than when you are viewing its occupant. Our obligation and duty as physicians is to smooth this difficult path as much as possible for our patients. Our psychologic approach must not diminish from or substitute for the best quality of modern scientific medical care. My message is that the intangible art of medicine is the reassurance and courage that we can and should deliver to all our patients. Without this support, our scientific actions are incomplete.

A positive placebo effect is neither intangible nor insignificant. It can return a patient to work and normal lifetime activity far more quickly. It can transform the unpleasantness of a surgical procedure into an interesting experience. It can greatly reduce or eliminate the need for sedatives, tranquilizers, and sleeping pills. It can cause your patients to be your loyal friends. It is the key to your sincere enjoyment of the practice of medicine.

5: Relation of the Primary Care Physician to the Patient, the Ophthalmologist, and Cataract Surgery

JAN D. SMITH

Introduction

Cataract surgery is one of the most frequently performed surgical procedures in the elderly patient. Constraints placed on physicians in hospitals by the regulatory authorities have made it necessary for most cataract procedures to be performed on an outpatient basis [1, 2]. Consequently, it is exceedingly rare for a patient who is to undergo cataract surgery to be admitted on the night prior to surgery.

Initially, ambulatory surgery was restricted to American Society of Anesthesiology (ASA) physical status I patients (normal healthy patient), or physical status II patients (patients with mild systemic disease). As experience was gained in handling more seriously ill medical patients, we now find that surgery is being performed on more ASA III (patients with severe systemic diseases limiting activity), and the occasional ASA IV patient (those patients with severe systemic disease which may be life threatening). These patients are considered acceptable surgical candidates provided their systemic diseases are under good control and stable [3,4].

The elderly patient

The elderly patient should not be considered as an old adult, but one who exhibits different physiologic and pharmacokinetic changes commensurate with age. Some of the changes noted with increasing age are discussed by Keating [5] (Table 5.1). These patients usually have complicated medical problems which impact on the course of surgery and anesthesia. All patients must be under the care of a primary care physician (internist or family physician) who must be in a position to adequately prepare the patient for surgery. This may require, for example, the stabilization of the patient's cardiac and/or respiratory status; control of their diabetic condition; and/or, regulation of their hypertension.

The preoperative evaluation

In many ambulatory clinics, patients are seen 2 or 3 days prior to their scheduled surgery. This allows for a complete preoperative evaluation to be performed and for the anesthesiologist to explain exactly what is needed to prepare the patient for surgery. Information that will be shared, will include rules regarding fasting; taking of medications; and, answering any questions that the patient may have. This preoperative visit may not always be feasible, and in some areas, the patient is seen for the first time on the day of surgery. If this occurs, it is imperative that there be an excellent working relationship between the primary care physician, ophthalmologist, and anesthesiologist so that each understands what is expected from the other [2].

A questionnaire which is given to patients by the surgeon at the time of their initial visit, together with an instruction sheet, should be returned ahead of time allowing problems to be identified. These can then be followed up and clarified by subsequent telephone calls. In some instances, this may require that the patient return to see either their primary care physician or make the effort to see the anesthesiologist prior to surgery. Families are instructed to inform the ambulatory surgery unit if there are

Table 5.1 Organ system changes with age. After [5]

Organ system	Physiologic change	Perioperative complication
Cardiovascular	↓ Myocardial contractility ↓ Cardiac output Autonomic dysautonomia ↑ Coronary artery disease ↑ Calcific aortic stenosis	Cardiac failure Pulmonary edema Orthostatic hypotension Myocardial infarction Syncope, angina
Pulmonary	↓ Vital capacity ↑ A–a gradient ↓ Oropharyngeal clearance	Atelectasis Hypoxemia Pulmonary infection
Genitourinary	↓ Glomerular filtration rate ↓ Tubular function ↓ Bladder tone	Drug clearance ↓ Volume depletion Urosepsis
Gastrointestinal	↓ Gastroesophageal tone Achlorhydria	Aspiration Change in gastrointestinal flora
Endocrine	↓ β-cell function ↑ Insulin resistance	Hyperglycemia Infection
Musculoskeletal	↓ Muscle/bone mass ↑ Degenerative joint disease	Fracture Mobility ↓

any changes in patient status or symptoms which may preclude the patient from coming in for surgery. Patients who arrive on the day of surgery having consumed tea, milk, or coffee, earlier that day, should either be cancelled or placed at the end of the days operating room schedule.

It is mandatory that a good preoperative history and physical examination be done by either the ophthalmologist or primary physician. If necessary, this in some instances, may be performed by the anesthesiologist.

Questioning should focus on the following points:
1 adverse reactions to anesthesia in patient or family;
2 drug therapy—allergies;
3 smoking, alcohol and drug abuse;
4 pulmonary problems such as bronchitis, emphysema, asthma, tuberculosis, shortness of breath, wheezing;
5 high blood pressure, heart attack, chest pain, cardiac murmur, other heart disease;
6 stroke, convulsions (frequency and therapy);
7 hepatitis, AIDS;
8 diabetes, renal and liver problems; and
9 bleeding tendencies, bruising, etc.

Examination of the patient must be informative. Vital signs must be noted and specific evaluation of the cardiac and respiratory system done. The anesthesiologist must carefully evaluate the airway. If the patient is edentulous and has dentures, the patient may proceed to surgery with dentures in place. Whenever possible, old records should be obtained and the previous medical history of the patient evaluated.

Despite the multiplicity of problems with which these patients present, many patients with significant multisystem disease will undergo cataract surgery. Unstable angina, hypertension or any other unstable medical condition is a contraindication to proceeding with surgery.

LABORATORY STUDIES

These are performed on a routine basis with additional tests being done when the medical condition so dictates. In the healthy elderly patient, the hematocrit, hemoglobin, electrocardiograph (EKG), electrolytes, glucose, and chest radiograph are the only routine tests needed. Patients taking diuretics need to have electrolyte determinations performed 48 h prior to surgery. Diabetic patients will have a glucose determination done the morning of surgery and patients receiving anticoagulants who have recently stopped their anticoagulants, or who are on anticoagulation therapy, will have a prothrombin/partial thromboplastin time (PT/PTT) done the morning of surgery. In those patients where aspirin has recently been ingested (3–5 days), a bleeding time is obtained. Patients on various medications such as theophylline, digitalis, or anticonvulsant drugs, should, if necessary, also have these levels confirmed within 48 h of surgery.

The presence of a signed operative consent must be verified and in some cases, preoperative medication, such as H2-blocking agents (cimetadine or ranitidine), may be given by mouth with a sip of water, 1 hour prior to surgery.

Most eye surgery is performed under a regional block with i.v. supplementation. In those patients who are felt to be uncooperative or confused, a general anesthetic may be administered. Other reasons for general anesthesia include patients who have difficulty in lying down due to musculoskeletal diseases or pain, who have hearing impairment, or who have a language barrier. Some patients may require general anesthesia because of the potential danger from bleeding due to a retrobulbar block. The mortality from eye surgery is low. Adler [6], concluded that the underlying systemic problems are the most important determinants of risk in these patients. It is thus important that these patients be brought to the operating room in an optimal stable state.

There are three situations which can be specifically addressed by the anesthesia staff in order to avoid intraoperative surgical difficulties [6]. These are: (a) preventing intraoperative coughing; (b) preventing movement; and (c) avoiding significant hypertension, especially diastolic pressures over 110 mmHg. Coughing causes intraocular pressure to rise and if the eye is open, could result in the eye contents being expelled and the eye destroyed. Consequently, every effort should be made to

suppress a cough and control its presence, with narcotics if necessary. If it is severe and surgery has to proceed, then it should be performed under general anesthesia. Patients who have uncontrollable movements or have difficulty in lying still, should also have their surgery performed under general anesthesia. Hypertension, with a diastolic pressure above 110 mmHg may increase the risk of bleeding into the eye. Therefore, efforts must be made to try and reduce the diastolic pressure to below 110 mmHg. Many patients are on maintenance diuretics and mannitol is given prior to surgery to lower intraocular pressure. These agents together may induce a brisk diuresis, which may produce orthostatic hypotension [6].

Specific medical problems

Heart disease

It is well recognized that factors leading to the development of perioperative myocardial infarction and heart failure are leading causes of postoperative death [7]. Associated cardiac problems—coronary artery disease, angina, congestive heart failure, peripheral vascular disease, hypertension, diabetes mellitus, and dysrhythmia, are frequently seen in the elderly patient presenting for cataract surgery. Goldman et al. [8], in their development of a risk index for use in patients over the age of 40, found nine risk factors that correlated with an increase in perioperative complications. These were:

1 age of 70;

2 a prior myocardial infarction within the past 6 months;

3 presence of an S_3 gallop;

4 distended jugular veins (congestive heart failure);

5 significant valvular aortic stenosis;

6 cardiac rhythm other than sinus or presence of premature atrial or ventricular contractions more frequently than 5/min;

7 the presence of intraperitoneal, intrathoracic or aortic surgery;

8 emergency surgery; and

9 poor general health. Poor general status

included a potassium level less than 3 mmol/l, a bicarbonate less than 20 mmol/l, BUN (blood, urea, nitrogen) greater than 50 mg%, creatine above 3 mg%, PO_2 less than 60 mmHg, a PCO_2 greater than 50 mmHg, and abnormal liver function studies.

These authors concluded that perioperative mortality could be significantly reduced if some of these abnormalities were corrected.

Advances in anesthesia, invasive monitoring and drug therapy have all contributed to a decrease in perioperative cardiac mortality. Tarhan et al. [9] showed that patients operated on within 3 months of an infarct, had a 37% reinfarction rate following subsequent surgery. This decreased to 16% if surgery was done 4–6 months after the myocardial infarction. The incidence of perioperative myocardial infarction stabilizes around 5% if surgery is done or delayed until 6 months or more after a myocardial infarct. Rao et al. [10], reported on a series of patients who had extensive surgery following myocardial infarction. These patients all had invasive cardiac monitoring. They found that perioperative reinfarction occured in 5.7% of patients who had an infarction within the previous 3 months, decreasing to 2.3% when surgery took place 4–6 months following the infarct. It is therefore strongly recommended, to delay elective surgery for at least 6 months after a myocardial infarction. Emergency surgery cannot be delayed and should proceed with appropriate monitoring.

There are an increasing number of patients who have sustained a previous myocardial infarct or who have undergone coronary artery bypass surgery and are now presenting for cataract surgery. In a study by Backer et al. [11], 195 patients were reviewed, all of whom had suffered a previous documented myocardial infarct and who subsequently underwent ophthalmic surgery. In 72% of these patients, cataract extraction was performed. Of these patients 21 underwent ophthalmologic surgery under general anesthesia. The remainder were performed under local or regional retrobulbar blocks. In none of these two groups was a perioperative myocardial infarct noted. It was concluded that local anesthesia and/or retrobulbar block for ophthalmologic surgery does not pose any special risks for reinfarction in patients with previous myocardial infarcts.

ANGINA

Those patients who present with stable angina are not at a substantially increased risk of developing cardiac complications following cataract surgery [7]. It is important to know their exercise tolerance, for if this is becoming compromised, it may indicate impending ventricular failure. These patients need to be under good symptomatic control and if necessary, their medications such as nitrates (i.v. or transdermal patch), β and calcium channel antagonists must be continued throughout the perioperative period [7].

Those patients with unstable angina generally have a poor prognosis. Non-urgent surgery should be postponed in patients with new onset or unstable angina until such time that the coronary ischemia has been stabilized. It may be necessary to perform a stress test, cardiac catheterization, or do coronary artery bypass surgery in these patients before they may be considered eligible for elective cataract surgery [7].

CONGESTIVE CARDIAC FAILURE

Congestive cardiac failure in the elderly is usually poorly tolerated. These patients stand a greater risk of developing complications such as hypoxemia, myocardial depression, volume overload, and pulmonary edema. Most of these patients have significant underlying coronary artery disease, hypertension, or valvular heart disease. Until recently, digitalis and diuretics have been the mainstay of therapy. New therapy now includes the use of vasodilators. These drugs decrease either the preload (venous capacitance), afterload (systemic resistance), or both. In the ambulatory setting, oral hydralazine plus nitrates provide good control by decreasing both afterload and preload. Recently, the introduction of angiotensin-converting enzyme (ACE) inhibitors such as captopril and enalapril, which block the conversion of angiotensin I to angiotensin II, have proven to be very beneficial in patients refractory to other forms of therapy [12].

It is thus imperative that patients with congestive heart failure be brought to the operating room in a stable physiologic state before surgery can be performed. This may entail cautious diuresis and optimization of drug therapy. Vigorous preoperative diuresis should be avoided as it may produce orthostatic hypotension.

VALVULAR HEART DISEASE

The prevalence of valvular *aortic stenosis* increases with age. It has been shown to be associated with a 13% perioperative mortality and if severe, patients will present with syncope, angina, and congestive heart failure [8]. The narrow outlet obstruction places an increased load on the left ventricle, impairing normal diastolic function. These patients tolerate hypovolemia and tachycardia extremely poorly. The echocardiogram is a highly sensitive method of making the diagnosis. In those patients with significant symptoms aortic valve replacement may need to be done prior to carrying out any other non-cardiac surgery. Patients with *mitral stenosis* also tolerate tachycardia very poorly. It produces a fall in cardiac output and may precipitate pulmonary edema. In these patients, control of ventricular rate is very important and surgery should not be performed if this is not well controlled.

An increasing number of patients with prosthetic cardiac valves present for cataract surgery. As these patients pose a definite risk of developing thrombotic complications they are usually on chronic anticoagulant (warfarin) therapy. In addition they may have the possibility of also developing bacterial endocarditis. There are some real concerns in operating on patients who are anticoagulated. Hall *et al.* [13] describe ophthalmic surgery in 42 patients on warfarin (coumadin) (49 operations) where the warfarin was not discontinued. Surgery was done under *local anesthesia* after patients had received their morning warfarin dose. PT/PTT levels were in the therapeutic anticoagulant range of $1-1\frac{1}{2}$ times control in 48% of patients. Three patients were noted to have blood in the anterior chamber on the first postoperative day. All cleared within 10 to 14 days. Excessive bleeding from the episcleral and wound vessels was not noted. In 1985, Stone *et al.* [14] presented the results of a questionnaire completed by cataract surgeons. Of the respondents 75% withheld warfarin prior to cataract surgery. Sequaelae were said to be severe in some patients with two documented deaths and other severe major cardiovascular complications. In those patients where warfarin was continued there were 22 episodes of bleeding with no adverse effects noted. Because the operative field is a relatively avascular one, the authors felt that intraocular surgery could be safely done on patients receiving anticoagulant therapy.

Another option as outlined by Tinker and Tarhan [15] is to discontinue the warfarin 3–4 days preoperative and then proceeding under heparin administered by constant infusion. This should be considered in those patients who have had previous thrombotic or embolic phenomenon.

If the patients give a history of a previous episode of bacterial endocarditis, then full antibiotic prophylaxis with ampicillin, and gentamicin, should be performed according to American Heart Guidelines [16]. As cataract surgery is "clean" surgery, it may be considered unnecessary to give patients with underlying valvular lesions endocarditis prophylaxis. This practice appears to be quite variable in the cataract surgery setting.

CARDIAC DYSRHYTHMIAS

Cardiac dysrhythmias, are frequent in the elderly patient [7]. The occasional premature ventricular contraction is not unusual in the normal healthy patient. However, in the presence of coronary artery disease, these may precipitate sudden ventricular fibrillation. Ventricular dysrhythmias that are not protracted and do not accompany left ventricular dysfunction, are usually benign. Following an acute myocardial infarction, in patients with acute myocardial ischemia, or hypokalemia, these patients are at greater risk for developing ventricular fibrillation [6].

Perioperative heart block rarely occurs in the asymptomatic patient [6]. If sinus bradycardia occurs during surgery, this usually responds to intravenous atropine 0.5–1 mg. Chronic bifascicular block is well tolerated. Important indications for preoperative pacemaker insertion are the presence of symptomatic bradycardia and advanced atrioventricular block [7].

HYPERTENSIVE CARDIOVASCULAR DISEASE

Hypertension is the most commonly encountered cardiovascular disease [7]. The prevalence of hypertension is estimated at 50% or more in those who are 55 years and over. Hypertension is considered to be one of the most important risk factors for the development of progressive cardiovascular disease. Uncontrolled hypertension due to non-compliance with therapy may be a major problem in preparing the patient for surgery. No patient should be referred for surgery unless their hypertension is under control. On the other hand, when the blood pressure is stable (<110 mmHg diastolic pressure) there is no further purpose in delaying surgery in the hope of achieving even better control [7].

Thiazide diuretics are the drug of choice for isolated systolic hypertension, effective, and well tolerated. These patients should have their electrolyte levels monitored at frequent intervals. For further control, hydralazine, β-adrenergic blocking drugs, calcium channel antagonists, clonidine and ACE inhibitors may all play a role [7].

A syndrome characterized by sympathetic over activity and rebound hypertension is seen 18–24 h following the abrupt withdrawal of clonidine—usually in patients taking more than 1.2 mg/day. Therapy may require the use of intravenous nitroprusside. Clonidine should be continued throughout the perioperative period and if patients cannot tolerate oral medications, transdermal clonidine should be commenced prior to surgery [7].

CARDIAC EVALUATION

How should patients with underlying cardiac disease be evaluated and which special tests may be of value? Normally, the routine resting 12-lead EKG is ordered and is inexpensive. It is of value in identifying frank changes, whether they be due to arrhythmias, changes in the ST configuration, or the presence of Q-waves. It is particularly valuable to compare previous tracings with the present one.

If symptoms and history so dictate, i.e. increasing angina, syncope, paroxysmal nocturnal dyspnea, or recent myocardial infarct, then a stress test or dipyridamole–thallium scintigraphy (non-exercise) may be indicated. Dipyridamole is administered to induce coronary vasodilation in areas of the coronary vascular bed which are not affected by atherosclerosis. This test identifies myocardium at risk levels [17].

Pulmonary disease

Chronic pulmonary problems are frequently encountered during the preoperative evaluation of elderly patients [18]. These include chronic obstructive pulmonary disease, asthma, and pulmonary embolization. A complete history and physical examination in these patients is especially important.

CHRONIC OBSTRUCTIVE PULMONARY DISEASE

This includes emphysema and chronic bronchitis and is characterized by small airway obstruction with decreases in expiratory flow rates, pursed lip breathing, use of accessory muscles of respiration, and wheezing on forced expiration. In patients with chronic bronchitis, sputum production is a prominent feature and these patients have a tendency to develop cor pulmonale early in the course of their disease. Patients presenting for surgery should be in optimal condition. If there are manifestations of infection (i.e. change in sputum color), then patients should be placed on antibiotics (ampicillin, tetracycline) for a course of 10–14 days. Smoking should be stopped for at least 8 weeks prior to surgery to be of any benefit [19]. Bronchodilators should be administered by the inhalation route, using metered dose inhalers or aerosols. Most patients will benefit from a treatment prior to surgery. In some patients theophylline levels need to be determined and drug dosage optimized. Corticosteroids may be of value in some patients and should be continued throughout the perioperative period. Pulmonary function studies enable one to categorize the severity of the disease and evaluate the response to bronchodilator therapy. Patients at risk include those with an FEV_1 (forced expiratory volume in 1 second) of less than 1 liter, and an $FEF_{25-75\%}$ (forced midexpiratory flow); less than 50% of predicted. Patients who are continuously hypoxemic (PaO_2 < 55 mmHg) despite therapy, should be placed on chronic low flow (1–4 l/min) of oxygen. This helps prevent the development of pulmonary hypertension. If patients are polycythemic, they should undergo prophylactic phlebotomy with restoration of the hematocrit to approximately 55%. In patients with chronic hypercapnia (PCO_2 elevation plus increase in HCO_3) further CO_2 retention should be guarded against [18].

ASTHMA

Asthma is a frequently seen complication. These patients must be well controlled in order to prevent the development of intraoperative bronchospastic attacks. All bronchodilator medication must be taken on a regular basis, and continued throughout the perioperative period. Whenever possible, theophylline levels should be measured 48 h prior to surgery and should be in the therapeutic range before proceeding with surgery. Patients can be followed on the basis of portable spirometry and peak flow measurements. Bronchodilator therapy and steroids should be continued right up to surgery and those patients on steroids should receive a steroid boost of 100 mg of hydrocortisone prior to surgery and 4 h after. This should also be done on all patients who have taken corticosteroids within the previous year.

RESTRICTIVE LUNG DISEASES

These patients with small lung volumes and low functional residual capacity due to numer-

ous causes such as interstitial fibrosis, generally do not pose a major risk during the perioperative period. Once again, preoperative pulmonary function studies need to be obtained as well as blood gases.

TUBERCULOSIS

Unfortunately, there is an increase in the prevalence of tuberculosis in the elderly patient population, most frequently due to reactivation. Patients known to have contracted tuberculosis and who are receiving therapy should have active surgery delayed for at least 2 months while active tuberculosis therapy is continued.

The preoperative preparation of patients with lung disease must be carefully orchestrated. This may include cessation of smoking and stabilization of bronchodilator therapy. In some patients, chest physical therapy and aerosol therapy will be of considerable benefit. The short-term use of antibiotics in select patients may be indicated.

THROMBOEMBOLIC DISEASE

Pulmonary embolism is a frequent cause of death in patients with many underlying diseases. Mortality has been shown to increase with age. Patients at risk are those who give a history of previous thromboembolism; venous thrombosis, cancer, have heart failure, or are to be immobilized from surgery. In those patients, low-dose heparin has been shown to prevent thrombosis. Other means of prophylaxis against venous thrombosis include intermittent pneumatic leg compression. In low-risk patients, such as patients presenting for cataract surgery, graduated compression stockings may be the most cost-effective measure [20].

Neurologic disease

DEMENTIA

Dementia is seen in 15% of patients over the age of 65 [21]. Derangement may vary from the mild forgetting of names to motor incoordination, ataxia, sensory loss, and ultimately progressive mutism. Alzheimer's disease is the most frequent cause of dementia in the elderly and these patients are unable to manage their affairs or take care of themselves.

Patients with *Parkinson's disease* pose a particularly challenging problem. The association of bradykinesia, tremor, and rigidity, as well as mood disorders, may make it very difficult to manage the patient under local or regional anesthesia. Drugs such as droperidol or metoclopramide should be withheld as they can exacerbate extrapyramidal symptoms [21, 22]. General anesthetics such as halothane which sensitizes the heart to catecholamines should be avoided as L-dopa can induce arrhythmias. Improvement in their disease may be seen with drug therapy, such as with Sinemet, a combination of both carbidopa and L-dopa. These drugs are the mainstay of Parkinson's disease therapy, have a short duration of action and should be discontinued the night before surgery. Bromocriptine, a dopamine antagonist, may also be used in treating patients with Parkinson's disease. It may produce hypotension by relaxing the vessels of the gastrointestinal and renal bed. Maintenance of a preoperative volume status is important.

STROKE

Millions of elderly Americans live with the effects of cerebrovascular insults [21]. These may be due to carotid artery disease where left hemispheric strokes may lead to aphasia and hemiplegia. Emboli from mural carotid thrombi or valvular disease may produce hemiplegia with visual defects. Patients with transient ischemic attacks need to be worked up before other forms of elective surgery can be done. Regardless of the type of stroke one should wait at least 2 weeks after the event before performing surgery [21]. In patients with embolic strokes who are on anticoagulants, they may be continued [13,14], or warfarin discontinued 3–4 days prior to surgery, proceeding with a constant heparin infusion [14].

SEIZURE DISORDERS

Patients with a history of a seizure disorder must be seizure free in order to be considered for ambulatory surgery. If necessary, anticonvulsant levels must be obtained prior to surgery and documented to be in the therapeutic range before proceeding. Most seizure disorders are controlled by phenobarbital and/or phenytoin [21].

Endocrine diseases

DIABETES MELLITUS

Diabetes mellitus is one of the most frequently seen diseases in the elderly patient presenting for cataract surgery [23]. The incidence of diabetes at age 60 years is 10% increasing to 20% by the age of 80. It is a diffuse disease with multisystem involvement and patients may present with coronary artery disease, hypertension, renal insufficiency, neuropathies, and disturbed gastric, bowel, and bladder function. Diabetic patients are classified into two groups, type I patients who are insulin dependent and type II, those who do not need insulin for control of their diabetes and are controlled by either diet, oral hypoglycemic drugs, or both. All diabetic patients need to be under good control and their associated systemic diseases must be stable if surgery is to be performed. If a patient has recently been admitted for the control of diabetes; or has had a recent episode of hypoglycemia, is especially brittle, then consideration should be given for the patient to be admitted preoperatively for stabilization and better control [4].

All diabetic patients should come in early on the morning of surgery. Insulin-dependent patients are asked to bring their insulin with them. The blood glucose level is obtained and infusion of dextrose 5% with lactated ringers is commenced at approximately 100 ml/h (2 ml/kg per h). If the blood glucose level is less than 150 mg/dl, then one-third of the routine insulin dose is given. If it is greater than 150 mg/dl, then one-half the routine insulin dose is administered. Blood glucose levels are monitored during surgery and additional regular insulin administered if necessary [4]. In the recovery room, the blood glucose level is checked and regular insulin administered if glucose levels are high. Diet-controlled diabetics can go through the perioperative period on a "no glucose, no insulin" regimen. Intravenous fluids contain no glucose and blood glucose levels are carefully monitored [22].

Patients on oral hypoglycemic drugs are instructed not to take their medicine on the day of surgery. Once again, a blood glucose check is performed. Insulin, if necessary, may be administered on a sliding scale or as a regular continuous infusion at 1–2 U/h. Oral hypoglycemic drugs currently in use have variable durations of action. Chlorpropamide, which has a long half-life (about 35 h) should be stopped 2–3 days prior to surgery. Short-acting agents such as tolazamide, or tolbutamide, have half-lives of approximately 7–8 h and should be stopped the night before surgery. Caution must be exercised in avoiding bladder distention, especially in those patients with associated autonomic dysfunction. Some of these patients may need to be catheterized and this should be done with a very careful aseptic technique. As many of these patients have gastroparesis, silent aspiration may occur [22].

THYROID

Thyroid function decreases with age. The presentation of hypothyroidism may be quite subtle and go unnoticed [23,24]. Therefore, one must be more alert to the possibility of this disease in the elderly. A history, which points to previous neck surgery, or the use of drugs such as lithium and amiodarone, should alert the physician to the possibility of hypothyroidism. Hypothyroidism is an easily treatable disease with either thyroid or L-thyroxone. These patients need to be worked up by their primary care physician and brought to the operating room when they are euthyroid.

There is also an increased incidence of hyperthyroidism in the elderly [23,24]. Once again, the manifestations are subtle but point to an anxious, nervous, hyperactive patient who invariably may be in atrial fibrillation and congestive heart failure. As the hyperthyroid state is considered to be detrimental to the cardiac status of elderly patients, rapid institution of a euthyroid state must be achieved. Cardiac symptoms can be attenuated with a judicious dose of β-adrenergic blocking agent such as propanolol. Drugs such as propylthiouracil and methimazole may help bring about a euthyroid state and once this has been achieved, definitive therapy with either surgery or radioiodine can be instituted. All elective surgery should be delayed until patients are euthyroid.

Hematologic problems

ANEMIA

With little supporting data, anesthesiologists and surgeons have continued to require that patients have a hemoglobin greater than 10 g before they are considered to be surgical candidates. Studies have now shown that surgery can be performed with safety in patients who have hemoglobin levels in the 6–7 g range provided oxygen transport and cardiac output can be maintained [25]. Nevertheless, it is important to determine the cause of the anemia, and if necessary, this should be worked up before surgery is planned.

POLYCYTHEMIA

Patients with polycythemia have an increased surgical mortality. The higher the hematocrit, the greater is the blood viscosity and the greater the risk for the development of venous thrombosis and bleeding. Patients should have the hematocrit decreased preoperatively by phlebotomies of 350–500 ml every other day until a hematocrit of approximately 55 is reached [25].

THROMBOCYTOPENIA

It is generally accepted that with a platelet count of greater than 50 000, surgery can be performed and that hemostasis will be satisfactory. If the platelet count is less than 20 000, the risk of bleeding from surgery is significant and surgery should be deferred until the platelet count can be raised [26]. All elective surgery should be deferred until a cause for the thrombocytopenia is found and corrected.

BLEEDING DISORDERS

Platelet defects which prolong bleeding time may be seen in patients taking aspirin. These drugs should be discontinued for 1 week prior to surgery. If emergency surgery must proceed, then platelet transfusions may be needed to decrease the bleeding time. There is also a recognized platelet defect associated with renal failure, which is usually corrected following dialysis or after the administration of deamino-D-arginine vasopressin (DDAVP) [27].

HEMOPHILIA

Hemophiliacs may undergo surgery. In these patients, i.m. injections should be avoided. DDAVP may elevate the Factor VIII level adequately to allow surgery to proceed without having to administer Factor VIII, thereby eliminating the potential hazards of giving infected blood products to a patient [28].

Other diseases

KIDNEY PROBLEMS

Preoperative problems encountered in patients with chronic renal failure are related to their associated hypertension, congestive cardiac failure, electrolyte and fluid imbalance, bleeding, and acidosis [29]. Generally, these patients develop a positive water balance, although, in some patients with chronic pyelonephritis there may be salt wasting, hypovolemia, and syncope. If hyperkalemia is a problem then surgery should be deferred until the potassium level is in the normal range.

An increasing number of elderly patients are being maintained on some form of dialysis. Patients with azotemia may have increased bleeding due to a platelet defect which can be corrected by the preoperative administration

of cryoprecipitate or DDAVP [28]. It is recommended that dialysis is best avoided in the 4 h prior to surgery and preferably done the day before.

Generally speaking, a normal BUN and creatinine excludes significant renal disease.

Many elderly males have manifestations of prostatism and have difficulty voiding. This may be a cause for restlessness and agitation and perioperative hypertension. Consequently, fluids need to be restricted during the perioperative period.

ARTHRITIS

In the elderly patient, there is an increase in the incidence of both osteo- and rheumatoid arthritis [30]. Pain may be quite severe making the conduct of surgery under monitored anesthesia care (MAC) difficult. Great care must be exercised in positioning these patients. The ability to establish an airway must be carefully evaluated as many of these patients have decreased neck mobility. Plans may need to be made to perform an awake fiberoptic intubation should general anesthesia be required. Rheumatoid arthritis is a systemic disease with pulmonary, cardiac, and other system involvement. Consequently, the stability of these organ systems must be ascertained during the preoperative evaluation. As many of these patients are on steroids they will need to be supplemented with hydrocortisone during the anesthetic procedure.

Infectious considerations

Acquired immune deficiency syndrome (AIDS)

AIDS is having its impact throughout all realms of society and the medical establishment [31,32]. The virus responsible has been isolated from seminal fluid, blood, tears, saliva, and synovial fluid [33]. The patient and health-care workers may be aware of HIV (human immunodeficiency virus) infection as the acute process may be asymptomatic. There is a definite risk to health-care workers. The most common exposure to the HIV virus has come about by needle sticks through the recapping of used needles.

It is estimated that there are over 1.5 million Americans who are HIV positive and the number continues to increase. It is thus recommended that all patients be considered potentially infectious to all health-care workers and that specific precautions be used. Current recommendations for preventing the transmission of the HIV virus include:

1 handling all sharp items with extraordinary care;

2 needles should not be recapped and should be disposed of in puncture proof containers;

3 barrier proof precautions and the wearing of gloves, gowns, mask and eye coverings whenever a health-care worker comes in contact with body fluids, mucous membranes, blood, or non-intact skin;

4 hands must be washed if contaminated;

5 resuscitation devices for airway management should be readily available to minimize the need for mouth to mouth respiration; and,

6 health-care workers with dermatitis should not be involved in direct patient care.

Health-care workers who are HIV positive or have AIDS pose a definite risk to patients who are immunocompromised and these workers should be removed from contact with those patients (see also Chapter 30).

Hepatitis

The most frequent causes of hepatitis are hepatitis B, hepatitis A, and hepatitis non-A, non-B. Hepatitis B, otherwise known as serum hepatitis, is transmitted by contaminated blood and blood products. A carrier state is common and hepatitis B virus may be transmitted through blood transfusions and from health-care workers. Hepatitis B is known to be an occupational hazard for health-care workers. Health-care workers who are unvaccinated and are directly exposed (e.g. needle stick) to patients who are known to be at a high risk or who are known to be hepatitis B surface antigen positive, should have an immediate dose of hepatitis B immunoglobulin to be followed by a hepatitis B vaccination series. If workers have already been vaccinated, hepa-

titis B surface antibodies should be verified and if inadequate, hepatitis B immunoglobulin administered together with a hepatitis B vaccine booster dose [32]. Surgery should be deferred in patients with acute viral hepatitis unless it is an absolute emergency. Patients who give a history of hepatitis exposure should be tested for hepatitis B surface antigen, liver enzymes, bilirubin, albumin, and PT/PTT.

Cirrhosis

The spectrum of the patient with cirrhosis is quite varied [34]. These patients, despite disturbed hepatic function, may be asymptomatic or have manifestations of liver failure. The latter are not candidates for cataract surgery. Patients with cirrhosis may have low serum albumin levels, prolongation of their PT/PTT and if the disease is far advanced, present with associated portal hypertension and thrombocytopenia. Patients with advanced liver disease must be carefully evaluated as the preparation for surgery may entail the correction of preoperative abnormal coagulation parameters, administration of vitamin K and, if necessary, fresh frozen plasma and platelets.

Drugs and the elderly

Polypharmacy is frequently encountered in the elderly. Most geriatric patients are taking at least two to three groups of medications and as these patients have a very narrow therapeutic window, the manifestations of drug toxicity occur frequently and should be looked for. Drug-related problems relate not only to drugs associated with the treatment of various systemic diseases, but also those used during the conduct of anesthesia for eye surgery (Table 5.2). The reader is referred to the review by McGoldrick [35], where problems with ocular drugs are discussed in greater detail.

Conclusion

Cataract surgery will continue to be a frequently performed surgical procedure in the ambulatory setting. For most patients it is safe and uncomplicated. However, it is important

Table 5.2 Side effects of ophthalmic eye drops. After [35]

Drug	Concentration (%)	mg/drop drug	Main side effect
Phenylephrine (Neosynephrine)	2.5–5	1.25–2.5	Hypertension
Epinephrine (Epifrin)	0.5–2	0.5–1	Hypertension
Timolol maleate (Timoptic)	0.25–0.5	—	β-adrenergic blockade
Cyclopentolate (Cyclogyl)	0.5–1	—	Hyperpyrexia, psychosis, seizures
Scopolamine (Isopto Hyoscine)	0.25	—	Excitation, disorientation
Atropine	0.5–1	0.1–0.5	Flushing, tachycardia
Tropicamide (Mydriacyl)	0.5–1	—	Psychosis, vasomotor collapse
Pilocarpine (Pilocar)	0.5–4	—	Hypertension, bronchospasm
Echothiophate iodide (Phospholine Iodide)	0.03–0.25	—	Anticholinesterase—prolongation of succinylcholine
Cocaine	4	1.5	Arrhythmias, hypertension

for the ophthalmic surgeon, primary care physician, and anesthesiologist to work closely together in preparing the patient for surgery. These patients have multiple medical problems and are on numerous medications. Patients must be in a stable medical condition before any form of surgery is to be performed.

References

1 Felts JA. Outpatient anaesthesia in the geriatric patient. *Clin Anaesth* 1986; **4**: 1025–34.

2 Wetchler BV. Outpatient anesthesia. *Prob Anesth* 1988; **2**: 9–17.

3 Meyers EF. Anesthesia for ophthalmic surgery in the aged. *Clin Anaesth* 1986; **4**: 979–1002.

4 Pasternak LR. Anesthetic considerations in otolaryngological and ophthalmological outpatient surgery. *Int Anesthesiol Clin* 1990; **28**: 89–100.

5 Keating HJ. Preoperative considerations in the geriatric patient. *Med Clin N Am* 1987; **71**: 569–83.

6 Adler AG. Perioperative management of the ophthalmology patient. *Med Clin N Am* 1987; **71**: 561–7.

7 Weitz HH, Goldman L. Noncardiac surgery in the patient with heart disease. *Med Clin N Am* 1987; **71**: 413–32.

8 Goldman L, Caldera DL, Nussbaum SR *et al.* Multifactorial index of cardiac risk in noncardiac surgical procedures. *N Engl J Med* 1977; **297**: 845–50.

9 Tarhan S, Moffit E, Taylor W *et al.* Myocardial infarction after general anesthesia. *JAMA* 1972; **220**: 1451–4.

10 Rao T, Jacobs K, El Etr A. Reinfarction following in patients with myocardial infarction. *Anesthesiology* 1983; **59**: 499–505.

11 Backer CL, Tinker JH, Robertson DM *et al.* Myocardial reinfarction following local anesthesia for ophthalmic surgery. *Anesth Analg* 1980; **59**: 257–62.

12 Arai AE, Greenberg BH. Medical management of congestive heart failure. *West J Med* 1990; **153**: 406–14.

13 Hall DL, Steen WH, Drummond JW. Anticoagulants and cataract surgery. *Ophthal Surg* 1988; **19**: 221–2.

14 Stone LS, Kline OR, Sklar S. Intraocular lenses and anticoagulation and antiplatelet therapy. *J Am Intraocul Implant Soc* 1985; **11**: 165–8.

15 Tinker JH, Tarhan J. Discontinuing anticoagulant therapy in surgical patients with cardiac valve prostheses. *JAMA* 1978; **239**: 738–41.

16 Shulman ST, Amren DP, Bisno AL *et al.* Prevention of bacterial endocarditis—a statement for health professionals by the committee on rheumatic fever and infectious endocarditis of the Council on Cardiovascular Disease in the Young. *Circulation* 1984; **70**: 1123A–7A.

17 Freeman WK, Gibbons RJ, Shub C. Preoperative assessment of cardiac patients undergoing noncardiac surgical procedures. *Mayo Clin Proc* 1989; **64**: 1105–17.

18 Tisi GM. Preoperative indentification and evaluation of the patient with lung disease. *Med Clin N Am* 1987; **71**(3): 399–412.

19 Gomez MN, Tinker JH. Smoking, anesthesia and coronary bypass operation: A witches' cauldron? *Mayo Clin Proc* 1989; **64**: 708–11.

20 Hull RD, Raskob GE, Hirsh J. Prophylaxis of venous thromboembolism. *Chest* 1986; **89**: 374S–83S.

21 Merli GJ, Bell RD. Preoperative management of the surgical patient with neurological disease. *Med Clin N Am* 1987; **71**: 511.

22 Brindle GT. Anesthesia in the patient with Parkinsonism. *Primary Care* 1977; **4**: 513–28.

23 Goldman DR. Surgery in patients with endocrine dysfunction. *Med Clin N Am* 1987; **71**: 499–509.

24 Kabadi UM. Thyroid disorders and the elderly. *Comprehensive Ther* 1989; **15**: 53–65.

25 Fellin F, Murphy S. Hematologic problems in the preoperative patient. *Med Clin N Am* 1987; **71**: 477–87.

26 McCullough J, Sleeper TA, Connelly DP *et al.* Platelet utilization in a university hospital. *JAMA* 1988; **259**: 2414–18.

27 Mannuc PM, Remuzzi G, Pusineri F. D-amino-8-D-arginine vasopressin shortens the bleeding time in uremia. *N Engl J Med* 1983; **308**: 8–12.

28 Richardson DW, Robinson AG. Desmopressin. *Ann Intern Med* 1985; **103**: 228–39.

29 Burke JF, Francos GC. Surgery in the patient with acute or chronic renal failure. *Med Clin N Am* 1987; **71**: 489–97.

30 Corman LC. Clinical spectrum and treatment of rheumatic syndromes in the elderly. *Med Clin N Am* 1989; **73**: 1371–81.

31 Gotta AW. AIDS and the implications for the anesthesiologist. *Adv Anesth* 1990; **7**: 75–82.

32 Bready L. Infectious disease and anesthesia. *Adv Anesth* 1988; **5**: 89–127.

33 Seifert MH. Transmission of human immuno-deficiency virus (HIV). *N Engl J Med* 1988; **318**: 1203.

34 Friedman LS, Maddrey WC. Surgery in the patient with liver disease. *Med Clin N Am* 1987; **71**: 453–76.

35 McGoldrick KE. Ocular drugs and anesthesia. *Int Anesthesiol Clin* 1990; **28**: 72–7.

6: How to Obtain the Best Visual Results: the Determination of the Correct Implant Power and Prediction of Postoperative Refractive Error

DONALD R. SANDERS, JOHN A. RETZLAFF & MANUS C. KRAFF

Introduction

In November, 1949, Ridley ushered in the era of intraocular lenses by implanting a plastic lens in a patient. At the same time, he unwittingly ushered in the subject of intraocular lens (IOL) power calculation as his patient's postoperative refraction was −24.00 + 6.00 × 30! [1] The dioptric power of those early lens implants was adjusted, eliminating the huge postoperative refractive errors, yet for primary implants, for almost two decades, the simplistic method of implanting the same strength implant ("standard lens") in every patient or using some simple modifications based on refraction was the rule.

In 1967, Fyodorov first presented his theoretic implant power formula based on geometric optics and utilizing keratometry and A-scan ultrasonography [2]. Since then, 20 years of refinements through experience, and the development of data-derived empiric models have led to our current high expectations for power prediction accuracy. Nevertheless, some interest has revived in the use of standard power implants [3,4]. Singh and Sommer [4] examined a series of 520 average posterior chamber intraocular lens (PCIOL) cases (<4.5 D of myopia or hyperopia) at the Wilmer Institute. The authors determined that 0.4% of eyes would have had >4 D of refractive error with a "predicted-emmetropic" lens, compared with 2.1% if a "standard" 20-D lens was used. They felt that this might be a reasonable trade-off given the difficulty and expense of axial length measurement and keratometry. However, with over a million IOLs implanted each year [5], use of a standard power lens would result in an excess of over 20 000 unhappy patients having >4 D of refractive error.

Until very recently, surgeons have been able to rely on a "comfort" zone of trying to place their patients between −0.75 D and −1.5 D postoperative refraction. If the power calculation is off on the hyperopic side then this would produce emmetropia. If it was wrong on the myopic side, good uncorrected near vision was possible. However with the reduction of postoperative astigmatism through small incision surgery, the ability to correct preexisting astigmatic errors and the advent of multifocal IOLs enabling good uncorrected near vision, the limiting factor for good visual results becomes the spherical component of the residual refraction. The objective must be to get as close to emmetropia as possible. With over a million IOL surgeries performed in the USA each year and the advent of multifocal lenses, the probability of emmetropic refraction must be increased, since accurate implant power calculation is now the major determinant of patient satisfaction. It is the purpose of this chapter to provide some insight into those factors which affect implant power accuracy: the choice of implant power calculation methods and the current hardware technologies and methodologies.

Development of implant power calculation

The choice of implant power calculation formulas has been a major source of controversy in the past. Formulas have developed along two lines: theoretic formulas and data-derived (empiric) regression formulas.

Theoretic formulas

The first theoretic implant power calculation formula was developed by Fyodorov and Kolonko in 1967 [2] and was introduced into the USA with the first English language publication by Colenbrander 6 years later, in 1973 [6]. Other early theoretic models were formulated by Thijssen [7], Van der Heijde [8], and Binkhorst [9], with Binkhorst's being the most popular. All of these formulas, were based on geometric optics as applied to schematic eyes; except for the value assumptions of various correction factors and theoretic constants, all of the formulas are identical and can be algebraically transformed to:

$$P = \frac{n}{L - ACD} - \frac{(n)(k)}{(n - k)\,(ACD)}$$

where P = implant power for emmetropia, n = aqueous and vitreous refractive index, ACD = estimated postoperative anterior chamber depth (in ml), L = axial length (in ml), and k = corneal curvature (in D).

In the early 1970s, as the first ultrasound instrument designed exclusively for axial length measurement (the DBR-300 by Sonometrics Inc.) was being developed, Binkhorst made his formula available for use to the ophthalmic community [6,10–13]. Hoffer's modification of the Colenbrander formula [14–17] was also published.

All of the theoretic formulas (except the Fyodorov formula) used a constant value for estimated postoperative anterior chamber depth (ACD). They differed with respect to the value assumptions of this constant, as well as of various other correction factors. Early efforts to predict postoperative ACD from preoperative measurements proved unsuccessful; thus, use of a fixed constant remained standard practice, although, over the years, the value assumptions have been refined.

Empirically derived formulas

In 1981, the first empiric models for IOL implant power calculations were published [18–22]. These models were essentially regression formulas, which described the relation-ships between emmetropizing implant power and measurable ophthalmic parameters using data. They didn't depend on the theoretic establishment of value assumptions for correction factors and constants.

The work of Retzlaff [19], and of Sanders and Kraff [21] coalesced with the collaborative refinement of the empirically derived SRK regression formula, which became the most widely used implant power formula throughout the world. During that period, these regression equations were demonstrated to be superior to the concurrent theoretic models [20,22,23].

Second generation formulas

During the 1980s, both the theoretic and empiric formulas were further refined, resulting in a "second generation" of available power calculation formulas. These second generation formulas are either modifications of the classic theoretic formulas, modifications of the SRK formulas or similar empirically derived approaches, or a combination of theoretic–empiric approaches. Overall, the impetus for the parallel development of second generation models for both the theoretic and empiric models was the dramatic shift to posterior chamber lenses, when it became evident that the early theoretic formulas tended to predict too large an emmetropia value in short eyes and possibly too small a value in long eyes, while the first regression formulas had the opposite tendency. Both types of models performed well for average eyes (with axial lengths between 22 and 24.5 mm).

SECOND GENERATION
THEORETIC FORMULAS

In 1981, Binkhorst recommended that estimated postoperative ACD be adjusted for different length eyes [12] (larger ACD for longer eyes and vice versa). Shammas (1982) [25], Hoffer (1982) [17], Olsen (1986) [26], and Holladay (1988) [27] followed with their own methods of predicting postoperative ACD. The Binkhorst and Hoffer adjustments are based on a correlation between measured postoperative

ACD and axial length. Olsen's adjustment involves a regression formula, derived by sophisticated analysis of a group of anterior chamber IOLs, and predicts postoperative ACD from corneal diameter, corneal curvature, preoperative ACD, and lens thickness.

Holladay's formula, which uses a sensory retinal thickness factor of 0.2 mm and the corneal refractive index of 1.333 recommended by Binkhorst adjusts expected postoperative ACD with a complex geometry-related equation relating ACD to both axial length and corneal curvature. He has demonstrated a high degree of prediction accuracy with his formula in several data sets including long, short, and average eyes.

Retzlaff has recently developed the SRK/T (for theoretic) formula [28]. This formula was developed in order to offer a theoretic approach under the umbrella of the SRK formulas, with some sort of definitive correlation between the empirically derived regression A-constants and the theoretic ACD determinations. After testing many models, the Fyodorov formula was chosen as the base, and the corneal height formula was chosen for ACD tailoring. The corneal height formula was first described in the implant power calculation literature by Fyodorov [29] in 1967 and recently advocated by Olsen and Holladay. The SRK/T formula gives predictions similar to Holladay's formula. Furthermore, the SRK/T formula can be personalized for a specific IOL and/or surgeon in two ways. One can input either an ACD value that one desires or an SRK A-constant, and the appropriate personalized ACD value will be calculated. Also, either an ACD value or an SRK A-constant can be derived from data.

SECOND GENERATION EMPIRIC FORMULAS

The SRK formula was reformulated in 1988 [30], resulting in the current second generation SRK II model. This formula was built upon, improved upon, and was meant to replace the SRK formula. For eyes with axial lengths between 22 mm and 24.5 mm, which constitute about 75% of cases, the emmetropia power predictions are identical to the SRK formula. For short eyes (axial length below 22 mm) which

tend to occur in 10% of cases, and long eyes (axial length of 24.5 mm and above), occurring in 14% of cases, emmetropizing powers are adjusted in a simple stepwise fashion illustrated below, where axial length = L, average keratometry (D) = k, and A-constant = A.

If $L < 20.0$, then $A1 = A + 3$.
If $20 \leq L < 21.0$, then $A1 = A + 2$.
If $21 \leq L < 22.0$, then $A1 = A + 1$.
If $22 \leq L < 24.5$, then $A1 = A$.
If $L \geq 24.5$, then $A1 = A - 0.5$.

SRK II emmetropia power (P) =

$A1 - 0.9 \times k - 2.5 \times L$
If $P \leq 14$, then $CR = 1.00$.
If $P > 14$, then $CR = 1.25$.

To find the predicted postoperative refraction (R) for a given implanted lens power (I),

$R = (P - I)/CR$.

To find the lens power required to be implanted (I) to produce a given refraction (R),

$I = P - (R \times CR)$.

The SRK II formula is easy to use, requiring no additional hardware or software, yet provides comparable or improved prediction accuracy over the second generation theoretic formulas [30].

Earlier, in 1984, Thompson et al. [31] described a new empiric intraocular lens formula also designed to improve results in axial myopes. Their formula was a linear regression equation for eyes with axial length below 24.5 mm and had quadratic or squared terms for both axial length and keratometry when axial length was greater than or equal to 24.5 mm. However, this formula was highly specific for the data set from which it was derived and there was no method for individually tailoring the formula for different types and manufacturers of IOLs.

Donzis et al. [32] developed what they termed the percentage change formula, which is a direct modification of the original SRK formula. It utilizes the SRK A-constants, but changes the relationship between axial length and power for emmetropia to a non-linear term whose magnitude is a function of the percentage deviation of a particular case's axial

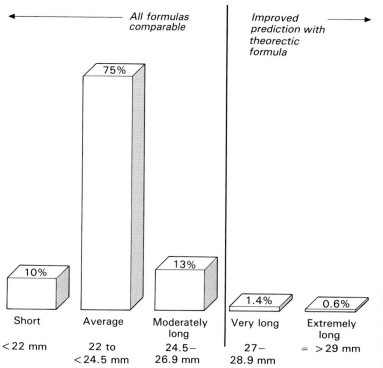

Fig. 6.1 Distribution of axial lengths in a sample of over 8000 intraocular lens surgeries performed at the Gimbel Eye Center, Calgary, Alberta Canada.

length from a mean value of 23.5 mm. The accuracy of this modified formula for extreme cases was tested by the authors in only four infant eyes, four short adult eyes, and six long adult eyes.

Both the TMB and Donzis–Kastl formulas have been evaluated more extensively in other data sets [30] and do not seem to maintain performance improvement when applied to other data.

ACCURACY OF THE CURRENT SECOND GENERATION FORMULAS

With the development of the second generation formulas, it appears that most of the researchers in this field are heading toward consensus in regard to predicted IOL power in a specific case. The predicted IOL powers are quite similar [28,30], even though the form of the formulas used are not. Also, even though in individual cases there may be differences in power prediction, over a series of cases the accuracy of the major formulas are similar.

We have evaluated the prediction accuracy of the major second generation formulas according to the distribution of axial lengths in a large series of cases ($n > 2000$) from various sources in the USA and from Dr Howard Gimbel in Canada (Fig. 6.1). Eyes with average axial lengths (between 22 and 24.5 mm) comprise 75% of these cases. It is generally accepted that both theoretic and regression derived formulas perform equivalently well for these eyes. One can expect that in 77–83% of these average cases, errors in emmetropia power predictions, no matter which formula is used, will be less than 1 D, and that errors of 2 D or more will occur in no more than 3–4% of cases (Fig. 6.2). Prediction accuracy for shorter eyes (axial length < 22 mm), which make up about 10% of the population, has been improved with the second generation formulas such that we can expect prediction errors of less than 1 D in 68–76% of cases (Fig. 6.3). This current level of accuracy approaches that for average eyes. Accuracy in eyes with longer axial lengths is summarized in Fig. 6.4. In the case of moderately long eyes (with axial length of 24.5–26.9 mm), making up 13% of the population,

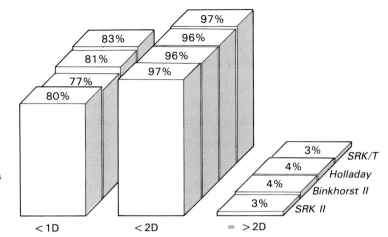

Fig. 6.2 Distributions of errors in prediction power using various formulas in a sample of cases (*n* = 1596) with average axial lengths. (US Series.)

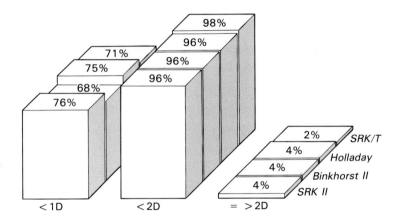

Fig. 6.3 Distributions of errors in prediction power using various formulas in a sample of cases (*n* = 201) with short axial lengths. (Combined US and Canadian Series.)

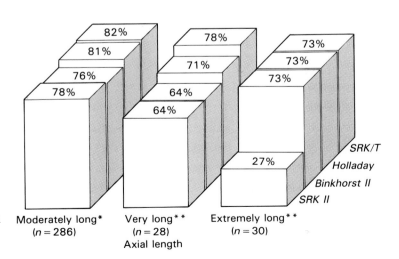

Fig. 6.4 Percentage of cases achieving prediction errors of less than 1 D using various formulas in a sample of cases with long axial lengths (* Combined US and Canadian Series; ** Canadian (Gimbel) Series.)

76–82% of cases have less than 1 D of prediction error. In general it is only when axial length reaches at least 27 mm (2% of the population) that important formula differences in prediction accuracy occur. For very long eyes accuracy drops slightly (to 64% of cases with <1 D error) for the Binkhorst II and SRK II formulas, but remains comparable to accuracy in average length eyes for the other second generation formulas. Prediction accuracy becomes unacceptable for the empiric SRK II formula when axial length is at least 29 mm (about 0.6% of the population) while accuracy remains fairly high (73% of cases with <1 D prediction error) for the second generation theoretic formulas.

Choosing a power calculation method

While regression-derived lens implant power formulas have an excellent record of accuracy [18–23], it is argued that theoretic formulas, because they are based on physiologic optics, may be more accurate than regression formulas when extended past the domain of a given database, as in unusually long or short eyes. However, theoretic formulas are complex and therefore difficult to use.

Along with proven accuracy, regression formulas are simpler to derive and manipulate than theoretic formulas. In addition, residual error, due to surgeon techniques, IOL design, etc., is combined into a single constant. In the case of the SRK and SRK II formulas, there are existing A-constants which were empirically derived and individualized by manufacturers and surgeons throughout the 1980s.

With the introduction of the second generation formulas, both theoretic and empiric, it appears that similar levels of prediction accuracy have been attained, even for shorter and moderately longer eyes. In cases with very long axial lengths (≥27 mm), it is advisable to use a second generation theoretic formula for maximum accuracy. For 98% of cases, however, the relative value of a given formula may be its relative cost and ease of use. Does use of the formula require the purchase of new computer hardware? Is the most current version of the formula in-built into your A-scan unit? How easy is it to "individualize" or "personalize" the formula constant(s) to your own practice?

Factors affecting the accuracy of power predictions

A number of factors affect the level of accuracy attained with any of the power calculation formulas.

Axial length measurement

The axial length of the eye, the distance from the corneal vertex to the vitreoretinal interface along the visual axis, must be measured precisely for accurate implant power calculation.

There are two basic methods of ultrasonic axial length determination: (a) the immersion, or water bath, technique; and (b) the applanation technique. With the immersion method, a small plastic eye cup is placed on the eye of a supine patient and filled with fluid. The ultrasound probe is placed in the solution but never comes into contact with the eye. With the applanation method, the patient is seated and an applanating cone is brought into contact with the anesthetized cornea.

Shammas has shown that measurements in the same patients with immersion and applanation A-scan correlate very well [33]; however, he and some others in the field feel that the immersion method may be more accurate, especially in patients with shorter eyes.

In current applanation ultrasound biometers, the ultrasound signals have been digitized, and cathode-ray tubes rather than oscilloscopes are used as a display. Algorithms have been developed to recognize the proper A-scan pattern and automatically record the axial lengths measured, rather than relying on the technician's pattern recognition ability. Water-tipped probes have often been superseded by solid-tipped probes. Power calculation software has been built into the ultrasound machines. While these changes have lowered the price and increased convenience of use, accuracy has not been improved. In the hands of experienced technicians, the earlier instruments may even be more accurate. Features to evaluate when choosing a biometer include ease of use, real-time pattern display, in-built power calculations, automatic mode, size, and, of course, price.

The ophthalmologist or a well-trained technician should carefully perform measurements using good quality, well-maintained equipment. To avoid errors which could lead to disastrous postoperative results, it is vital to perform preoperative measurements on *both* eyes. The importance of this cannot be emphasized too much.

Technicians performing axial length measurements should be taught the importance of obtaining accurate measurements. In addition to measuring *both eyes*, the following measurements guidelines are advised. Remeasure axial length if:

1 the difference between the two eyes is more than 0.5 mm;

2 the axial length measurement seems wrong when compared with refraction; and

3 dealing with a problem patient: if there is poor cooperation or fixation it is best to have another technician remeasure the A-scan without prior knowledge of the previous A-scan results.

Keratometry

The use of a manual keratometer requires some technical experience. A potential source of serious error in manual keratometry is failure by the technician to calibrate the eyepiece to his or her eye. Readings may be in error by as much as 1 D due to this failure to calibrate. Such a 1 D error translates to a 0.9 D error in calculated implant emmetropia power. Autokeratometers are not subject to this error, so, in this respect, are "technician-proof." Autokeratometers are also rapid and produce hard copy. Their accuracy has been documented and these keratometers are valuable in high volume practices.

Another possible source of error when using manual keratometers is the index of refraction figure used to convert the radius of curvature scale to diopters of power.

In general, we recommend remeasuring keratometry if (a) the corneas are extremely flat or steep; (b) the difference in average keratometry between the two eyes is greater than 1 D; (c) the difference in corneal cylinder between right and left eye is more than 1 D; or (d) the corneal cylinder does not correlate well with the refractive cylinder.

Surgical technique

Changes in surgical technique should be accompanied by a reevaluation of individualized power calculation constants, such as the SRK II A-constants and Holladay surgeon factors, and optimized ACD values.

PLACEMENT OF THE IOL

Posterior chamber IOLs may be implanted in the ciliary sulcus or the capsular bag. Sometimes, one loop is in each location. Placement of implants into the capsular bag places the implant further back in the eye, decreasing the effective power of the lens. There is usually a 0.5–1.5 D loss of effectivity by placing the implant in the capsular bag as opposed to the ciliary sulcus. A higher power lens should be used when the implant is placed in the capsular bag. This should be borne in mind if the surgeon switches to capsulorhexis which in most cases would guarantee in-the-bag placement.

ORIENTATION OF THE IMPLANT OPTIC

Plano–convex optic

Some surgeons implant plano–convex posterior chamber lenses with the plano surface forward. Such "flipping" of the implant *decreases the effective power of the lens* by about 0.75 D, even if the position of the lens is unchanged. An additional 0.5 D loss of effectivity occurs because the principal plane of the lens is usually displaced further back into the eye. Thus, a total loss of effectivity of 1.25 D is expected by turning the lens around. In practice, if an implant power formula predicts an 18 D lens power for emmetropia using a plano–convex lens with the convex side forward, then a 19.25 D implant power will be required if the same lens is implanted plano side forward.

Meniscus optic

Flipping a meniscus optic implant might produce marked mechanical difficulties and is not recommended. However, if such an optic were flipped, the principal plane of the lens would be displaced posteriorly and the effective power decreased as with convex–plano optics.

Biconvex optic

Flipping a non-angulated biconvex optic superficially would seem to have no effect on the effective power of the implant. This is probably true if the anterior and posterior biconvex curves are equal (1:1), as they sometimes are. However, some manufacturers use the ratio of 1:3, mimicking the natural crystalline lens, and flipping these lenses would change their effective power. In general biconvex designs have lower effective powers than other optic designs thus usually more power is needed. This translates into larger SRK A-constants and ACD values.

POSTOPERATIVE CHANGE IN
CORNEAL CURVATURE

Modern microsurgical techniques have a tendency to steepen the cornea postoperatively. This is especially true in corneas where the horizontal meridian is steeper preoperatively than the vertical one ("against-the-rule" astigmatism). Suturing of a cataract incision has a tendency to steepen the vertical meridian; with preoperative "against-the-rule" astigmatism, the cornea will become more spherical and the average "k" will be steeper after surgery. With small incision surgery and horizontal suture closure corneal curvature is changed minimally

Manufacturer variation in implant power labeling

Although Olson and Water [34] found no evidence of implant power mislabeling *per se*,

there was ample evidence for industry-wide variation in methods of calculating implant power. They found variations, due to different methods of calculating among companies studies, to be *as much as 0.95 D*. We have found differences, in certain cases, to be substantially higher than 1 D. To add to these difficulties, seemingly minor variations in manufacturing technique and lens design may change implant power required for emmetropia.

Final selection of implant power

After the measurements are obtained and the chosen implant power formula is applied, the surgeon, armed with the calculated emmetropizing and ametropizing values for the patient, must make the final decision of what strength implant to actually place in the patient's eye. The decision should be made in a quiet environment so distraction does not cause failure to actually select the intended IOL power due to things such as looking at the wrong line on the power calculation sheet, writing down the wrong number, or using the wrong A-constant or ACD. Adequate lead time of at least 24–36 h is needed so that measurements may be repeated when indicated, and implants of unusually high or low strength can be ordered and received prior to surgery. The entire patient chart should be available for a quick overview in which data from *both* eyes are checked for consistency and reasonableness.

The following factors should be considered when making the choice of an implant:
1 fellow eye refraction and cataract, if any;
2 emmetropia, isometropia, iseikonia;
3 one diopter myopia, monovision;
4 patient's lifestyle: active patients are usually best served by near emmetropia; sedentary patients may prefer myopia; and
5 hedging: even under ideal circumstances, the actual postoperative refraction will be more than 1 D different from the calculated postoperative refraction over 10% of the time. The surgeon should consider the effects of this sort of variation in either direction.

Points 3 and 4 may become moot with the advent of quality bifocal and multifocal IOLs.

Each of our patients deserves an unhurried,

thoughtful decision regarding what implant they will have for the rest of their life.

Making the proper implant power decision does not guarantee that the correct implant will end up in the patient's eye—mix-ups, unavailability of the required power or style of IOL, and confusion regarding alternate implant power can all ruin a properly made decision. Effective implementation of the implant power decision includes posting the power and style of the IOL selected beside the patient's name on the operating room wall, not using too many different style IOLs, and developing clear instructions for the staff for selecting an alternate anterior chamber IOL during a capsule rupture or vitreous loss situation.

Analyzing and correcting power calculation surprises

Large, unexpected postoperative refractive errors require forthright, vigorous action. If an error is identified, such as discovering an 18 D rather than the planned 24 D IOL was implanted, a lens exchange must be considered. First, a contact lens and/or spectacle correction with or without a slab off should be tried. The health of the eye, especially corneal endothelium, should be considered.

The situation is even more difficult when no error can be identified; remeasurement of axial length and corneal curvature confirm the original measurements and all investigation indicate the correct, and desired power lens implant in fact was used during the surgery. A mislabeled lens implant or a subtle posterior pole staphyloma with aberrant foveal location are possibilities. B-scan might be helpful. Determination of the power of the lens implant *in situ* should be considered.

If lens exchange is planned, the calculated functional axial length and the resultant new emmetropia IOL power should be calculated.

References

1 Ridley H. Intraocular acrylic lenses: A recent development in the surgery of cataract. *Br J Ophthalmol* 1952; **36**: 113.

2 Fyodorov SN, Kolonko AI. Estimation of optical power of the intraocular lens. *Vestnik Oftalmol* 1967; **4**: 27.

3 Olson RJ. Intraocular lens power calculations: an extra edge or expensive waste? *Arch Ophthalmol* 1987; **105**: 1035–6.

4 Singh K, Sommer A. Intraocular lens power calculation: a practical evaluation in normal subjects at the Wilmer Institution. *Arch Ophthalmol* 1987; **105**: 1046–50.

5 Stark WJ, Sommer A, Smith RE. Editorial. Changing trends in intraocular lens implantation. *Arch Ophthalmol* 1989; **107**: 1442–4.

6 Colenbrander MC. Calculation of the power of an iris-clip lens for distance vision. *Br J Ophthalmol* 1973; **57**: 735–40.

7 Thijssen JM. The emmetropic and iseikonic implant lens: computer calculation of the refractive power and its accuracy. *Ophthalmologica* 1975; **171**: 467–86.

8 Van Der Heijde GL. The optical correction of unilateral aphakia. *Trans Am Acad Ophthal Otolaryngol* 1976; **81**: 80–8.

9 Binkhorst RD. The optical design of intraocular lens implants. *Ophthal Surg* 1975; **6**: 17–31.

10 Binkhorst RD. Pitfalls in the determination of intraocular lens power without ultrasound. *Ophthal Surg* 1976; **76**: 69–82.

11 Binkhorst RD, Loones LH. Intraocular lens power. *Trans Am Acad Ophthal Otolaryngol* 1976; **81**: 70–79.

12 Binkhorst RD. *Intraocular Lens Power Calculation Manual: A Guide To The Author's TI58/59 IOL Power Module*, 2nd edn. New York: Binkhorst, 1981.

13 Binkhorst RD. Biometric A-scan ultrasonography and intraocular lens power calculation. In: *Current Concepts in Cataract Surgery. Proceedings of the Fifth Biennial Cataract Surgical Congress*. St Louis: CV Mosby, 1987: 175–82.

14 Hoffer KJ. Mathematics and computers in intraocular lens calculation. *AIOISJ* 1975; **1**: 14.

15 Hoffer KJ. Biometry of 7500 cataractous eyes. *Am J Ophthalmol* 1980; **90**: 360–8.

16 Hoffer KJ. Accuracy of ultrasound intraocular lens calculation. *Arch Ophthalmol* 1981; **99**: 1819–23.

17 Hoffer KJ. Preoperative cataract evaluation: intraocular lens power calculation. *Int Ophthal Clin* 1982; **22**: 37–75.

18 Gills JP. Minimizing postoperation refractive error. *Contact Intraocul Lens Med J* 1980; **6**: 56–9.

19 Retzlaff J. A new intraocular lens calculation formula. *AIOISJ* 1980; **6**: 148–52.

20 Retzlaff J. Posterior chamber implant power calculations: regression formulas. *AIOISJ* 1980; **6**: 268–70.

21 Sanders DR, Kraff MC. Improvement of intraocular lens power calculation using empirical data. *AIOISJ* 1980; **6**: 263–7.

22 Sanders DR, Retzlaff J, Kraff MC. Comparison of empirically derived and theoretical aphakic refraction formulas. *Arch Ophthalmol* 1983; **101**: 965–7.

23 Sanders DR, Retzlaff J, Kraff MC *et al*. Comparison of the accuracy of the Binkhorst, Colenbrander and SRK implant power prediction formulas. *AIOISJ* 1981; **7**: 337–40.

24 Binkhorst RD. *Intraocular Lens Power Calculation Manual: A Guide To The Author's TICC-40 Programs*, 3rd edn. New York: Binkhorst, 1984.

25 Shammas HJF. The fudged formula for intraocular lens power calculations. *AIOISJ* 1982; **8**: 350–2.

26 Olsen T. Prediction of intraocular lens position after cataract extraction. *J Cataract Refract Surg* 1986; **12**: 376–9.

27 Holladay JT, Praeger TC, Chandler TY, Musgrove KH. A three-part system for refining intraocular lens power calculations. *J Cataract Refract Surg* 1988; **14**: 17–24.

28 Retzlaff JA, Sanders DR, Kraff MC. Development of the SRK/T™ intraocular lens implant power calculation formula. *J Cataract Refract Surg* 1990;

16: 333–40.

29 Fyodorov SN, Kolonko AI. Estimation of optical power of the intraocular lens. *Vestnik Ofthalmol* 1967; **4**: 7.

30 Sanders DR, Retzlaff J, Kraff MC. Comparison of the SRK II formula and other second generation formulas. *J Cataract Refract Surg* 1988; **14**: 136–41.

31 Thompson JT, Maumenee AE, Baker CC. A new posterior chamber intraocular lens formula for axial myopes. *Ophthalmology* 1984; **91**: 484–8.

32 Donzis PB, Kastl PR, Gordon RA. An intraocular lens formula for short, normal and long eyes. *CLAO J* 1985; **11**: 95–8.

33 Shammas HFJ. A comparison of immersion and contact techniques for axial length measurements. *AIOIS J* 1984; **10**: 444–7.

34 Olson RJ, Water SW. The clinical use, accuracy and reliability of the VeriVu Lensometer. *Arch Ophthalmol* 1980; **98**: 2060.

7: Diagnosing Visual Loss in Cataract Patients: Is the Cataract Really the Cause?

KEVIN G. SMITH & ROBERT L. TOMSAK

Introduction

One of the most important clinical problems faced by ophthalmologists is the patient who is evaluated for visual loss and in whom cataract is thought to be the most likely cause. The question should always be asked: Is the decreased acuity fully explained by the cataract or is there another condition contributing to all or part of the visual loss?

Unfortunately, this question is sometimes avoided or forgotten resulting in an unhappy patient and a chagrined ophthalmologist postoperatively. Of course it is impossible to eliminate all visual surprises following cataract surgery, especially in cases when the lens is so dense that the fundus cannot be visualized. Likewise, there are some instances when cataract extraction is performed with full knowledge that vision will be improved, but to subnormal levels, because of pre-existing ocular pathology. Our belief is that the surgeon can give better informed consent to his or her patients if the potential for subnormal postoperative vision is recognized. Of course, if cataract is not the cause for visual loss, we would hope that appropriate diagnostic tests, consultations, or both would be obtained before cataract surgery is performed. Therefore, our goal in this chapter is to present some guidelines to help diagnose conditions which may cause decreased visual acuity other than cataracts and which mainly involve the realm of neuro-ophthalmology. We will emphasize the clinical approach and diagnostic technique and will provide occasional case examples from our practice to illustrate important points.

The history

Paradoxically, the history is the most important part of the visual loss assessment but costs the least and yields the most information. Yet its importance is too often minimized and its performance is repeatedly done with the least amount of skill and enthusiasm than any other part of the evaluation, except perhaps the refraction. Perhaps a careful history is so often neglected because repeated visualization is all that is needed for most diagnoses and because ophthalmology is such a procedure-oriented specialty.

There are many important questions, other than those that directly relate to the history of visual loss, that may suggest specific non-cataract diagnoses. Many times patients do not volunteer information that seems to them unimportant until they are specifically asked. Some of these questions include the following: Is there any history of prior ocular trauma? Has one eye always been "weaker" than the other (suggesting amblyopia)? Is the patient taking, or have they taken, systemic medications with potential optic nerve or retinal toxicity like ethambutol, amiodarone, or phenothiazines? Is the vision better with hard contact lenses than with spectacles? An affirmative answer would suggest a corneal disorder like keratoconus. Have they had problems with headache, weight loss, muscle pain or joint stiffness, thus raising the possibility of giant cell arteritis? Do they have problems with memory, reading comprehension, management of finances, or spatial orientation (such as becoming lost in familiar places), which would suggest a dementing illness like Alzheimer's disease (AD)? Is there a family history of unexplained visual loss in relatives, which indicates an hereditary disturbance like Leber's optic neuropathy?

It is well known that patients correctly remember only a small percentage of the information communicated to them by physicians, so it is very useful to obtain records from any previous examiners.

Quality of visual loss

The quality of visual loss is often very useful to know, for example is it loss of central vision, peripheral vision, or both? Is color perception troublesome, indicating macular or optic nerve disease? Is vision worse in daylight (e.g. cone dystrophy) or worse at night (e.g. retinitis pigmentosa, etc.)?

Temporal profile of visual loss

An approach to the history of the visual loss, is outlined with examples in Table 7.1. However, since most patients with visual loss from cataract present with slowly progressive visual loss affecting one or both eyes, the differential diagnosis of this particular temporal profile deserves further amplification.

OPTIC NERVE AND RETINAL DISEASE

From a neuro-ophthalmologic perspective, visual loss of gradual onset is the hallmark of a compressive lesion affecting the prechiasmal or chiasmal visual pathways [1]. Common causes include pituitary tumors, aneurysms, craniopharyngiomas, meningiomas, and gliomas.

For example, we recently examined a 64-year-old woman with progressive loss of vision in her right eye for a period of 4 months. She had gone blind 30 years previously in the left eye from metastatic endophthalmitis, but denied any other prior eye problem. Examination showed a visual acuity of counting fingers at 1 m (3 ft) with the right eye. The left eye was completely blind. Intraocular pressures were normal, and a large relative afferent pupillary defect was present in the left eye (OS).

Table 7.1 Temporal profile of visual loss, with examples

Visual loss of sudden onset
Unilateral transient visual loss
    Amaurosis fugax
    Retinal migraine
    Subacute angle closure glaucoma
    Visual loss in bright light from macular disease
    Uhthoff's symptom
    Transient visual obscurations in papilledema
Bilateral transient visual loss
    Migraine
    Posterior circulation transient ischemic attacks
Non-progressive unilateral sudden visual loss
    Anterior ischemic optic neuropathy
    Retinal arterial or vein occlusions
    Central serous choroidopathy
    Traumatic retinopathy or optic neuropathy
Non-progressive bilateral sudden visual loss
    Cortical infarction
    Pituitary apoplexy
Visual loss of sudden onset with progression
    Optic neuritis
    Sudden discovery of a chronic problem
      (e.g. tumor)

Visual loss of gradual onset
Tumor compression of anterior visual pathways
Degenerative or toxic retinal diseases
Degenerative or toxic optic nerve disease
Dysthyroid optic neuropathy
Low-tension glaucoma
Dementia (e.g. Alzheimer's disease)

Other
Functional visual loss

Confrontation visual fields, confirmed by kinetic perimetry, showed complete loss of the *temporal* and upper nasal field in the right eye (OD), involving fixation. Dilated examination showed moderate nuclear lens sclerosis OD and diffuse optic atrophy with a large optic cup, suggestive of glaucomatous optic atrophy. Diffuse chorioretinal scarring was present OS, consistent with prior endophthalmitis.

Comment. The lens changes in this patient were not commensurate with the severity of the loss of vision. Glaucoma was considered a possibility because of the appearance of the optic disc, but was discarded from the differential diagnosis because of a lack of prior history, normal intraocular pressure, and especially because the *nasal* visual field was primarily spared. Ischemic optic neuropathy was excluded because of the progressive character of the visual symptoms. Because of these considerations, a compressive lesion affecting the intracranial right optic nerve and chiasm was suspected and a computerized tomography (CT) scan was done. This confirmed a large cystic parachiasmal tumor which proved to be a craniopharyngioma at neurosurgery.

Granulomatous involvement of the optic nerve from sarcoid or tuberculosis can also cause chronic progressive visual loss. Compression of the optic nerve at the orbital apex from ocular dysthyroidism may occur with minimal periocular signs or ocular motility disturbances. Hereditary or degenerative diseases of the optic nerve or retina, for example hereditary optic neuropathies and cone/rod dystrophies, also need to be included in the differential diagnosis. For example, the familial optic atrophies are bilateral and are usually discovered in the first 2 decades of life although vision may become most troublesome later in life. Nystagmus as well as other neurologic and endocrine abnormalities may be present.

Low-tension glaucoma is often confused with a compressive optic neuropathy. Here glaucomatous disc and field changes develop in the presence of normal intraocular pressure. Low tension glaucoma is bilateral in the majority of patients and women in their sixth decade of life are most often affected. A prior history of cardiovascular shock is present in a small percentage of these patients. The condition may be static or progressive.

Toxic and nutritional amblyopias also are bilateral and usually progressive. The nutritional form of the disease is characterized by a history of dietary indiscretion, gradual painless onset of visual impairment over weeks to months, impairment of color vision, cecocentral scotomas, and development of optic atrophy late in the disease. Other conditions that lead to nutritional deficiency states such as jejunoileal bypass and ketogenic diet have also been associated with bilateral optic neuropathy.

Certain medications have definitely been proved toxic to the optic nerve in certain situations. These include ethambutol, isoniazid, chloramphenicol, amiodarone, and diiodohydroxyquin. Retinal toxins include chloroquin and phenothiazines.

Cone dysfunction syndromes [2] can be especially difficult to diagnose, as illustrated by the following case. A 68-year-old man complained: "I can't see . . . my vision's better in the dark . . . just give me a little sunlight and I've had it!" His visual function had diminished in both eyes over a period of 2 years. An ophthalmologist measured his vision at 20/50 OD and 20/70 OS, and recommended cataract extraction OS because of nuclear lens sclerosis. The surgery was performed but the patient complained: "My vision's twice as bad." A retinal consultant found distance acuities of 20/100 OD and 20/200 OS, but noted that near acuities were at the 20/40 level. The macular areas showed fine, diffuse pigment mottling of minimal degree and the patient was referred for a neuro-ophthalmologic consultation.

A key historical point was that he could see the colors of traffic lights at dawn, dusk, or in darkness, but could not discern them in daylight. As part of the examination, the patient was allowed to dark-adapt prior to testing visual acuity. Best corrected vision was found to be one letter on the 20/50 line in both eyes (OU). Near vision with dim over the shoulder illumination was J2 OU, and he missed only four color plates OD and only two OS. However, after performing a photostress test (see below) it took over 1 min for him to be able to discern the 20/400 "E" at distance. The fundus indeed showed a fine pigmentary disturbance in both macular areas with absence of the foveal reflexes. An electroretinogram confirmed the diagnosis of cone dystrophy.

Comment. This man's chief complaint was hemeralopia, or "day blindness," which is a classic symptom for cone dysfunction. The fact that the patient's vision was better after dark adaptation and the strongly positive macular photostress test made the diagnosis even more likely. Full-field electroretinography confirmed a cone dysfunction syndrome, although in certain cases, focal electroretinography is required to prove the form of this disease that is limited to the fovea [3].

VISUAL DISORDERS OF HIGHER CORTICAL
FUNCTION

Visual disturbances due to problems of higher
cortical function can be extremely elusive,
especially in the early stages of a dementing
illness like AD. These patients can have excellent visual acuities and apparently normal peripheral fields and still be visually incapacitated.
As an example, consider a 55-year-old man
who had the chief complaint: "It's my vision."
He had problems with reading comprehension and had had three rear-end automobile
accidents during the last 2 years because of
difficulties in judging depth. He could no
longer balance his checkbook and had turned
this responsibility over to his wife. Conversa-
tionally he appeared completely normal and
had a preserved sense of homor. Ophthalmologic examination, including visual field
examination, was completely normal. More
detailed neuropsychologic testing showed that
he had impaired visual searching and picture
interpretation, had marked problems with
reading comprehension, had clear-cut problems with drawing even simple geometric
figures, and had problems with calculation.
Thus, although his primary visual functions
and social skills were spared, higher cortical
functions associated with vision were pro-
foundly impaired leading to his visual disability. His neurologic disabilities fulfilled the
criteria for clinically probable AD which are: (a)
dementia with deficits in two or more areas
of cognition; (b) progressive worsening; (c)
no disturbance of consciousness; (d) onset
between the ages of 40 and 90; and (e) absence
of any other systemic or brain diseases which
could cause dementia [4].

Disorders of the visual system in AD can be
divided into those affecting *basic visual functions*
(e.g. contrast sensitivity, visual fields, visual
evoked potentials), *eye movements* (e.g. abnormal pursuit, saccades or fixation, including
abnormal visually guided movements), and
complex visual functions. Of a series of 30 patients
with AD [5], complex visual findings were as
follows:

1 disturbances of visuospatial perception: five
patients (17%) had prominent difficulties finding objects, looking at them, and reaching for
them;

2 visual localization problems: seven additional
patients (23%) had less severe difficulties
visually finding objects;

3 environmental disorientation: five patients
(17%) had problems finding their way in familiar surroundings not due to a general spatial
agnosia;

4 spatial alexia: three patients (10%) easily lost
their place while reading, not due to language
disturbances or general spatial agnosia;

5 visual agnosia: three patients (10%) had
problems recognizing common objects when
visually presented;

6 facial identification problems: one patient
had prosopagnosia; and

7 visual hallucinations: three patients (10%)
had formed hallucinations.

Other syndromes of cortical visual dysfunction, which usually occur in demented patients
or in those who have suffered strokes, include
Anton's syndrome (cortical blindness with
denial of visual disability), and Balint's syndrome (oculomotor apraxia, optic ataxia or
problems with visually guided reaching, and
simultanagnosia) [6]. Office testing to screen
for some of these disorders is discussed in the
examination section which follows.

FUNCTIONAL VISUAL DISTURBANCES

The possibility of non-organic (e.g. functional)
visual disturbances always needs to be considered when evaluating any patient with
visual loss, especially if the immediate cause is
not apparent [7]. Functional visual problems
are estimated to represent from 1 to 5% of an
average ophthalmologist's practice. The two
major categories of functional visual disturbance are conversion reaction (i.e. hysteria)
and malingering. For present purposes, malingering means a conscious pretense of ocular
disease for some personal gain and is most
often seen with compensation neurosis. In
general, malingerers exaggerate their behavior
and become hostile when confronted. Conversion reaction visual disturbances are much
more common in clinical neuro-ophthalmologic
practice. The psychodynamics of this form of

functional behavior are beyond the scope of this discussion. It must be emphasized that one of the most difficult situations to deal with is a case in which there is organic visual loss with a superimposed functional component.

Different tests are necessary for different types of functional visual disturbances. For example, if a person claims total blindness in one or both eyes important tests might include examination of the pupils, elicitation of optokinetic nystagmus, and the use of a large mirror held close to the face to induce eye movement via a pursuit reflex. If the patient claims some vision then it is often useful to test for a disparity in distance acuity versus near acuity as well as to test for the presence of stereopsis.

Visual field testing is extremely important in the evaluation of functional visual disturbances and usually have one of four abnormal patterns: (a) tubular contraction; (b) spiral; (c) star-shaped; or (d) isopter inversion, meaning that a larger, brighter stimulus results in a smaller isopter than does a smaller, dimmer stimulus.

The use of visually evoked potentials (VEP) to diagnose functional visual loss can be frustrating. If the VEP is normal, then useful information is gained. However, it is known that factitious abnormalities in the VEP are easily induced by normal subjects who fix eccentrically on the target or who converge and accommodate and thus blur their vision. Thus an abnormal VEP *is not* always diagnostic of an organic visual disturbance.

Patterns of visual field loss

For simplicity, visual field defects can be classified in one of three groups: prechiasmal, chiasmal, and retrochiasmal [8,9]. Unilateral prechiasmal lesions affect the visual field in one eye only; chiasmal lesions affect the fields of both eyes in a non-homonymous fashion (i.e. bitemporal), and retrochiasmal lesions give homonymous field defects with variable degrees of congruity depending on their location. Any defect in the field of vision is called a scotoma, originating from the Greek word meaning darkness. Loss of central vision, resulting in a central scotoma, is usually quickly

noticed and reported. Peripheral visual field defects like homonymous hemianopia may be asymptomatic, or they may be referred to the eye with the larger homonymous visual field defect. If a central scotoma is present, it is usually due to disease involving the central retina or optic nerve anywhere along its intraocular, intraorbital, intracanalicular, or intracranial course. In the case of predominantly one-sided involvement of the optic chiasm a central scotoma may be associated with a contralateral silent temporal hemianopia, also called a junctional scotoma. Therefore, it is imperative that the visual function of each eye is separately assessed in history taking as well as during the examination (see examination section below).

In general, scotomas due to macular disease are positive, meaning that they are perceived as a black or grey spot in the visual field. Patients with macular visual loss may also complain of distortion of images so that straight edges or geometric figures appear crooked or distorted. This symptom is called metamorphopsia and is almost always caused by a retinal problem; only rarely does metamorphopsia represent a disorder of higher cortical function.

Optic nerve lesions characteristically produce negative scotomas, or areas of absent vision not otherwise perceptible, often in conjunction with decreased color and light brightness appreciation. On occasion paradoxic photophobia or glare is a prominent symptom of optic nerve damage. Photopsias (light flashes) may be perceived with retinal or optic nerve disease and imply an active or irritative etiology; they may also be a result of migrainous cortical phenomena and are therefore non-localizing unless they are clearly correlated with eye movement which implicates the retina or optic nerve. Aside from ocular diseases, deficits of bilateral central visual function can also be produced by chiasmal lesions or by bilateral lesions in the macular visual cortex; the possibility of feigned or hysterical visual loss must also be kept in mind. The importance of carefully examining the visual field in cases of visual loss cannot be overemphasized.

Smith [10] has developed a set of general

Table 7.2 General rules of visual field interpretation

Lesions of the retina and optic nerve produce field defects in the ipsilateral eye only, unless the lesions are bilateral

True bitemporal hemianopia is caused only by a lesion at the optic chiasm

Retrochiasmal lesions produce homonymous visual field defects

Anterior retrochiasmal lesions produce incongruous homonymous visual field defects

Posterior retrochiasmal lesions produce congruous visual field defects

Temporal lobe lesions give slightly incongruous homonymous hemianopias involving the upper quadrant

There is no localizing value to a complete homonymous hemianopia except that the lesion is retrochiasmal and contralateral to the visual field defect

A unilateral homonymous hemianopia does not reduce visual acuity

rules of visual field interpretation (Table 7.2) and some further comments about these rules may be useful.

Rule 1. Optic nerve lesions produce prechiasmal visual field abnormalities that are often characteristic. Ischemic optic neuropathy usually leads to inferior altitudinal defects, optic neuritis usually manifests as a cecocentral scotoma, and compressive lesions often give abnormalities in the peripheral field as well as centrally. Binasal hemianopias are the result of local ocular disease the majority of the time; these diseases include ischemic optic neuropathy, glaucoma, optic nerve drusen, congenital optic nerve pits, optic nerve hypoplasia, and sector retinitis pigmentosa. Less often hydrocephalus, ectatic parasellar arteries, or basal tumors cause binasal field defects.

Rule 2. True bitemporal hemianopias are the hallmark of chiasmal disease, the common causes are discussed above. Less commonly, ischemia, radiotherapy, or demyelination can cause chiasmal syndromes. Bitemporal defects that cross the vertical midline (pseudo-

bitemporal hemianopias) are virtually always due to a congenital anomaly causing rotation or tilting of the optic discs.

Rule 3. Homonymous hemianopia is present in the same hemifield or visual quadrant of each eye. The only retrochiasmal exception to this rule is the monocular temporal crescent syndrome, in which only unpaired visual fibers residing in the contralateral anterior medial occipital lobe are affected. The most common occipital lobe lesions causing homonymous hemianopias are infarcts.

Rule 4. Incongruous hemianopias are seen in more anterior lesions, for example affecting the optic tract or temporal lobe.

Rule 5. Congruous homonymous hemianopias have patterns that are identical in each affected visual field; they are usually seen in visual field defects resulting from occipital lobe infarcts.

Rule 6. Even a complete unilateral homonymous hemianopia is not justification for decreased visual acuity since the remaining macular cortex in the opposite hemisphere is still functioning. However, if input to both macular cortices are abnormal, then central acuity often is diminished, but the acuities should be equal in both eyes. If the visual acuities are unequal, another explanation for the visual asymmetry needs to be sought.

The examination

Measurement of visual acuity

The measurement of best corrected visual acuity is extremely important in the evaluation of visual disability, especially when cataract is thought to be the primary cause. A tedious refraction may be required, often with the use of supplementary aids like the pinhole, stenopaic slit, potential acuity meter, etc. Once the best refraction is obtained, the physician needs to urge the patient to read the next smallest line possible, thus forcing them to "guess." Only when this has been done is the true best corrected visual acuity obtained.

Streak retinoscopy often brings out evidence of subtle nuclear lens sclerosis or posterior subcapsular changes.

The direct ophthalmoscope, or Hruby lens on the slit-lamp biomicroscope, are also useful for judging the visual significance of cataracts. Both these methods use relatively large portions of the pupil. Therefore, the view that the examiner has in observing the fundus correlates well with the patient's view. By contrast, the indirect ophthalmoscope requires a smaller area of the pupil and a significant lens opacity, such as a posterior subcapsular cataract, can be missed while still obtaining an adequate view of the fundus.

Smith [10] advises using a multiple pinhole disc with the center pinhole slightly enlarged to minimize diffraction. In older patients, placing the pinhole device in a trial frame minimizes problems with head movement or hand tremor. Another aid in the elderly patient is to securely place their head against the examining chair headrest so that they are more stable. Since the pinhole is unable to compensate for high refractive errors, spherical manifest refraction over the pinhole may be needed. If the patient sees significantly better with the pinhole, an optical or refractive aberration is confirmed. If vision is worse using the pinhole then a central scotoma or posterior subcapsular lens opacity is suggested, assuming the visual axis is lined up well and the patient is actually looking through one of the holes.

A disparity between the best corrected distance and near visual acuity is often indicative of a specific problem. For example, the most common cause of distance acuity being better than near acuity is uncorrected presbyopia. Other conditions in which distance vision is often better than near vision include supranuclear disorders of downgaze like Parkinson's disease and progressive supranuclear palsy. Common causes of near acuity being better than distance acuity are myopia or congenital nystagmus. In the latter disorder, convergence required for near vision dampens the nystagmus amplitude, thus resulting in more consistent foveation and better binocular near acuity than distance acuity.

When measuring near vision the reading card should be held at the specified distance of 35 cm (14 in) so as to control for image size variation on the retina. If a non-standard distance is used it should be clearly specified in the medical record.

Two types of near cards are readily available; one has numbers and other figures while the other has written text. Both are useful, but in neurologic or neuro-ophthalmic practice a near card with text measures not only *visual acuity* but also *reading ability*. A disparity between these measurements may reveal a disturbance of higher cognitive functions, specifically alexia.

Visual field testing

Evaluation of the visual fields should be considered a vital sign of neuro-ophthalmology. Numerous techniques are available ranging from confrontation testing to sophisticated threshold static perimetry. For the purposes of this discussion, simple techniques are emphasized and the more complicated methods briefly summarized.

THE HISTORY VISUAL FIELD

The first assessment that should be performed is the "history visual field." This involves asking the patient to observe the examiner's face or another part of the environment with each eye and to report if anything is missing or blurred. For example, a patient with optic neuritis and a central scotoma might look at a face and report that the eyes and nose are missing. Another patient with ischemic optic neuropathy and an inferior altitudinal visual field defect might state that everything below the nose is absent. Similarly, half the face would be missing with an homonymous hemianopia.

CONFRONTATION TESTING

Confrontation testing should then be done. Although many methods have been advocated, a simple, thorough examination can be done by finger counting in quadrants coupled with hand comparison [10,11]. The steps are as follows: (a) the patient covers one eye and fixates on the center of the examiner's face; (b) hold up fingers sequentially in each of the four quadrants of the visual field and ask the patient to count how many he or she sees; (c) if this last stage is completed normally, double simultaneous finger counting can be done, first in both upper right and left quadrants of the visual field, and then in both right and left lower quadrants; the patient is asked to total the number of fingers shown with each hand. This stage of confrontation testing often brings out evidence of extinction, hemineglect, or problems with calculation; (d) lastly, both hands are held open in the right and left upper and lower quadrants and the patient is asked to compare the quality of the images. For example, a patient with a subtle bitemporal hemianopia might be able to pass steps a–c, but, when shown hands on either side of the vertical midline, state that the hands in both temporal hemifields are not as clear as the ones held in the nasal hemifields.

A major advantage to the finger-counting method over kinetic methods of confrontation testing is that the Riddoch phenomenon is eliminated. Simply, the Riddoch phenomenon is a dissociation between the visual perception of form and movement so that the patient has the ability only to perceive moving targets in a hemianopic visual field. This phenomenon usually occurs with homonymous hemianopias that have resulted from injuries to the occipital cortex. Thus, a hemianopia may be missed if the examiner only uses a moving target such as wiggling fingers in the far periphery.

Confrontation methods using colored objects can also be useful in detecting visual field abnormalities. Confrontation testing is also useful for patients with constricted visual fields. Normally, as the distance from the examiner to the patient increases, the visual field expands, or "funnels"; with psychogenic visual field constriction the field remains the same size even at longer distances, or "tunnels" [9].

AMSLER GRID EXAMINATION

Measurement of the central 20° of visual field can be done using the Amsler grid chart. The chart is held in good light at a distance of 30 cm

from the eye with the patient wearing reading glasses, if needed. The following questions are asked: (a) Can you see the spot in the center of the square? (b) While looking at the center, can you see the entire square or are any sides or corners missing? and (c) While looking at the center, are any small squares missing or distorted? If any positive responses to these questions are given, the examiner should ask the patient to draw the abnormal areas on the chart. This can then be kept in the medical record.

Patients with a central scotoma often report the center of the grid as missing or blurred; those with hemianopic defects will say that one-half of the grid is missing; others with macular disease may report that some of the lines are wavy or distorted (metamorphopsia) and if this symptom is of recent onset, a choroidal neovascular membrane must be excluded.

OTHER METHODS OF VISUAL FIELD TESTING

Numerous other methods for examining the visual field are available but are beyond the scope of this chapter. Fortunately, excellent texts about these other methods are available [8,9] and only an overview will be given in this section.

The normal visual field has a temporal extent of 100°, a nasal extent of 60°, a superior extent of 60°, and an inferior extent of 75° from fixation. Neurologic diseases may affect any or all parts of the visual field; hence, a neurologic visual field examination is not complete unless the entire field of vision is examined. This can only be done with some type of perimeter; the tangent screen which only measures the central 30° of visual field at a distance of 1 m is not adequate in isolation but often is combined with a perimetric examination as well as the other methods discussed above. Remember that many popular programs used on computer-driven machines are limited to the central 30°.

Examination of the pupils

Examination should include measurement of pupillary size, the direct and consensual reaction to light, the accommodative reaction, and the presence or absence of an afferent pupillary defect [12]. If anisocoria is found, the presence of ptosis should be looked for, keeping in mind the possibility of Horner's syndrome or third cranial nerve paresis. This information should be recorded in an easily understood format. The abbreviation PERRLA (*p*upils *e*qual *r*ound and *r*eactive to *l*ight and *a*ccommodation) usually means that an all too cursory pupil examination was performed.

The measurement of pupil size and light reaction should be made in constant dim illumination with the patient fixating at an immobile distance target. When measuring the light reaction, or looking for the afferent pupillary defect, the brightest light available should be used. The reaction to a near object is best brought out by having the subject look at his or her own finger or thumb at a distance of 15–30 cm (6–12 in). Using this method, a near pupillary response can be observed in a completely blind person because of proprioceptive influences.

The observation of a relative afferent pupillary defect (Gunn pupil or Marcus Gunn pupil), is an invaluable indication of a conduction defect in the optic nerve. Indeed, many neuro-ophthalmologists regard this as the most important pupillary abnormality of all. It is a sign that must be checked for before the patient is dilated, preferably by the physician and not by the technician. This difference in pupillary reaction is best brought out by alternately illuminating one pupil and then the other, hence the name "swinging flashlight test." The swinging light test can also be considered as a comparison of the direct and consensual response in the same eye. Normally these pupillary responses are equal; in an eye with an optic nerve conduction defect the direct response will be less than the consensual response, hence the term "relative" afferent pupillary defect (RAPD) (Fig. 7.1). There is one important caveat: the swinging light test brings out an asymmetry of optic nerve conduction. Thus if both nerves are injured to the same extent, for example in glaucoma, an obvious afferent pupillary defect will not be observed. Furthermore, severe macular or retinal disease

can produce a Marcus Gunn pupil, but these problems are virtually always apparent on fundoscopic examination. By contrast, minimal optic nerve disease commonly yields an obvious afferent pupillary defect [13].

Light brightness comparison

Light brightness comparison can be thought of as a subjective "swinging flashlight test." The subjective appreciation of light intensity is often impaired in optic nerve disease but not with macular problems. The test is done by directing a bright light into both eyes in succession and the patient is asked to estimate the percentage difference in subjective brightness. For example, the examiner might ask a question like: If this light (normal eye illuminated) was worth $1 in terms of light brightness or intensity, what would this one be worth (abnormal eye illuminated)? The patient is then often able to semiquantitate the difference in perceived brightness.

Photostress test

Some disorders that affect the macula are very difficult to observe with the direct ophthalmoscope (see the case of cone dystrophy detailed above). Fortunately, the photostress test is an excellent method for determining if a reduction in visual acuity is due to an abnormality in central retinal function [11]. The test is performed by first measuring the best corrected visual acuity with each eye. Thereafter, the eye with faulty vision is occluded and the normal eye is subjected to a bright light for a period of 10 seconds. Immediately thereafter the patient is instructed to read the next larger line and the recovery period is timed. The same procedure is done with the fellow eye and the results are compared. The upper limit is 50 seconds of normal for visual recovery. In diseases that affect the macula, it is not unusual for the recovery period to take several minutes.

Color vision testing

Disordered color perception, especially if asymmetric between the eyes, is a good indication

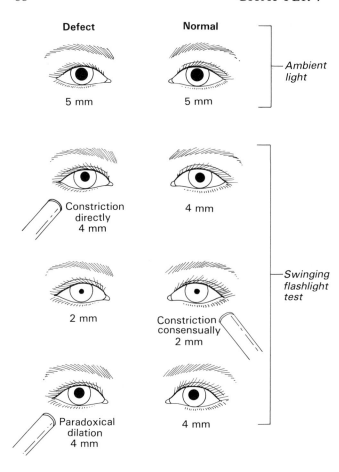

Fig. 7.1 Relative afferent pupillary defect (RAPD), right eye. Patient has right optic neuropathy. Top: pupils are of equal size in ambient light. Second row: some direct and consensual pupillary response is elicited by direct light stimulation of the *abnormal* right eye. Third row: better direct and consensual pupillary response is observed by direct light stimulation of the *normal* left eye. Bottom row: when the light stimulus is swung back to illuminate the right eye, the right pupil dilates resulting in a positive "swinging flashlight test," equivalent with a right relative afferent pupillary defect.

of optic nerve dysfunction; symmetric acquired color vision defects should raise the possibility of a retinal degeneration like cone–rod dystrophy. However, it must be remembered that congenital color vision anomalies occur in approximately 8% of men and 0.5% of women. Techniques for measuring color vision range from the simple to the sophisticated. Holding a brightly colored object in front of each of the patient's eyes individually and asking for a comparison of both brightness and color intensity is a useful office and bedside technique for the detection of central color defects. If a patient has a dense nuclear sclerotic cataract, color discrimination is helpful in predicting macular, but not foveal, dysfunction. When testing a patient monocularly if one or two quadrants are relatively color desaturated then a retinal or chorioretinal problem is suspect. Also, testing with colored objects on each side of fixation can often detect a subtle bitemporal hemianopia.

More formal estimates of color vision can be made with standard pseudoisochromatic color charts (Ishihara or Hardy–Rand–Rittler) or with sorting tests like the Farnsworth–Munsell or Sahlgren's saturation test.

Strabismus/amblyopia evaluation

Testing for subtle strabismus or amblyopia is often neglected in the adult patient. Fortunately, most patients are astute enough to realize that they have a "lazy eye," but there are patients with small angle tropias who are completely unaware of their impairment. If a small suppression scotoma is suspected, it can be verified with a 4 prism diopter test. Testing stereo acuity and watching for the "crowding" phenomenon, where visual acuity is better with isolated optotypes rather than whole lines, are useful techniques in the evaluation of amblyopia [14].

Office tests for cognitive disturbances

Numerous sophisticated neuropsychologic tests [6,15] are available to evaluate cognition as it relates to visual function, but most of these are impractical for the ophthalmologist to learn and administer. However, we have found that a few simple tasks will often highlight visual perceptual disturbances quickly and without the need for complex equipment or training.

One can simply show patients an advertisement from a magazine, point to common objects for them to identify, ask them to describe the theme of the scene, and ask them to read text. This procedure quickly screens for agnosias, disorders of visual synthesis, and alexias. Patients with visual neglect or problems with visually guided movements will often ignore entire parts of the picture or leave out important details of the scene. If the patient is a golfer, ask if they have trouble finding the ball after hitting it.

Simultanagnosia (i.e. the inability to "see the forest for the trees") can be evaluated by drawing a series of lines or dots randomly on a blank page and asking the subject to cross out all the lines or to circle all the dots.

Constructional impairments can be screened for by drawing a circle on a blank sheet of paper and asking the patient to complete the picture so that it is a clock with all the numbers and with the hands at a particular time.

Face identification problems (prosopagnosia) can be screened for by showing pictures of famous people (e.g. the President, actors, etc.)

Environmental orientation can ordinarily be assessed by asking if the person gets lost in familiar places, for example driving home from work. Or, do they have trouble finding their car in a large parking lot? Office testing can be done by drawing an outline of the map of the USA and asking the subject to locate certain states or cities like New York, Chicago, and Dallas. If a visuoperceptual abnormality is obvious, then neurologic consultation is clearly indicated before cataract surgery is performed.

Other tests

A number of other tests, such as fluorescein angiography, electroretinography, visual evoked potentials, potential acuity metering, laser interferometry, etc., may be needed in selected patients, but are beyond the scope of this discussion.

Acknowledgments

The authors thank Dr Eric Mass for his helpful comments and Ms Nancy Burgard for preparing Fig. 7.1.

References

1 Miller NR. *Walsh and Hoyt's Clinical Neuro-ophthalmology*, vol 1. 4th edn. Baltimore: Williams and Wilkins, 1985.

2 Zervas JP, Smith JL. Neuro-ophthalmic presentation of cone dysfunction syndromes in the adult. *J Clin Neuro-ophthalmol* 1987; **7**: 202–18.

3 Berson E. Electrical phenomena in the retina. In: Moses RA, Hart WM Jr, eds. *Adler's Physiology of the Eye: Clinical Application*. 8th edn. St Louis: CV Mosby, 1987: 506–67.

4 McKhann G, Drachman D, Folstein M, Katzman R, Price D, Stadlan EM. Clinical diagnosis of Alzheimer's disease: report of the NINCDS-ADRDA Work Group under the auspices of Department of Health and Human Services Task Force on Alzheimer's Disease. *Neurology* 1984; **34**: 939–44.

5 Mendez MF, Tomsak RL, Remler B. Disorders of the visual system in Alzheimer's disease. *J Clin Neuro-ophthalmol* 1989; **10**: 62–9.

6 Kirshner HS. *Behavioral Neurology: A Practical Approach*. New York: Churchill Livingstone, 1986.

7 Kramer KK, La Piana FG, Appleton B. Ocular malingering and hysteria: diagnosis and management. *Surv Ophthalmol* 1979; **24**: 89–96.

8 Anderson DA. *Perimetry With and Without Automation*. 2nd edn. St Louis: CV Mosby, 1987.

9 Ellenberger C Jr. *Perimetry: Principles, Technique and Interpretation*. New York: Raven Press, 1980.

10 Smith JL. *The Optic Nerve*. Miami, Neuro-ophthalmology Tapes, 1977.

11 Glaser JS. *Neuro-ophthalmology*. Hagerstown: Harper and Row, 1978.

12 Smith JL. *The Pupil*. Miami, Neuro-ophthalmology Tapes, 1976.

13 Thompson HS, Corbett JJ, Cox TA. How to measure the relative afferent pupillary defect. *Surv Ophthalmol* 1981; **26**: 39–42.

14 von Noorden GK. *Binocular Vision and Ocular Motility: Theory and Management of Strabismus*. 3rd edn. St Louis: CV Mosby, 1985.

15 Strub RL, Black FW. *The Mental Status Examination in Neurology*. 2nd edn. Philadelphia: FA Davis, 1985.

8: Management and Care of the Cataract Patient: Pre- and Postoperative Care from the Standpoint of the Technician and Surgical Counselor

WILLIAM A. BOROVER

Once the patient's cataract has been identified, the ophthalmologist generally explains the options to the patient and then a technician/surgical counselor orchestrates the pre- and postoperative particulars. Because the news and a decision whether or not to have surgery is traumatic, the ophthalmic staff who prepares the patient well, assists the ophthalmologist in rendering the best possible care.

This excellence in care begins with a patient's bill of rights. This bill of rights includes the following.

1 Each patient has a right to considerate and respectful care.

2 Each patient has a right to every consideration of privacy concerning his or her particular medical care regimen. Case discussion, consultation, examination, and treatment are confidential and should be conducted discretely. Those not directly involved in care must have permission of the patient to be present.

3 Each patient has the right to be provided with complete information concerning diagnoses, treatment, and prognoses. If it is not medically advisable to give such information to the patient, the information should be made available to the appropriate person on the patient's behalf.

4 Each patient has a right to refuse treatment and to refuse any participation in experimental research, if the patient so wishes.

5 Each patient has a right to participate in decisions regarding health care except when such participation is contraindicated for medical reasons.

6 Each patient has a right to continuity of care.

7 Each patient has a right to examine and receive an explanation of related fees regardless of the source of payment.

The technician/surgical counselor who embraces the patient's bill of rights adopts a philosophy of believing that it is the responsibility of the ophthalmologist to render patient care and services in accordance with these bill of rights. Additionally, the surgical counselor believes that it is essential to meet the psychologic and sociologic needs, as well as the physiologic needs of the patient and family.

When this philosophy is translated into providing the highest quality of care in a hazard-free environment within an atmosphere of patient advocacy, this bill of rights has been fulfilled.

Surgical counseling

The role of the surgical counselor is to ensure that the patient has been advised and understands the bill of rights as it applies to them and to test for comprehension. The best communication is a combination of audio and visual. Thus, the surgical counselor who first explains that a cataract is the clouding of the crystalline lens of the eye and then demonstrates that concept through utilization of a physical model and/or video, this develops the greatest chances for communication success. When an accompanying staff member stays with the patient during a video viewing, the incidence of comprehension rises.

Patients frequently feel uncomfortable with technical vocabulary or with their own perception of their ability to understand foreign material. Therefore, the surgical counselor who

Dear Patient,

As assignment is not routinely taken on elective surgeries, Medicare requires that I give you financial information before surgery when my charges are $500.00 or more. The following information concerns the surgery we have discussed. These estimates assume that you have already met the $75.00 annual deductible.

Surgery procedure: 66984 Cataract Removal with Intraocular Lens Implantation

Estimated charge	Medicare approves	Medicare pays	Supplement pays	Out of pocket
1,735.00	1,471.30	1,177.04	294.26	263.70

Preoperative tests: HIGHLIGHT THOSE WHICH PERTAIN TO THIS PATIENT

DBR (IOL power calculation) 76519

150.46	73.50	58.80	14.70	76.96

Endo cell count 92286

101.51	79.00	63.20	15.80	22.51

B-scan 76512

125.00	103.70	82.96	20.74	21.30

*Total out of pocket expense to you: _____

You will also be billed separately for the surgery center fee, anesthesia preoperative appointment, anesthesia standby during surgery, cardiogram and the reading, and the lens implant. There may be additional charges that we cannot anticipate such as laboratory work that may be indicated due to the use of certain medications, the presence of (or suspicion of) diabetes, or the abnormal results of any of the preoperative tests. A "short-term" overnight stay in the hospital is subject to a different Medicare deductible and therefore may affect your total. Charges made by any doctor other than your surgeon are not reflected on this estimate.

Medicare requires that we obtain your signature so that it is documented that this information has been given to you.

Date _____ Patient Signature _____

Fig. 8.1 Samples of financial aspects of surgery. If the patient does not have supplemental insurance, their total out-of-pocket expense would include both the supplemental payment and out-of-pocket columns for the procedures involved.

informs and reassures simultaneously gains the confidence of the patient, helps bond further with the ophthalmologist, and communicates all in one. A sample script for this is as follows:

Step 1. "Dr Borover has asked me to go over the particulars of your cataract surgery and even though you may already be aware of this information, please allow us to explain it once again. As the eye begins to age, the normally crystalline lens of the eye (demonstrate) begins to become cloudy. This clouding is called a cataract. What Dr Borover can do is surgically remove this cataract and replace it with an artificial lens implant which acts just like the original lens of your eye and focuses clear light once again."

Step 2 (testing for comprehension). "Can you see the model of the clouded lens in an eye?"

Step 3 (wait for patient comprehension affirmation). For example: "Yes, I see it."

Step 4. Continue with next phase of counseling and/or scheduling.

Added reinforcement for the patient in the form of an in-office brochure (with large print and good graphics) enhance this process even more.

Once the patient understands the clinical aspect of their surgery, there is frequently a concern regarding the financial aspects of this procedure.

Financial counseling

Whether or not the ophthalmologist participates in Medicare as a participating provider or as a non-participating provider, the patient

Cataract surgery—physicians surgery center

Our office will submit Medicare and/or private insurance for all charges for cataract surgery and preoperative tests. *Dr   accepts Medicare assignment* effective April 1, 1992, on outpatient surgery, Medicare pays 80% of the allowable fee, the 20% is approximately $302.00. There are preoperative tests required in the office and the hospital the day before surgery. Office preoperative tests will be approximately $600–$700. Medicare will pay 80% of the allowable charge and the 20% (approximately $110.00) will be the patient's responsibility. However, our office will be happy to submit the claims to your supplemental insurance. Our office and the surgery center will file these charges to your insurance companies. Although we will be submitting your insurance forms for prompt reimbursement, only you and your insurer can resolve any differences that may arise over a claim. Additional fees may be charged for other procedures required at the time of the surgery as determined by your physician.

Out of pocket expenses to you are:

1	Medicare deductible (if not already met)	$ 75.00
2	20% of cataract exc. with implant approx.	300.00
3	20% of office preop tests approx.	110.00
4	20% of anesthesiologist charges approx.	80.00
5	20% interpretation fees for EKG and blood work approximately	15.00
6	Physicians surgery center approx. 20%	198.00
	Total out of pocket expenses	$778.00

After your surgery, Dr   will be scheduling you for periodic follow-up examinations. In our office we abide by Medicare guidelines established for follow-up examinations for all of our surgery patients. Therefore, there will be no charge for any follow-up examinations within 90 days from your surgery. *Please note* that any additional testing or procedures required during that period will be charged at the normal fee.

I have read the explanation of charges for outpatient surgery and have gone over it with the office manager. I understand fully with regards to the charges stated.

_____   _____

Date   Patient signature

Fig. 8.2 Sample of financial aspects of surgery.

who is most informed regarding all financial aspects of their surgery, achieves the highest level of confidence and the lowest level of stress. It is the role of the technician/surgical counselor to cover these subjects in a consistent and efficient manner. Specifically, these subjects should include the estimated charge, the Medicare approved charge, the Medicare payment, the patient's supplemental, or secondary, insurance payment, and the patient's projected out-of-pocket expense. In addition, it should include the estimated, Medicare approved, Medicare payable, supplemental, and expense for any and all diagnostic, or preoperative, charges. Thus, the patient can understand and comprehend their total out-of-pocket expense (Figs 8.1 to 8.4).

Many times a patient has difficulty in understanding and comprehending the aspects of their surgery. Because the fear usually paralyzes the patient, the surgical counselor must make every effort to help the patient understand, both intellectually, as well as emotionally.

Role of surgical counselor

Because cataract surgery is usually an elective procedure, the patient who decides that the proposed surgery is of great benefit is the patient who psychologically does best with that surgery. In this regard, the surgical counselor needs to have an understanding of how elective surgical decisions are made.

Patients arrive at a decision to have cataract surgery when they believe that the benefit outweights the risk. The decision to have surgery or not have surgery is purely emotional,

---

Explanation of costs for Medicare patients

Dr   or Dr   has recommended that you have cataract surgery with intraocular lens implant.

We cooperate with Medicare and accept Medicare assignment. Medicare sets the fees for those who cooperate with them. Since Medicare sets the fee for any service we provide to Medicare patients, we have no choice in the matter. We must accept the fee they set and collect the 20% copayment from the patient or from the patients secondary insurance company. Also, if the patient has not met the Medicare annual deductible, we are required to collect it as well.

The only legal way any doctor can provide service without collecting the 20% copayment is if the patient has supplemental insurance which will pay it or if you state you can not afford it. We are required, then, by Medicare law to do the following:

    1 Collect your part from your secondary insurance.
    2 Collect your part from you in cash, or
    3 Have you sign a statement that you do not have secondary insurance and
       cannot afford to pay your part.

Total amount patient or secondary insurance must pay for cataract surgery with intraocular lens implant (20% copayment):

Surgery	$386.16
Lens	$72.76
Facility fee	$117.32
Total	$576.24

There could be additional diagnostic tests performed which you or your supplemental insurance will be charged for the 20% copayment. You will also have to purchase some prescription medications from your pharmacist or the Dallas Eye Surgicenter.

Please mark the box below which applies to you:

I have an insurance policy which supplements my Medicare coverage. I hereby assign those benefits to the Dallas Eye Institute. Should any payments be sent to me, I will forward them to the Dallas Eye Institute. I must meet my annual Medicare and supplemental insurance deductible as well as any remaining balance my supplemental insurance does not cover, if any.

I *do not* have supplemental insurance; however, I am able to and will pay the 20% copayment, plus and deductible that may apply.

I *do not* have supplemental insurance, and I am unable to pay the 20% copayment or deductible.

....

Signature   Printed name

....

Date   Witness

Fig. 8.3 Sample of financial aspects of surgery.

where the two emotions that exist are (a) the desire for gain (wanting to be better off); and (b) the fear of loss (risk). When the desire for gain is higher than the risk of loss, then the patient decides to go ahead and submit to surgery. The surgical counselor can use several techniques to assist the patient in decision making. The techniques are: (a) gaining attention; (b) presenting the aspects of the procedure; (c) asking questions; (d) summarizing; and (e) inviting the patient to make the decision. Because the patient is frequently distracted with thoughts and concerns of worry, the surgical counselor must have their full attention before explanation can begin. When the surgical counseling process is done in a private atmosphere, the patient is more relaxed and can pay attention easier. A cold or hot beverage may help him or her relax as the surgical counselor begins the process. One way of gaining attention is by asking questions which require the patient to talk. These

Dear Patient,

This information is provided to advise you of the financial arrangements for your surgery. The following are estimates only, your specific costs may vary:

	Estimate	Medicare pays	You pay
History and physical, including lab and EKG tests to make sure you are in good physical condition for your surgery.	$160.00	$128.00	$32.00
A-scan to determine the correct prescription for your lens implant	$75.00	$60.00	$15.00
Surgery			
Surgeon's fee: This is the fee for performing the surgery.	$1500.00	$1200.00	$300.00
After surgery			
Postoperative examinations, to monitor the progress of your vision after surgery, are included in the Surgeon's fee.	-0-	-0-	-0-
Other fees			
These are fees which you should be aware of, but which are from providers outside of our office.			
Operating room fee: This is the charge for using the operating room for your surgery	$1500.00	$1200.00	$300.00
Anesthesia fee: This is the fee for the anesthesiologist who attends to you during surgery.	$350.00	$150.00	$200.00
Lens implant: This is the cost of the lens which is implanted in your eye during surgery.	$500.00	$400.00	$100.00

*Your supplemental insurance may pay all or some of these costs, depending on your policy.

Please do not hesitate to ask if you have any questions.

Office Manager (or other employee—not from the doctor)

Fig. 8.4 Surgery fee explanation. Modify this sample to fit your practice's policies and situation.

questions are of two types; open-ended and close-ended. Open-ended questions are questions which encourage the patient to talk in sentences. For example, they begin with the words, how, when, why, what, where, and who. For example: "How long have you noticed a decrease in your vision? Did you find it coming on gradually or rather quickly?" Close-ended questions begin with a verb and require a Yes or No answer. For example: "Would you like your surgery early in the morning? Do you want your family to be present?" The technique of using open-ended questions to get the patient to relax and talk about themselves and their concerns, along with close-ended questions to make decisions and move the conversation along is an effective method of assisting patients in decision making.

When the surgical counselor summarizes, the patient is once again allowed the opportunity to hear, in summary, what has just transpired. For example: "As I understand it, then, you are interested in having your surgery early in the morning so that you can be home in the afternoon and you would like to have your family present. You should be at the surgery center early enough to have all your paperwork completed. You also have indicated to me that you understand that this elective procedure

---

Acknowledgment of non-covered services

My physician advised me that based on Medicare B guidelines the
following services may be denied as not medically necessary. Therefore,
I acknowledge and accept liability for payment of these services.

Service date	Procedure code/description	Charge
_____	_____	_____
_____	_____	_____
_____	_____	_____
_____	_____	_____

Patient signature	Patient's Medicare number	Date
_____	_____	_____

Provider signature	Physician's Provider number	Date
_____	_____	_____

Patient name		Provider name
_____		_____

Fig. 8.5 Acknowledgment of non-covered services.

does have some risk, which has been discussed with you in detail and that there is a 90% chance that things will be just fine and your vision will be improved."

The final phase in this surgical counseling technique is to invite the patient to make the decision by saying: "Can we go ahead and schedule that date for you and reserve your surgery time?"

These techniques can be used not only for the preoperative surgical counseling but also the diagnostic sessions and postoperative sessions.

Preoperative diagnostics

Once the surgical decision has been made and the patient has approved their surgical dates, the preoperative diagnostics of ultrasound and keratometry, along with any other prognostic testing of macular function, can be scheduled. These testings can be accomplished at the time of surgical scheduling or at an alternative time. The key to the most efficient surgical scheduling systems lies in a staff flexibility to be able to accomplish the presurgical testings of A-scan and any other testing, such as retinometry, specular microscopy, inferometry, etc., at a time convenient both to the practice and the

patient. It is most efficiently carried out on the same day as surgical approval is given. When such preoperative testing and associated functions are explained to the patient, the patient is encouraged and more cooperative. This is best accomplished by utilizing an actual script for the technician which emphasizes communication to the patient. For example:

Mr Borover, the doctor, has requested me to take some specific measurements so that he may choose the best course of action for your surgery and implant. As you have now learned, the artificial lens implant will take the place of the cataractous lens which will be removed. Since this lens needs to be calculated for the proper power, the doctor will be using this very sophisticated measurement instrument, using ultrasound. It is called by the nickname "A-scan." He has instructed me exactly how he wanted this to be accomplished for your eye and I would like to tell you a little bit about what you can expect.

Basically, we will first place a drop in your eye which may sting a bit but won't hurt. This test will take only a few minutes of time and when the results are printed out, the doctor will take those results and analyze them for the calculation of the precise implant lens power for your eye. I am now turning the machine on and am ready to place a drop in your eye [etc.] . . .

When patients are advised about what is happening with this being reinforced as the action is occurring, and then reinforced once again after the action, the highest level of communication and cooperation is achieved. The formula for this is to explain, explain, and explain.

"I" problems

Frequently, the ophthalmic staff tends to work somewhat independently and, in this regard, begins to develop a very close bonding with their own skills and job descriptions. Whereas there is great pride in "job ownership," it sometimes separates the patient from the ophthalmologist. When staff members speak in the first person ("I want you to do this," or "I need to take this measurement"), the staff member inadvertently drives a wedge between the patient and the ophthalmologist. In cases where patients were unhappy with the ophthalmologic care, they often spoke in terms of the doctor not being there to take measurements or to counsel them. In questionnaires circulated to patients, one of the largest responses regarding patient care was that other people took care of them and that the doctor

was only with them for a short while. This perception can be changed with the elimination of the first person and by inserting the doctor's name. For example:

Incorrect dialogue: "I need to take this measurement today and so will need to have you sign the consent form."

Correct dialogue: "Dr Borover has asked me to gather this information for him today. In order to do that, he would like you to sign the consent form. If you would then be kind enough to find a comfortable chair over there, we can begin."

Learning to consistently reinforce the doctor and continue the bonding process eliminates "I" problems.

Psychology of surgical patients

Dr Eric Berne, in his book, *Games People Play*, described the human personality as a combination of child, parent, and adult. These three personalities coexist as ego states within each surgical patient. The technician/surgical counselor who recognizes these can effect improved communication. When the technician/surgical counselor and the patient are interacting, therefore, there are six personalities at work, i.e. two children, two parents, and two adults.

The most effective communication is along straight linked lines (child to child, parent to parent, and adult to adult) (Fig. 8.6). Cross-link lines of communication, such as child to adult and parent to adult are less effective (Figs 8.7 to 8.9).

The cross-link communication of parent to child is the least effective! Parent to child communication, when initiated by the surgical counselor, is frequently interpreted by the patient as condescending and is resented.

The key to understanding the psychology of the patient during the surgical counseling and preoperative period is to always attempt communication on a straight linked basis and, above all, avoid parent to child remarks.

The greatest cause of disappointment in the surgical patient results from a combination of fear, disappointment, and frustration; fear of the unknown, disappointment from an expectation standpoint, and frustration in

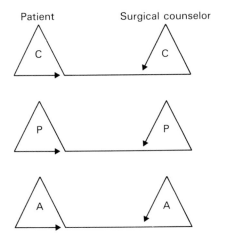

Fig. 8.6 Effective straight-linked lines of communication. C, child; P, parent; A, adult.

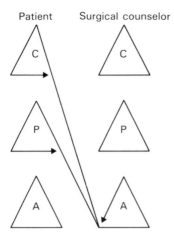

Fig. 8.7 The effective cross-linked lines of communication.

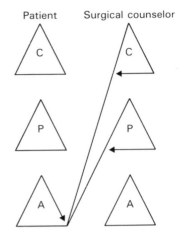

Fig. 8.8 Less effective lines of communication.

being either unable to understand or unable to communicate. It is the role of the technician/surgical counselor to neutralize these emotions and replace them with positive and secure ones. For example, ophthalmic personnel speak a language which is highly technical. It is easy to forget that the patient lacks the relevant education and exposure to these technical terms. When communicating with the patient, it is better to use replacement words, such as those listed in Table 8.1.

Quality assurance

It is the role of the technician/surgical counselor to ensure quality for all the areas of the pre- and postoperative surgical procedure. The highest level of quality assurance occurs where the surgical counselor can document a check-list of all pertinent items to be monitored. A basic guideline will allow the ophthalmologist and his or her support staff to create and monitor a quality assurance program with regard to the management and care of the cataract patient:

1 patient medical records are clearly maintained and in proper alphabetical or numerical order;

2 patient's date of birth and year of the surgery are on the medical record;

3 documentation and signatures are legible;

4 erasures or white-outs are not used and

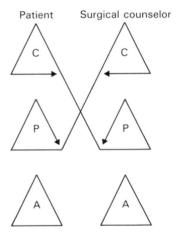

Fig. 8.9 Seldom effective lines of communication.

errors are not scribbled over. Any change or corrections are signed;

5 informed consents are signed;

6 orders are signed. Verbal orders are signed and countersigned;

7 physical examination has been completed and signed;

8 pre-anesthesia assessment has been documented and signed by a physician or CRNA;

9 results of ordered diagnostics and assessment tests are documented with the specific implant type and power clearly noted, both pre- and postoperatively;

Table 8.1 Replacement words in surgical counseling

Technical word	Replacement word
A-scan	Eye length measurement
IOL	Cataract lens replacement
ASC	Outpatient surgery department
Ks or keratometry	Front of the eye curvature measurement
Cataract	Cloudy lens
Consent form	Your permission
Pain	Discomfort

10 medication, treatment, and other procedures have been administered under orders of the ophthalmologist; and
11 the surgical chart has been completed.

In addition, the technician/surgical counselor can create a chart review to ensure quality is continuing. This should include, but is not limited to, the following question.
1 Is the chart dated?
2 Is the chief complaint documented?
3 Is the history of the patient's eye problems documented?
4 Has preoperative telephone call been made?
5 Has the patient's personal physician been notified? Is his, or her, name, address, and telephone number on the chart?
6 Have any special laboratory tests been required?

7 Is the contemplated implant type and power noted on the chart and available for surgery?

Finally, the ophthalmologist's surgical scheduling staff should monitor the compliance of the patient regarding antibiotic drops, smoking, aspirin, anticoagulants or other medications, appropriate clothing to be worn for surgery, etc.

When a good-quality assurance program is administered, along with carefully thought out systems of checks and balances, the cataract patient is given every opportunity to have his or her surgery and its surrounding protocols carried out in the safest and most efficient manner. Combining this with compassion and understanding and with a determined effort for effective communication, these are the hallmarks of excellence in ophthalmology.

9: Evaluation of Visual Function Prior to Cataract Surgery

GARY S. RUBIN & WALTER J. STARK

Preoperative evaluation of visual function once consisted solely of a visual acuity measurement. Now there are a multitude of tests ranging from simple glare and contrast sensitivity tests to sophisticated laser interferometers and electrophysiologic instruments. Some of these tests are available as commercial instruments suitable for the private ophthalmology practice, and these will be the focus of attention in this chapter. However, several important tests available only through specialized laboratories will be briefly discussed. Our purpose is not to present a thorough evaluation of the pros and cons of individual instruments or a "buyer's guide." Instead, the goal is to discuss in more general terms when and how each type of instrument might aid in the preoperative evaluation of visual function.

There are a variety of reasons for assessing visual function prior to cataract surgery. In this chapter we will concentrate on two of them:
1 to assess the level of visual disability due to cataract; and
2 to predict visual function following cataract surgery.

Assessing visual disability due to cataract

For much of this century visual disability has been defined primarily as a loss of visual acuity. Acuity tells us about the eye's ability to resolve fine detail at high contrast but may not adequately describe one's ability to see large, low contrast patterns like faces or nearby objects. In addition, acuity tests are usually conducted in a darkened examination lane with moderately bright test targets. The results may not generalize to other situations such as high ambient lighting (e.g. outdoors in bright sunlight) or dim illumination (e.g. night driving). For these and many other reasons, many people now argue that visual acuity testing should be supplemented by other tests of visual function. In the evaluation of cataracts, the two most frequently discussed alternatives are *contrast sensitivity* and *glare sensitivity* tests.

Contrast sensitivity tests

In recent years, contrast sensitivity testing has been widely promoted as an important adjunct to or even replacement for visual acuity. Whereas visual acuity tests measure how large an object must be in order for the patient to discern the critical details, contrast sensitivity measures how much a pattern must vary in luminance for it to be seen.

Contrast sensitivity was originally developed as a research tool, and for theoretic reasons most investigators use sinewave grating patterns consisting of alternating light and dark bars which have a sinusoidal luminance profile. Sinewave gratings vary in spatial frequency (bar width) and contrast. By measuring the lowest detectable contrast across a wide range of spatial frequencies, a contrast sensitivity function is derived as illustrated by the curves in Fig. 9.1.

In a normal healthy human eye, contrast sensitivity and visual acuity typically vary in the same fashion. But various types of visual dysfunction including cerebral lesions, optic neuritis, glaucoma, diabetic retinopathy, and

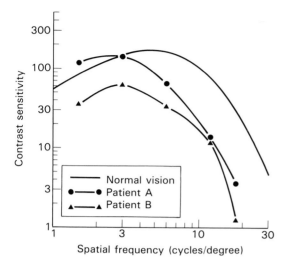

Fig. 9.1 Contrast sensitivity functions for two cataract patients.

amblyopia, may cause a reduction in contrast sensitivity despite near normal Snellen acuity. Similarly, in patients with mild to moderate cataracts, it has been shown [1,2] that visual acuity does not correlate well with contrast sensitivity, particularly at low spatial frequencies. The two cataract patients in Fig. 9.1 both have visual acuities of 20/30. Both show a loss of contrast sensitivity at high spatial frequencies (narrow bars). But Patient B also shows a loss of sensitivity at low and mid frequencies.

While it is clear that contrast sensitivity and visual acuity need not go hand in hand, what does contrast sensitivity loss tell us about a patient's visual disability? Photographic simulations of the world as seen though a cataract suggest that the loss of contrast sensitivity makes the world appear hazy or washed out [1]. Loss of contrast sensitivity at low spatial frequencies makes it difficult to recognize faces [3] and navigate safely and efficiently through unfamiliar environments [4]. Unfortunately, none of these disabilities has been tied in a precise, quantitative fashion to loss of contrast sensitivity. However, there have been several quantitative studies of reading performance in patients with impaired vision due to cataract and other forms of vision loss. One such study [5] indicates that patients with normal contrast

sensitivity can tolerate substantial reductions in the contrast of printed text with little effect on reading speed. But patients with reduced contrast sensitivity require high contrast text in order to read well, and may be severely handicapped by low contrast text such as that found with colored letters on colored papers.

Traditional methods for measuring contrast sensitivity require relatively expensive and sophisticated equipment—typically a computer-controlled video display—and employ time-consuming psychophysical procedures. More recently, several contrast sensitivity tests have been developed for clinical use. These include plate tests with photographically reproduced sinewave gratings and various low contrast optotype tests.

There is considerable controversy about whether it is necessary to measure contrast sensitivity at several spatial frequencies using sinewave gratings, or whether a single global measure of contrast sensitivity is adequate for clinical purposes. In visually impaired patients anterior segment disorders, there may be a general loss of contrast sensitivity across a wide range of spatial frequencies, or the sensitivity loss may be confined to the mid to high spatial frequencies. Both types of loss are illustrated in Fig. 9.1. It has been shown [5] that overall changes in contrast sensitivity and changes near the peak of the function are more important than subtle bumps and wiggles in the curve. Thus, global tests of contrast sensitivity provide as much useful information as tests which measure the entire function.

The Pelli–Robson Letter Sensitivity Chart is a commercially available test that provides a single, global measure of contrast sensitivity. The chart is illustrated in Fig. 9.2. Letters of constant size are arrayed in triplets of decreasing contrast. When viewed at the recommended test distance, the letters subtend 3° of visual angle, equivalent to a 20/720 Snellen letter. These large letters have been shown to provide a reliable measure of peak contrast sensitivity even for patients with visual acuities down to 20/400.

In summary, contrast sensitivity tests provide important information about visual function that might be missed by visual acuity tests

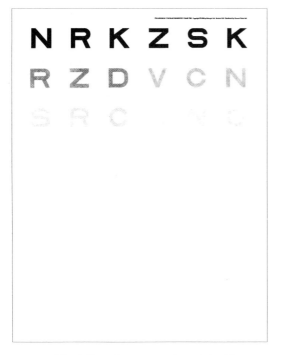

Fig. 9.2 The Pelli–Robson Letter Sensitivity Chart.

alone. For preoperative evaluation of cataracts it is important to be able to state precisely and confidently how contrast sensitivity loss translates into functional disability. Although we are not at that point yet, ongoing research is helping to clarify the relation between contrast sensitivity and functional ability.

Glare sensitivity tests

Cataract patients frequently report vision problems associated with glare. "Glare" can refer to a variety of phenomena. Most commonly these are divided into discomfort and disability glare. *Discomfort glare* refers to the photophobic sensation one experiences when the overall illumination is too bright, for example when leaving a darkened movie theater on a sunlit afternoon. Any disorder which alters the dynamics of light and dark adaptation, or reduces the light level at which the photoreceptors become saturated may cause problems due to discomfort glare. Specific tests have been developed to evaluate

adaptation and saturation, but these generally evaluate retinal and neurologic function and are outside the scope of this chapter.

Disability glare refers to the reduced visibility of a target due to the presence of a light source elsewhere in the field. Light from the glare source is scattered and creates a veiling luminance which reduces the contrast and thus the visibility of the target. This effect is illustrated in Fig. 9.3. Any disorder which increases intraocular light scatter may cause problems due to disability glare. These include keratoconus, corneal edema, cataract, and capsular opacification.

Most disability glare tests are simple in concept. A conventional visual function test, usually acuity or contrast sensitivity, is administered in the presence of a glare source. The glare source can be a spot, bar, or ring of light, or an extended bright background. A disability glare score can be obtained from the glare test alone, but it is usually preferable to compare performance with and without the glare source in order to factor out differences between patients on the basic visual function being tested (e.g. visual acuity).

Like contrast sensitivity, glare tests provide information about visual function that cannot be found in visual acuity tests alone. A study of 186 normal, cataractous, and aphakic patients [6] showed that differences in glare sensitivity between groups of patients could not be accounted for by differences in visual acuity. The dissociation between visual acuity and glare sensitivity is particularly evident in cases of posterior subcapsular cataract [2,7].

The application of glare testing to preoperative visual evaluation has been aimed at two problems: (a) predicting visual acuity outdoors in bright sunlight; and (b) measuring visual disability related to night driving. Several studies have compared commercial glare testers' ability to predict outdoor visual acuity, however there is no consistency in the results. The Miller–Nadler glare tester [6] measures contrast sensitivity for identification of a Landolt C in the presence of a bright square glare source. One study [8] found the test to be a good predictor of visual acuity facing the sun, accounting for 64% of the variance in a sample

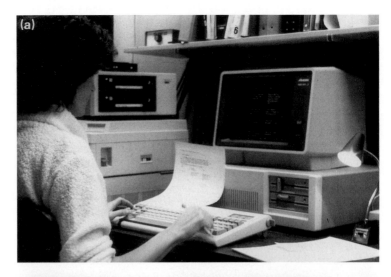

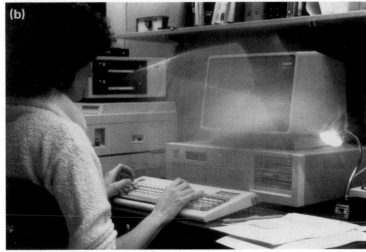

Fig. 9.3 Demonstration of disability glare. Photograph (b) was taken through a simulated cataract which scatters light from the glare source (desk lamp), reducing the visibility of the target (computer monitor).

of 84 cataractous eyes. The brightness acuity tester (BAT) [9] is a brightly illuminated hemispherical cup held in front of the eye through which a conventional eye chart is viewed. It is generally found to be a better predictor of outdoor acuity than the Miller–Nadler instrument [9,10]. However one study compared the BAT with the Miller–Nadler test [11] and reported that neither instrument was very good at predicting acuity facing the sun (each accounting for less than 25% of the variance in a sample of 47 eyes).

Many of the commercial glare testers provide a glare source that simulates the headlight of an oncoming automobile. Unfortunately, there are no quantitative data comparing how well such tests predict visual disability under night driving conditions. It is important to remember that pupil dilation under dim ambient illumination may change the amount of intraocular light scatter depending on the size and location of opacities in the lens.

Although glare tests have been in existence for over 50 years and the principles underlying disability glare are well understood, the field of *clinical* glare testing is still in its infancy. There are no standards specifying what aspect of visual function to test (visual acuity or contrast sensitivity), the configuration of the glare source, or the levels of illumination. But it is generally agreed that we need to understand better the role of disability glare in visual function before setting such standards [12]. As in the case of contrast sensitivity testing, the clinician is left in a quandary. Research and clinical wisdom confirm that visual acuity does not adequately characterize the cataract patient's functional disability. Alternative tests are available, but their role in patient evaluation remains unclear.

Predicting visual function following cataract surgery

The vast majority of cataract surgeries are "successful." Prior to surgery the patient may not even be able to see the largest letters on the acuity chart. After removal of the crystalline lens and its replacement with an intraocular lens the patient has 20/20 vision. What was once considered miraculous is now commonplace. Occasionally, there is disappointment when the physician's or patient's expectations are not met. In order to avoid these disappointments the physician searches for a method to accurately predict postoperative visual function.

Most often these predictions are limited to postoperative visual acuity. It is often assumed that if there is little predicted improvement in visual acuity, then the removal of the cataract is unwarranted or unnecessary. This assumption is mistaken. It should be clear from the first part of this chapter that there are aspects of visual function besides visual acuity which play an important role in the patient's functional ability. For patients with age-related macular degeneration (AMD), functional impairment in general orientation and mobility tasks is more closely related to contrast sensitivity than visual acuity [3]. While these patients often show less improvement in visual acuity following cataract surgery than patients without maculopathy, they still report significant improvement in their ability to perform such tasks [13]. Reading ability is more closely tied to visual acuity, but many maculopathy patients with reduced acuity can read with sufficient magnification. However, cataracts in addition to maculopathy may make it impossible to read [14]. Even if

removing the cataract has a minimal effect on visual acuity, it can still have a profound effect on the patient's ability to function independently. Unfortunately, there are no commercial tests of potential visual function other than those which try to predict postoperative visual acuity, so our discussion will be limited to potential acuity tests.

Commercially available potential acuity tests include the potential acuity meter (PAM), laser and white-light interferometers, the blue field entoptoscope (BFE), and tests based on the visual evoked potential (VEP). Comparative evaluations of these tests are complicated by differences in the criteria used to judge their predictions. The most obvious criterion is *accuracy*. How close are the predicted acuities to the actual postoperative acuities? Or, how well does the instrument predict the number of lines of improvement in acuity? Another criterion is *predictive value*. How good is the test at predicting which patients will meet a criterion for success such as 20/40 acuity or better, or at least four lines of improvement?

Criteria based on a prior definition of success or failure are quite familiar to those who study medical decision making. It is well known that the apparent value of a test will depend on the sample of patients to which it is applied. Consider the following numerical examples. Two potential acuity tests are administered to groups of 100 cataract patients. The results of the tests are represented by 2 × 2 tables in Figs 9.4 and 9.5.

The tables are divided into two rows according to the predictions of the tests. For this example, the top row is predicted success, defined as 20/40 or better acuity. The bottom row is predicted failure, worse than 20/40 acuity. The two columns categorize the postoperative results. The left column is postoperative success, again defined as a final acuity of 20/40 or better. The right column is failure, i.e. a final acuity worse than 20/40. Each cell contains a number indicating the number of patients who fall into the appropriate category, and the standard name given to that category. In Fig. 9.4, 80 of the patients who were predicted to have postoperative acuities of 20/40 or better actually did so. They are referred to as

Outcome

	Success	Failure
Prediction — Success	True positive 80 (90)	False positive 3 (10)
Prediction — Failure	False negative 10 (0)	True negative 7 (0)

Fig. 9.4 Results of a potential acuity test administered to 100 cataract patients, 90% of whom had successful surgeries.

Outcome

	Success	Failure
Prediction — Success	True positive 60 (70)	False positive 3 (30)
Prediction — Failure	False negative 10 (0)	True negative 27 (0)

Fig. 9.5 Results of a potential acuity test administered to 100 cataract patients, 70% of whom had successful surgeries.

"true positives." Three of the patients who were predicted to have 20/40 or better acuity turned out to have acuities worse that 20/40. They were "false positives." At first glance, the test looks like a good one. There were very few false positives and relatively few false negatives. The test accurately predicted the final outcome for 87% of the patients ([80 true positives + 7 true negatives] ÷ 100 patients total). Another way to evaluate the test is to compute it's "predictive value." The positive predictive value (PPV) indicates how accurate the test is in predicting success. The negative predictive value (NPV) indicates how accurate the test is in predicting failure. In our example, the PPV is 96% (80 ÷ [80 + 3]) and the NPV is 41% (7 ÷ [10 + 7]). The test is good at predicting success, but bad at predicting failure. What if we had simply ignored the test and predicted success for all 100 patients? The numbers in parentheses in Fig. 9.4 show the results. By ignoring the test we would accurately predict the final outcome for 90% of the patients. The PPV would be 90% and the NPV would be 0%.

A second example is illustrated in Fig. 9.5. The only difference is that 20 fewer patients are predicted (correctly) to be successful and all 20 are predicted (correctly) to fail. The accuracy of the test remains 87%. The PPV is 95% and the

NPV is 73%. This test is also fairly accurate, very good at predicting success, and better than the previous test at predicting failure. If we had ignored the test and predicted success for all patients we would have been accurate in only 70% of the cases; the PPV would be 70% and the NPV would be 0%.

These examples are meant to illustrate two problems in evaluating potential acuity tests. The first is that there are many ways to measure how well a test predicts patient outcome. To decide which measure is best one could assign values (positive or negative) to each of the cells in the table in Figs 9.4 and 9.5, and compute a single index of the test's "expected value." But to do this one would have to decide such things as whether it is worse to incorrectly predict success (false positive) or failure (false negative). Such analyses have not been attempted for the prediction of postoperative acuity.

The second problem is that the apparent value of a test may be strongly influenced by the patient sample to which it is applied. In the first example 90% of the patients had a successful outcome. It is very difficult in this case for any test to provide increased accuracy or predictive value. In the second example, only 70% of patients had successful outcomes. Here there is more room for improvement in both accuracy and predictive value. The first case was deliberately chosen to be representative of the general cataract practice where the vast majority of procedures are successful. The second case may be more representative of the referral practice where there is a greater risk of poor outcome due to ocular pathology.

With these qualifications in mind, we will briefly review each of the major types of potential acuity tests.

BFE

By viewing a bright empty field illuminated with blue light one sees small white dots that move along arcuate paths in a pulsating manner. The BFE phenomenon is attributed to light which passes through leukocytes between red blood cells in perifoveal retinal capillaries. Only diffuse illumination at the retina is required to see the effect, but one must have intact retinoneural function. Therefore it should be well suited to testing the integrity of the visual system behind media opacities. The BFE can only make a binary classification of patients—either they see the white dots or they don't. It does not lend itself to a quantitative evaluation of retinal function. In addition it is sometimes difficult to explain the phenomenon to the patient. These disadvantages are offset by the claim that the BFE can penetrate dense cataracts which interfere with other types of tests.

Early investigations using a commercial prototype BFE appeared promising. However subsequent studies have shown it to be of limited usefulness. Recent evaluations of the BFE [15] indicate that a positive test (seeing the white dots) is a reliable predictor of good postoperative acuity, but a negative test is not a reliable predictor of bad postoperative acuity. To put this in the terms described above, the test is prone to false negatives. In one study [16], 25 patients with dense cataracts were predicted to have poor outcomes. However 20 achieved final acuities of 20/40 or better. Thus the test does not make quantitative predictions of postoperative acuity and its qualitative assessment appears to have poor predictive value.

VEP

There are many types of VEP tests. The one most commonly used for preoperative evaluation of cataracts is the steady-state VEP. A bright uniform field is flickered on and off at a constant rate, typically around 10 times per second. The cortical potential is measured with scalp electrodes. Although commercial VEP test equipment is available, interpretation of the results usually requires a level of expertise found only in specialized laboratories. The test can make quantitative predictions of postoperative acuity, but these predictions tend to be less precise than those produced by interferometers or the PAM.

The two principal advantages of the VEP are its low rate of false negatives and ability to penetrate dense cataracts. The low false negative rate means that patients with abnormal VEPs are likely to have poor postoperative acuity. In a review of eight studies [15], 84% of the patients who were predicted to have poor outcomes fulfilled that prediction. Unlike other tests, the rate of false negatives did not increase for dense cataracts [17]. However, the VEP is more susceptible than most tests to false positives. 23% of patients with normal VEPs continue to have poor acuity following surgery.

Proponents of VEP testing advocate its use primarily in cases of dense cataract where additional ocular pathology is suspected. The discussion above indicates that a normal VEP is not a reliable predictor of good postoperative acuity. But an abnormal VEP is a reliable indicator that the pathology is severe enough to prevent good postoperative acuity. Nevertheless, an improvement from 20/400 to 20/60, while not qualifying as a good outcome by the definition used in these studies, would mean a substantial improvement in the patient's ability to perform visual tasks.

Interferometers

There are two types of clinical interferometers. Laser interferometers use a low-power helium–neon laser to form a red and black sinewave grating at the retina. White light interferometers use ordinary incandescent light and diffraction gratings to produce a black and white moiré grating at the retina. Despite their differences, laser and white-light interferometers produce similar results in clinical tests. Both types of interferometers produce grating patterns with large depths of field that are largely unaffected by optical characteristics of the eye such as refractive error and spherical aberration.

Initially, interferometers were used to investigate the retinal limits to visual resolution in normal eyes. But it quickly become apparent that the technique was a potentially powerful tool for evaluating retinal integrity in eyes with degraded optical properties due to corneal or lenticular opacities. Early reports were very optimistic. For example, Green and Cohen [18] reported that in a series of 51 patients, interferometry never overestimated postoperative visual acuity by more than two lines (false positives), and all patients who were predicted to achieve good acuities did so. However, they recognized that interferometric acuity sometimes underestimated postoperative acuity (false negatives).

It has since become clear that interferometry is susceptible to both false negatives and false positives. In some studies [15], over half of the patients who were predicted to have poor postoperative acuities contradicted the prediction. False negatives are a particular problem when preoperative acuity is worse than 20/200. Although the test is insensitive to certain types of optical aberrations, it does require that sufficient light reach the retina unscattered to form the interference grating. In dense cataracts this becomes more of a problem. Even if the examiner locates a "window" in the cataract, any light scattered by lenticular opacities will add speckle noise and reduce the grating's visibility. In some studies [18,19], over one-quarter of the patients have been unable to see any gratings, making it impossible to predict postoperative acuity.

Most of the criticism of interferometry has been directed at the false positives. Averaging across all previous studies [15], 11% of patients who had good preoperative interferometric acuity failed to achieve good postoperative Snellen acuity. A number of conditions have been identified which lead to false positive predictions. AMD presents a particular problem. Two studies [20,21] of AMD patients with *clear* media reported false positive interferometric acuities in one-third to one-half of the measurements. Amblyopia presents another problem since it is well known that grating acuities overestimate letter acuities in many of these individuals.

Unlike the blue field and VEP tests, interferometry can give a precise, quantitative prediction of postoperative acuity. How accurate are these predictions? The numbers vary widely from study to study, but in general, accuracy to within ±2 Snellen lines are found in the majority of patients [22,23].

PAM

The PAM projects an acuity chart onto the retina through a small aperture. The small aperture gives the image a large depth of field and allows the examiner to direct the beam around opacities in the lens. Early evaluations of the PAM were very optimistic [24]. Although a number of patients achieved better postoperative acuities than the test predicted, there were almost no false positives. However, it was subsequently recognized that false positives may be a problem for this test, but not to the same extent as for interferometry. On average, fewer than 5% of patients who are predicted to have good postoperative acuity fail to do so [15]. As an advantage over interferometry, the PAM does not produce false positives for patients with amblyopia [24], and false positives for AMD patients are less frequent [21]. However, false positives are reported for patients with macular edema.

False negatives with the PAM are uncommon if preoperative acuity is 20/200 or better. Interestingly, one study reported much higher rates of false negatives for posterior subcapsular cataracts than for nuclear sclerosis [25]. Accuracy of postoperative predictions are limited to about ±2 Snellen lines [26].

Summary and new directions

If one is interested in evaluating potential acuity in patients with dense cataracts, the VEP offers the distinct advantage of making few false negative predictions. Patients who have abnormal VEPs are unlikely to achieve good postoperative acuity. But a normal VEP gives little information about what to expect following cataract surgery. For patients with mild to moderate cataracts, the PAM has the edge over interferometry. Accuracy of prediction is probably no better, but the PAM is less likely to make false positive predictions. If the test indicates a potential acuity of 20/40 or better, then the outcome is quite likely to be good, unless macular edema is documented.

Several new tests have been developed to assess potential acuity which require the patient to judge the displacement of a test stimulus. It has been found that normal observers are quite sensitive to small displacements, and that displacement sensitivity is more resistant to optical degradation than standard acuity tasks. Although promising results have been reported for both a vernier alignment test [27] and an oscillatory displacement test [28], no commercial instruments are available.

Up to this point, the discussion has treated the various potential acuity tests as isolated predictors of postoperative acuity. Several investigators have begun to investigate how to combine multiple test results optimally. One study [29] demonstrated that the VEP combined with interferometry gave significantly better predictions of postoperative acuity than either test alone. Another approach is to combine potential acuity tests with clinical judgement. In one study [30], an objective clinical index was developed which incorporated the patient's age, preoperative acuity, current medications, and newspaper reading ability. The index was good at predicting success but poor at predicting failure. This is just the opposite from the PAM and interferometer. The authors make the intriguing suggestion that the prediction be done in two stages. First the patient is tested with a standard instrument. If the results are positive, the test can be trusted. But if the results are negative the test should be followed with the clinical assessment. If the results are still negative, then it is much more likely that final acuity will be poor.

However, one should be cautious about using this or any potential *acuity* test to rule out cataract surgery. Even if the outcome is an acuity worse than 20/40, the benefits in improved glare and contrast sensitivity may justify the procedure.

In everyday practice, the cataract surgeon is confronted with difficult decisions particularly when faced with patients who have good acuity despite mild cataracts or patients whose loss of vision may be due to ocular disease besides cataract. In general, cataract surgery is indicated when reduced visual function interferes with the patient's daily activities, and examination suggests that the cataract is the cause of the reduced vision. Glare and contrast sensitivity testing will become increasingly useful for documenting visual disability, especially as the tests become more standardized. However, one must avoid using these tests to pressure patients into having their cataracts removed. Potential acuity tests are valuable in determining the degree to which cataracts limit vision. Because none of these tests are foolproof, however, they should be used to complement rather than supersede a careful, conventional ophthalmic examination including tonometry, check of the pupils, confrontation field testing, and, if there is a mature cataract, B-scan ultrasonography.

References

1 Hess R, Woo G. Vision through cataracts. *Invest Ophthalmol Vis Sci* 1978; **17**: 428–35.
2 Elliott DB, Gilchrist J, Whitaker D. Contrast sensitivity and glare sensitivity changes with three types of cataract morphology: are these techniques necessary in a clinical evaluation of cataract? *Ophthal Physiol Opt* 1989; **9**: 25–30.
3 Lennerstrand G, Ahlstrom CO. Contrast sensitivity in macular degeneration and the relation to subjective visual impairment. *Acta Ophthalmol* 1989; **67**: 225–33.
4 Marron JA, Bailey IL. Visual factors and orientation–mobility performance. *Am J Optom Physiol Opt* 1982; **59**: 413–26.
5 Rubin GS, Legge GE. The psychophysics of reading. VI. The role of contrast in low vision. *Vis Res* 1989; **29**: 79–92.
6 Hirsch RP, Nadler MP, Miller D. Clinical performance of a disability glare tester. *Arch Ophthalmol* 1984; **102**: 1633–6.

7 Abrahamsson M, Sjostrand J. Impairment of contrast sensitivity function (csf) as a measure of disability glare. *Invest Ophthalmol Vis Sci* 1986; **27**: 1131–6.

8 Hirsch RP, Nadler MP, Miller D. Glare measurement as a predictor of outdoor vision among cataract patients. *Ann Ophthalmol* 1984; **16**: 965–8.

9 Holladay JT, Prager TC, Trujillo J, Ruiz RS. Brightness acuity test and outdoor visual acuity in cataract patients. *J Cataract Refract Surg* 1987; **13**: 67–9.

10 Neumann AC, McCarty GR, Locke J, Cobb B. Glare disability devices for cataractous eyes: A consumer's guide. *J Cataract Refract Surg* 1988; **14**: 212–16.

11 Prager TC, Urso RG, Holladay JT, Stewart RH. Glare testing in cataract patients: instrument evaluation and identification of sources of methodological error. *J Cataract Refract Surg* 1989; **15**: 149–57.

12 American Academy of Opthalmology. Contrast sensitivity and glare testing in the evaluation of anterior segment disease. *Opthalmol* 1991; **97**: 1233–7.

13 Berenth-Petersen P. Cataract surgery: outcome assessments and epidemiologic aspects. *Acta Ophthalmol Suppl (Copenh)* 1985; **174**: 3–47.

14 Legge GE, Rubin GS, Pelli DG, Schleske MM. Psychophysics of reading. II. Low vision. *Vis Res* 1985; **25**: 253–66.

15 Odom JV, Chao GM, Weinstein GW. Preoperative prediction of postoperative visual acuity in patients with cataracts: a quantitative review. *Doc Ophthal* 1988; **70**: 5–17.

16 Skalka HW. Blue field entoscopy and VEP in preoperative cataract evaluation. *Ophthal Surg* 1981; **12**: 642–5.

17 Odom JV, Chao GM, Hobson R, Weinstein GW. Prediction of post cataract extraction visual acuity: 10 Hz visually evoked potentials. *Ophthal Surg* 1988; **19**: 212–18.

18 Green DG, Cohen MM. Laser interferometry in the evaluation of potential macular function in the presence of opacities in the ocular media. *Am Acad Ophthalmol Otol* 1971; **75**: 629–37.

19 Bernth-Peterson P, Naeser K. Clinical evaluation of the Lotmar Visometer for macula testing in cataract patients. *Acta Ophthalmol* 1982; **60**: 525–32.

20 Bloom TD, Fishman GA, Traubert BS. Laser interferometric visual acuity in senile macular degeneration. *Arch Ophthalmol* 1983; **101**: 925–6.

21 Fish GE, Birch DG, Fuller DG, Straach R. A comparison of visual function tests in eyes with maculopathy. *Ophthalmology* 1986; **93**: 1177–82.

22 Spurny RC, Zaldivar R, Belcher CD, Simmons RJ. Instruments for predicting visual acuity. *Arch Ophthalmol* 1986; **104**: 196–200.

23 Miller ST, Graney MJ, Elam JT, Applegate WB, Freeman JM. Predictions of outcomes from cataract surgery in elderly persons. *Ophthalmology* 1988; **95**: 1125–9.

24 Minkowski JS, Palese M, Guyton DL. Potential acuity meter using a minute aerial pinhole aperture. *Ophthalmology* 1983; **90**: 1360–8.

25 Carpel EF, Henderson V. The influence of cataract types on potential acuity meter results. *J Cataract Refract Surg* 1986; **12**: 276–7.

26 Severin TD, Severin SL. A clinical evaluation of the potential acuity meter in 210 cases. *Ann Ophthalmol* 1988; **20**: 373–5.

27 Enoch JM, Williams RA, Essock EA, Barricks M. Hyperacuity perimetry: assessment of macular function through ocular opacities. *Arch Ophthalmol* 1984; **102**: 1164–8.

28 Whitaker D, Elliott D. Towards establishing a critical displacement threshold technique to evaluate visual function behind cataract. *Clin Vis Sci* 1989; **4**: 61–9.

29 Davis ET, Sherman J, Bass S. Presurgical prediction of postsurgical visual function in cataract patients. Digest of topical meeting on noninvasive assessment of the visual system, Washington, DC. *Optical Society of America* 1990; **3**: 147–50.

30 Graney MJ, Applegate WB, Miller ST *et al*. A clinical index for predicting visual acuity after cataract surgery. *Ophthalmology* 1988; **105**: 460–5.

10: The 20/100 Surprise: Poor Vision after Cataract Surgery

JAMES A. KIMBLE & JAMES B. BYRNE JR

CASE HISTORY

A 71-year-old woman had cataract surgery on her left eye. Her 20/400 vision did not improve. She was not given an explanation of why the acuity was poor. After 3 months, she was referred to us for evaluation.

Visual acuity in the left eye was 20/400. There was a clear cornea, well-centered posterior chamber implant, and a clear posterior capsule. The refractive error was minimal. The macula had a small disciform scar arising from age-related macular degeneration.

The patient was surprisingly relieved when we informed her of this untreatable diagnosis. She said, "At least now I know what it is. Why did my ophthalmologist have to wait 3 months to let me find out the cause of the trouble?"

When a patient sees poorly after technically successful cataract surgery, it is a disappointment for the surgeon and a major calamity for the patient. This chapter is intended to help the ophthalmologist diagnose the cause of this situation, which we call the "20/100 surprise." The unhappy patient's acuity can range from 20/25 to light perception; 20/100 is our estimate of the "average."

Uncovering the diagnosis is important so that proper treatment can begin as soon as possible, while maintaining a good surgeon–patient relationship. A treatable cause of poor vision after surgery, overlooked or ignored, can become a source of permanent eye damage and ill will between surgeon and patient.

Unfortunately, many of the conditions causing a 20/100 surprise are untreatable. Even here, the operating surgeon will maintain the patient's confidence if he or she diagnoses the condition promptly with as few tests and delays as possible, and discusses the problem fully with the patient and family.

Optical conditions

Optical problems which can reduce vision after cataract surgery include irregular astigmatism, corneal edema, a severely decentered implant, posterior capsular opacity, and vitreous hemorrhage. Most of these conditions can be seen with a slit-lamp, but the amount by which they reduce vision may be difficult to estimate.

Irregular astigmatism is not visible with the slit-lamp unless an obviously tight suture is detected. Keratoscopy is very sensitive but cumbersome to perform on every patient. The retinoscope is an ideal instrument for detecting this optical problem. Irregular astigmatism will produce a "scissors" reflex which is not ameliorated by neutralizing lenses. An approximate retinoscopic refraction can be performed rapidly by the physician, and the quality of the retinoscopic reflex is an excellent indicator of the quality of the eye's optical system.

The retinoscope is also useful for judging to what extent corneal edema, a decentered lens, or a cloudy posterior capsule are interfering with the patient's vision. Practice in using the retinoscope for this purpose, in addition to refracting, will allow the ophthalmologist to develop the necessary experience to judge the significance of optical irregularities. For example, diffuse opacities such as corneal edema or vitreous hemorrhage make the retinoscopic reflex dim. A cloudy posterior capsule makes the reflex irregular, with dark

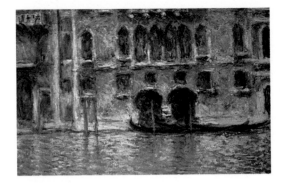

Plate 2.1 Monet. *Palazzo de Mula, Venice*. Oil on canvas, 1908. National Gallery of Art, Washington DC.

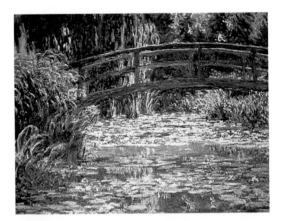

Plate 2.2 Monet. *The Japanese Footbridge at Giverny*. Oil on canvas, 1900. Art Institute of Chicago.

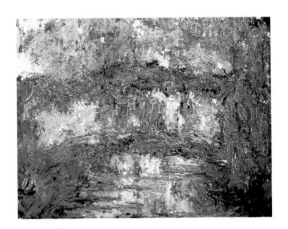

Plate 2.3 Monet. *The Japanese Footbridge at Giverny*. Oil on canvas, 1923. Marmottan Museum, Paris.

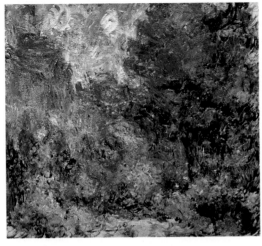

Plate 2.4 Monet. *The House from the Garden*. Oil on canvas, not dated. Marmottan Museum, Paris.

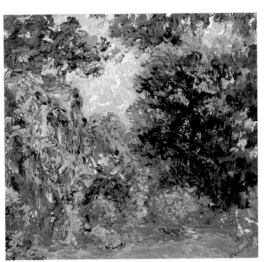

Plate 2.5 Monet. *The House from the Garden*. Oil on canvas, 1922. Marmottan Museum, Paris.

[facing page 110]

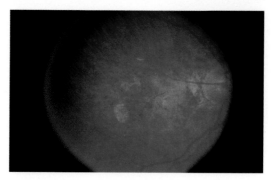

Plate 10.1 Geographic atrophic age-related macular degeneration, photographed through a moderate cataract prior to surgery. There are three discrete areas of retinal pigment epithelial atrophy. An easily seen oval of atrophy is temporal and a little inferior from the center of the macula. Two other areas are more difficult to see, superior-temporal and superior-nasal from the center. The areas of atrophy are easily seen on the corresponding angiogram, Fig. 10.1.

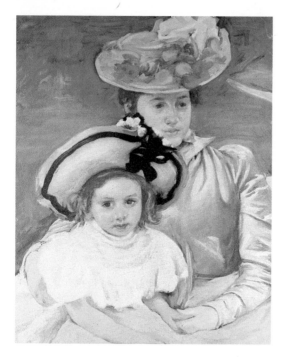

Plate 2.6 Cassatt. *Young Mother and Daughter.* Pastel on paper, 1901. Memorial Art Gallery of the University of Rochester, New York.

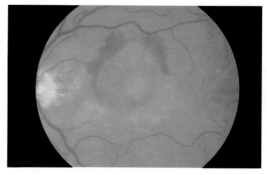

Plate 10.2 Exudative age-related macular degeneration. Subretinal choroidal neovascularization is producing serous detachment of the retinal pigment epithelium surrounded by subretinal hemorrhage. The neovascularization is demonstrated in Fig. 10.2.

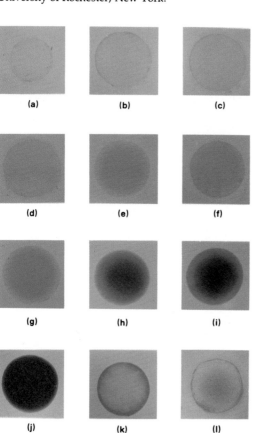

(a) (b) (c)

(d) (e) (f)

(g) (h) (i)

(j) (k) (l)

Plate 3.1 (*Left*) The increasing yellow–brown color of the normal lens as it ages: from 6 months (a) through 8 years (b), 12 years (c), 25 years (d), 47 years (e), 60 years (f), 70 years (g), 82 years (h), 91 years (i), 70-year-old brown nuclear cataract (j), 68-year-old cortical cataract (k), and 74-year-old mixed nuclear and cortical cataract (l).

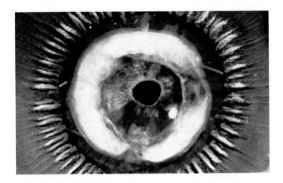

Plate 12.1 Gross photograph from behind an autopsy eye showing placement of a modified J-loop Sinskey-style intraocular lens with both loops in the ciliary sulcus. Centration is excellent. A complete Soemmering's ring is present, but the central vision axis remains clear.

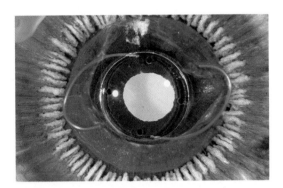

Plate 12.2 Gross photograph from behind an autopsy eye showing a perfectly centered modified J-loop posterior chamber lens implanted in the lens capsular bag. An iridectomy is present at 12 o'clock. Note the C-shaped bend of the loops. Cortical clean-up was extremely thorough, and the lens capsular bag shows only a faint gray Soemmering's ring.

Plate 12.5 (*Right*) Gross photograph from behind of an autopsy eye containing a Simcoe C-loop style posterior chamber intraocular lens. The optic is well centered and, because of extremely thorough cortical clean-up, almost no residual lens substance is present.

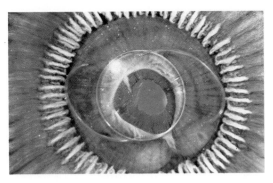

Plate 12.3 Gross photograph from behind an autopsy eye showing a Sinskey-style modified J-loop posterior chamber intraocular lens implanted within the lens capsular bag. The optic is well centred, the visual axis is clear, and there is only minimal regeneration of cortex in scattered areas. There is moderate haziness or opacity at the margins of the anterior capsulectomy, but this does not encroach upon the visual axis.

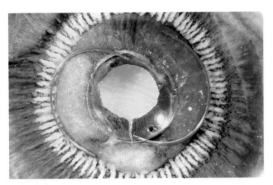

Plate 12.4 Gross photograph from behind an autopsy eye showing in-the-bag placement of a Simcoe C-loop style posterior chamber intraocular lens. The optic is well centered and the loops conform to the circumference of the lens capsular bag. There is moderate retention of cortical material throughout several clock hours in the periphery, but the central visual axis remains clear.

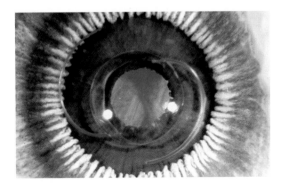

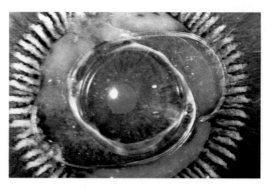

Plate 12.6 Gross photograph from behind an autopsy eye showing a one-piece all-PMMA style posterior chamber intraocular lens (Arnott–Jaffe style), with both loops implanted in the capsular bag. The modified C-style loops show moderate compression in order to conform to the diameter and shape of the capsular bag. The central visual axis shows a few scattered opacities, but is otherwise unremarkable. The optic is well centered and is surrounded by a ring of cortical material representing retained and regenerate cortex—this residual cortex being peripheral to the visual axis.

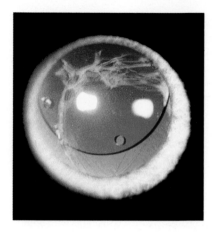

Plate 12.8 Clinical photograph of the sunrise syndrome (upward deviation). The inferior loop was implanted in the capsular bag and the superior loop in the ciliary sulcus. The unequal pressures exerted on the loops caused an upward decentration of the lens optic. Note that a large portion of the optic edge and a positioning hole are visible within the pupil. (Courtesy of Douglas D Koch MD, Houston, Texas.)

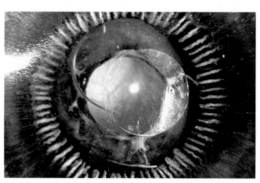

Plate 12.7 Gross photograph from behind an autopsy eye showing a C-loop posterior chamber intraocular lens implanted asymmetrically with one loop in the ciliary sulcus (upper left) and the opposite loop (with the Lester notch) in the capsular bag. Notice the extensive upward decentration of the lens optic so that the optic edge and a positioning hole are within the pupillary aperture. Such decentration is very common with such symmetrically implanted intraocular lenses.

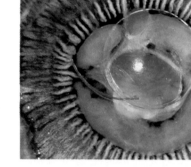

Plate 12.9 Gross photograph from behind an autopsy eye showing a Sinskey-style posterior chamber intraocular lens with both loops in the ciliary sulcus. Note the marked decentration of the intraocular lens, primarily in an axis perpendicular to the longitudinal direction of the loops. Note also extensive posterior capsular opacification and epithelial pearl formation.

Plate 12.10 (*Right*) Gross photograph from behind an autopsy eye with a modified J-loop Sinskey-style posterior chamber intraocular lens in which both loops were implanted in the ciliary sulcus. The optic is badly decentered so that a positioning hole is situated in the pupil. There is marked fibrosis of the posterior capsule and there is epithelial pearl formation.

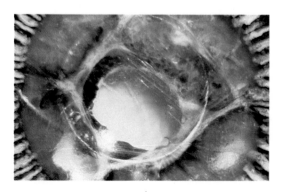

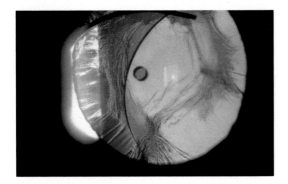

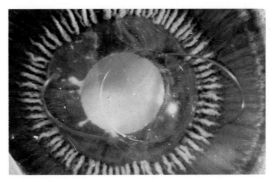

Plate 12.11 Clinical photograph showing a posterior chamber intraocular lens that is horizontally displaced to the left so that the edge of the lens, a positioning hole, and one of the loops are within the visual axis. Ruptured and stretched zonular fibers are seen on the right. This is an unusual case of horizontal displacement (east–west syndrome), which is most frequently caused by asymmetric loop fixation rather than zonular rupture as seen here.

Plate 12.13 Gross photograph from behind an autopsy globe showing the presence of a moderately dense layer of epithelial cells. Note the folds in the capsule which are caused by a fibromyometaplasia of residual lens epithelial cells.

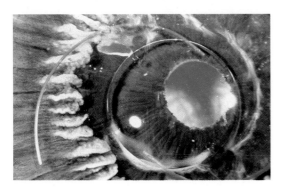

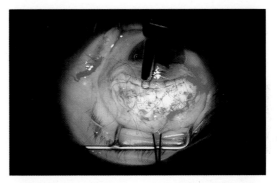

(a)

Plate 12.12 Gross photograph from behind an autopsy globe containing a modified J-loop posterior chamber intraocular lens in which the loop on the left was implanted in the capsular bag and the loop on the right extended through the zonules and landed in the pars plana. This caused an extreme amount of decentration to the right so that the left edge of the optic in this photograph and the positioning holes are in the pupil. Note an apparent tear of the posterior capsule seen superiorly in this photograph.

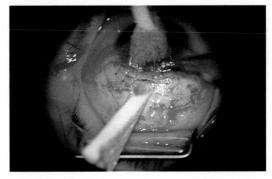

(b)

Plate 15.1 Combined cataract extraction and guarded posterior lip sclerectomy. (a) Modified Gass punch is used at the end of the cataract procedure to excise posterior sclera. (b) Appearance of corneoscleral wound after performing the sclerectomy.

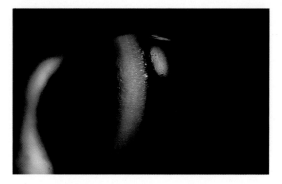

Plate 24.1 Slit-lamp appearance of Fuchs' dystrophy with characteristic 'beaten metal' appearance of Descemet's membrane.

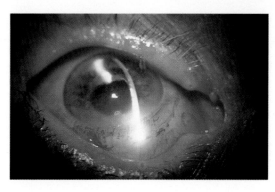

Plate 24.4 Superior corneal edema is seen in this patient with stripped Descemet's membrane. The membrane is visible folded on itself in the anterior chamber. (Courtesy of S Arthur Boruchoff MD.)

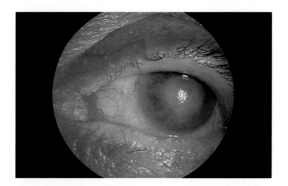

Plate 24.2 Advanced corneal edema with stromal neovascularization and fibrosis.

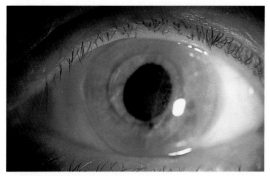

Plate 24.5 Corneal edema associated with a closed loop anterior chamber lens.

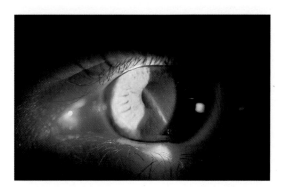

Plate 24.3 Endothelial scar from forceps delivery. Visual acuity 20/200 secondary to amblyopia.

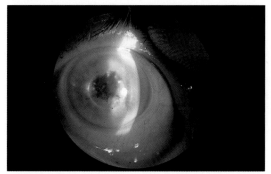

Plate 24.6 Corneal edema associated with a 'sputnik' style iris plane lens.

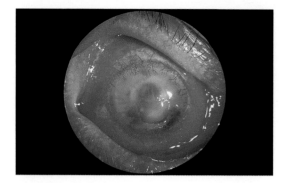

Plate 24.7 Severe corneal edema with an epithelial defect is seen in this patient with uveitis, glaucoma, and hyphema syndrome. The anterior chamber lens is visible superiorly.

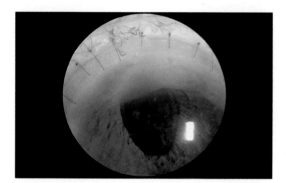

Plate 24.8 Fluorescein staining is seen in a patient with epithelial ingrowth following cataract surgery.

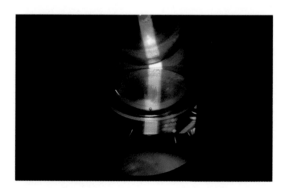

Plate 24.9 Gonioscopy demonstrates membrane obscuring structures of superior chamber angle.

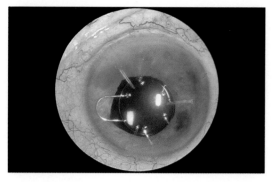

Plate 24.10 Displaced 'sputnik' style lens.

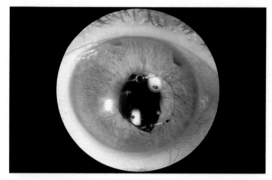

Plate 24.11 Displaced iris clip lens.

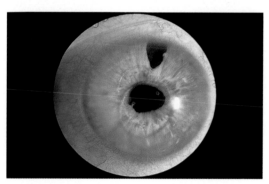

Plate 24.12 Iris clip lens displaced into anterior chamber with corneal decompensation.

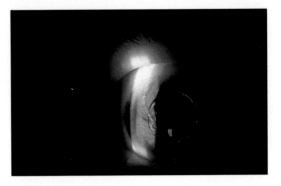

Plate 24.13 McCannal sutures used to secure an iris clip lens.

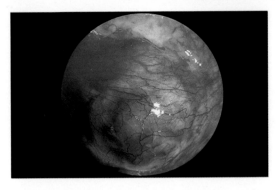

Plate 24.15 Postoperative appearance of a Gundersen flap for pseudophakic cornea edema in an eye with poor visual potential.

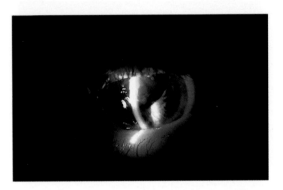

Plate 24.14 An area of endothelial/vitreous touch is seen superiorly with localized bullous keratopathy.

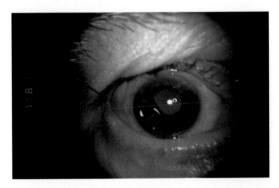

Plate 26.1 Peaking of pupil with vitreous strand to wound, easily visualized through undilated pupil.

opacities against the red of the fundus. A clear central space of only 2 or 3 mm, however, can permit normal visual acuity.

The clarity of the direct ophthalmoscopic image may also be used in this way to determine the quality of the eye's optical system, but in our hands is not quite as sensitive as retinoscopy.

Discussion of treatment of optical conditions reducing postoperative vision is beyond the intent of this chapter.

Endophthalmitis

Endophthalmitis, particularly in its chronic form, may occasionally present as reduced vision in the postoperative patient. This topic is covered in Chapter 20.

Retinal disease

Retinal disease is the most common cause of 20/100 surprises. Because many retinal diseases are not treatable, we will emphasize, not only postoperative diagnosis but also prevention of postoperative surprises by detecting these conditions before surgery. Depending on the patient's visual needs and ability to understand the situation, extraction of a dense cataract may still be indicated, expecting less than a 20/20 outcome. Postoperative acuity of 20/100 may be acceptable as long as it is not a "surprise."

History

Prevention of unpleasant postoperative surprises begins with the history. The ophthalmologist should ask the patient when and how rapidly the vision decreased. The comments of previous examiners are sometimes remembered vividly by the patient.

CASE HISTORY

A 68-year-old man had a cataract extraction in the right eye, and the vision did not improve beyond 20/80. The upper part of his macula had white, sclerotic veins, and there were venous shunt vessels temporal to the macula. Fluorescein angiography confirmed the presence of a superior macular branch vein occlusion.

Careful questioning prompted the patient to recall that his vision had decreased 10 years earlier. An ophthalmologist told him he had a "busted blood vessel in the back of his eye." This was probably the time at which his branch vein occlusion occurred. The physical signs at the time of cataract extraction were minimal and would not have been visible ophthalmoscopically through the cataract.

The patient's perception of his or her vision loss is important information that the ophthalmologist should listen to carefully. Most patients can distinguish between generalized blurring and metamorphopsia, for example. The patient can describe scotomata in many instances, indicating their relative position in the visual field and whether they involve the point of fixation. Sometimes we, in a referral practice, are tempted to spare the patient the necessity of repeating a precise description of the visual complaint. All but the most impatient, however, will be happy to explain the symptoms in detail to a sympathetic ear. The description may be rambling, but it can be gently steered back in the right direction to give the ophthalmologist a good idea of the nature of the problem before the physical examination is even begun. The slow, gradual onset of reduced vision from cataract is the story most often heard, of course. Detecting significant variations from this typical history will serve ophthalmologists well in preventing 20/100 surprises.

Age-related macular degeneration (ARMD)

ARMD is common in the cataract age group. Non-exudative "dry" ARMD can allow good vision after cataract surgery. Drusen alone usually do not cause vision loss greater than 20/50. If no other macular abnormality is present, drusen found preoperatively are not a reason to avoid surgery. If there is poor vision after cataract surgery, drusen alone should not be accepted as the only cause.

Drusen do cause significant vision loss when they are so frequent and closely spaced as to be confluent. A small retinal pigment epithelial detachment may actually occur, and the acuity can be significantly reduced in the absence of

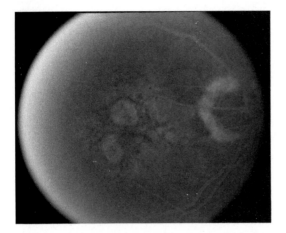

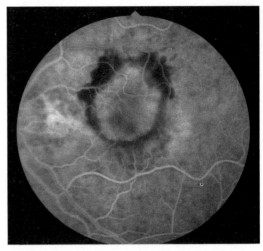

Fig. 10.1 This fluorescein angiogram of a patient with geographic atrophic age-related macular degeneration corresponds with Plate 10.1. The areas of geographic atrophy of the retinal pigment epithelium appear here as easily seen window defects. Angiography is not usually necessary to see these areas, and we do not recommend its routine use.

Fig. 10.2 Intravenous fluorescein angiogram of subretinal choroidal neovascularization in the macula, surrounded by hemorrhage. Hyperfluorescence occurs early in the angiogram and increases in the later phases. The corresponding color photograph is Plate 10.2.

any other macular disease. In this situation, the drusen are usually large and "soft" in appearance.

Geographic atrophy is the most severe form of dry ARMD. It creates a dense scotoma and can produce profound visual loss if the central macula is involved. If the atrophy spares the central fovea, the patient can see well even with extensive areas of retinal pigment epithelium (RPE) loss.

CASE HISTORY

A 72-year-old white woman had 20/400 vision with eccentric fixation in the right eye. Cataract extraction and intraocular lens implantation did not improve her vision.

Examination showed a large area of atrophy of the retinal pigment epithelium in the macula of the right eye (Plate 10.1 and Fig. 10.1).

These areas of atrophy are visible with the indirect ophthalmoscope, even through a fairly advanced cataract. Since there is no treatment available, prevention of these surprises is of great importance. This is one of the areas in which use of the indirect ophthalmoscope is

indispensable to the highest quality practice of ophthalmology. RPE atrophy is difficult to appreciate with the direct ophthalmoscope or with other high magnification examination techniques, such as the macular contact lens.

We have no numerical data but have a distinct impression that geographic atrophic ARMD tends to be bilateral. The acuity can be asymmetric, however, with the fovea being involved on one side only.

Exudative ARMD

CASE HISTORY

A 68-year-old white woman had 20/20 vision in the right eye following cataract and intraocular lens implantation 1 year ago. She has only a few drusen in the macula.

She had cataract and implant surgery in her left eye because of 2/200 visual acuity. Her vision did not improve following surgery. There was an oval area of elevation of the retinal pigment epithelium surrounded by subretinal hemorrhage (Plate 10.2).

Fluorescein angiography showed a hyperfluorescent area in the macula, including the central fovea.

Fluorescence increased in the late venous phase of the angiogram (Fig. 10.2).

This patient has exudative or "wet" ARMD. The subretinal neovascularization arises from the choroid and grows through defects in Bruch's membrane. Exudation and hemorrhage under the RPE or sensory retina produce visual loss. Treatment is possible at the stage in which the subretinal neovascular membrane is outside the fovea, yet producing visual distortion and metamorphopsia.

The physical findings with subretinal neovascularization include hemorrhage in or under the retina, hard exudate, subretinal fluid, and a faintly visible gray (occasionally pink) view of the membrane itself. These findings may be subtle. Whether before or after surgery, we recommend evaluation of the macular area with a magnified stereoscopic view. This requires either the Volk +90 or +78 D lens, or the Goldmann macular contact lens. Our routine is to use the Volk lens first, so that gonioscopic solution will not be placed on the cornea in case angiography is necessary. Recognition of the physical findings in subtle cases is enhanced by a high index of suspicion, familiarity with the various presentations of subretinal neovascularization, and experience in the use of these examining techniques.

Timely recognition of the presence of subretinal neovascularization is important. The subretinal membranes grow towards the fovea at unpredictable rates. Laser treatment is less successful once neovascularization is within the foveal avascular zone. Even outside the foveal avascular zone, the outcome depends upon distance of the membrane from the fovea when treatment is initiated. Patients who develop scotoma or metamorphopsia should be evaluated and offered treatment the same or next day whenever possible.

Cystoid macular edema (CME)

CME (Irvine–Gass–Norton syndrome) commonly results in decreased central visual acuity after an interval of good vision following cataract surgery. Decreased vision results from the accumulation of serous fluid in cystic spaces within the macula. Blurring of vision is the most common symptom and usually occurs between 2 and 12 weeks postoperatively. Some cases develop months to years after surgery.

Many cases will improve over time without treatment, but a small percentage of patients will develop chronic macular edema with permanently decreased central vision. Irvine *et al.* [1] showed that there is angiographic evidence of fluid accumulation in the macula in 50–70% of patients who undergo "uneventful" or uncomplicated intracapsular cataract extraction. Gass [2] suggests that this response is so common as to represent "a normal physiologic response to intracapsular cataract extraction." Allen and Jaffe [3] showed a 50–70% lesser prevalence after extracapsular cataract extraction (ECCE). A distinction must be made between angiographic evidence of fluorescein leakage and biomicroscopic evidence of macular edema. Of patients with perifoveal fluorescein leakage upon angiography 90% will not show any biomicroscopic evidence of edema or any decrease in visual acuity.

Clinically significant CME, causing a measurable decrease in visual acuity, occurs after approximately 0.5–5% of ECCE with intraocular lens (IOL) procedures. Less than 2% of patients will develop permanent loss of central acuity caused by chronic macular edema.

The pathogenesis of CME is unknown. Macular edema is associated with signs of intraocular inflammation including conjunctival injection, aqueous and/or vitreous cell and flare, photophobia, optic disc edema, perivascular cuffing, and fluorescein angiograpic evidence of leakage from the disc, retinal vessels, and intraretinal capillaries. One currently popular explanation for these findings is that intraocular inflammation causes the increased release or decreased clearance of chemical substances, presumably prostaglandins and leukotrienes, which drift back to the macula and produce increased capillary leakage within the macula. The clinical response to anti-inflammatory treatment supports this hypothesis.

Distortion of the pupil, and/or traction on the vitreous base and ciliary body appear to worsen this inflammation. The incidence is higher with rupture of the posterior capsule, vitreous loss, and with pupillary distortion by vitreous incarcerated in the operative wound. CME is more common and more severe in blue than brown eyes and more common in white than in black patients. Vitreous traction on the macula may play a role in a minority of cases.

The duration of CME seems to be involved in the effectiveness of treatment. Early treatment is more likely to result in visual recovery and a better final visual outcome than delayed treatment. Prolonged cystic distortion of the macula can result in permanent structural and functional damage.

DIAGNOSIS

The diagnosis of CME is based upon a typical history of decreased central vision developing after an interval of good vision following cataract surgery. Biomicroscopic examination of the macula usually is sufficient to reveal cystic accumulation of fluid in the fovea. Fluorescein angiography is helpful in making the diagnosis in difficult cases. Typical findings on angiography include diffuse parafoveal leakage with late accumulation of dye in a "flower petal" pattern centered in the fovea. Recall, however, that a very large percentage of patients appear to have "CME" on angiography but do not truly suffer from the syndrome because they have neither decreased vision nor macular edema. Fluorescein angiography is not a substitute for thorough examination and should not be a routine examination.

PROPHYLACTIC TREATMENT

Avoidance of trauma to the iris and pupillary margin, minimizing iris damage and the release of chemical mediators of inflammation, is probably important. Preoperative treatment with topical steroids or non-steroidal anti-inflammatory medications has been shown to decrease the amount of intraocular inflammatory substances released during surgery. Topical prednisolone acetate, subconjunctival or sub-Tenon's injections of corticosteroids, systemic steroids, and topical or oral non-steroidal anti-inflammatory drops have all been shown to lower the incidence of angio-

graphically proven CME after cataract extraction. It has not been proven that any of these treatments reduce the incidence of clinically significant macular edema. These same medicines have been less helpful in treating established cases of CME.

Primary capsulotomies increase the incidence of angiographically proven CME from 5.6 to 21.5%, when the angiogram was performed 1 week postoperatively. There was no significant difference in visual acuity between these two groups when tested 3 weeks postoperatively.

TREATMENT

The treatment of established aphakic CME is unsatisfactory. Anti-inflammatory agents such as antiprostaglandins and corticosteroids may result in some temporary improvement in visual acuity, yet there is no evidence that they shorten the duration or reduce the incidence of developing chronic CME.

Corticosteroids have been shown effectively to reduce macular edema secondary to ocular inflammation. They have also been helpful in the treatment of aphakic CME, but the effect has been temporary in many cases.

Oral non-steroidal anti-inflammatory medications have some theoretic role in the treatment of CME. Ketorolac has been shown to help improve vision in a small number of patients with macular edema.

Hyperbaric oxygen has also been shown to have a beneficial effect on eyes with established CME. Thus far, the number of eyes studied has been small.

SURGICAL TREATMENT

Vitrectomy has been shown to be effective in improving CME in eyes with vitreous strands to the wound, distorted pupillary margins, and iris distortion by IOL haptics or synechiae. Some patients with vitreous incarceration, particularly those with complaints of irritation and photophobia and those with many vitreous opacities, do obtain relief of symptoms and improvement in acuity following vitrectomy. YAG vitreolysis of strands causing pupillary distortion has also been shown to be effective in certain cases.

Vitrectomy has also been effective in improving vision in patients with chronic uveitis, vitreous opacities, and epimacular membrane.

Photocoagulation has been shown to reduce macular edema and improve visual acuity in patients with perifoveal vascular leakage syndromes such as diabetes mellitus. However, there is no evidence that photocoagulation is effective in the treatment of aphakic CME.

Epiretinal membranes

Epiretinal membranes, preretinal gliosis, macular pucker, cellophane maculopathy, and epimacular proliferation (EMP) are all terms used to describe a thin layer of fibrous tissue which covers and sometimes distorts the macula. Such membranes are fairly common, being present at autopsy in 2% of all eyes of persons over 50 years of age and 20% of eyes in persons over 75 years of age [4]. Significant membranes causing macular pucker occur in 3–8.5% of eyes after retinal detachment surgery [5–8].

Most are asymptomatic and most have normal or near normal vision. The most common symptom experienced by persons with macular distortion from epimacular membranes is metamorphopsia. Distortion of the fovea results in corresponding distortion of the retinal image transmitted to the brain and visual changes. Perimacular vessels damaged by the distorting force sometimes become permeable, causing macular thickening or cystic foveal edema. Mild visual loss is common. Severe cases develop progressive foveal distortion and visual loss.

The diagnosis is made by the clinical appearance of a transparent glistening membrane on the macular surface which may be recognized by its "wrinkled cellophane" appearance and the vascular tortuosity or macular distortion it induces. The fovea may be dragged away from its normal location or even detached from the RPE. These membranes are difficult to photograph and are sometimes easier to see with red-free light. Fluorescein angiography plays a limited role in making the diagnosis but can be helpful in evaluating the impact a membrane is having on the retina. Patients with pronounced symptoms of metamorphopsia and perifoveal leakage, demonstrated angiographically, may be considered for early intervention before permanent foveal damage occurs.

In some cases, the fovea itself appears to have been spared by the surface membrane creating a foveal pseudohole. Eyes with pseudoholes usually have normal vision and no foveal leakage on angiography. True macular holes cause dense central scotomata and window defects angiographically.

While the vast majority of patients with epimacular membranes do not require treatment, those with significant foveal distortion can sometimes be helped by vitrectomy and epimacular membrane removal. All eyes being considered for vitrectomy and epimacular membrane removal require careful assessment to be certain that the membrane is responsible for the majority of the visual loss. Postcataract macular edema, subretinal neovascularization, macular hole, or capillary non-perfusion must be excluded as contributing factors.

Traumatic maculopathy

Patients with traumatic maculopathy can usually recall the injuring event when asked specifically to describe the onset of their visual loss. The few patients who forget or fail to mention significant ocular trauma prior to surgery will frequently be able to recall their injuries when confronted postoperatively with decreased vision and scarring in the fovea. Common etiologies include blunt trauma, ball and sport injuries, fist fights, and orbital trauma.

Any combination of retinal and RPE changes, including choroidal ruptures, pigmentary macular changes, subretinal scarring, and macular holes can be seen in the posterior pole and periphery. Peripheral scarring from subretinal hemorrhage and vitreous-base avulsion help to confirm the diagnosis. Changes limited to one eye help to differentiate traumatic changes from macular degeneration and other disorders.

No treatment is available at this time to reverse traumatic macular damage.

Photic retinal injury

It has become apparent in recent years that visible light, even in the absence of ultraviolet (UV) or infrared radiation, can damage the retina. The cornea absorbs most light energy of 300 nm and less. The natural lens is responsible for preventing light made up of 300–400 nm from reaching the retina. Removal of the lens combined with ocular akinesia and prolonged exposure to intense microscope light create a high-risk setting for photic retinal injury. Cataract extraction procedures are the most common setting where such damage occurs. The first report of retinal injury by an operating microscope was published in 1983. The incidence of retinal injury, noted angiographically, has been reported to be as high as 7% after ECCE with IOL implantation. None of the patients in this study were symptomatic.

The most common symptoms of macular burn are erythropsia and visible scotomata seen soon after surgery. Early findings may be subtle and include a pale oval-shaped retinal lesion in the posterior pole which is hyperfluorescent on angiography. This same lesion will become variably pigmented over a period of weeks to months.

Prevention of photic retinal toxicity requires attention to minimizing retinal exposure. Filtering wavelengths below 400–450 nm, using paraxial rather than coaxial illumination whenever a red reflex is not needed, minimizing brightness and exposure time, and covering the visual axis with an opaque barrier can all help to prevent macular burns.

Retinal vascular occlusions

Any interruption of the normal retinal blood supply can affect visual function. The classic findings seen after arterial and venous occlusions may resolve with time, leaving only subtle evidence of their occurrence. Most of these clues can be difficult or impossible to see through a cataractous lens. Any history of sudden visual loss or decreased vision out of proportion to the opacification of the lens should raise the suspicion of vascular occlusive disease as a contributing factor.

With branch retinal vein occlusion, vision can range from normal to 20/400, depending on the amount of macular edema and damage to perifoveal capillaries. With time, the typical hemorrhages and edema resolve, leaving small vascular anomalies, arteriovenous anastomoses, and macular atrophy or edema. Angiography reveals the vascular changes, poor capillary perfusion, and if edema is present, late staining of the fovea.

Central retinal artery occlusion is best identified by a history of sudden profound visual loss. Visible changes are usually limited to optic atrophy and narrowed arterioles. Angiography reveals delayed and slow arterial filling.

Diabetic retinopathy

Diabetic retinopathy rarely presents as a postoperative surprise. Significant macular edema, macular ischemia, and proliferative scarring are frequently more easy to evaluate and treat after a cloudy lens has been removed. Patients with macular exudates or scarring and those suspected of having macular damage should be warned preoperatively not to expect excellent visual recovery. Limiting patient's expectations in advance is definitely easier than explaining a poor operative result.

Retinal detachment

Any history of curtain-like visual loss or decreased acuity out of proportion to the lens opacification should alert the clinician to the possibility of retinal detachment. An afferent pupillary defect, low intraocular pressure, or the presence of pigment cells in the vitreous also increases the likelihood that the retina is detached. In the absence of a view of the retina to sufficiently ascertain whether the retina is attached and the macula and optic nerve head are grossly normal, preoperative ultrasonography can be helpful.

Optic nerve diseases

Chronic open-angle glaucoma

Chronic open-angle glaucoma produces damage to the optic nerve that is, with rare exceptions, irreversible. Again, prevention of surprises is important. Because the intraocular pressure may be normal much of the time, tonometry alone is not adequate in detecting glaucoma prior to cataract surgery. Careful inspection of the optic nerve for evidence of glaucomatous damage should be performed whenever possible.

The patient may recall hearing about elevated eye pressure in the past. Perimetry may be possible even in the presence of cataract, although subtle field defects will not be detectable. The optic nerve can be inspected through many cataracts with indirect ophthalmoscopy and a +20D lens or with biomicroscopy at the slit-lamp. Evaluation of the fellow eye is valuable because of the usual bilateral occurrence of glaucoma.

If the vision is poor after cataract surgery, glaucoma should be easy to evaluate. Glaucoma rarely reduces visual acuity until late in its course, when findings are dramatic. The intraocular pressure may be falsely decreased to normal levels for some time after surgery, however. Detailed perimetry should be possible, and the optic disc and nerve fiber layer can be inspected closely.

Optic atrophy

Optic atrophy, if it occurs due to a compressive lesion of the visual pathways, usually does not produce a distinctive visual history. There may be endocrine changes in the history if a pituitary adenoma is compressing the chiasm asymmetrically. If anterior ischemic optic neuropathy has occurred in the past, the patient may recall the abrupt onset of reduced vision.

Before surgery, optic atrophy will be difficult to see ophthalmoscopically unless it is severe and the cataract is mild. Careful pupil examination will disclose a relative afferent defect on the affected side. Such a defect should not be attributed to a dense cataract, which cannot produce a conduction defect in the absence of optic nerve atrophy.

Evaluation of optic atrophy, whether discovered before or after cataract surgery, involves attention to the afferent visual pathways, including the optic nerve and chiasm. Perimetry is the primary diagnostic tool here. Both eyes should be evaluated carefully.

CASE HISTORY

A 63-year-old woman had 2/200 vision in the left eye. After cataract surgery, there was no improvement in acuity. She had optic atrophy in the left eye; the right eye had 20/20 vision with a normal optic disc.

Confrontation visual fields were normal in the right eye and produced no response in the left eye. Goldmann perimetry on the right eye showed a small superotemporal defect respecting the vertical midline.

Neuroradiologic studies showed a meningioma at the chiasm, compressing the left nerve more than the right nerve.

Anterior ischemic optic neuropathy

Anterior ischemic optic neuropathy can occur in elderly patients either before or after cataract surgery. When it has occurred prior to surgery, it will produce optic atrophy in the affected eye, as discussed above.

Anterior ischemic optic neuropathy occurring in the days of weeks following cataract surgery may represent a distinct entity, at least in the view of some researchers [9]. Intraocular pressure within the first few hours or days after surgery may precipitate ischemic optic neuropathy in an eye that is predisposed to it by anatomic or vascular factors. Prevention of postoperative pressure "spikes" is a goal that is difficult to achieve. During surgery, removal of viscoelastic materials from the anterior chamber is probably the most important maneuver.

Preoperative and postoperative use of medications such as acetazolamide and β-blocker drops have been advocated. Intraocular use of acetylcholine or carbachol may also be effective. The best regimen is not yet known.

Damage to the optic nerve from the tip of the retrobulbar needle may present as ischemic optic neuropathy. The current trend toward safer local anesthetic placement should make this source of surprise even rarer.

Table 10.1 Prevention of postoperative surprises

Detailed history of prior visual acuity and a description of vision loss

Careful preoperative examination to reveal any evidence of retinal detachment, macular scarring, vascular changes in the posterior pole, or diabetic changes

Preoperative antibiotics and/or lavage of conjunctival surfaces with saline or antiseptic solution to minimize resident flora

Bacterial cultures and prosthesis removal in monocular patients

Minimally traumatic surgical technique

Perioperative steroids or non-steroidal anti-inflammatory agents

Avoid primary capsulotomies and vitreous loss

Minimize coaxial light exposure of the retina

Amblyopia

Strabismic amblyopia seldom produces a post-operative surprise. Usually, the patient is aware of a history of strabismus during childhood, and there is often visible misalignment of the eyes prior to surgery. If there is poor vision after cataract surgery and amblyopia is suspected, it is necessary that it be a diagnosis of exclusion. Occasionally, sensory tests, such as the +4 D base-out prism test, will demonstrate a sensory pattern that is diagnostic of strabismus.

Instrumentation

We have not discussed the potential acuity meter, the laser interferometer, and other psychophysical or electrophysiologic testing. These methods fail to detect poor vision frequently enough that they cannot be relied upon prior to surgery to predict surprises. As in all of medicine, a careful history and physical examination by the surgeon prior to operation is the best way of detecting potential visual problems. When postoperative surprises do occur, history and physical examination, once again, will give the answer in the vast majority

Table 10.2 Evaluation of patients for decreased vision after "successful" cataract surgery

Detailed history of visual loss
Amblyopia
Trauma
Sudden visual loss from ischemia
Metamorphopsia from epimacular proliferation or
   subretinal neovascularization
Good postoperative vision followed by blurring
   suggests cystoid macular edema

Examination
Visual axis
   Astigmatism
   Lens centration
   Capsular clarity
   Vitreous opacities
   Retinoscopy
Ophthalmoscopy—both indirect ophthalmoscope
   and high magnification stereoscopic exam (macular
   contact or 90 D lens)
   Optic nerve
      pallor
      cupping
      swelling
      pupillary response, bright light comparison, or
         visual fields if abnormality suspected
   Vessels
      arteriolar narrowing or Hollenhorst plaques
      abnormal perifoveal vessels or shunt vessels
      vein occlusions
   Macula
      drusen—probably not causing severe visual loss
      pigmentary changes
      subretinal scarring, hemorrhage, fluid, or retinal
         exudate
      surface wrinkling
      macular hole
Fluorescein angiography if examination suggests
   Abnormal circulation
      arteriolar obstruction
      abnormal vessels
      venous occlusion
   Macular edema
      subretinal neovascularization
      cystoid macular edema
      photic maculopathy

of cases. Fluorescein angiography will be helpful in diagnosing selected cases.

Summary

Table 10.1 summarizes our approach to the prevention of 20/100 surprises. Even the most careful surgeon, however, may occasionally need the recommendations in Table 10.2 for evaluating patients with poor results.

References

1 Irvine AR, Bresky R, Crowder BM, Forster RK, Hunter DM, Kulvin SM. Macular edema after cataract extraction. *Ann Ophthalmol* 1971; **3**: 1234–40.

2 Gass JDM. *Stereoscopic Atlas of Macular Diseases: Diagnosis and Treatment*, vol. 1. St Louis: CV Mosby, 1987; 368.

3 Allen AW, Jaffe NS. Cystoid macular edema—a preliminary study. *Trans Am Acad Ophthalmol Otolaryngol* 1976; **81**: 133–4.

4 Ryan SJ. *Retina*, vol. 2. St Louis: CV Mosby, 1989: 789.

5 Hagler WS, Aturaliya U. Macular puckers after retinal detachment surgery. *Br J Ophthalmol* 1971; **55**: 451–7.

6 Lobers LA Jr, Burton TC. The incidence of macular pucker after retinal detachment surgery. *Am J Ophthalmol* 1978; **85**: 72–7.

7 Michels RG. Vitrectomy for macular pucker. *Ophthalmology* 1984; **91**: 1384–8.

8 Tannenbaum HL, Scheppens CL, Elzeneiny I, Freeman HM. Macular pucker following retinal detachment surgery. *Arch Ophthalmol* 1970; **83**: 286–93.

9 Hayreh SS. Anterior ischemic optic neuropathy. IV. Occurrence after cataract extraction. *Arch Ophthalmol* 1980; **98**: 1410–16.

11: The Best Operation for the Cataract Patient: Specific Techniques and Future Considerations

H. JOHN SHAMMAS & RICHARD P. KRATZ

In a patient with a cataract, the ophthalmologist has first to make a decision on whether the patient needs surgery or not. It is generally agreed that cataract surgery is indicated when the patient cannot function adequately due to the poor sight produced by the cataract.

Once this is done, the ophthalmologist has to decide on the following:

1 whether the cataract should be removed by phacoemulsification, planned extracapsular cataract extraction (ECCE), or intracapsular cataract extraction (ICCE);

2 whether an implant should be inserted at the time of surgery; or

3 whether the cataract procedure should be combined with a trabeculectomy, in the presence of glaucoma, or with a corneal transplant, in the presence of corneal clouding.

The decision for each surgery is individualized to yield the best results for the patient.

The cataract operation

ICCE, where the lens is removed with its capsule, has lost its popularity with the introduction of modern extracapsular techniques. ICCE is still performed by some ophthalmologists and is indicated in certain cases such as lens dislocation.

ECCE removes the nucleus by phacoemulsification or planned ECCE, leaving an intact posterior capsule and allows the insertion of a posterior chamber intraocular lens (IOL).

Phacoemulsification cataract extraction

ADVANTAGES

1 Phacoemulsification requires an incision of 3 mm chord (3.1 mm arc) versus 10.5 mm chord (12 mm arc) for a planned ECCE;

2 it is a closed system in which the surgeon has total control;

3 there are no reported expulsive hemorrhages. The small incision may be instantly closed if there is a sudden increase in intraocular pressure; and

4 the small incision allows rapid healing with little chance of wound leak and iris prolapse. The refraction stabilizes rapidly with minimal induced astigmatism.

DISADVANTAGES

1 Phacoemulsification requires special training and is machine-dependent;

2 there are increased costs because of the disposables; and

3 it is not suited for all types of cataracts such as very hard nuclei, hypermature cataracts, and subluxed lenses.

OCULAR REQUIREMENTS FOR A SUCCESSFUL PHACOEMULSIFICATION

A careful preoperative evaluation is necessary to choose the cases that are best handled by this technique. The procedure is as follows:

1 the cornea is examined for any signs of endothelial dystrophy. Emulsifying the nucleus in the posterior chamber causes less endothelial damage than emulsifying it in the anterior chamber or at the iris plane;

2 the pupil is dilated with 2.5% phenylephrine and 1% cyclopentotate eyedrops. A well-dilated pupil facilitates phacoemulsification and decreases the risks of iris injury during surgery. A pupil that does not dilate well will make phacoemulsification a more difficult procedure with a higher rate of complications; and

3 the nucleus consistency is evaluated through a dilated pupil. A mildly sclerotic nucleus is easily removed by phacoemulsification. Emulsification of a hard nucleus requires more ultrasound energy and is more difficult to perform. A hypermature cataract with a liquified cortex and a very hard, small nucleus is best removed by planned ECCE.

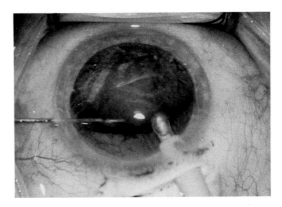

Fig. 11.1 The cataract is removed by phacoemulsification. The nucleus is manipulated with a spatula inserted from a side port while the phaco tip is emulsifying portions of the nucleus.

SURGICAL PROCEDURE (Fig. 11.1)

The original technique of phacoemulsification in the anterior chamber is now rarely used due to the increased incidence of endothelial damage. For the past few years, phacoemulsification of the nucleus at the iris plane has been the standard procedure. Recently, the introduction of capsulorhexis or continuous tear anterior capsulotomy is allowing a safe and successful phacoemulsification of the nucleus within its bag in the posterior chamber.

PHACOEMULSIFICATION AT THE
IRIS PLANE

A small fornix-based conjunctival flap is dissected superiorly and the bleeders are cauterized. A scleral groove is made 2 mm posterior and parallel to the limbus; the groove should be as large as the IOL optic diameter that has to be inserted at the completion of the cataract removal. A scleral pocket is dissected all the way to clear cornea. Through a 1 mm stab incision, a cystotome or a curved needle is used to perform an anterior capsulotomy. The anterior chamber is maintained with viscoelastic material.

The incision is then enlarged to 3 mm to allow the insertion of the phaco tip into the anterior chamber. The nucleus is centrally hollowed out like a bowl; the cortical attachments keep the nucleus in place and facilitate the sculpting procedure. A small spatula is then introduced through a side port at 2 o'clock to engage the nuclear bowl at 6 o'clock and to press the inferior nucleus posteriorly and inferiorly. Subluxed anteriorly, the superior pole is engaged with the phaco tip. Emulsification of the nucleus starts superiorly and the spatula keeps the nuclear material in the iris plane away from the endothelium and the posterior capsule. The nucleus is repeatedly rotated with the spatula presenting different portions of the nucleus to be emulsified at the iris plane until completion.

Cortical clean-up is performed with a 0.3 mm irrigation and aspiration tip. The posterior capsule is cleaned with a capsule polisher or under low vacuum. The incision is then enlarged to allow the insertion of the IOL.

PHACOEMULSIFICATION IN THE
POSTERIOR CHAMBER

Emulsification of the nucleus within the capsular bag is best performed after a capsulorhexis or continuous tear capsulotomy. The circular tear can be performed with a bent needle or with forceps leaving a central opening of 5–6 mm with smooth edges.

The nucleus is hydrodissected by injecting balanced salt solution under the anterior capsular rim to separate the anterior cortex from the nucleus, separating it from the posterior capsule and cortex.

The nucleus is then slowly emulsified within the capsular bag. A second instrument introduced through the side port assists in rotating the nucleus and keeping it away from the cornea. Two main techniques are used to successfully emulsify the nucleus in the posterior chamber: the first one creates a nuclear bowl by removing the bulk of the nuclear tissues while the posterior pole of the bowl protects the posterior capsule from inadvertent injury; the bowl is then reduced to a nuclear plate and totally removed. The second technique creates a deep central vertical groove within the nucleus. The nucleus is then rotated 90° and a second groove is performed. Using the phaco tip and the spatula inserted through a side port, the nucleus is broken into four quadrants that are safely emulsified.

The cortical clean-up is carried out with the irrigation and aspiration tip.

Planned ECCE

Planned ECCE is safe to use on all types of cataracts, regardless of nuclean hardness, pupil size, or endothelial status. The only disadvantage of the procedure is that it requires a 10.5 mm chord incision (12 mm arc) which increases the risks of wound leak, iris prolapse, and induced astigmatism.

A fornix-based conjunctival flap is dissected superiorly, and the bleeders are lightly cauterized. A limbal groove is made between the 10 and 2 o'clock positions, going half the depth of the sclera. A 1 mm stab incision into the anterior chamber is made superiorly. A U-shaped capsulotomy is performed with an irrigating cystotome or a bent needle; using side-to-side movements, multiple small cuts are made, making sure that each new cut connects with the adjacent one in a continuous tear technique.

An 8/0 silk suture is placed superiorly and looped through the groove; the preplaced suture is a means of immediate wound closure

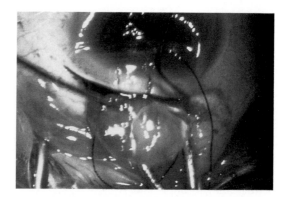

Fig. 11.2 The nucleus is being expressed and speared out of the eye in planned extracapsular cataract extraction.

in the presence of positive vitreous pressure. The wound is enlarged from 10 to 2 o'clock and using a curved McPherson forceps, the anterior capsule is grasped and cut with scissors.

The nucleus is expressed out of the eye by applying pressure slightly behind the scleral lip superiorly and counterpressure to the limbus inferiorly with a muscle hook or a bent spear. The nucleus can also be hydrodissected by allowing balanced salt solution to flow under it or looped out of the eye (Fig. 11.2).

The cortical material is removed with an automated or manual irrigating and aspirating system and the posterior capsule is cleaned with a capsule polisher (Fig. 11.3). The wound is partially closed with 10/0 nylon sutures, leaving a 6–7 mm opening to allow for the insertion of the IOL.

Implant surgery

Alternatives to implant surgery

When the crystalline lens of the eye is removed by cataract surgery and no implant is used, alternate methods to restore vision are needed:
1 cataract glasses are thick and heavy. They increase the size of objects by about 25% and clear vision is only obtained through the central part of the glasses. Furthermore cataract glasses cannot be used if only one eye is being operated for the cataract; or
2 hard or soft contact lenses are another alter-

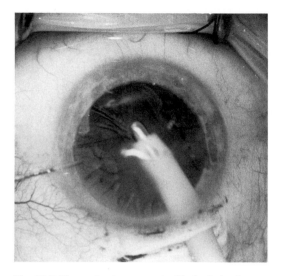

Fig. 11.3 The cortex is removed with the irrigation and aspiration tip whether the nucleus has been removed by phacoemulsification or by planned extracapsular cataract extraction. The irrigation and aspiration tip is aimed towards the superior cortical layers, stripping them gently, leaving an intact and clear posterior capsule.

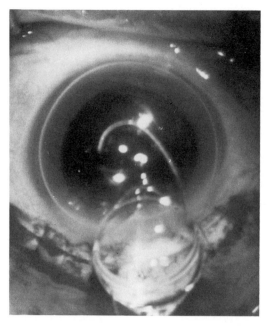

Fig. 11.4 The posterior chamber implant is inspected prior to inserting it in the eye. Note that the wound is partially closed and that the anterior chamber has been deepened with an air bubble to facilitate lens insertion.

native. The apparent size of objects is increased by about 8%, but handling a contact lens is difficult for some individuals and not everyone can tolerate them. For near tasks, reading glasses may be required in addition to contact lenses.

Indications for implant surgery

With implant surgery, an IOL is placed inside the eye permanently with no apparent change in the size of objects seen.

Through the years, implant surgery has evolved from inserting a Binkhorst iris-supported lens or a Choyce Mark VIII anterior chamber lens to inserting a posterior chamber lens in the capsular bag, avoiding any contact with the surrounding uveal tissue.

Implant surgery is now the standard for all cases. Occasionally, the ophthalmologist is faced with a dilemma if implant surgery has been unsuccessful in the first eye. Sometimes in very high myopia (over 10 D), a simple cataract extraction will restore emmetropia; however, even in such cases, we favor the use of a very low power implant; an implant placed in the

capsular bag has the added advantage of preventing postoperative forward movement of the vitreous and its complications.

Iris-supported lenses that fit in the pupillary area are rarely used nowadays due to their high rate of complications. We will only discuss the insertion of posterior and anterior chamber lenses.

Inserting a posterior chamber lens (Fig. 11.4)

A posterior chamber lens has loops attached to a central optical portion. The optical portion is commonly made of polymethylmetacrylate (PMMA) that has been rendered ultraviolet absorbent. It can have a plano–convex, biconvex, or meniscus configuration with a diameter ranging from 5 to 7 mm; it can have positioning holes, tabs, or laser ridge. The loops are commonly made of prolene or PMMA; they can be flat or angulated with an overall length of 12–14 mm. The loop configurations vary from "J" and modified "J" to "C" and modified "C." All

PMMA lenses perform well and are considered relatively safe. Silicone and hydrogel foldable lenses are gaining in popularity since they can be inserted through a small incision following phacoemulsification.

The posterior chamber lens is inserted behind the iris, preferably in the capsular bag. The following technique is recommended for in-the-bag insertion of a posterior chamber lens after an uneventful extracapsular cataract extraction by phacoemulsification or planned ECCE where the posterior capsule is left intact. Small amounts of viscoelastic material are injected in the anterior chamber and between the anterior capsule rim and posterior capsule to separate the bag. The implant is inserted through the wound into the eye and the lower loop is placed in the capsular bag inferiorly. The superior loop is then maneuvered with forceps to place it in the capsular bag superiorly. An alternative is to place the tip of a hook in the superior positioning hole pushing the implant inferiorly and rotating it clockwise to place the superior loop in the bag.

A posterior chamber lens should not be inserted if the surgery has been complicated by a wide rupture of the posterior capsule with or without vitreous loss. In such cases, it is safer to use an anterior chamber lens.

Inserting an anterior chamber lens

The rigid anterior chamber lens has been successfully used for many years but it has lost its popularity to the one-piece, Z-shaped flexible lens which reduces the incidence of postoperative tenderness and pupil ovaling associated with the rigid lens.

The anterior chamber lens is inserted in front of the iris with footplates resting in the angle. It is used after ICCE or in the presence of a large capsular rupture with or without vitreous loss during an extracapsular extraction. The following technique is recommended for its insertion. The corneal diameter is measured from "white" to "white" and 1 mm is added to this measurement to determine the size of the implant. A small amount of viscoelastic material is injected into the anterior chamber to keep it formed with a flat iris diaphragm. A Sheets' glide is placed over the iris and the implant is inserted over the glide until the lower footplates are positioned in the inferior angle. The glide is then removed and the superior footplates placed in the angle superiorly.

Wound closure (Fig. 11.5)

The wound is best sutured with 9/0 or 10/0 nylon sutures to provide a well-sealed incision. The incision may be corneal, limbal, or scleral and vary from 3 mm for a phacoemulsification with no lens implant to an 11 mm for a planned ECCE or ICCE, with or without lens implantation.

Interrupted sutures are commonly used for wound closure. Small bites are taken on the corneal side and larger bites on the scleral side to avoid induced postoperative astigmatism. Each suture is tied with a 3/1/1 knot, that is buried within the tissues to avoid postoperative irritation.

Alternatives to the interrupted sutures include the "X" sutures and the "shoelace" suture. These methods are commonly used to close smaller wounds, i.e. 3–7 mm after phacoemulsification with or without lens implantation.

Combined procedures

Corneal transplant–ECCE–lens implant

In the presence of a cataract with marked epithelial dystrophy causing corneal edema, the surgeon has the choice of:
1 performing a corneal transplant first, followed a few months to a year later by cataract and implant surgery. The main advantage is that the final refraction is more predictable; the power of the corneal transplant is known at the time of cataract surgery, and any induced astigmatism from the corneal transplant procedure can be corrected during the second surgery. The disadvantages are that it requires two surgeries and a long period of visual rehabilitation;
2 removing the cataract first followed by a corneal transplant. This procedure can be done if the cornea is still relatively clear; or

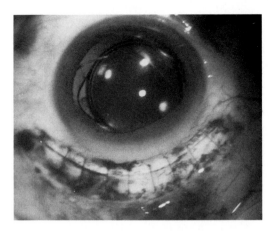

Fig. 11.5 The wound is closed with interrupted 10/0 nylon sutures at the end of surgery. Note the smaller bites on the corneal side and the longer bites on the scleral side.

3 combined corneal transplant–ECCE–lens implant surgery with the main advantage of avoiding a second surgery and the long rehabilitation period. The procedure requires removal of the corneal button, anterior capsulotomy with scissors or a cystotome, extraction of the nucleus, and manual removal of the cortical material. The implant is inserted in the bag under direct visualization and the anterior chamber is filled with viscoelastic material. The new corneal button is applied over the eye and sutured in place with 10/0 nylon sutures.

Trabeculectomy–ECCE–lens implant

In the presence of glaucoma with a cataract, it is important to control the intraocular pressure by medications or laser trabeculoplasty prior to cataract surgery. If the glaucoma cannot be controlled, the surgeon has the opportunity to decrease and control the intraocular pressure by performing a triple procedure of trabeculectomy, ECCE, and lens implantation.

With this procedure, a trabeculectomy flap is dissected at 12 o'clock and the limbal groove is continued on either side of the flap. The cataract is removed by phacoemulsification or planned ECCE followed by lens implantation. The deep scleral layers within the trabeculectomy site are cut with scissors and the

edges are lightly cauterized. The scleral flap is closed with 10/0 interrupted nylon sutures.

Future considerations

A more controlled cataract removal

In experienced hands, the best intraoperative control is obtained with phacoemulsification. This is a closed system where there is no "moment of truth" and no reported expulsive hemorrhage. It only requires a 3 mm incision whereas intracapsular and planned ECCE requires a 10–12 mm incision.

IMPROVEMENT IN THE PHACO UNITS

Phacoemulsification units are becoming more sophisticated allowing more power and control than the original units. The surgeon can use:
1 the irrigation only, to maintain a deep anterior chamber during the anterior capsulotomy or at any other desired moment;
2 irrigation and aspiration for removal of cortical material. The vacuum can be set to either minimal (low vac.) or maximal (high vac.). The rate of aspiration can be either preset or controlled by varying the pressure on the footplate; or
3 phacoemulsification for removal of the nucleus. The power can be preset to 50 or 70%, or controlled by the surgeon; it is decreased for a soft lens and increased for a hard lens. If the nucleus is driven away from the tip, the ultrasound mode is changed to pulse which tends to hold the nucleus against the tip.

Hopefully the future will see smaller handles, requiring even smaller incisions. Different modalities of energy such as laser and magnetic resonance are being experimented with to replace ultrasound.

IMPROVEMENT IN THE SURGICAL TECHNIQUES

The changes in the phaco units and the introduction a few years ago of viscoelastic material are allowing for continuous improvement in the surgical techniques. Although emulsification at the iris plane is a safe procedure, more control is obtained with capsulorhexis and emulsification of the lens within the capsular bag.

Newer techniques call for a very small incision in the anterior capsule and removal of the cataract leaving the bag intact. Different chemical materials are being used experimentally to prevent postoperative proliferation of the lens epithelial cells.

New implant designs

A small incision produces less astigmatism, less complications, and promotes rapid healing. Thus if a cataract can be removed through a 3 mm incision, it is advantageous to enlarge the wound the least possible to allow for the insertion of an IOL.

Regular PMMA IOLs require enlargement of the wound for a total of 6–7 mm depending on the size of the implant's optics. Some surgeons are favoring the use of oval implants that require only a 5 mm incision.

Foldable implants such as silicone and hydrogel lenses are gaining in popularity since they can be inserted through a 3.5–4.5 mm incision. However, long-term follow-up on these lenses is not yet available.

Different designs of bifocal IOLs are also being investigated.

A better astigmatic control

The best astigmatic control for a 6–7 mm incision is obtained with a shoelace running suture whilst checking the amount of induced astigmatism at the end of surgery with a surgical keratometer such as the Terry Keratometer. The postoperative healed incision will usually result in a flattening of that meridian of about 1.5–2 D, thus surgery performed at 12 o'clock would reduce a 2 D with-the-rule astigmatism to approximately plano.

Smaller incisions of 4–5 mm are closed with either one "X" suture or a single horizontal suture. Checking the keratometric readings at the end of surgery is always helpful to avoid induced astigmatism. Interrupted sutures can be cut about 9 weeks after surgery to relieve with-the-rule astigmatism.

Some surgeons have recommended moving the scleral flap to control large amounts of astigmatism while others have recommended the use of "T" cuts for large cylinders; unfortunately the "T" cuts are unpredictable. As of 1989, excimer trials have begun and show a promise of correcting any amount of residual astigmatism or ametropia.

Sutureless surgery

New techniques call for dissecting a scleral flap, starting 3–4 mm behind the limbus. The anterior chamber is entered through clear cornea, creating a posterior corneal lip.

At the end of surgery, this corneal lip acts like a valve that hermetically seals the wound. No sutures are needed.

Further reading

1 Colvard DM, Maxocco TR, Kratz RP, Davidson B. Clinical evaluation of the Terry Surgical Keratometer. *AIOISJ* 1980; **6**: 249–51.
2 Davison JA. Modified J-loop intraocular lens insertion after posterior chamber iris-plane phacoemulsification: A safe, easy method. *AIOISJ* 1981; **7**: 368–72.
3 Davison JA. Bimodal capsular bag phacoemulsification. A serial cutting and suction ultrasonic nuclear dissection technique. *J Cataract Refract Surg* 1989; **15**: 272–82.
4 Faulkner GD. Folding and inserting silicone intraocular lens implants. *J Cataract Refract Surg* 1987; **13**: 678–81.
5 Friedberg HL, Kline OR, Freidberg AH. Comparison of the unwanted optical images produced by 6 mm and 7 mm intraocular lenses. *J Cataract Refract Surg* 1989; **15**: 541–4.
6 Galand A. A simple method of implantation within the capsular bag. *AIOISJ* 1983; **9**: 330–2.
7 Ginidi JJ, Wan WL, Schanzlin DJ. Endocapsular cataract surgery. I. Surgical technique. *Cataract* 1985; **2**: 6–10.
8 Johnson SH, Kratz RP, Olson PF. Emulsification of the nucleus: the bimanual technique. In: Abrahamson IA, ed. *Cataract Surgery*. McGraw Hill, New York, 1986: 55–73.
9 Keates RH, Rothchild EJ, Bloom R. Endocapsular triple procedure. A new triple procedure technique. *J Cataract Refract Surg* 1989; **15**: 332–4.
10 Kratz RP, Johnson SH, Olson PF, Farley MK. Phacoemulsification associated with intraocular lenses. In: *Surgery of the Eye*. New York: Churchill Livingstone, 1988: 131–40.
11 Kratz RP, Mazocco TR, Davidson B, Colvard DM.

The Shearing intraocular lens: a report of 1000 cases. *AIOISJ* 1981; **7**: 55–7.

12 Kronish JW, Forster RK. Control of corneal astigmatism following cataract extraction by selective suture cutting. *Arch Ophthalmol* 1987; **105**: 1650–5.

13 Lindstrom RL, Harris WS, Doughman DJ. Combined penetrating keratoplasty, extracapsular cataract extraction and posterior chamber lens implantation. *AIOISJ* 1981; **7**: 130.

14 Mazocco TR, Kratz RP, Davidson B, Colvard DM.

Phacoemulsification and posterior chamber lens implantation in open angle glaucoma. *AIOISJ* 1981; **7**: 250–1.

15 Maloney WF, Grindle L, Sanders D, Pearcy D. Astigmatism control for the cataract surgeon: A comprehensive review of surgically tailored astigmatism reduction. *J Cataract Refract Surg* 1989; **15**: 45–54.

16 Newman AC, Cobb B. Advantages and limitations of current soft intraocular lenses. *J Cataract Refract Surg* 1989; **15**: 257–63.

12: Update on Implantation of Posterior Chamber Intraocular Lenses

DAVID J. APPLE, ROBIN C. MORGAN, JULIE C. TSAI
& EDWARD S. LIM

The return to Harold Ridley's [1] original concept of intraocular lens (IOL) implantation in the posterior chamber occurred in 1975 when John Pearce of England [2] implanted his rigid tripod design. Steven Shearing [3] of Las Vegas introduced a major lens design breakthrough in early 1977 with his flexible J-loop posterior chamber lens. William Simcoe of Tulsa publicly introduced his C-looped posterior chamber lens shortly after Shearing's J-loop design appeared, and Robert Sinskey of Santa Monica followed by Richard Kratz of Newport Beach and others introduced various modified J-loop designs that are in widespread use today. These flexible loop designs, as well as more recently introduced modified or short C-loop designs, account for the largest number of IOLs implanted today. These modern IOL styles, which are lightweight and provide better fixation, have greatly increased the safety and efficacy of the IOL implantation [4].

One obvious major theoretic advantage a posterior chamber IOL (PCIOL) has over an anterior chamber IOL (ACIOL) is its position behind the iris, away from the delicate structures of the anterior segment including the cornea, the aqueous outflow channels, the iris, and the ciliary body (Fig. 12.1). The only type of IOL that has no direct contact with uveal tissues is a PCIOL implanted entirely within the lens capsular bag.

As posterior chamber lens implantation evolved, the type of fixation achieved in the early years depended largely on chance or on the surgeon's individual preference. In general, the loops were anchored in one of three ways:
1 both loops were placed in the ciliary region

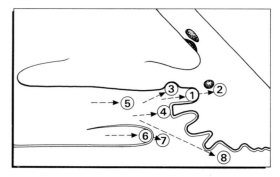

Fig. 12.1 Schematic illustration showing possible placement sites of PCIOL loops. *Site 1*: loop in the ciliary sulcus. *Site 2*: loop after erosion into the ciliary body stroma in the region of the major iris arterial circle. *Site 3*: loop in contact with the iris root. *Site 4*: loop attached to a ciliary process. *Site 5*: loop in aqueous without tissue contact (can cause windshield wiper syndrome because of inadequate fixation). *Site 6*: loop in the lens capsular bag. *Site 7*: loop ruptured through the lens capsular bag (a rare occurrence). *Site 8*: loop in the zonular region between the ciliary sulcus and the lens capsular bag. The loop may penetrate the zonules (zonular fixation) or extend as far posteriorly as the pars plana (pars plana fixation).

[5–13] (Plate 12.1 and Fig. 12.2). We now know from autopsy studies that true ciliary sulcus fixation of *both* loops was, and still is, achieved much less often than was previously assumed;
2 both loops were placed within the lens capsular bag. Capsular fixation evolved from the original work of Cornelius Binkhorst, who advocated and popularized the use of extracapsular cataract extraction (ECCE) used in conjunction with his two-loop iridocapsular IOL and its modifications (cited in [4]). In the early years of posterior chamber implantation

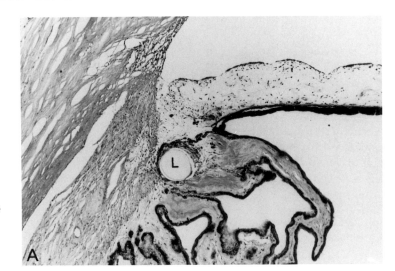

Fig. 12.2 Photomicrograph of an eye showing a loop (L) situated in the ciliary sulcus. The loop has migrated into the substance of the ciliary body stroma. (Hematoxylin and eosin stain; original magnification ×20.)

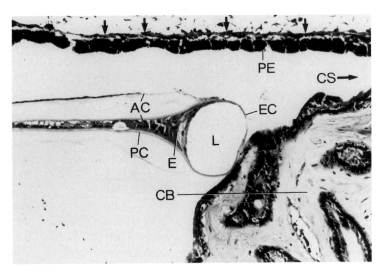

Fig. 12.3 Photomicrograph of a capsule-fixated PCIOL loop (L) in an autopsy eye. The intraocular lens was well tolerated and the patient had good visual acuity until the time of death. The loop (L) is firmly secured between the equatorial–posterior capsule (PC) and an abundant flap, rim or anterior capsule (AC). Note the artifacticious lamellar splitting of the anterior capsule that occurred during tissue processing. The ciliary sulcus (CS) is situated to the right. The dilator muscle of the iris (small arrows) is particularly clear in this picture. This muscle and the sphincter muscle are responsible for the constant movements of the pupil, one of the major factors in the pathogenesis of chafing defects. Note the residual lens epithelial (E) cells adjacent to the lens loop. Equatorial capsule (EC), posterior capsule (PC), ciliary (CB), and iris pigment epithelium (PE). (Hematoxylin and eosin stain; original magnification ×20.)

capsular or in-the-bag fixation (Plates 12.2 to 12.6 and Fig. 12.3) was intentionally performed by only a handful of surgeons, widespread use did not occur until the mid-1980s; or

3 one loop (usually the leading or inferior loop) was placed in the capsular bag and the other loop (usually the trailing or superior loop) was placed in a variety of locations *anterior* to the anterior capsular flap (Plate 12.7). This has been the most common type of fixation since the late

1970s when the flexible PCIOLs were intro- duced. Retrospective analysis of clinical cases, autopsy studies, and experience with animal implantations have shown that this asymmetric fixation occurs in most implantations when an IOL is simply inserted behind the iris, without specific intended placement of the loops. The direction of the IOL as it enters the posterior chamber is usually the deciding factor in deter- mining where the loop is fixated. The IOL passes through the pupil in an oblique fashion during the insertion process. Typically the leading or inferior loop passes into the equa- torial fornix of the capsular bag at 6 o'clock. Then, as the superior or trailing loop is in- serted, often without good visibility, the loop springs into a site behind the iris but anterior to the anterior capsular flap at 12 o'clock.

Another cause of asymmetric fixation is the "pea-pod" effect in which a loop exits from the capsular bag, either during intraoperative manipulations such as dialing, or postopera- tively. The major causes of "pea-podding" are the pressure of a radial tear in the anterior capsule or too scanty an anterior capsular flap after a large capsulectomy. An abundant anterior flap is necessary to secure permanently the loop in the equatorial fornix (Fig. 12. 3).

Since the introduction of viscoelastic agents, and with the trend toward smaller anterior capsulectomies that leave an adequate rim of anterior capsule to provide sufficient equatorial support for the loops, easier, more consistent and more permanent in-the-bag IOL placement is now possible.

In actuality, as Fig. 12.1 schematically illus- trates, there are several loop-fixation sites possible with modern flexible-loop PCIOLs. These fixation sites have been confirmed histologically by analyses of postmortem globes implanted with PCIOLs. When the loops fixate directly on the surface of the ciliary sulcus, they are secured in the angle formed by the junction of the posterior iris root and the anterior margin of the ciliary processes or pars plicata. This site is theoretically the ideal place- ment area for uveal fixation because a fibrous encapsulation around the loop often develops, enhancing fixation and preventing deep loop erosion into the ciliary body. However, fixation

of both IOL loops at this site is achieved in fewer than one in five cases [9,12].

The loops may migrate or erode through the ciliary epithelium and into the stromal tissues of the ciliary body. This is actually the most common form of uveal fixation. The loops may encroach upon or compress the major iris circle and other vessels in the ciliary vascular plexus. At times a loop may migrate through the ciliary body stroma, become embedded in the ciliary muscle, or may even come to rest on or near the supraciliary space adjacent to the sclera. When such a migration occurs, this may play a role in the pathogenesis of such lens malpositions (Plates 12.8 to 12.11) as the "sunrise syn- drome," particularly after asymmetric im- plantation of the IOL loops.

When both loops are secured in the lens capsular bag, one achieves the only type of fixation in which IOL contact with uveal tissues is avoided. Fixation of iris support, irido- capsular, anterior chamber, or uvea-fixated posterior chamber IOLs, by definition, implies direct contact of the loop or haptic with delicate ocular tissues.

If IOL loops are either intentionally or in- advertently placed in front of the capsular bag, as occurs in as many as 8% of cases [12], the loop may be positioned so that it is neither in the ciliary sulcus nor in the lens capsular bag. The loop may slide between these structures and become entangled in the zonules or may pass through the zonules to settle as far pos- teriorly as the pars plana (Plates 12.12 and 12.13). This may be clinically significant as a case of zonular rupture and lens decentration.

The multiple fixation sites shown in Fig. 12.1 which designate a loop that is placed anterior to the anterior capsular flap (sites 1–5 and 8 in Fig. 12.1) have led the authors to use not only the term sulcus fixation, but also the terms "uveal, ciliary, or ciliary region, zonular or pars plana fixation" to designate the placement site of any IOL placed in front of the anterior capsule. The more frequently used clinical term "ciliary sulcus fixation" is too often used in a general sense when the loops may be fixated behind the iris, anywhere in front of the ante- rior capsular flap. Simply placing the loops behind the iris and allowing them to land or settle where they may (termed "self-fixation" by S. Obstbaum, personal communication), can cause a needless complication. For example, the incidence of decentration caused by asymmetric loop fixation is clearly higher than in cases where symmetric fixation is accomplished [11,12,14].

The excellent success rate now achieved with PCIOL implantation is associated with improved IOL designs and improved surgical techniques, including meticulous placement of loops. Explanation of PCIOLs for a complication is now rarely required—particularly for well-implanted capsule-fixed IOLs.

From the earliest phases of our studies at the Center for Intraocular Lens Research in Charleston, South Carolina, on human eyes obtained postmortem with PCIOLs, evidence accumulated that capsular bag fixated IOLs demonstrated subtle but measurable advantages. For example, two major factors that we analyzed were decentration and posterior capsular opacification (PCO)—two complications that still remain (1989) relatively common complications of PCIOL surgery (Plates 12.8 to 12.13). These studies included our initial analyses in 1984–85 [5–7], a subsequent autopsy study on 75 eyes in 1986 [9–11], a study on 222 eyes in 1988 [12], and our most recent report on 425 eyes later in 1988 [13].

The various advantages of capsular bag fixation noted in our initial publications in 1984–85 [6,7] have been supported by our more recent observations in a much larger series of cases [4]. These advantages are summarized as follows:

1 positions the IOL in the proper anatomic site;

2 as easy to place both loops symmetrically in the capsular bag as in the ciliary sulcus;

3 intraoperative stretching or tearing of zonules by loop manipulations in front of the anterior capsular leaflet is avoided;

4 low incidence of lens decentration and dislocation;

5 no evidence of spontaneous lens dislocation into the vitreous cavity;

6 IOL is positioned a maximal distance behind the cornea;

7 IOL is positioned a maximal distance from the posterior iris pigment epithelium, iris root, and ciliary processes;

8 reduces postoperative pigment dispersion into the anterior chamber caused by iris chafing;

9 no direct contact by, or erosion of, IOL loops or haptics into ciliary body tissues;

10 avoids chronic uveal tissue chafing and reduces probability of long-term blood–aqueous barrier breakdown;

11 surface alteration of loop material is less likely;

12 safer for IOL implantation in children and young individuals;

13 may reduce posterior capsular opacification; and

14 easy to explant, if necessary.

At present we have accessioned approximately 1300 eyes obtained postmortem with all types of IOLs. Approximately two-thirds of these globes contained PCIOLs. We have recently reviewed and updated the clinico-pathologic data on these cases and have verified to our satisfaction the efficacy and the advantages of capsular bag fixation, particularly in terms of achieving optimal centration. In this chapter we provide several examples from our most recent series of accessioned cases to illustrate the impact that type of fixation may have in overall long-term IOL centration.

There are several causes of PCIOL decentration:

1 asymmetric loop insertion [12], one loop in the lens capsular bag, one loop in the ciliary region (sunrise syndrome or east–west syndrome) (Plates 12.7, 12.8, 12.12 and 12.13);

2 escape of a loop initially placed in the lens capsular bag, either intraoperatively, during rotation or dialing of the IOL, or postoperatively because of a too large anterior capsulectomy that does not leave enough anterior capsular flap to hold the lens in place (pea-pod effect);

3 sliding or slippage of a loop that is sandwiched between the iris and anterior capsular flap but not securely fixated in the ciliary sulcus (Plate 12.10);

4 perforation of a loop through the iris or displacement through an iridectomy;

5 optic migration during pupillary capture;

6 distorting or bending of a loop during insertion, usually during excessive flexion or pronation of the superior loop, causing a difference in loop length and subsequent asymmetric fixation. Permanent loop distortion is most likely to occur in three-piece IOLs with polypropylene loops that do not have memory retention qualities;

7 pressure or traction exerted on the loop and/or optical component of the IOL by proliferating residual lens epithelial cells and their derivatives. A fibrous or myoepithelial metaplasia of these cells produces a cicatricial contraction of the capsular bag. This phenomenon may be exacerbated by an asymmetric anterior capsulotomy;

8 loop disinsertion at the site where the loop is staked into the loop–optic junction; or

9 loop fracture.

It is important to minimize these complications by careful surgical technique and special attention to precise loop placement. Otherwise clinically significant signs and symptoms may occur. These may include undesirable visual complications such as glare, halo, monocular diplopia, or other visual aberrations. These may occur because of the presence of optic edges or other lens elements such as positioning holes within the pupillary aperture. It is well documented that these phenomena may be clinically significant [14]. Even in eyes in which postoperative vision is adequate—as determined by a Snellen visual acuity test—the subjective symptoms experienced by the patient may be troublesome. The symptoms may be exacerbated in conditions such as dim light when pupillary dilatation occurs [14].

The best means of decreasing such visual aberrations is to decrease the incidence of optic decentration by symmetric loop placement.

With the use of viscoelastic agents and a well-controlled anterior capsulectomy that leaves a large enough anterior capsular flap for good loop support, symmetric placement of both loops in the lens capsular bag is not difficult in most instances. As surgeons gain experience with various implantation techniques, including modern capsulorhexis procedures, a more carefully controlled operation is possible during all stages of IOL implantation. A traumatic removal of lens substance without damage to the capsular–zonular apparatus is possible, Behind-the-iris, uncontrolled, asymmetric implantation (one loop fixated in the capsule and the opposite loop in the ciliary region) may seem technically easier but the potential for intraoperative and postoperative complications is increased. Intraoperative tearing of zonules by loops that are manipulated or dialed in front of the anterior capsular flaps, as well as rupture through the zonules, can be avoided by placing the loops within the capsule.

Other means to address the problem of visual aberration caused by optic components in the pupil include increasing the effective optical zone of the optic by increasing the diameter of the optic, or eliminating or reducing the number of positioning holes.

Published studies have reported the diameter of the evacuated and crushed capsular bag to be approximately 10.3–10.8 mm. These measurements on crushed or flattened capsular bags are not totally relevant to in-the-bag IOL implantation. In most cases, the bag does not completely collapse and flatten to a larger diameter after ECCE. In general, a lens opened with a relatively small anterior capsulotomy—especially if done with a circular continuous tear capsulorhexis—retains its original shape and diameter. A large series of autopsy eyes with PCIOLs was analyzed, and the mean capsular bag diameter was 9.6 mm (standard deviation 0.4 mm) (S. Ohmi, personal communication). The diameter of the ciliary sulcus was 11 mm (standard deviation 0.5 mm).

The original Shearing PCIOL measured 12.5 mm in diameter, and it was not as flexible as today's modified J-loop and C-loop designs. If the lens was too small for the eye or if a loop eroded into the ciliary body, the IOL became decentered and "wind-shield wiper" syndrome and other undesirable IOL movements occurred. These problems prompted most lens designers to increase the total lens diameter. Most flexible-looped IOLs in current use measure from 13.75 to 14.5 mm in diameter. These IOLs were sized to ensure consistent ciliary region fixation, to provide a snug fit and thus prevent the IOL from dislocating. In general, when such IOLs are used with capsular fixation, the flexible loops must bend or crimp sufficiently to conform to the much smaller diameter of the capsular bag. The loop tip may even extend to the edge of or over the optic in such cases.

Most lenses designed specifically for in-the-bag placement, have a smaller total diameter (10.5–13 mm). As more surgeons now prefer capsular bag implantation, use of these smaller diameter IOLs has increased. It is likely that this trend will help reduce the incidence of problems associated with severe bending and crimping of lens loops, capsular distortion, and the spring effect that can occur when the loop is exposed to contractile forces within the capsular bag.

Park *et al.* [10] examined autopsy eyes to determine the configuration of the posterior chamber lens loops within the ciliary sulcus region and within the capsular sac. In general, the final configuration of the lens loops of all IOL styles assumed a C-shape that conformed to the circular capsule. There was significant compression and bending of J-loop or modified J-loop loops (Plates 12.2 and 12.3). The distal portion of J-loop or modified J-loop IOLs frequently exerted a one-directional force that caused stretching and ovaling of the capsular sac. This resulted in the formation of folds or striae parallel to the long axis of the lens. These changes may occasionally cause such clinically significant problems as glare or a Maddox-rod effect.

There is now a definite trend among manufacturers to produce lenses with more C-shaped or rounded loops (Plates 12.4 to 12.6). These subtle modifications are adaptations of the original Simcoe C-loop and variations of the original Sinskey and Kratz designs. Modified or short C-loop lenses are now widely used because surgeons find these IOLs easy to insert and the loops conform to the circular shape of the capsular sac.

Posterior capsular opacification (Elschnig pearls, or so-called secondary cataract) is a significant postoperative complication [4]. Evidence is accumulating that placement of a well-designed posterior chamber lens in the lens capsular sac provides a gentle but taut radial stretch on the posterior capsule [15,16].

The original Anis IOL was designed to create a symmetric radial stretch on the capsule. Similar disc-like prototype IOLs have been tested also to achieve this goal [16]. Of the present open-loop flexible IOLs, the one-piece, all-PMMA (polymethylmetacrylate), posterior chamber designs appear to be especially effective in providing a symmetric stretch. This may aid in minimizing posterior capsular opacification by reducing the folds in the capsular sac and holding the posterior capsule firmly against the posterior surface of the IOL optic. This is sometimes termed the "no space, no cells" concept [4]. If IOL loops are placed in front of the anterior capsule, i.e. if the loops are not in place to expand or stretch the capsule at the equatorial fornix, there is no mechanical means to prevent shrinkage and/or corrugation of the capsule. In such cases, as the bag shrinks, traction on the zonules with stretching or rupture may occur.

Regardless of the IOL style used and independent of the subtleties of any surgical techniques, there are two vital tools available to surgeons today that make precise loop or haptic placement possible. First, the introduction of Healon in the early 1980s provided a new horizon to intraocular surgery (visco surgery). This was the most important breakthrough in IOL implantation surgery since the introduction of flexible J-loop and C-loop posterior chamber IOLs in the mid-1970s. The tissue-protective properties of viscoelastic agents give a surgeon the ability to move and manipulate the tissues of the eye, to control the configuration of the various chambers and structures of the eye during surgery, and to insert the IOL more easily into the desired location. Second, attention to the size, shape, and quality of the anterior capsulotomy can enhance one's ability to achieve optimal haptic placement. The intercapsular technique [17] as well as the recently popularized technique of the circular continuous tear capsulorhexis [18] (at present used mostly by phacoemulsification surgeons) greatly increase the facility to achieve accurate and permanent loop placement.

We have emphasized that precise, symmetric placement of PCIOL loops or haptics in the desired location is important. Although lens capsular bag implantation of PCIOLs is aesthetically desirable and certainly physiologically more appropriate, one should not in any way construe this discussion as an exhortation for in-the-bag placement in every case. Ciliary or sulcus fixation has provided excellent clinical results for a long time. As we previously stated, "sulcus fixation is good but in-the-bag implantation is better" [19].

Acknowledgments

Emily Hindman typed and edited the manuscript. Sandra Brown and Catherine Barry assisted in preparation of the photographs. Supported in part by an unrestricted grant from Research to Prevent Blindness, Inc., New York.

References

1 Ridley H. Intra-ocular acrylic lenses. *Trans Ophthalmol Soc UK* 1951; **71**: 617–21.

2 Pearce JL. Pearce-style posterior chamber lenses. *J Am Intraocul Implant Soc* 1980; **6**: 33–6.

3 Shearing SP. Evolution of the posterior chamber intraocular lens. *J Am Intraocul Implant Soc* 1984; **10**: 343–6.

4 Apple DJ, Kincaid MC, Mamalis N, Olson RJ. *Intraocular Lenses. Evolution, Designs, Complications and Pathology*. Baltimore: Williams and Wilkins, 1989.

5 Apple DJ, Gieser SC, Isenberg RA. *Evolution of Intraocular Lenses*. Salt Lake City: University of Utah Printing Service, 1985.

6 Apple DJ, Mamalis N, Loftfield K et al. Complications of intraocular lenses. A historical and histopathological review. *Surv Ophthalmol* 1984; **29**: 1–54.

7 Apple DF, Reidy JJ, Googe JM et al. A comparison of ciliary sulcus and capsular bag fixation of posterior chamber intraocular lenses. *J Am Intraocul Implant Soc* 1985; **11**: 44–63.

8 Apple DF, Cameron JD, Lindstrom RL. Loop fixation of posterior chamber intraocular lenses. *Cataract* 1984; **2**: 7–10.

9 Apple DJ, Park SB, Merkley KH et al. Posterior chamber intraocular lenses in a series of 75 autopsy eyes. Part I: Loop location. *J Cataract Refract Surg* 1986; **12**: 358–62.

10 Park SB, Brems RN, Parsons MR et al. Posterior chamber intraocular lenses in a series of 75 autopsy eyes. Part II: Postimplantation loop configuration. *J Cataract Refract Surg* 1986; **12**: 363–6.

11 Brems RN, Apple DJ, Pfeffer BR, Park SB, Piest KL, Isenberg RA. Posterior chamber intraocular lenses in a series of 75 autopsy eyes. Part III: Correlation of positioning holes and optic edges with the pupillary aperture and visual axis. *J Cataract Refract Surg* 1986; **12**: 367–71.

12 Hansen SO, Tetz MR, Solomon KD et al. Decentration of flexible loop posterior chamber intraocular lenses in a series of 222 postmortem eyes. *Ophthalmology* 1988; **95**: 344–9.

13 Gwin TD, Apple DJ. *A study of posterior chamber intraocular lens fixation and loop configuration: An analysis of 425 eyes obtained postmortem*. Presented at the American Society of Cataract and Refractive Surgery Meeting, Los Angeles, California, March 27, 1988.

14 Apple DJ, Lichtenstein SB, Heerlein K et al. Visual aberrations caused by optic components of posterior chamber intraocular lenses. *J Cataract Refract Surg* 1987; **13**: 431–5.

15 Hansen SO, Solomon KD, McKnight GT et al. Posterior capsular opacification and intraocular lens decentration. Part I: Comparison of various posterior chamber lens designs implanted in the rabbit model. *J Cataract Refract Surg* 1988; **14**: 605–14.

16 Tetz MR, O'Morchoe DJC, Gwin TD et al. Posterior capsular opacification and intraocular lens decentration. Part II: Experimental findings on a prototype circular IOL design. *J Cataract Refract Surg* 1988; **14**: 614–23.

17 Baikoff G, Colin J, Sourdille PH. Technique d'implantation extra-capsulaire (English abstract). *Bull Soc Ophthalmol Fr* 1979; **79**: 901–2.

18 Neuhann T. Theorie und Operationstechnik der Kapsulorhexis. *Klin Monatsbl Augenheilkd* 1987; **190**: 542–5.

19 Apple DJ. Intraocular lenses: Notes from an interested observer (special article). *Arch Ophthalmol* 1986; **104**: 1150–2.

13: Anesthesia for Cataract Surgery

LEE HOFFER

Introduction

Restoration of satisfactory vision is a major concern for individuals suffering from the formation of cataracts. Their quest for resolution of this visual impairment is often associated with a deep-seated anxiety, more so if they are still active and independent. Their anxiety is also increased if a spouse or other individual(s) is dependent upon them, or if vision is impaired in the other eye. In addition to anxiety, the effects of the normal aging process must also be considered since more than 90% of patients undergoing cataract surgery are 50 years of age or older. A discussion of the physiology of aging and the concurrent anesthesia-related problems is beyond the scope of this chapter. There are good discussions on this topic in most current textbooks of anesthesiology. In addition, several multi-author monographs and a recent refresher course are also available (see [1–5]).

In the last decade, there have been numerous changes in cataract surgery. Many factors have influenced these changes including:
1 an increase in the geriatric population;
2 improvements in the quality of lenses;
3 refinements in the surgical procedures;
4 alterations in health care expenditures including major reductions in Medicare reimbursements;
5 advancements in anesthesia care; and
6 the marked rise in ambulatory surgery.

In the USA 30–50% of all surgical procedures are currently performed on an ambulatory basis, and it is predicted that during the decade of the 1990s this will rise to 60–70%. Ambulatory surgery is done in a variety of clinical settings that range from hospital based to completely independent and free-standing centers [6–7].

In addition, some ophthalmologists perform cataract surgery in their office suites. However, patient safety may be severely compromised in such situations because monitoring and resuscitative equipment is frequently inadequate, and a full complement of emergency drugs and equipment is seldom available. Ancillary medical personnel are usually not trained in the Advanced Cardiac Life Support (ACLS) Program or the management of medical crises which often compounds any associated perioperative complications. Such crises may include respiratory distress, cardiac arrest, acute hypertension, diabetic coma, aspiration, or hyperthermia.

In the USA most cataract surgery is performed on an ambulatory basis. To provide optimal care in an ambulatory center, several key factors are vital:
1 the medical and nursing staff and other personnel must function as a well-coordinated, efficient, health care team;
2 the patient should sense that all of the personnel are interested in him or her as a person and that the care rendered is individualized;
3 the surgical schedule should proceed as planned;
4 the ophthalmologist's skills should not be compromised by fatigue or other factors;
5 the patient's anxiety and other concerns should be handled in a personalized manner; and
6 the anesthesia care must be individualized

for the patient and his or her unique medical problems.

In our institution, the vast majority of cataract procedures are performed at a full-service, free-standing ambulatory surgery center located approximately 8 km (5 miles) from the main hospital. Anesthesia services at both facilities are provided by the same anesthesia group. Patients with severe or unstable medical problems are scheduled at an area hospital. In addition, the ophthalmologists and other surgeons maintain privileges at the ambulatory center as well as one or more of the area hospitals.

Preoperative evaluation and preparation

Since cataract surgery is an elective procedure, there is usually ample time to evaluate the patient properly prior to surgery. At our center, the patient is scheduled for a preoperative visit 2–5 days prior to the procedure. Generally, the patient has a brief history and physical examination form (Fig. 13.1) completed by the patient's family physician before this visit.

During the preoperative visit, staff nurses interview the patient, discuss the sequence of events on the day of surgery, and give the patient a booklet and written instructions to take home. The patient also completes a preoperative questionnaire (Fig. 13.2). The patient is then evaluated by an anesthesia provider, and appropriate laboratory tests and diagnostic studies are obtained before the patient leaves the center.

The anesthesia evaluation includes a review of:

1 any drugs, foods, or substances to which the patient may be allergic;
2 current medications;
3 previous surgical procedures and significant hospitalizations;
4 any history of anesthetic problems encountered by the patient or a blood relative;
5 any dysfunction in major physiologic systems and current medical problems;
6 social habits such as ethanol, tobacco, or other substance abuse;

7 exercise, physical activity, and stress tolerance; and
8 the results of previous laboratory and diagnostic studies which may be available.

A brief physical examination may also be done as indicated. This information is noted on the top of the anesthesia record (Fig. 13.3). The primary objective of this preoperative evaluation is to optimize the patient's medical and physiologic condition and to help alleviate any anxiety the patient may have concerning surgery and anesthesia. The preoperative visit and anesthesia evaluation minimizes cancellations on the day of surgery and the resultant frustrations for everyone involved.

Because of various logistic problems at different institutions, some anesthesiologists conduct the preoperative evaluation immediately prior to surgery; interview the patient via telephone; make a preoperative appointment for the patient at the anesthesiologist's office; or rely on a review of questionnaires which the patient and the family physician have mailed to the center prior to the date for the procedure.

Many patients scheduled for cataract surgery are older and may have one or more coexisting disease(s) such as hypertension, diabetes mellitus, athrosclerotic cardiovascular disease, chronic pulmonary disease, and musculoskeletal problems such as arthritis. Medical management of these diseases often includes the administration of multiple medications exclusive of the ophthalmologic preparations. It is therefore imperative that the anesthesiologist review all medications prior to surgery if untoward drug interactions are to be avoided.

Also prior to surgery a physical status (PS) classification is assigned to each patient by the anesthesiologist. This classification system was established by the American Society of Anesthesiologists in 1963 and is an assessment of the relative risk for surgery and anesthesia care. A PS 1 denotes a normal healthy patient; PS 2 is a patient with mild systemic disease; PS 3 is a patient with a severe, systemic disease that limits activity but is not incapacitating; PS 4 is a patient with an incapacitating systemic disease that is a constant threat to life; and PS 5 is a moribund patient not expected to survive 24 h with or without the operation. Since the

AULTMAN CENTER FOR
ONE DAY SURGERY
CANTON, OHIO
HISTORY & PHYSICAL

Patient's Name _____

Procedure Planned _____ Procedure Date _____

1 **Disease History:** Do you have or have you had any of the following/If *none* please mark:

Lung
( ) Bronchitis
( ) Emphysema
( ) Asthma
( ) TB

( ) Sinusitis
( ) Recent Cold or
    Respiratory Infection
( ) *None*

Vascular
( ) High Blood Pressure
( ) Heart Attack
( ) Heart Murmur
( ) Circulation Problem
( ) Heart Disease

( ) Sicklecell
( ) Bleeding Problems
( ) *None*

Systemic
( ) Convulsions
( ) Glaucoma
( ) Hepatitis
( ) Fainting
( ) *None*

( ) Diabetes
( ) Glandular Trouble
( ) Kidney or Bladder Problems
( ) Alcohol
( ) Stomach or Bowel Problems

2 **Drug History:** In the last six months have you taken any of the following drugs/If *none* please mark:

( ) Steroids
( ) Aspirin
( ) Insulin
( ) Oral Diabetes

( ) Birth Control Pills
( ) Tranquilizers
( ) Thyroid
( ) None

( ) Antibiotics
( ) Narcotics
( ) Heart Medication
( ) SPECIFY "YES" ANSWERS or any other medications: _____

( ) Anti-Coagulants (blood thinners)
( ) Arthritis or Joint Medicine
( ) Blood Pressure Medicine

3 **Personal History**
Present Illness/Why are you having surgery: _____

Yes No
( ) ( ) Allergies/Specify _____
           Type of Reaction _____
( ) ( ) Physical Limitation/Explanation: _____
( ) ( ) Previous Hospitalizations/Where _____ When _____
           Reason _____
( ) ( ) Previous Surgery/Where _____ When _____
           Type _____
( ) ( ) Previous Anesthesia/Type_____ Complications_____

4 **Females Only**
Last menstrual period/Date_____ IUD (intrauterine device) Yes ( ) No ( )
Have you ever been pregnant/ Yes ( ) No ( ) Now ( ) # of children _____ # of miscarriages _____

5 **Physical Examination:**
H.E.E.N.T.:   Abnormal Findings:

Heart:

Lungs: Impression:

Abdomen:

Signature and Date of examination _____

ONLY IF INDICATED:

If History and Physical examination performed more than seven (7) days prior to surgery:

( ) Patient's condition unchanged and may proceed with proposed surgery.

( ) Patient's condition has changed/Specify _____

Signature and Date _____

Form No. 1   8/89

Fig. 13.1 Typical history and physical examination form.

**AULTMAN CENTER
FOR ONE DAY SURGERY
CANTON, OHIO**

**PREOPERATIVE
QUESTIONNAIRE**

Check "YES" or "NO" and fill in the answers as best you can. There will be opportunity to discuss your answers with a member of the Anesthesia Care Team.

YES NO

☐ ☐ 1. Have you ever received anesthesia before? (include numbing medicine)

☐ ☐ 2. Did you ever have a problem with anesthesia? If so, what was the problem? _____

_____

☐ ☐ 3. Have you had a yellow jaundice or a fever after anesthesia?

☐ ☐ 4. Has any blood relative of yours had problems with anesthesia?

☐ ☐ 5. Are you allergic to anything? If yes, what?_____

☐ ☐ 6. Do you smoke? If yes, how much a day? _____ No. of Years? _____

☐ ☐ 7. Do you drink alcohol? If yes, how many drinks a day? _____

☐ ☐ 8. Did you ever take a drug for fun? If yes, what? _____ How often? _____

☐ ☐ 9. Have you ever been treated in a drug or alcohol detoxification program?

☐ ☐ 10. Are you taking medicine at home? If yes, what? (Include eye drops, over-the-counter medicine, prescriptions) _____

☐ ☐ 11. (a.) Have you ever had a blood transfusion?

☐ ☐ (b.) If yes, did you have a problem with it? If yes, what? _____

☐ ☐ 12. If you are a woman, do you think you are pregnant?

☐ ☐ 13. Do you feel comfortable with having your operation and going home the same day?

☐ ☐ 14. Have you or your child been exposed to **any** communicable diseases in the last 21 days? (ex.: measles, chickenpox, strep throat, etc.)

Place a checkmark **before** each of the following that you **have ever had:**

☐ heart failure   ☐ asthma   ☐ stomach ulcers   ☐ muscle weakness or paralysis

☐ high blood pressure   ☐ frequent bronchitis   ☐ hiatus hernia   ☐ muscle cramps

☐ irregular heart beats   ☐ pneumonia   ☐ frequent indigestion   ☐ numbness

☐ heart attack   ☐ emphysema   ☐ hepatitis or yellow jaundice   ☐ convulsions or epilepsy

☐ chest pain or angina   ☐ chronic cough   ☐ thyroid trouble or goiter ☐ kidney disease or nephritis

☐ heart murmur   ☐ fainting spells   ☐ diabetes   ☐ back trouble or broken back

☐ unexplained shortness of breath   ☐ bleeding tendencies   ☐ unexplained weight loss   ☐ mental health problem

☐ varicose veins   ☐ limited movement in any joints

Is there anything that has **not** been asked that you think we should know about you? ☐ Yes ☐ No

If yes, what? _____

_____

_____

| DATE | PATIENT OR GUARDIAN SIGNATURE | RELATIONSHIP IF NOT PT. | THIS SPACE FOR OFFICE USE ONLY |
| | | | DATE REVIEWED   INTERVIEWER |

FORM NO. 19 11/84

Fig. 13.2 Preoperative questionnaire.

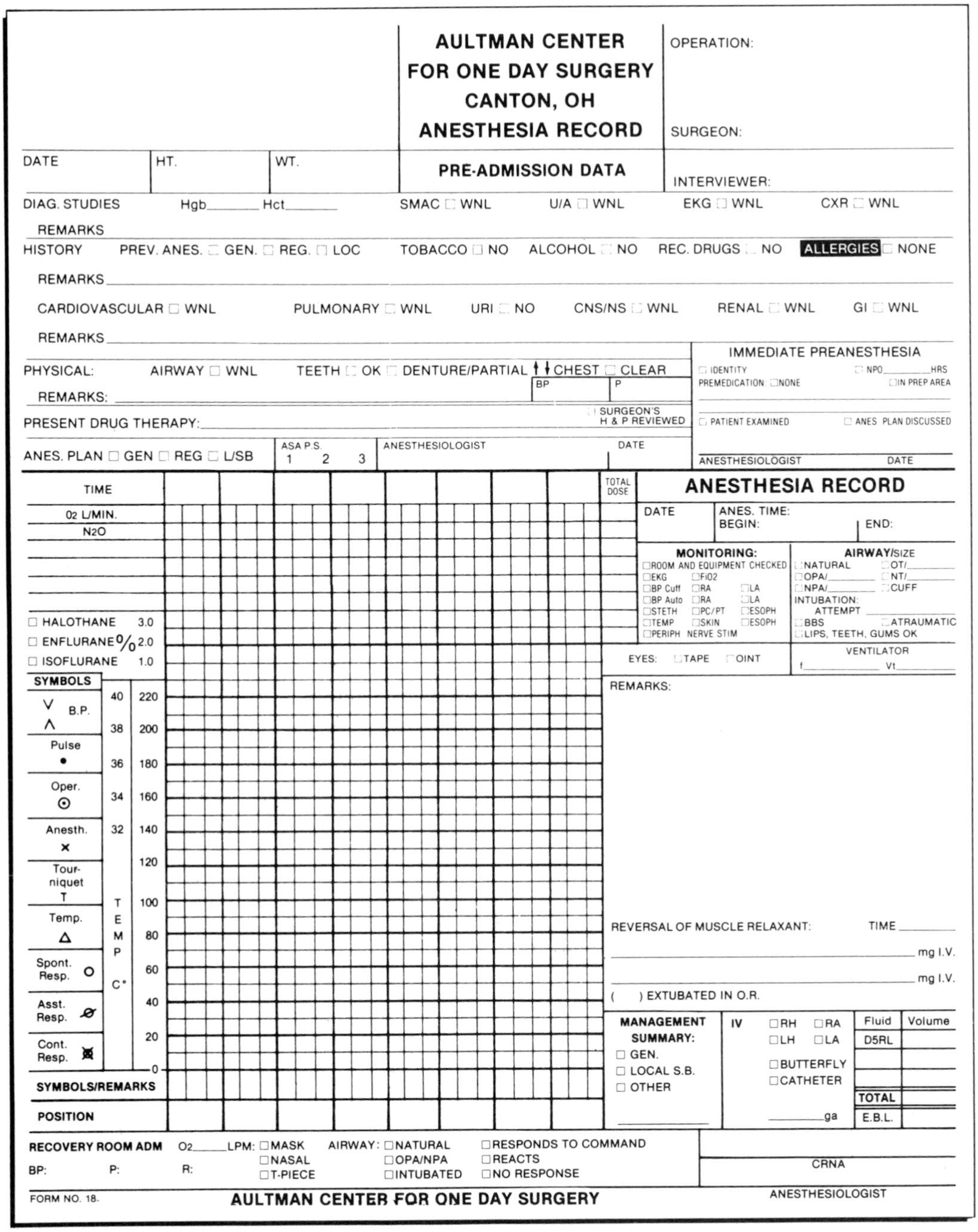

AULTMAN CENTER FOR ONE DAY SURGERY CANTON, OH ANESTHESIA RECORD

OPERATION:

SURGEON:

PRE-ADMISSION DATA

INTERVIEWER:

DATE | HT. | WT.

DIAG. STUDIES   Hgb_____ Hct_____   SMAC ☐ WNL   U/A ☐ WNL   EKG ☐ WNL   CXR ☐ WNL

REMARKS

HISTORY   PREV. ANES. ☐ GEN. ☐ REG. ☐ LOC   TOBACCO ☐ NO   ALCOHOL ☐ NO   REC. DRUGS ☐ NO   **ALLERGIES** ☐ NONE

REMARKS_____

CARDIOVASCULAR ☐ WNL   PULMONARY ☐ WNL   URI ☐ NO   CNS/NS ☐ WNL   RENAL ☐ WNL   GI ☐ WNL

REMARKS_____

PHYSICAL: AIRWAY ☐ WNL   TEETH ☐ OK ☐ DENTURE/PARTIAL ↑↓ CHEST ☐ CLEAR

REMARKS:

PRESENT DRUG THERAPY:_____

BP | P

IMMEDIATE PREANESTHESIA
☐ IDENTITY   ☐ NPO_____ HRS
PREMEDICATION: ☐ NONE   ☐ IN PREP AREA

SURGEON'S H & P REVIEWED

☐ PATIENT EXAMINED   ☐ ANES. PLAN DISCUSSED

ANES. PLAN ☐ GEN ☐ REG ☐ L/SB   ASA P.S. 1 2 3   ANESTHESIOLOGIST   DATE

ANESTHESIOLOGIST   DATE

TIME

TOTAL DOSE

ANESTHESIA RECORD

O2 L/MIN.

N2O

DATE | ANES. TIME: BEGIN: | END:

☐ HALOTHANE   3.0
☐ ENFLURANE %   2.0
☐ ISOFLURANE   1.0

MONITORING:
☐ ROOM AND EQUIPMENT CHECKED
☐ EKG
☐ BP Cuff   ☐ RA   ☐ LA
☐ BP Auto   ☐ RA   ☐ LA
☐ STETH   ☐ PC/PT   ☐ ESOPH
☐ TEMP   ☐ SKIN   ☐ ESOPH
☐ PERIPH NERVE STIM

AIRWAY/SIZE
☐ NATURAL   ☐ OT/_____
☐ FIO2   ☐ NT/_____
☐ OPA/_____
☐ NPA/_____   ☐ CUFF
INTUBATION:
ATTEMPT
☐ BBS   ☐ ATRAUMATIC
☐ LIPS, TEETH, GUMS OK

EYES: ☐ TAPE   ☐ OINT

VENTILATOR
f_____   Vt

SYMBOLS

V / ∧ B.P.
Pulse •
Oper. ⊙
Anesth. ×
Tourniquet T
Temp. △
Spont. Resp. O
Asst. Resp. ⌀
Cont. Resp. ⌀

40 220
38 200
36 180
34 160
32 140
120
T 100
E
M 80
P 60
C° 40
20
0

REMARKS:

REVERSAL OF MUSCLE RELAXANT: TIME_____

_____ mg I.V.
_____ mg I.V.

(   ) EXTUBATED IN O.R.

SYMBOLS/REMARKS

POSITION

MANAGEMENT SUMMARY:
☐ GEN.
☐ LOCAL S.B.
☐ OTHER

IV   ☐ RH   ☐ RA
☐ LH   ☐ LA
☐ BUTTERFLY
☐ CATHETER
_____ ga

Fluid | Volume
D5RL |

TOTAL
E.B.L.

RECOVERY ROOM ADM   O2_____LPM: ☐ MASK   AIRWAY: ☐ NATURAL   ☐ RESPONDS TO COMMAND
☐ NASAL   ☐ OPA/NPA   ☐ REACTS
BP: P: R: ☐ T-PIECE   ☐ INTUBATED   ☐ NO RESPONSE

CRNA

FORM NO. 18.   **AULTMAN CENTER FOR ONE DAY SURGERY**   ANESTHESIOLOGIST

Fig. 13.3 Anesthesia record.

assignment of a physical status classification is a clinical judgement by the anesthesiologist, there may be some variation between different anesthesiologists. The majority of elderly patients scheduled for cataract surgery who have significant coexisting diseases are usually classified as either a PS 3 or PS 4. Essentially all of the ambulatory surgery centers in the USA will accept PS 1, 2, 3, and "selected PS 4" patients. The "selected PS 4" indicates that a patient may, for example, have severe ischemic heart disease that is stable with mild exertion and routine daily activity or may have severe pulmonary disease that requires periodic supplemental oxygen. Such selected patients usually tolerate cataract surgery performed under regional anesthesia with a minimum of difficulty. Obviously, if these same patients are medically unstable, then they should be stabilized first or the procedure should be performed in a hospital facility where more extensive support capabilities are readily available.

During the preoperative visit, patients are instructed to avoid oral intake after midnight on the evening preceding surgery. If the procedure is scheduled later in the afternoon, they may be allowed to have a clear liquid breakfast. Patients are generally instructed to take their usual morning doses of antihypertensive, cardiovascular, pulmonary, and other significant medications on the morning of surgery. Diuretics are usually withheld the morning of surgery because of the logistic difficulties involved with frequent perioperative urination and to avoid the intraoperative problems associated with the relative hypovolemia.

Patients with diabetes mellitus should be scheduled as early as feasible in the morning. If they are maintained on oral medications few problems are experienced, though oral medications are withheld on the morning of surgery. For those individuals who are insulin dependent, a variety of perioperative management plans have been suggested. The primary goal is to maintain the blood glucose in the approximate range of 100–200 mg/dl. The effects on different organ systems and the perioperative management of diabetic patients was recently reviewed by Ammon [8]. At our center, the patient is instructed to withhold their morning dose of insulin and to bring their insulin with them to the center. The blood glucose is checked when the intravenous catheter is inserted, and based on the blood glucose level, one-half to two-thirds of their usual morning dose of insulin is given. Having the patient use their own insulin decreases the risk of errors and minimizes any variation from different sources of insulin. At the discretion of the anesthesiologist, the

intravenous solution may or may not contain glucose. After surgery, blood glucose is usually checked when the patient arrives in the postanesthesia care unit (PACU) and it is often repeated prior to discharge from the center.

Patients with coronary artery disease or a history of a recent myocardial infarction are of particular concern for any surgical procedure. Several studies have shown that approximately 50% of patients over 65 years of age have significant coronary artery disease. The classic studies of Goldman [9] identified a number of conditions which increase the risk of perioperative cardiac problems. Steen [10], Rao [11], and others evaluated the risk of perioperative reinfarction in patients with a history of a recent myocardial infarction. If surgery was performed within 3 months after the infarction, the risk of perioperative reinfarction range from 5.7 to 37%. For surgery performed 3–6 months after the infarction, this risk decreased to 2.3–16%. For 6 months or more after the initial insult, the incidence of perioperative reinfarction was 5–6%. If a perioperative reinfarction occurred, the mortality was greater than 50%. Without a prior history of myocardial infarction, the risk of perioperative myocardial infarction is approximately 0.13% in patients undergoing a similar operation.

Several studies, however, seem to indicate that ophthalmic procedures do not carry the same risk of morbidity or mortality as other surgical procedures although a direct correlation is difficult because of the variations in the patient's physical status, choice of local or general anesthesia, and the type of surgery. Backer et al. [12] retrospectively reviewed 10 278 ophthalmic procedures and found that the reinfarction rate with local anesthesia was less than for other procedures under general anesthesia. Older studies indicated similar results. Lang [13] analyzed 14 889 ophthalmic cases over a 2-year period (1977–79) and found only two deaths (unrelated to anesthesia or surgery) within 48 h of the procedure. In addition, Snow and Sensel [14] and Lynch et al. [15] reviewed the morbidity and mortality of local versus general anesthesia for cataract surgery and found no significant differences except that nausea and vomiting occurred more frequently in the patients who had general anesthesia. In older studies, Breslin [16] reviewed the mortality associated with all ophthalmic procedures reported for the period from 1931 to 1971. Some of these reports included perioperative periods up to 30 days after surgery. The overall death rate per 1000 varied from 0.62 to 3.95. Myocardial infarctions and pulmonary embolisms were major causes of death. However, this data cannot be easily compared to current procedures because of significant improvements in the procedure, perioperative care, prophylactic use of antibiotics, and anesthesia care. In summary, there seems to be less morbidity and mortality associated with ophthalmic procedures than with other surgical procedures.

At the conclusion of the anesthesia preoperative evaluation, the anesthesiologist may consider the use of preoperative medications such as sedatives, H_2-antagonists, or gastrokinetic agents. Most anesthesiologists do not routinely prescribe preoperative sedation for ambulatory patients, but on an individual basis intravenous medications such as fentanyl or midazolam may be given after the patient arrives at the facility.

Selection of anesthesia

Anesthetic objectives for cataract surgery include safety, adequate analgesia, prevention of untoward changes in intraocular pressure, blunting of the oculocardiac reflex, appropriate perioperative monitoring, awareness and management of potential drug interactions, and avoidance of perioperative coughing, vomiting, or retching.

It is estimated that more than 95% of adult cataract procedures in the USA are currently done with regional (or local) anesthesia as opposed to general anesthesia. In contrast, Adams [17] states than general anesthesia is popular for cataract surgery in the UK. General anesthesia does offer several advantages as it eliminates the apprehension about being awake during the procedure, and it allows a relaxed atmosphere for the surgeon with minimal

time constraints. In addition, it negates the difficulties that patients with respiratory or cardiovascular disease may have in lying supine for prolonged periods of time. However, with general anesthesia there is a greater incidence of postoperative nausea and vomiting as well as a prolonged recovery time.

The selection of anesthesia is made by the anesthesiologist on an individual basis after careful consideration of various factors. These factors include:

1 the patient's preference;
2 the patient's ability to cooperate (e.g. a language barrier or previous neurologic problems);
3 conditions such as a severe chronic cough that cannot be controlled and may create major intraoperative problems for the operating surgeon;
4 the inability to assume a suitable recumbent position for the procedure;
5 unique requirements of the ophthalmologist; and
6 age of the patient. (Regional anesthesia may be precluded in most pediatric patients because of decreased cooperation during the procedure.)

General anesthesia

As noted above, general anesthesia is employed less frequently than regional anesthesia. If selected, a variety of anesthetic techniques have been utilized with good success. Neuromuscular blockade is required for intubation of the trachea and may be continued throughout the procedure. A curved oral RAE endotracheal tube maximizes surgical access and minimizes the risk of kinking the endotracheal tube. Anesthesia can be maintained with halogenated agents, nitrous oxide and narcotics, intravenous infusions, or a combination of these techniques. A smooth emergence from general anesthesia is important to minimize the risk of coughing, vomiting, or retching with a resultant potential for ocular damage. At the end of the procedure, intravenous lidocaine (1.5 mg/kg) is frequently used and the patient is extubated at a deep plane of anesthesia to minimize these risks.

Regional anesthesia

There are a variety of retrobulbar, peribulbar, and infiltration techniques in use today that fit in the category of regional anesthesia. Specific details of these techniques are adequately described in textbooks of ophthalmology and anesthesiology. Usually a mixture of drugs is employed to obtain the desired effects. Combinations of lidocaine and bupivicaine contribute to the speed and duration of the block; epinephrine (1:100000) may be added for localized vasoconstriction and prolongation of the block; and hyaluronidase may be used to facilitate localized spread of the anesthetic. Typical mixtures include: lidocaine 2% with epinephrine 1:100000 and 150 U of hyaluronidase; or lidocaine 2%, bupivacaine 0.75% (1:1 ratio) with epinephrine 1:100000 and 150 U hyaluronidase. Approximately 8 ml is used. The ophthalmologist usually administers the anesthetic block, although in some facilities it is done by the anesthesiologist in the preoperative area preceding the cataract procedure. In our center, the regional block is performed by the ophthalmologist in the operating room prior to final positioning and surgical preparation. This ensures that appropriate monitoring and anesthesia equipment as well as emergency drugs, equipment, and personnel are immediately available should any untoward complications occur.

Most of the local anesthetic effects are resolving by the time the patient is discharged from the facility (1–1.5 h following completion of the procedure). It is felt that this practice optimizes the patient's safety because it minimizes the duration of the block, and decreases the risk of corneal abrasion or damage postoperatively. In addition, this reduces the patient's discomfort from a prolonged block.

Many anesthesiologists provide some intravenous sedation during the administration of regional anesthesia. We have seen a large number of patients who have had one cataract procedure performed elsewhere and received no concurrent sedation or may have had some preoperative medication such as meperidine or diazepam. Nearly all of these patients stated that the pain and discomfort of the block was the most terrifying and unpleasant aspect of the whole procedure. Therefore, it is felt that concurrent intravenous sedation of short duration is a critical aspect of good patient care. The objectives of this sedation are:

1 a safe, repeatable, and easily titratable technique;
2 total amnesia for administration of the regional block;
3 no movement by the patient;
4 little obtundation of the patient's cardiovascular and respiratory systems;
5 a rapid onset;
6 a short duration of effect;
7 no discomfort on injection;
8 minimal side effects or interactions with other drugs; and
9 a fairly distinct endpoint as to when the local anesthetic can be injected.

Several agents have been employed for sedation. Thiopental, diazepam, or midazolam can be used, but they do not always have a well-defined endpoint, and depressant effects on the central nervous, cardiovascular, and respiratory systems are more pronounced and variable. In addition, the residual effects are prolonged. Current studies are being conducted with a new anesthetic agent propofol (Diprivan), and initial reports are quite promising.

We have found that methohexital comes close to satisfying all the objectives listed above. Some patients may experience a mild burning sensation with injection, but a small dose of lidocaine preceding the methohexital will usually obtund this discomfort. Hiccups and coughing can occur with large doses of methohexital, particularly if injected rapidly, but this has rarely been a problem in the dose range employed.

The technique that works very well at our center is as follows: the initial dose to be given depends upon the age and clinical status of the patient. For a healthy patient below 60 years of age, 0.5–0.6 mg/kg is used; 0.4 mg/kg from 60–75 years; and 0.3 mg/kg for patients over 75 years of age. The dose is reduced for patients with significant coexisting diseases. If additional methohexital is required, it is titrated in 5 or 10 mg increments depending upon the age and status of the patient. The slower circulation time of the geriatric patient must also be considered in the speed of onset.

When the patient is in the operating room and the necessary positioning, baseline vital signs, monitoring, and preparation are complete, the flow rate of the intravenous fluid is increased. Then the initial dose of methohexital is slowly injected i.v. as close to the patient as possible to optimize the onset of the effects. Usually patients are not told that "they are going to sleep now."

As the injection is begun, the patient is asked a series of questions by the anesthesiologist. It is important that these questions relate to basic information that require no concentration or thought by the patient. Each subsequent question is usually based upon the patient's reply. This seems to provide an easy transition as the loss of consciousness occurs. A typical sequence of questions is: Where are you from? Were you born there (or here)? (Most patients were born outside of the town where they now reside.) How long did you live there before you moved? Do you have any children? Where do they live? Do you have any grandchildren (or great-children)? How many are boys or girls? Questions about where they work (or previously worked) are also useful.

We have found that the time from the start of injection of methohexital until the patient no longer responds to a question is about 35–65 s. When no verbal response can be elicited, this is usually a good endpoint where the patient will

not move or respond to the block. Additional increments are given if needed. Occasionally, a patient may respond during the block, but the amnesia provided by the methohexital is profound enough so that the patient has no recall.

Our studies have shown that the duration of effect is quite consistent. From the beginning of the injection, the patient will usually respond coherently to conversation in 3.5–5.5 min and thereafter will have very few clinical effects from the methohexital. In one case, a healthy male about 48 years of age lost consciousness in the middle of a sentence and when he awoke, he completed the sentence without missing more than two or three words.

Although the retrobulbar block is widely used, it can induce local and systemic effects which may result in blindness or even death. It is rare, but the most common complication is puncture of blood vessels in the retrobulbar space with a resultant hemorrhage. If this occurs, there is usually a palpable increase in intraocular pressure, a rapid onset of a profound oculomotor blockade, proptosis, and closing of the upper eyelid. Other complications include:

1 stimulation of the oculocardiac reflex;

2 intravascular injection;

3 perferation into the globe with or without intraocular injection and possible retinal detachment;

4 occlusion of the central retinal artery secondary to retrobulbar hemorrhage or compression of the vessel from inadvertent injection of the local anesthetic inside the dura surrounding the retinal arteries which, in turn, results in compressive occlusion of the vessel;

5 direct needle injury to the optic nerve; or

6 inadvertent brainstem anesthesia which may be delayed for some time after completion of the retrobulbar block. These complications are summarized in Table 13.1.

Table 13.1 Complications of retro- and peribulbar blocks

Retrobulbar hemorrhage
  Increased intraocular pressure, oculomotor
  blockade, proptosis

Oculocardiac reflex

Intravascular injection

Perforation of globe
  With or without intraocular injection
  Possible retinal detachment

Central retinal artery occlusion
  From hemorrhage or compression of vessels

Trauma to optic nerve

Brainstem anesthesia

Monitoring

It is very important that there be good rapport and interaction between the patient, the anesthesiologist, and the nursing staff, as well as any relatives or friends who accompanied the patient to the facility. Thoughts and concerns about the procedure frequently weigh heavily upon the elderly patient's mind and subtle changes in the patient's level of anxiety are often manifested via the autonomic nervous system as exacerbations in blood pressure or heart rate, or symptoms of coronary insufficiency. Often reassurance and discussion of their concerns can provide relief and calm the patient, but occasionally small doses of a sedative such as midazolam may be needed. In some cases small doses of vasodilators that affect the coronary arteries (such as intravenous nitroglycerin) may be used.

Prior to surgery, routine vital signs are usually taken at 15-min intervals while the dilating drops are instilled into the eye. Intraoperative monitoring for cataract procedures under regional anesthesia usually includes the inspired oxygen concentration (F_IO_2), electrocardiogram (ECG), blood pressure, heart rate (commonly derived from the ECG, pulse oximeter, or non-invasive blood pressure monitor), and a pulse oximeter. In addition, a precordial stethescope provides an early indication of changes in the respiratory pattern and the cardiac rate and rhythm. Temperature monitoring should be readily available.

At our center, a strip chart recording is made of the initial ECG in the operating room. This recording is automatically annotated with the date, time, and heart rate. It provides a baseline reference that can be used for comparison of any subsequent ECG changes. Should any sig-

nificant changes occur perioperatively, these ECG recordings can be included in the patient's medical record for documentation.

Periodic verbal contact with the patient is also maintained, but caution must be used so that the patient does not talk during the critical phases of the procedure when movement of the head and eye must be minimized. Some facilities also monitor expired carbon dioxide. Bowe *et al.* [18] have inserted a cannula (such as a cut off intravenous catheter) through one side of the standard nasal oxygen prongs and have connected this to an end tidal carbon dioxide monitor ($P_{ET}CO_2$). If general anesthesia is utilized, additional monitoring is necessary as recommended by the American Society of Anesthesiologists. This would include a low pressure disconnect and $P_{ET}CO_2$ monitoring.

Monitoring in the PACU includes the routine vital signs about every 15 min. Verbal interchange is also important for assessment of the patient's psychologic and physiologic status. Additional monitoring such as cardiac, pulmonary, or blood glucose may be initiated based upon the clinical judgement of the anesthesiologist.

Positioning

In the geriatric population, positioning and comfort are important since these patients often have musculoskeletal and other organ system problems. In our ambulatory facility, the

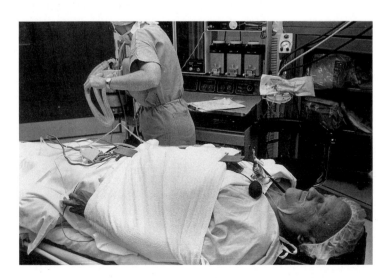

Fig. 13.4 Positioning and support of the patient's arms for cataract surgery.

patient is put on a Stryker ophthalmology cart in the preoperative area, and the back of the cart is raised to approximately 45° while the dilating medications are instilled in the patient's eye. Two large bath towels are folded and used as a pillow under the head. A large regular pillow is placed under the knees to minimize any strain on the back or the sciatic nerves. The patient is transported to the operating room on this same Stryker cart.

In the operating room, the head of the cart is lowered, and the patient is positioned so that the top of their head is flush with the end of the Stryker bedframe. A flat, 2.5 cm (1 in) thick, vinyl-covered foam pad with a central hole for the occiput is placed under the head. Because of kyphosis or lordosis, some patients may be uncomfortable with their head in this position, and folded towels are placed under the foam pad. The objective is to have the frontal plane of the face parallel to the cart. Some ophthalmologists further stabilize the head by running a strip of 5 cm (2 in) adhesive tape across the patient's forehead and securing the ends to the Stryker cart. The position of the pillow under the knees is rechecked. This pillow minimizes the stress on the vertebral column and the musculoskeletal system, and enhances the patient's comfort.

Positioning and support of the arms is also important. This is usually accomplished by wrapping a large towel around each arm to form a sling from approximately the mid humerus to the hand. The elbows are flexed so that the hands are resting comfortably at the patient's side or on the abdomen. This technique is shown in Fig. 13.4. The ends of the towels are overlapped along the sternum and upper abdomen and secured with two large spring-loaded "Zimmer" plastic clips. Utilization of the bath towels (originally used as a pillow under the head in the preoperative area) for support of the arms in the operating room minimizes the handling and laundry expense. If the patient is obese and the bath towels are not long enough to form a sling under the arms, then a sheet or blanket can be used in a similar manner.

There are several advantages to supporting the arms in this manner:

1 the arms are comfortably supported since the tapered upper body segment of the Stryker ophthalmology cart allows little space to rest the arms;

2 potential damage to the ulnar nerve is minimized because the elbow can be supported and not allowed to rest heavily on the operating room cart;

3 it eliminates the need for the armboards that come with the Stryker cart and thereby allows the operating team closer access to the operative field;

4 if the patient relaxes or goes to sleep, there is minimal movement of the arms which could inadvertently disrupt the position of the eye under the microscope;

5 the towels significantly restrict movement of the patient's hands which could contaminate the sterile field; and

6 it provides ready access to the patient's hand by the anesthetist for placement of the pulse oximeter probe, evaluation of radial pulses, access to the i.v. site which is usually located on the hand or wrist, and assessment of capillary refill in the nail beds.

A typical procedure

The aforementioned discussion described various aspects of the anesthesia evaluation as well as perioperative care and management of the cataract patient. Implementation of these concepts in an integrated manner can be illustrated by describing the sequence of events that take place on the day of surgery for a typical cataract patient at our ambulatory center.

The patient is scheduled to arrive at the center 1 or 1.5 h before the procedure. A staff nurse confirms the patient's identification and takes him or her to a dressing room in the preoperative area. The patient changes into an open-backed hospital gown and robe. To retain modesty, the patient's undergarments are not removed. The patient's clothing is placed in a "pass through" locker which has a second keyed-alike door in the backside of the locker. This second door opens into another dressing room in the phase II recovery area. The locker key is attached to a clipboard holding the patient's chart. After changing clothes, use of the bathroom is encouraged. The patient then removes the bathrobe and gets onto a Stryker ophthalmology cart in the preoperative area. The patient is covered with a warm blanket. Folded bath towels are used for a pillow, and a regular pillow is placed under the patient's knees. The back of the bed is raised to approximately 45° for the patient's comfort. Information on the identification band is verified with the patient, and the band is secured on his or her wrist. Allergies, *non per os* (NPO) status, and medications taken that morning are verified and the initial vital signs recorded.

The anesthesiologist performs a brief preoperative physical examination of the respiratory and cardiovascular systems, confirms any medications that the patient was instructed to take that morning, and verifies other pertinent medical data as necessary. An 18 or 20 gauge intravenous catheter is placed in the hand, wrist, or forearm on the operative side. (Because of the support equipment location in the operating room, the anesthetist is positioned on the operative side of the patient, and the anesthesia machine is located at the foot of the cart.) The relatives or friends accompanying the patient are invited into the preoperative area to sit with the patient. Overhead lighting above the patient is extinguished to aid ocular dilation.

As prescribed by the ophthalmologist, dilating medications are instilled by the nurse. For the usual regimens, medications are instilled every 5–15 min. There is some variation in the protocols of the different ophthalmologists and either 1 or 1.5 h are allowed for the preoperative preparation of the cataract patients. This usually requires one nurse essentially dedicated to the preoperative preparation of these patients.

When the preceding case is finished, the ophthalmologist usually comes to the preoperative area, speaks to the patient, family or friends, answers any questions, and examines the eye. The ophthalmologist then goes to speak with the family or friends of the preceding patient.

When it is time for surgery, another warm blanket is placed over the patient since the operating rooms are cooler than the rest of the facility. The patient is transported to the operating room on the Stryker cart. In the operating room: the wheels on the cart are locked; the head of the cart is lowered to the horizontal position; the patient is moved cephalad until the top of the head is at the edge of the frame of the cart and the pillow under the knees is repositioned; a special 2.5 cm (1 in) thick, vinyl-covered foam head rest is placed under the patient's head in lieu of the two folded bath towels; the cart is adjusted to the appropriate height with the cephalad end slightly elevated; nasal oxygen cannulae (2–3 l/min) are placed and secured with adhesive tape; ECG electrodes, non-invasive blood pressure monitor, pulse oximeter probe, and a precordial stethescope are appropriately connected; and the initial vital signs are taken and recorded. The two bath towels removed from under the head are used to form a sling around each arm and secured across the chest.

While the surgeon is preparing for the retrobulbar block, the flow rate of the i.v. solution is increased, and the precalculated dose of methohexital is titrated into the i.v. injection port closest to the patient while the anesthesiologist begins a series of basic questions. The lack of verbal response usually corresponds to loss of consciousness and an adequate depth of anesthesia for the surgeon to do the regional block with minimal response from the patient. Additional aliquots (5–10 mg) of methohexital may be needed to achieve loss of verbal response. Occasionally the patient's chin may need to be elevated for 2–3 min to prevent the tongue from obstructing the airway.

As soon as the surgeon has completed the block, the operating room cart is rotated 90° to position the eye appropriately under the microscope, and the face and eyes are prepped by the operating room nurse. The anesthetist is located at the operative side of the patient and has ready access to the patient's hand, i.v., pulse oximeter probe, and precordial stethescope. The patient nearly always awakens while the face and eyes are being prepped.

After the prep is completed, a Mayo stand is positioned above the patient's neck and chest and a disposable eye drape is appropriately

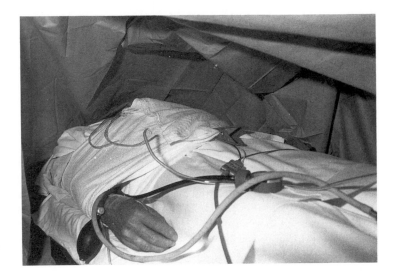

Fig. 13.5 Sterile drapes placed over Mayo stand allows air circulation and limited access to the patient.

positioned around the eye and over the top of the Mayo stand. This arrangement creates a "pyramid" over the patient's mouth and minimizes the feeling of claustrophobia. It permits air circulation and allows limited access for the anesthetist to the patient's airway, thorax, and upper arms in the event that repositioning of the blood pressure cuff or precordial stethescope is necessary. This arrangement is shown in Fig. 13.5. During the procedure which typically requires 50–65 min, routine vital signs are taken every 5 min, and monitored anesthesia care is provided. Usually no additional sedation is given intraoperatively, but if necessary small doses of midazolam (0.5–1 mg) or methohexital (5–15 mg) may be titrated intravenously. Perioperative anxiety is probably the most common problem seen in the patient for cataract surgery.

Although it occurs infrequently, hypertension is probably the second most common problem seen intraoperatively. This can be secondary to anxiety or pre-existing hypertension. If anxiety or other causes are ruled out as the etiology, then it is commonly treated with hydralazine, labetalol, or other vasodilators.

On rare occasions, other problems may occur after beginning the surgical procedure which make it very difficult for the surgeon to continue the operation. Such problems include:

1 periodic apnea from excessive sedation or complete apnea secondary to migration of the local anesthesia from the retrobulbar block to the respiratory center;

2 uncontrollable coughing (usually associated with chronic lung disease or tobacco abuse);

3 claustrophobia not responding to verbal reassurance or i.v. anxiolytic medications; or

4 excessive tremors associated with musculoskeletal dysfunction.

These situations should be immediately evaluated and alternate anesthetic management considered. The urgency and options should be quickly communicated to the surgeon. One solution that can be expeditiously implemented is to proceed to general anesthesia. The surgeon can easily cover the eye and maintain sterility with a sterile drape and the patient can be gently ventilated with a mask. General anesthesia can be induced with i.v. anesthetic agents and endotracheal intubation accomplished. Sterility of the surgical field can be maintained if disposable ophthalmic sterile drapes are routinely utilized. (These drapes have an adhesive plastic segment surrounding the eye.) After induction of general anesthesia is complete and the patient stabilized, the "old" sterile drapes can be removed and the eye can be redraped in a sterile fashion so that the surgical procedure can be continued. The selection of muscle relaxants for intubation must be made with caution. During certain portions of cataract surgery, the eye is open and may be vulnerable to extrusion of the vitreous humor. Therefore, at such times succinylcholine should not be used unless the other potential benefits of rapid paralysis outweigh this possible risk.

At the completion of the procedure, an eyeshield is secured over the eye and the patient is transferred to a regular recovery room bed. The surgeon also gives the patient the medications for postoperative use at home. The patient is transported by the anesthetist and a nurse to phase I PACU. Postoperative recovery takes place in two areas of the PACU. The first area is called phase I. In phase I the patients are resting on full size recovery room beds and gradually recover from anesthesia and surgery. During this recovery, the head of the bed is periodically elevated and movement and conversation is encouraged. When they are able, patients sit on the side of the bed, and then walk with assistance to the second area.

Since the only sedation or medication which the patient has received was the methohexital given when the retrobulbar block was done approximately 1 h earlier, the patient is usually awake, alert, and oriented. Routine vital signs are taken every 15 min during the recovery phase.

When the patient is ready to leave the phase I PACU, he or she is assisted from the bed. Use of a rest-room or bathroom is encouraged, and the patient walks to the second recovery area (phase II). The total time spent by the patient in phase I is usually 30–45 min. In the phase II area, the patient sits in a recliner and is offered their choice of coffee, tea, cola, fruit juice, or an English muffin. The patient's relatives or friends may also join the patient at this time.

While in phase II, some of the ophthalmologists have a patient care coordinator who carefully reviews with the patient and family or friends the exact instructions for postoperative care and activities. A staff nurse also reiterates the individualized follow-up instructions from the ophthalmologist. In addition, a set of individualized written instructions are given to the patient which contain the phone numbers to call if any problems should occur after the patient leaves the facility.

Except for problems related to the preexisting conditions, postoperative complications such as nausea, vomiting, or hiccups are extremely rare among cataract patients. When the patient is ready for discharge, the i.v. is discontinued. The patient is assisted into the dressing room and he or she changes back into street clothes.

After the subsequent case, the ophthalmologist usually speaks with the patient again in phase II. Just prior to leaving the facility, the anesthesiologist evaluates the patient and gives discharge instructions for the next 24 h. These instructions can be summarized as the five Ds:

1 no *d*riving or operating hazardous machines;
2 no *d*rinking of alcoholic beverages;
3 *d*ietary precautions;
4 no major *d*ecisions; and
5 to contact their *d*octor or the center if there are any problems or questions.

The total elapsed time from completion of the procedure until the patient leaves the facility is approximately 1–1.5 h.

The patients are usually questioned about their recall of the procedure and if they remember going to sleep during the regional anesthesia block. About 95% of the patients initially deny going to sleep at all, but when the sequence of questions in the operating room is reviewed and they also have no recall of the needle placement, they agree they must have been asleep for "a few minutes." It is believed that this smooth, subtle titration of methohexital is very effective and that it is a great benefit for the typically anxious geriatric patient.

The patient is encouraged to stop at a restaurant on the way home for a late breakfast or lunch, and approximately 50–60% of the patients do so. Psychologically, it is felt that this helps the patient to feel that the operation is over, that they can resume near normal activity, and it creates a positive attitude toward their recovery period.

In conclusion, we have briefly reviewed anesthesia care and management for cataract surgery, and have described some of the other aspects for patient care which are utilized effectively for these patients in an ambulatory surgery center. Although the procedure can be done with only local anesthesia, it is felt that use of anesthesia services greatly enhances patient safety, allies the patient's anxiety, and in general, markedly contributes to a more pleasant perioperative experience for the patient.

References

1 Davenport HT, ed. *Anaesthesia and the Aged Patient*. Oxford: Blackwell Scientific Publications, 1988.

2 Felts JA. Anesthesia and the geriatric patient. *Clin Anaesthesiol* 1986; **4**: 799–1050.

3 McLeskey CH. Perioperative geriatrics. *Prob Anesth* 1989; **4**: 527–652.

4 Muravchick S. The aging patient, an age related disease. *ASA Refresher Courses in Anesthesiology*, vol. 16. American Society of Anesthesiologists. Philadelphia: JB Lippincott, 1988: 145–53.

5 Stephen CR, Assaf RAE, eds. *Geriatric Anesthesia: Principles and Practice*. Boston, Massachusetts: Butterworths, 1986.

6 Wetchler BV, ed. *Anesthesia for Ambulatory Surgery*, 2nd edn. Philadelphia: JB Lippincott, 1991.

7 White PF, ed. *Outpatient Anesthesia*. New York: Churchill Livingstone, 1990.

8 Ammon JR. Perioperative management of the diabetic patient. *ASA Refresher Courses in Anesthesiology*, vol. 16. American Society of Anesthesiologists. Philadelphia: JB Lippincott, 1988: 1–15.

9 Goldman L, Caldera DL, Nussbaum SR *et al.* Multifactorial index of cardiac risk in non-cardiac surgical procedures. *N Engl J Med* 1977; **297**: 845–50.

10 Steen PA, Tinker JH, Tarhan S. Myocardial reinfarction after anesthesia and surgery. An update: Incidents, mortality, and predisposing factors. *JAMA* 1978; **239**: 2566–70.

11 Rao TLK, Jacobs KH, El-Etr AA. Reinfarction following anesthesia in patients with myocardial infarction. *Anesthesiology* 1983; **59**: 499–505.

12 Backer CL, Tinker JH, Robertson DM, *et al.* Myocardial reinfarction following local anesthesia for ophthalmic surgery. *Anesth Analg* 1980; **59**: 257–62.

13 Lang DW. Morbidity and mortality in ophthalmology. In: McGoldrick K, Bruce RA, Oppenheimer P, eds. *Anesthesia for Ophthalmology*. Birmingham, Alabama: Aesculapius, 1982: 195–204.

14 Snow JC, Sensel S. A review of cataract extraction under local and general anesthesia at MEEI. *Anesth Analg* 1966; **45**: 742.

15 Lynch S, Wolf GL, Berlin I. General anesthesia for cataract surgery: a comparative review of 2217 consecutive cases. *Anesth Analg* 1974; **53**: 909–13.

16 Breslin PP. Mortality in ophthalmic surgery. *Int Ophth Clin* 1973; **13**: 215–26.

17 Adams AP. Anaesthesia for ophthalmic surgery. In: Nunn JF, Utting JE, Brown BR, Jr., eds. *General Anaesthesia*, 5th edn. London: Butterworths, 1989: 948–57.

18 Bowe EA, Boysen PG, Broome JA, Klein EF Jr. Accurate determination of end-tidal carbon dioxide during administration of oxygen by nasal cannulae. *J Clin Monit* 1989; **5**: 105–10.

14: Ophthalmic Anesthesia: Local vs. General, Retrobulbar vs. Peribulbar

DAVID B. DAVIS II & MARK R. MANDEL

General anesthesia for cataract surgery was commonly used in the USA until the mid-1970s when local anesthesia became the dominant form of anesthesia. General anesthesia still remains a very common method of anesthesia for cataract and intraocular lens (IOL) surgery outside of the USA. However, with the introduction of outpatient surgery to the European continents, general anesthesia is now being replaced by local anesthesia.

General anesthesia has some inherent advantages over local anesthesia.

1 the patient is asleep. For a very few adults, the fear of surgery under a local anesthetic is extremely disturbing, and they resist all urging to have local anesthesia. However, for young adults and children, general anesthesia is usually *required*;

2 the patient is usually immobile with no tendency to move. An injection such as a retrobulbar, which has vision-threatening complications, is not necessary. Some ophthalmic surgeons and anesthesiologists feel they have better control over the patient under these conditions;

3 the surgeons are free to discuss the case as they see fit, without concern about the patient's emotional response; and

4 general anesthesia is still extremely useful in perforating injuries of the globe, where a retrobulbar block would be contraindicated.

In most cases, the disadvantages of general anesthesia seem to outweigh the advantages. These include:

1 putting the patient at greater systemic risk with a higher mortality and morbidity;

2 patients inadequately anesthetized or paralyzed may tend to buck or cough, suddenly increasing the intraocular pressure, and creating an emergency situation;

3 recovery from general anesthesia is not always quick and ambulation may be delayed. This is especially true in older individuals. In addition, some patients have postoperative lightheadedness, disorientation, and pharyngitis. Some become nauseated and vomit, often requiring additional medication with possibly more side effects, and further delaying physical rehabilitation. This may present a problem for the patient undergoing outpatient surgery;

4 when a patient having undergone ocular surgery under general anesthesia awakens, he or she normally will have ocular pain since no local anesthetic had been given. Therefore, these patients will require pain medication earlier and more often than when local anesthesia is utilized; and

5 in order to relieve the post-general anesthesia ocular pain, some physicians administer a retrobulbar block while the patient is under general anesthesia. This practice compounds the potential disadvantages of *both* methods of anesthesia.

Retrobulbar anesthesia has been used quite safely and effectively for over 100 years [1,2]. It has proven to be an excellent source of local anesthesia for major ocular surgery. Therefore, why should anyone consider changing from this effective, well-established, and familiar technique with a relatively low incidence of complications? Anytime the rate of serious complications can be reduced by even a small fraction without compromising the effectiveness

Table 14.1 Complications of retrobulbar injections

Side effects
  Pain upon injection
  Retrobulbar hemorrhage

Sight-threatening complications
  Optic nerve damage
  Central retinal artery occlusion
  Embolization of injectate into retina/choroid

Life-threatening complications
  Cardiac arrest
  Respiratory depression
  CNS depression
  Seizures

of a technique, this should be considered. Retrobulbar anesthesia, although extremely safe, has potentially devastating consequences. The peribulbar block offers a safer, less painful, and equally effective means of obtaining ocular anesthesia and akinesia [3,4].

Complications of retrobulbar anesthesia

Table 14.1 lists the complications of retrobulbar anesthesia. The problems associated with retrobulbar injections can be classified into three levels of concern:
1 *side effects* such as pain upon injection and the need to cancel a case due to retrobulbar hemorrhage;
2 *sight-threatening complications* such as optic nerve damage, central retinal artery occlusion, embolization of material into retinal and choroidal circulation, and globe perforation; and
3 *life-threatening disasters* such as cardiac arrest, respiratory and central nervous system (CNS) depression.

Receiving a retrobulbar injection is not a painless event, especially upon penetration of the muscle sheath. Although not serious, pain can be considered a "side effect." In many cases, in order to alleviate the pain of the retrobulbar and/or seventh nerve block or to create an amnesic state, the anesthesiologist may administer substances such as alfentanil hydrochloride, fentanyl citrate, methohexital sodium, and sodium pentobarbital. While these are generally safe drugs, whilst not used in excessively high doses, no systemic drug is without potential problems, especially in older adults who are frequently on multiple medications. The peribulbar block is not painful, does not require a seventh nerve block, and does not necessitate the use of powerful and potentially dangerous sedatives.

Retrobulbar hemorrhages necessitating cancellation of surgery and postponement to a later date occur with an incidence of 1% when blunt needles are used to 5% when sharp needles are used [5]. These are not only disappointing to the patient and frustrating for the surgeon, but potentially serious in that optic nerve function can be permanently compromised [6–8]. Although not *usually* sight impairing, it is not uncommon for a patient to lose confidence in their physician and not return for future surgery.

Optic nerve and/or retinal ischemia is a well-known complication that may be due to mechanical trauma from the volume of the injection [9], direct trauma to the nerve from the retrobulbar needle [10], intra-arterial injection with subsequent ischemia [11,12], a retrobulbar hemorrhage [6–8], or possibly vasospasm [13]. Although optic nerve or retinovascular ischemia are not commonly reported occurrences, these complications are probably more frequent than the literature reports.

Perforations of the globe are not uncommon in high myopes who have large eyes with thin sclera, but also occur in otherwise normal eyes [14–16]. Intravitreal injection with secondary retinal toxicity, retinal detachment, or macular trauma may result in permanent loss of vision.

Contralateral amaurosis is a reported complication [17,18]. This is felt to be due to direct invasion of the dural sheath by the local anesthetic with distribution of the anesthetic into the optic chiasm or the contralateral optic nerve. Although this has cleared in each reported case, it is conceivable that permanent contralateral blindness could occur. Transient central retinal artery occlusion together with contralateral amaurosis following retrobulbar injection has been recorded [19].

CNS effects [20–22] and respiratory depression [23–25] are not uncommon. Frank cardiac or pulmonary arrest are less commonly reported but do occur [26,27]. The cause is felt to be due to either an intravascular injection or to the introduction of the local anesthetic into the optic nerve sheath and subsequently into the cerebrospinal fluid (CSF) [28–31]. Grand mal seizures have also been described following retrobulbar anesthesia [32].

Peribulbar anesthesia

History

Although the above sight-threatening complications are uncommon, if they occur to a one-eyed patient, his or her life may be ruined forever. If only one vision-threatening complication in 5000 cases could be prevented without sacrificing the efficacy and therapeutic value of the procedure, then one should consider alternatives to retrobulbar anesthesia. Peribulbar or periocular anesthesia affords us that alternative.

Charles Kelman MD first began using what he describes as a "modified retrobulbar injection" in 1973. Originally this was not considered a "peribulbar" approach. However, Kelman noted that he did not achieve amaurosis in these patients (personal communication). This indicates that the anesthetic was deposited primarily outside of the muscle cone, and that optic nerve function remained intact. At the Medical-Surgical Eye Center in California, in 1982 we first began utilizing peribulbar anesthesia and after many modifications, have used it exclusively for the past 9 years. In our personal experience with over 4000 consecutive cases, the side effects have been mild and we have yet to encounter any significant complication. This technique is performed for all of our cataract surgery, penetrating keratoplasty, intraocular surgery, and for the occasional difficult radial keratotomy patient in whom topical anesthesia is not deemed adequate. It is also useful for panretinal photocoagulation and cyclodestructive procedures.

Modifications of periocular or peribulbar anesthesia have been propounded by Spencer Thornton MD, Leroy Bloomberg MD, Jaswant Pannu MD, Jack Weiss MD, Barry Galman MD, Howard Friedberg MD, and others.

Table 14.2 Advantages of peribulbar injection

Less pain
No need for additional seventh nerve block
Less intraoperative posterior pressure
Easily taught
No intraoperative or postoperative amaurosis

Advantages

The complications that are seen in retrobulbar injections are greatly minimized in peribulbar anesthesia because the injection is deposited entirely outside the muscle cone. The muscles themselves are not engaged and the needle is further from the globe, optic nerve, dural sheaths, and optic foramen than with standard retrobulbar anesthesia.

In addition to the lower incidence of sight- and life-threatening complications, Table 14.2 lists the secondary advantages of peribulbar injection. These include:

1 less pain upon injection and therefore the need for less systemic medication and no need for an additional painful seventh nerve block;

2 less intraoperative posterior pressure because the anesthetic material seems to diffuse into a wider orbital area creating a softer eye during surgery;

3 the fact that an anesthesiologist or first year ophthalmology resident is more easily taught this technique than the standard retrobulbar injection; and

4 no intraoperative amaurosis which is a marked advantage in the one-eyed patient who would otherwise experience temporary total blindness following the case.

Disadvantages

There are disadvantages to the peribulbar technique. It is a new procedure, requires a larger volume of anesthetic which is an unusual concept to surgeons used to small retrobulbar volumes, and it takes longer to achieve full lid and globe anesthesia and akinesia (Table 14.3).

Every new technique has an intrinsic learning curve which can be frustrating to the surgeon. As with retrobulbar anesthesia, each attempt will not result in total akinesia. When

Table 14.3 Disadvantages of peribulbar injection

New procedure
Larger volume of anesthetic
Longer to achieve full anesthesia and akinesia
Eyelid ecchymosis

first learning the technique, incomplete block may occur in 30–40% of trials. However, once mastered, this rate is significantly less.

The peribulbar block requires a large (but safe) volume of anesthetic. In retrobulbar anesthesia, 2–3 cm^3 of anesthetic is deposited into the cone, whereas in peribulbar, 6–10 cm^3 are placed in the *periconal* space. After depositing the volume of fluid into the orbit, the lids initially become quite tense. We list this as a "disadvantage" because, if not expected, it is alarming to the surgeon as it mimics a retrobulbar hemorrhage. However, after placement of an ocular compression device, the area quickly becomes soft, and one realizes that no hemorrhage has occurred.

An additional disadvantage of the peribulbar injection is that it requires more time to take effect. In a well-placed retrobulbar injection adequate effect may be present within 3–5 min. However, with the peribulbar block, anesthesia and akinesia typically occur after 8–12 min. If one plans accordingly, this does not create a problem and can be accomplished by either the surgeon or an anesthesiologist in a surgical facility or a hospital outpatient department.

Some surgeons report a need for a second injection 1–5% of the time and the need for a third injection in about 5% of cases. This disadvantage is offset by the second and third injections being placed outside the cone away from the globe, and the need for only small amounts of additional injectable drug.

The side effect of the peribulbar procedure reported to date is periorbital ecchymosis which does not cause intraoperative or postoperative problems. This is probably related to the initial superficial intraorbicularis injection. However, with newer needle points, the rate of ecchymosis does not appear to be any greater with peribulbar than with retrobulbar injection. Physicians utilizing a conjunctival cul-de-sac approach note little or no lid ecchymosis.

We are aware of the need to cancel surgery in two cases following peribulbar injection. In one case, a large lid hemorrhage occurred in a patient on Coumadin therapy. There was no permanent damage in this case (G. Elian MD, personal communication). Paul N. Arnold MD experienced one case of "retrobulbar hemorrhage" out of 2804 cases which precluded surgery (personal communication).

Robert H. Fier MD reported to us one case of orbital hemorrhage out of 2540 injections. This was in an 83-year-old hypertensive patient. There was posterior pressure during lens insertion, however, the case was completed without complication with a 20/20 visual result. A 1–1/2 in 23 gauge needle was used (personal communication). Dr Fier stated that he did not check for amaurosis, so it is not known definitely if this was a true peribulbar or a retrobulbar injection. Spencer Thornton MD has developed a new "hypotraumatic" peribulbar needle produced by Alcon (Alcon no. 8065-4206-01) which he feels reduces ecchymosis in all types of injections. To date, this also seems to be the case in our small series, using his needle. We are aware of one anecdotal case of disturbing glare from the operating microscope light experienced by a prominent ophthalmologist undergoing cataract surgery. In our hands in over 4000 cases, and by others contacted by us utilizing the peribulbar technique, no patient has ever complained about the microscope light causing undue discomfort. In our postanesthesia questionnaire, all patients are questioned about this and pain upon injection.

One of our patients with a long-standing dense unilateral cataract developed a 3 prism D esotropia postoperatively. His muscle status prior to the cataract surgery is unknown. Howard Fine MD (personal communication) noted a "small but significant increase in vertical muscle imbalance," but this has not been seen by others.

Complications

The reported complications include two cases of respiratory depression reported by Jaswant Pannu MD (in 1800 cases) following superior-

Table 14.4 Complications of peribulbar injection
(personal communications)

Respiratory depression (Pannu, Thornton)
Globe perforation (Kimble)

---

temporal periocular injection utilizing a 1–1/2
in needle. Spencer Thornton MD has noted one
similar case (in over 3000 cases), again utilizing
a 1–1/2 in needle superior-temporally (personal
communication). We have always recommended a needle no longer than 1–1/4 in in
length and presently we utilize a 7/8 in needle.
Dr Pannu felt that the length of the needle
allowed insertion of the point into the optic
foramen.

We are aware of four cases of globe perforation during peribulbar anesthesia. Two of these
are attributed to long, thin, 27 gauge flexible
needles, which are not recommended in either
peribulbar or retrobulbar anesthesia [14].
Of note, however, Robert C. Hamilton MB,
FRCPE, anesthesiologist in Calgary, Alberta,
Canada has performed over 15 000 retrobulbar
or peribulbar injections with a 1 in 27 gauge
needle without a known globe perforation (personal communication). In the third perforation
case, a sharp 22 gauge 1–1/2 in needle was
utilized. In the fourth case, a sharp 1 in 23 gauge
needle was used in the superior-temporal
region by an anesthesiologist who learned the
technique by "hear-say" (personal communication). Again, we have always recommended
the "blunted" type needles [32], and now
prefer the Thornton needle, 23 or 25 gauge.

The senior author (Davis) in an uncontrolled
study on animal eyes using Thornton needles,
Atkinson needles, the new Vistec retrobulbar
needle, and standard disposable sharp needles
found that perforation occurred easily and with
little resistance with *any* sharp nedle, especially
a 27 and 25 gauge. The next easiest to perforate
was the Vistec needle (25 and 23 gauge). Both
the blunted Atkinson 25 and 23 gauge needles
and the Thornton 25 and 23 gauge required
definite effort to perforate. The Thornton
needle would penetrate the sclera about 0.1–
0.2 mm easily, but then required force to complete the penetration.

The Vistec was one of the smoothest feeling needles in penetrating skin tissue (in
human patients) compared to the Thornton and
Atkinson, which is an advantage if you are *not*
injecting near the globe.

Technique

The technique has two parts: an initial superficial injection and a deep peribulbar injection. Robert Hustead MD, anesthesiologist in
Wichita, Kansas, introduced us to an almost
painless injection technique which we employ
for the superficial injection.

Although we use midazolam hydrochloride
in very low dosages (maximum: 0.5–1 mg),
many patient receive absolutely *no* sedation
and rarely complain of discomfort with our
technique. Nine milliliters of buffered saline
solution (BSS) taken from the sterile 15 cm³ BSS
vial used in eye surgery is mixed with 1 cm³
of 1% lidocaine with epinephrine in a 10 cm³
syringe. This and the peribulbar injection to be
given later are warmed to body temperature in
a heating pad. Care must be taken to avoid
raising the temperature of the medications over
100°.

The superficial injection of the mixture of 9:1
BSS/lidocaine is given at the junction of the
lateral one-third and medial two-thirds of the
lower lid just above the orbital rim using a 1/2
in 27 gauge needle (Fig. 14.1a). A total of 2 cm³
is given. First, a small skin wheal is raised and
then approximately 0.5 cm³ is deposited in the
orbicularis. The needle is then directed almost
straight posteriorly to the full 1/2 in needle
length, avoiding the globe, and an additional
1 cm³ of this dilute mixture is deposited in the
anterior orbit. Because the pH of this mixture is
more physiologic than 1% lidocaine alone, it
does not cause burning or stinging. James Gills
MD and others utilize sodium bicarbonate buffered lidocaine and find that this, too, gives no
stinging or burning. We have had no experience with this technique.

Some surgeons prefer to anesthetize the
conjunctiva with dilute proparacaine and then
administer the dilute BSS/lidocaine injection
subconjunctivally rather than through the lid.

After approximately 1 min of holding press-

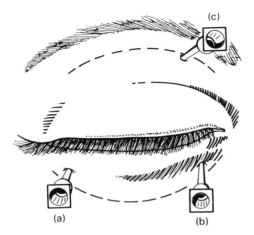

Fig. 14.1 (a) Sight of inferior temporal injection. (b) Sight of inferior nasal injection. (c) Sight of superior nasal injection.

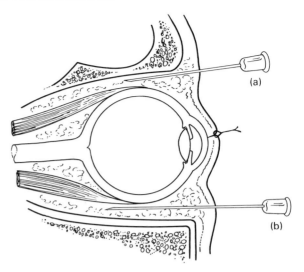

Fig. 14.2 (a) Injection at or just anterior to equator. Bevel towards globe. (b) Injection just posterior to equator. Bevel towards globe.

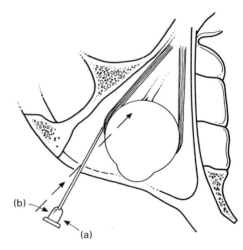

Fig. 14.3 Superior view. (a) Approximate direction of peribulbar injection. (b) Approximate direction of retrobulbar injection.

ure over the injection site to diminish the incidence of ecchymosis, the deep injection is given, using a modified point 23 or 25 gauge 7/8 in needle. A 3/4 or 1 in needle is also satisfactory. A mixture of $6.5\,cm^3$ bupivicaine 0.75%, $3.25\,cm^3$ lidocaine 1% without epinephrine, and $0.1-0.25\,cm^3$ hyaluronidase is prepared in a $10\,cm^3$ syringe. The mixture is warmed to body temperature. A total of $6-8\,cm^3$ is very slowly given. Because the initial superficial injection of the BSS/lidocaine combination was administered, the second injection is usually not uncomfortable. James Gills MD also buffers this injection with sodium bicarbonate, rendering it even more comfortable (personal communication). Pain also is diminished as the needle does not penetrate the rectus muscles. The peribulbar needle is introduced at the same location as the skin injection (Fig. 14.1a), depositing approximately $1\,cm^3$ in the orbicularis. It is advanced just anterior to the equator of the globe, staying slightly further away from the globe than a retrobulbar injection. The bevel side should be directed towards the globe. The patient is instructed to look straight ahead, not up or up-and-in. The needle, rather than passing under the globe and into the cone, is angled slightly laterally and less superiorly than a retrobulbar injection. Two to three milliliters are deposited slowly at or just anterior to the equator (Fig. 14.2a and Fig. 14.3), and the

needle is slowly advanced past the globe, just past the equator, remaining outside of the cone (Fig. 14.2b and Fig. 14.4). An additional 4–$7\,cm^3$ of anesthetic is then administered. The injection is given slowly, stopping when the superior lid fold disappears. By injecting slowly, further discomfort is reduced. The exact amount given varies with each patient and depends upon the volume of the orbit. This

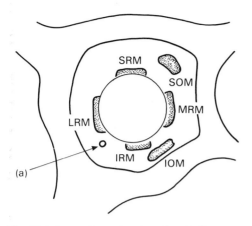

Fig. 14.4 Approximate location of peribulbar needle (a) at cross-section of globe equator.

block can also be given through the inferior conjunctival cul-de-sac.

Following peribulbar injection, if slight proptosis and bulging of the superior-nasal lid fold is observed, one can be almost assured of proper placement of anesthetic and that complete akinesia and anesthesia will result from a single injection.

No seventh nerve block is given. In over 4000 cases we have had to give a supplementary lid block on only 12 occasions (0.27%) by injecting an additional $1-2\,cm^3$ of the bupivicaine/lidocaine mixture into the inferior or superior orbicularis.

Immediately following this injection, the "super pinkie" is placed on the eye for approximately 15–30 min. The super pinkie is applied with moderate pressure and moderate spring-back of the ball. Unlike the Honan balloon, the pressure cannot be quantitated. It is most important that the lid be kept closed while the pressure device is in place to assure that no corneal abrasion occurs. We tape the lids closed and place three 4 × 4 sterile pads beneath the super pinkie. Although we do not feel it is essential, we have a family member or technician gently elevate the ball off the globe for 10 s every 3 min.

Although we prefer 30 min of pressure, we have found that 10–20 min seems to be adequate in all but the most unusual cases. Any ocular compression device used correctly

is probably effective. We performed a prospective evaluation of intraocular pressure drop in 100 consecutive cases using our technique. The average decrease in intraocular pressure following the use of the super pinkie was 7.5 m of mercury, as tested with the Tonopen.

Ten minutes following the block, ocular motility is evaluated. The peribulbar block has a more delayed onset than retrobulbar anesthesia and it is not uncommon after 8–10 min to still see some minor movement. This will usually disappear. However, in the event of significant action of one or more muscles, an additional injection may be required. When one begins to perform peribulbar anesthesia, there is a need in a significant number of cases to give a second injection.

We have found that, if an incomplete block exists, the medial rectus or the superior rectus will usually demonstrate the residual activity. In that case, the block can be repeated either in the superior-nasal or inferior-nasal quadrant (Fig. 14.1b, c) or through the nasal conjunctiva cul-de-sac or caruncle [21]. We prefer the inferior-nasal location, since this area may be anatomically safer.

For supplementation, the preinjection of BSS/lidocaine is given at the junction of the medial one-third and lateral two-thirds of the lower lid at the inferior orbital rim. This is followed by several milliliters of peribulbar anesthetic delivered just slightly anterior to the equator and then just slightly posterior to the equator inferior-nasal to the globe. If a superior injection is desired, it is given in the lid fold between the supraorbital notch and trochlea. The needle is advanced essentially parallel with the roof of the orbit, staying away from the globe.

As in the rare retrobulbar injection we have found that with an occasional peribulbar injection we have been unable to entirely eliminate the residual ocular movement in one direction. Surgery proceeded without an increase in intraoperative intraocular pressure in all of these cases. We cannot explain why residual muscle activity should be less important in peribulbar than retrobulbar anesthesia, but our and many others experience in giving local anesthesia seems to bear this out (S.

Thornton, J. Pannu, D. Benson, B. Galman, and L. Bloomberg, personal communication).

Modifications of technique

We modify the peribulbar injection for glaucoma patients. Instead of giving the entire bolus in a single injection, the anesthetic is deposited in graded doses of 2–3 cm³ each time, to avoid raising the intraocular pressure. Following the initial 2–3 cm³, either the ocular compression device is placed with only mild pressure, or digital massage is administered. The aim here is to attempt to prevent the intraocular pressure from rising to levels which could damage the optic nerve. After about 5–7 min, the block is reevaluated and the pressure of the eye rechecked. If the block is not adequate, additional 2–3 cm³ aliquots are given followed by mild pressure until akinesia and anesthesia is achieved. In patients who have a functioning glaucoma filtering bleb, it is quite easy to collapse the anterior chamber with excessive pressure from the compression device. In these cases, we use extremely light pressure from the ball and observe the chamber at 5–7 min intervals. If there is any tendency for the chamber to collapse from the fluid being forced into the bleb, the compression device is discontinued.

Variations of technique

There are many variations of the peribulbar technique which work well. Kelman utilizes a 1–5/8 in 25 gauge needle through the superior fornix, depositing 4–5 cm³ of anesthetic superiorly. To date, he has performed over 9600 of these injections without serious complication (personal communication). He bends the needle at the hub to a 70° angle. The injection is delivered transconjunctivally through the superior fornix ". . . all the way back until I can feel the top of the needle hit the bony roof of the orbit. The needle is always held parallel to the plane of the operating room floor." He then injects 4–5 cm³ of a mixture of 2% mepivacaine hydrochloride and hyaluronidase.

Pannu now utilizes a 5/8 in needle with a mixture of bupivicaine 0.75%, lidocaine 4%,

and hyaluronidase. Approximately 8–10 cm³ of the mixture is given in the infratemporal quadrant. The needle is directed away from the globe, muscle cone, and optic foramen towards the lateral wall of the orbit. He no longer utilizes the supratemporal approach. If supplement is needed, he injects through the conjunctiva directly around the muscle.

Thornton now gives the injection in the superior-temporal area just lateral to the temporal edge of the superior rectus muscle using a 3/4 in 27 gauge Thornton needle. He initially directs the needle 45° upward toward the orbital roof until the roof is "gently touched at the level of the equator of the globe" and then redirects it posteriorly to behind the globe outside of the muscle cone. Five to six milliliters of bupivicaine 0.75%, lidocaine 2%, and hyaluronidase are given. He emphasizes that the opening of the needle should always be directed towards the globe. Twenty minutes of pressure is applied.

Bloomberg employs a 1 in 25 gauge needle, injecting along the orbital floor both inferior-temporally and inferior-nasally. He previously used a 3/4 in needle, but because of the high cost of these needles he now uses the 1 in. He administers a total of 10 cm³ etidocaine hydrochloride 1% with epinephrine and hyaluronidase. He applies pressure with the Honan balloon for 20 min.

Galman and Friedberg use a 7/8 in needle with an inferior-temporal approach followed by digital massage for 4–5 min. Six to seven milliliters of bupivicaine 0.75% and mepivicaine 2% with hyaluronidase is used. They note a reinjection rate of less than 5%, and have noticed that 100% akinesia does not always occur, but "a small amount of residual eye movement has not caused any problems during surgery."

Weiss uses a 25 gauge 5/8 in needle at the inferior-temporal location. Five milliliters of a 50/50 mixture of bupivicaine 0.75% and lidocaine 2% with hyaluronidase is given. The Honan device is applied for 10 min.

To date, the following surgeons have used periocular technique without a significant complication in the following number of cases: Charles Kelman MD over 9600; Barry Galman

MD and Howard Freidberg MD over 1000; Spencer Thornton MD over 3300 except for the single case of CNS involvement (surgery was later performed without problem); Rand Institute, over 3000 cases; Leroy Bloomberg MD over 1350; Jack Weiss MD over 800 cases; Larry R. Smith CRNA over 2006 cases; Robert H. Fier MD over 2540 cases; and our study over 3600 cases (personal communications, Summer, 1989).

Paul H. Arnold MD has performed 2804 cases (personal communication). He has noted seven cases of intraoperative suprachoroidal hemorrhage, none of which has progressed to expulsive hemorrhage. In six cases, a posterior chamber IOL was inserted and all had 20/40 postoperative vision or better. One case required a vitrectomy and placement of an anterior chamber IOL with a final vision of 20/80.

We are presently conducting a multicenter prospective detailed study of peribulbar anesthesia with a goal of 15 500 consecutive peribulbar injections. Those included to date are: David B. Davis II MD and Mark R. Mandel MD, The Medical Surgical Eye Center, Hayward, California; Leroy Bloomberg MD, Bloomberg Eye Center, Newark, Ohio; Spencer Thornton MD, Baptist Hospital, Nashville, Tennessee; Mario Oyarzun MD, Conception, Chile; Larry Smith CRNA, Heart of Texas Outpatient Cataract Center, Brownwood, Texas; Jack L. Weiss MD, Cornea Consultant, San Diego, California; Robert H. Fier MD, Stuart, Florida; Dewey Benson DO, FAAOS, Franklin, Michigan; and Albert Neumann MD, Neumann Eye Center, DeLand, Florida.

From the inception of the formal prospective study to March 30, 1991, the group has performed 15 600 consecutive peribulbar injections. The only complication in this study are one case of respiratory depression reported by Thornton. There was one globe perforation, one retrobulbar hemorrage, one no anesthesia, two expulsive hemorrages (in PPKs), and one AION. A 95% or better block (akinesia) was present in over 95% of cases, and supplemental blocks varied from 2 to 30%, depending upon surgeon and the exact technique. Ptosis appears to occur no more frequently than with the peribulbar anesthesia, but this part of the study is in its initial phase.

Summary

Although peribulbar injection is quite simple, it too, like all other techniques, must be properly taught and practiced. There is a proper area into which to place the anesthetic. Depositing anesthetic outside of this area gives a less than desirable result, while injecting central to the area may give retrobulbar effects and increase the potential for complications. We have noted a true retrobulbar effect in less than three in 100 cases, as noted by the patient having no perception of the microscope light during surgery. This we try to avoid. Because they are flexible and the surgeon cannot completely control the direction of the tip, we especially recommend against the use of long, thin, ultrasharp 27 gauge needles, and also recommend a modified point type needle (i.e. Thornton).

We also feel that whether one utilizes retrobulbar or peribulbar anesthesia, needles longer than 1 in are unnecessary and serve only to increase the danger of complications.

We have also noted that most of the complications that were communicated to us occurred also with injections in the superior-temporal area.

Although we do not feel than any technique where a needle is introduced into the orbital area is completely safe and without some danger, we feel that peribulbar is considerably safer than retrobulbar anesthesia. Presently, this is being borne out by a large prospective series. Because the needle is not directed towards the globe or into the area of the optic nerve and dural sheaths, there is less chance for serious sight-threatening or life-threatening complications.

References

1 Atkinson WS. The development of ophthalmic anesthesia. *Am J Ophthalmol* 1961; **51**: 1–11.
2 Knapp H. On cocaine and its use in ophthalmic and general surgery. *Arch Ophthalmol* 1884; **13**: 402–48.

3 Davis DB II, Mandel MR. Posterior peribulbar anesthesia: An alternative to retrobulbar anesthesia. *J Cataract Refract Surg* 1986; **12**: 182–5.

4 Weiss JL, Deichman CB. A comparison of retrobulbar and periocular anesthesia for cataract surgery. *Arch Ophthalmol* 1989; **107**: 96–8.

5 Feibel RM. Current concepts in retrobulbar anesthesia. *Surv Ophthalmol* 1986; **30**: 102–85.

6 Ellis PR. Retrobulbar injections. *Surv Ophthalmol* 1974; **18**: 425–30.

7 Goldsmith MO. Occlusion of the central retinal artery following retrobulbar hemorrhage. *Ophthalmologica* 1967; **153**: 191–6.

8 Krauchar MR, Seelenfreund MD, Freilich DB. Central retinal artery closure during orbital hemorrhage from retrobulbar injection. *Trans Am Acad Ophthalmol Otolaryngol* 1974; **78**: 64–70.

9 McLean EB. Inadvertent injection of corticosteroid into the choroidal vascular. *Am J Ophthalmol* 1975; **80**: 835–7.

10 Paulter SE, Grizzard WS, Thompson LN *et al.* Blindness from retrobulbar injection into the optic nerve. *Ophthal Surg* 1986; **17**: 334–7.

11 Ellis PR. Occlusion of the central retinal artery after retrobulbar corticosteroid injection. *Am J Ophthalmol* 1978; **85**: 352–6.

12 Klein ML, Jampol LM, Condon PI *et al.* Central retinal artery occlusion without retrobulbar hemorrhage after retrobulbar anesthesia. *Am J Ophthalmol* 1982; **93**: 573–7.

13 Cowley MD, Campochiaro PA, Newman SA *et al.* Retinal vascular occlusion without retrobulbar or optic nerve sheath hemorrhage after retrobulbar injection of lidocaine. *Ophthal Surg* 1988; **19**: 859–61.

14 Bettman JW. A retrospective look at twenty-two medicolegal claims. How they might have been avoided. *Surv Ophthalmol* 1983; **28**: 55–60.

15 Giles CL. Bulbar perforation during periocular injection of corticosteroids. *Am J Ophthalmol* 1974; **77**: 438–41.

16 Ramsay RC, Knobloch WH. Ocular perforation following retrobulbar anesthesia for retinal detachment surgery. *Am J Ophthalmol* 1978; **86**: 61–4.

17 Antoszyk AN, Buckley EG. Contralateral decreased visual acuity and extraocular muscle palsies following retrobulbar anesthesia. *Ophthalmology* 1986; **93**: 462–5.

18 Friedberg HL, Kline OR Jr. Contralateral amaurosis after retrobulbar injection. *Am J Ophthalmol* 1986; **101**: 688–90.

19 Brad RD. Transient central retinal artery occlusion and contralateral amaurosis after retrobulbar anesthetic injection. *Ophthal Surg* 1989; **20**: 643–6.

20 Ahn JC, Stanly JA. Subarachnoid injection as a complication of retrobulbar anesthesia. *Am J Ophthalmol* 1987; **103**: 225–30.

21 Hamilton RC. Brainstem anesthesia following retrobulbar blockade. *Anesthesiology* 1985; **63**: 688–90.

22 Meyers EF. Brain-stem anesthesia after retrobulbar block. *Arch Ophthalmol* 1985; **103**: 1278–9.

23 Rodman DJ, Notaro S, Peer GL. Respiratory depression following retrobulbar bupivicaine: three case reports and literature review. *Ophthal Surg* 1987; **18**: 768–71.

24 Smith JL. Retrobulbar bupivicaine can cause respiratory arrest. *Ann Ophthalmol* 1982; **14**: 1005–6.

25 Wittpenn JR, Rapoza P, Sternberg P Jr *et al.* Respiratory arrest following retrobulbar anesthesia. *Ophthalmology* 1986; **93**: 867–70.

26 Rosenblatt RM, May DR, Barsoumian K. Cardiopulmonary arrest after retrobulbar block. *Am J Ophthalmol* 1980; **90**: 425–7.

27 Ruusuvaara P. Respiratory arrest after retrobulbar block. *Acta Ophthalmol* 1988; **66**: 223–5.

28 Javitt JC, Addiego R, Friedberg HL *et al.* Brainstem anesthesia after retrobulbar block. *Ophthalmology* 1987; **94**: 718–24.

29 Kobet KA. Cerebral spinal fluid recovery of lidocaine and bupivicaine following respiratory arrest subsequent to retrobulbar block. *Ophthal Surg* 1987; **18**: 11–13.

30 Nichol JMV, Acharya PA, Ahlen K *et al.* Central nervous system complications after 6000 retrobulbar blocks. *Anesth Analg* 1987; **66**: 1298–302.

31 Meyers EF, Ramirez RC, Boniuk I. Grand mal seizures after retrobulbar block. *Arch Ophthalmol* 1978; **96**: 847.

32 Kimble JA, Morris RE, Witherspoon CA *et al.* Globe perforation from peribulbar injection. *Arch Ophthalmol* 1987; **105**: 749.

15: Cataract Surgery and Glaucoma

THOMAS STANK, MARIANNE E. FEITL & THEODORE KRUPIN

The incidence of visually significant cataract in the elderly population has been estimated at 4–19% [1]. The miotic effect of cholinergic medications and the cataractogenic nature of glaucoma surgery raises the incidence of visually significant cataract even higher in the glaucomatous population. Furthermore, reduced visual acuity in the glaucomatous eye may be due to extensive optic nerve damage and associated visual field damage, as well as macular abnormalities, and not due to a cataract. Cataract surgery in a glaucomatous eye is associated with higher intraoperative and postoperative complications when compared to cataract extraction in non-glaucomatous eyes. Therefore, the ophthalmologist should consider medical or laser therapy alternatives to reduce miosis and improve vision prior to cataract removal. Finally, when confronted with cataract removal in the glaucomatous eye, one should formulate a logical surgical approach designed to minimize the risks and maximize the benefits of cataract removal.

Surgical alternatives

The first question to be answered when considering cataract surgery on a glaucomatous eye is whether the patient is suffering from miotic-induced decrease in vision. Often, an assessment of visual function, e.g. visual acuity, visual field examination, and potential acuity meter (PAM) testing; an appraisal of the appearance of the optic nerve and macula; and the clarity of view of the posterior pole with the direct ophthalmoscope after pupillary dilation, will answer this question.

Several alternatives exist if the patient is having miotic-induced decrease in vision. Substitution of the miotic therapy with either a β-adrenergic antagonist, an epinephrine compound, or a systemic carbonic anhydrase inhibitor may provide adequate intraocular pressure (IOP) control while eliminating the miosis. Other forms of miotic drug delivery systems, such as pilocarpine gel or Ocusert therapy, may have a sufficient therapeutic response with reduced pupillary miosis and a subsequent increase in vision.

Argon laser trabeculoplasty (ALT) prior to cataract surgery has several clinical indications. If successful in lowering IOP, ALT may eliminate the need for miotic therapy and thereby improve visual function. Laser treatment may stabilize IOP control, thereby eliminating the need for a combined cataract and filtration or a staged filtration procedure with later cataract removal. Some clinicians feel the success rate of ALT is higher in phakic versus pseudophakic eyes and therefore recommend that ALT be performed prior to cataract surgery [2]. However, our experience indicates that the ability of ALT to lower IOP in the pseudophakic eye is more dependent upon the type of glaucoma which is present. Eyes which have open-angle glaucoma prior to the cataract removal and postoperatively have an open iridocorneal angle, have a high success rate if ALT is performed after the eye is pseudophakic. However, secondary glaucoma which develops after the cataract surgery has a very low response to ALT.

The concomitant use of topical neosynephrine 2.5% with the miotic therapy may

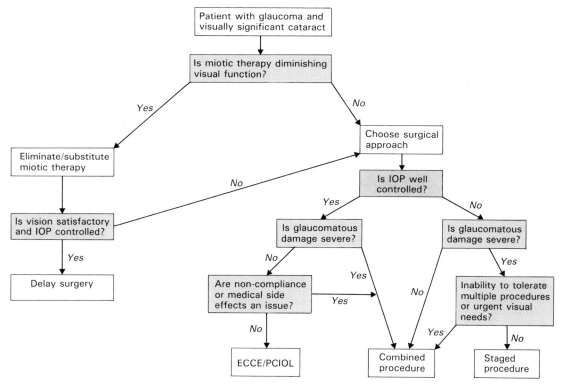

Fig. 15.1 Schematic representation of the factors involved in the decision process relating to the management of coexisting cataract and glaucoma.

reduce pupillary miosis while not affecting IOP control. In addition, laser pupilloplasty or sphincterotomy can be attempted to enlarge the pupil. Failing all of the above maneuvers, miotic therapy may still be required to control the IOP with its associated reduction in vision. The ophthalmologist must then select a surgical approach to best manage the cataract and the glaucoma.

Surgical approaches

There are three approaches to cataract surgery in the glaucomatous eye including: (a) a primary extracapsular cataract extraction (ECCE) either with or without a posterior chamber implant (PCIOL); (b) combined cataract and filtration surgery; and (c) a filtration procedure followed later by cataract removal. Factors

influencing the type of operation chosen are the level of glaucoma control, the severity of visual field loss, stability of glaucomatous optic nerve damage, visual status of the fellow eye, compliance and tolerance of the current glaucoma medical regimen, and the ability of the patient to tolerate multiple surgical procedures. These factors are considered for each patient and are used to guide the type of surgery to be performed (Fig. 5.1).

Extracapsular cataract extraction with posterior chamber implant (ECCE/PCIOL)

We feel that the majority of patients with coexisting glaucoma and cataract are best managed by ECCE/PCIOL. Potential benefits of cataract surgery alone include improved vision and stable or possibly improved long-term control of the IOP. Indications include well-controlled IOP and mild to moderate glaucomatous damage. The patient should be compliant with their current medical regimen and tolerating the medications well. The surgeon should be confident that the optic nerve could safely tolerate a potential postoperative IOP rise.

Combined filtration and cataract surgery (combined surgery)

Patients with cataract, uncontrolled IOP, and extensive glaucomatous damage may benefit from a combined rather than a two-step (see below) procedure, particularly if they have urgent visual needs (e.g. poor sight in their fellow eye), or if they are unable to tolerate two separate surgical procedures. In addition, patients having side effects from their glaucoma treatment or who are non-compliant, are good candidates for combined surgery. Finally, we feel combined surgery is indicated in patients with controlled IOP and moderate to severe glaucomatous damage since the procedure minimizes the risk of a postoperative increase in IOP which may not be tolerated by a severely damaged optic nerve.

Staged filtration and cataract procedures (staged procedure)

A staged procedure is an alternative approach to the glaucoma patient with a cataract. Indications include uncontrolled glaucoma and severe glaucomatous damage. The filtration surgery is performed to control the IOP with cataract removal 4–6 months later. The major disadvantage is prolonged visual rehabilitation and the risks associated with two separate procedures.

Surgical techniques

ECCE/PCIOL

Preoperative evaluation must note the size of the maximally dilated pupil, the presence of posterior synechiae, the type of the glaucoma

(especially pseudoexfoliation), and the location of an iridectomy or a filtration bleb if previous surgery has been performed. Miotic therapy should be discontinued the day before surgery in an attempt to increase pupil size. Phospholine iodide can cause an intensive postoperative inflammatory response. This medication should be stopped at least 3 weeks before surgery and pilocarpine used in its place. Prior to surgery we administer topical cycloplegics and mydriatics to produce a maximum-sized pupil. Topical flurbiprofen sodium can be given in an attempt to maintain pupil dilation during surgery.

Operative techniques vary greatly between individual surgeons. We perform a fornix-based conjunctival flap and a posterior limbal site for the cataract incision. Cataract surgery in the glaucomatous eye requires special attention regarding management of the pupil and nucleus expression. Phacoemulsification through a small pupil will not be covered in this chapter.

MANAGEMENT OF THE PUPIL

Chronic miotic therapy frequently results in a small and rigid pupil with posterior synechiae. The pupil may not respond to dilation. In this situation, we will make a 3–5 mm entry into the anterior chamber and perform a peripheral iridectomy. Lysis of the posterior synechiae is performed using a smooth cyclodialysis spatula which is inserted through the peripheral iridectomy. The peripheral iridectomy is converted into a radial iridectomy using Vannas scissors. An inferior, and occasionally lateral, sphincterotomy is also performed to create a sufficiently sized pupil for the surgery. Instillation of a viscoelastic agent behind the iris will assist in enlarging the pupil. We routinely close the sector iridectomy at the conclusion of the cataract removal (see below).

CAPSULOTOMY

We presently perform a "can opener" style anterior capsulotomy using a bent 25 gauge needle. The surgeon must be conscious of the visual axis and the center of the lens. The presence of a sector iridectomy can lead to opening the anterior capsule too superiorly with possible extension of the capsule tear to the equator of the lens. Limited pupil enlargement may require performing the inferior 180° of the capsulotomy behind the iris. Instillation of a viscoelastic substance behind the iris to create a space in front of the lens, or a two-handed technique to retract the iris, facilitates performing a capsulotomy with at least an 8 mm diameter. The lens nucleus is rocked from 3 to 9 o'clock and from 6 to 12 o'clock with the 25 gauge needle to facilitate expression (see below). The dissected anterior capsule is removed from the anterior chamber.

LIMBAL WOUND

The wound is enlarged to a chord length of 11 mm with corneal scissors. A larger wound is necessary in the glaucomatous eye due to the rigid iris and limited size of the pupil and capsulotomy.

LENS REMOVAL

Nucleus removal can be associated with a higher incidence of vitreous loss in the glaucomatous eye. The rigid iris and limited pupil size resists mechanical "pushing" of the nucleus out of the eye. In addition, eyes with pseudoexfoliative glaucoma may have weak zonules which can rupture following external pressure on the globe. Therefore, we use the minimum external pressure necessary to rotate the superior pole of the nucleus forward where it can be hooked and rotated out of the anterior chamber. This technique of "pulling the nucleus out" is in contrast to the method of "pushing the nucleus out" used in standard cataract surgery.

Cortical material is removed using irrigation–aspiration techniques. A two-handed technique can be used to retract the iris and enhance visualization during this stage. Care must be taken not to be too aggressive removing cortex in the superiorly exposed area of the sector iridectomy. This can result in damage to the superior capsule or zonules and vitreous loss.

INTRAOCULAR LENS

Glaucomatous eyes often have irregular, eccentric pupils postoperatively due to the necessary operative manipulations of the pupil and to the rigid nature of the iris. Therefore, we prefer a 7 mm, no hole optic with poly-methylmetacrylate (PMMA) haptics. This design minimizes the postoperative risk of edge glare, iris/lens capture, and lens decentration. The IOL is placed into the capsular bag except in exfoliative eyes where sulcus fixation is used. The haptics are rotated to the horizontal position.

CLOSURE OF THE IRIDECTOMY

We routinely reapproximate the sector iridectomy with a 9/0 prolene suture on a tapered, non-cutting needle (Ethicon BV 100–4). This double-armed suture is 5 cm (2 in) long. One side of the cut iris sphincter muscle is fixated using a fine toothed forceps and one arm of the suture is placed through the iris from the anterior to the posterior surface. The opposite side of the cut sphincter muscle is fixated and the second arm of the suture passed in a similar fashion. The suture is tied, placing the knot under the iris. Our reason for closure of the iridectomy is to prevent possible iris capture of the IOL and subsequent intraocular inflammation.

WOUND CLOSURE

The corneal–scleral incision is closed using 10/0 nylon sutures. The viscoelastic substance is aspirated from the anterior chamber. The conjunctival flap is closed at both ends so that it covers the limbal wound. Subconjunctival antibiotics (e.g. gentamicin 40 mg) and corticosteroids (e.g. dexamethasone 2 mg or triamcinolone 40 mg) are given.

OPERATIVE COMPLICATIONS

Intraoperative complications unique to the glaucomatous eye are increased bleeding and a higher incidence of vitreous loss. Hemorrhage may be more common due to glaucoma therapy-induced alterations of the blood–aqueous barrier and to the greater operative manipulations of the iris. The increased occurrence of vitreous loss has been attributed to abnormal lens zonules and to the technical complexities associated with a small, non-reactive pupil.

POSTOPERATIVE COMPLICATIONS

Inflammation

Postoperative inflammation is more common in the glaucomatous eye, again due to the increased operative manipulations. Intense anterior chamber reaction, including a fibrinoid reaction, is not uncommon. Topical corticosteroids are used more frequently and for longer periods of time. Our routine is to administer either topical dexamethasone phosphate 0.1% or prednisolone phosphate 1% every 2h while awake for the first postoperative week and then slowly taper the drops over 6–8 weeks. Occasionally we will use short (5–7 days) durations of oral prednisone.

Hyphema

The incidence of postoperative hyphema has been reported to be 8.3% in glaucomatous eyes versus 2.5% in non-glaucomatous eyes [3,4]. However, in a recent study of 46 eyes with open-angle glaucoma who underwent ECCE/PCIOL, the incidence of hyphema was 2% [5]. All eyes in this study had a peripheral iridectomy. The hyphema resolved spontaneously and did not alter the outcome of the cataract procedure.

Early increase in IOP

Significant early postoperative increases in IOP occur in 10–55% of normal eyes following ECCE/PCIOL [6–10]. The onset of the pressure rise can be as early as 3h with the maximum increase occurring 16–24h after surgery [10, 11]. Postoperative increases in IOP occur more frequently and to higher levels in eyes with pre-existing glaucoma: 62–69% of glaucomatous eyes have a pressure rise greater than 7–10 mmHg on the first postoperative day [6,12]. For this reason, a "triple procedure" of ECCE/PCIOL and filtration surgery (see below) has been recommended [6,7,13].

The exact mechanisms responsible for the postoperative increases in IOP are unknown. This complication, which also occurs following intracapsular cataract surgery with or without the use of α-chymotrypsin, is more common since the introduction of viscoelastic agents during surgery [14]. These agents block trabecular outflow pathways as their mechanism for induced rises in IOP. The glaucomatous eye with an already reduced outflow facility, may not be able to tolerate additional outflow facility compromise by viscoelastic agents, even though the bulk of these agents are aspirated from the anterior chamber. Other substances such as cortical material, iris debris, and red blood cells, may also compromise outflow facility. Postoperative use of pilocarpine gel [10] and the operative administration of carbachol intracamerally [15] have both been shown to maintain stable IOP at 24–48h postoperatively in non-glaucomatous eyes. Topical β-blockers and oral carbonic anhydrase inhibitors may lower a postoperatively increased IOP, but hyperosmotic agents are usually the most rapid and effective treatment of this complication.

These transient increases in IOP following ECCE/PCIOL pose a threat to an already compromised glaucomatous optic nerve. Savage *et al.* have reported that 9.7% of glaucomatous eyes had worsening of visual field after cataract surgery [3]. Cashwell and Deok [16] described one case of loss of central fixation ("snuff-out") in a series of 54 glaucoma patients undergoing ECCE/PCIOL. This patient had a significant postoperative pressure rise and extensive visual field loss preoperatively. In addition, the increased IOP may be sufficiently high to result in a retinal vascular occlusion. It is extremely important to monitor IOP within the first 24–48h following cataract surgery in glaucomatous eyes to detect and treat an increased IOP.

Cystoid macular edema

Cystoid macular edema occurs in 1–3% of non-glaucomatous eyes following ECCE/PCIOL

[17]. This complication is more common after cataract surgery in glaucomatous eyes. In our study, 11.6% of glaucomatous eyes had visually significant angiographically confirmed cystoid macular edema [5]. This complication resolved spontaneously in all eyes by 7 months postoperatively. The increased incidence of this complication in the glaucoma patient may be explained by the greater operative manipulations and the increased postoperative inflammation. Glaucoma patients need to be warned of this possible complication and subsequent delayed visual rehabilitation following cataract surgery.

LONG-TERM RESULTS

Glaucoma control

Cataract surgery in glaucomatous eyes may have a beneficial effect on the long-term control of IOP. Several investigators have reported postoperative reductions in both IOP and the number of medications required to achieve pressure control following ECCE/PCIOL [3,5, 6,18]. This effect on IOP is not related to an inadvertent filtration bleb or a cyclodialysis cleft. The mechanisms for this positive effect on IOP are unknown and may relate to altered anatomic relationships and outflow mechanisms, rate of aqueous humor formation or composition, or increased drug penetration and effectiveness in the aphakic or pseudophakic eye. The effect persists in many eyes for years after cataract surgery.

Visual acuity

Postoperative visual acuity is similar to results obtained after ECCE/PCIOL in nonglaucomatous eyes [3,5,6]. In our study, 72% of eyes had a visual acuity of 6/12 or better. Failure to obtain this level of postoperative vision was related to either extensive glaucoma damage or macular degeneration.

Combined surgery

Many techniques have been described to combine a filtration procedure with the cataract

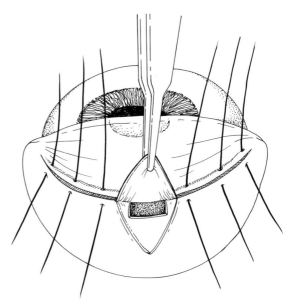

Fig. 15.2 Schematic of the limbal incision for a combined cataract extraction and trabeculectomy.

removal. Most commonly a trabeculectomy or a guarded posterior lip sclerectomy is performed as part of the combined procedure; however, trabeculotomy, a full-thickness sclerostomy, or a cyclodialysis have also been used. These latter procedures will not be described in this chapter.

COMBINED TRABECULECTOMY (Fig. 15.2)

Many techniques have been described for combining a trabeculectomy with the ECCE/ PCIOL. We prefer using a limbus-based conjunctival flap to reduce the chance of a postoperative wound leak at the limbus. However, many surgeons use a fornix-based conjunctival flap presumably without problems. We dissect the trabeculectomy scleral flap (triangular or rectangular) into clear cornea and then make a corneoscleral groove for the cataract removal to both sides of the scleral flap. A corneal paracentesis tract at a site distant from the wound is performed. Entry is made into the anterior chamber through the corneal base of the scleral flap dissection bed. Surgery is then modified depending upon the size of the pupil.

Large pupil

If the pupil is of sufficient size to perform the cataract surgery, then the anterior capsulotomy and nucleus dislocation are performed. The trabeculectomy block is excised and the corneoscleral wound enlarged with scissors. Nucleus removal, cortex aspiration, and IOL insertion are performed as described above. The corneoscleral wound is closed using 10/0 nylon sutures which are placed on either side of the trabeculectomy flap and along the wound to adequately close it. An iridectomy is performed at the base of the trabeculectomy flap and the scleral flap is closed with 10/0 nylon sutures. The anterior chamber is deepened either through the paracentesis tract or the corneoscleral wound. The conjunctival flap is closed using an 8/0 or 9/0 suture on a tapered needle (Ethicon BV 130–5).

Small pupil

A miotic pupil requires that the corneoscleral wound be enlarged to either side of the trabeculectomy block in order to provide sufficient working room in the anterior chamber. A peripheral iridectomy is performed at the base of the trabeculectomy block. Pupillary enlargement is achieved by lysing posterior synechiae with a smooth cyclodialysis spatula, converting the iridectomy to a sector opening, and inserting a viscoelastic agent behind the iris as previously described. The corneoscleral wound is enlarged to at least 11 mm and the anterior capsulotomy, nucleus removal, cortex removal, and lens insertion performed. The iridectomy is sutured. Closure of the corneoscleral and conjunctival wounds are as previously described.

COMBINED POSTERIOR LIP SCLERECTOMY

We presently prefer using a guarded posterior lip sclerectomy for combined surgery. This procedure is performed at the conclusion of the cataract removal and requires less operative manipulation. In our experience the early postoperative results are similar to a combined trabeculectomy procedure.

The initial corneoscleral incision is made posteriorly with a long posteriorly beveled shelf. Cataract removal and IOL implantation are performed as described with attention to the pupil size. The corneoscleral wound is closed except for a 3 mm area over the region of the iridectomy. A 10/0 nylon suture is placed across this wound opening, 1 mm to either side of the limiting sutures, and is looped out of the wound. A punch is inserted into the 2 mm opening to excise a piece of the posterior scleral lip (Plate 15.1). If iris tissue is present at the base of the excised posterior lip, it is removed. The remaining 10/0 nylon suture is pulled up, tied, and cut. The excised posterior lip sclerectomy should be partially covered by the anterior portion of the corneoscleral wound. Surgery is completed as previously described.

Several scleral punches are commercially available. We have recently described a modified version of the Gass punch (Fig. 15.3) [19]. This punch allows a controlled and fully visualized removal of the posterior scleral lip. With any device, care must be taken not to direct the punch too far posteriorly or extensive bleeding can occur from the ciliary body or processes. If required, the punch sclerectomy can be enlarged by using cautery to retract the scleral side of the wound.

OPERATIVE COMPLICATIONS

Hemorrhage may be more common with combined surgery than cataract surgery alone in the glaucomatous eye. This occurs if the excised trabeculectomy or the posterior lip tissue is too posterior. The incidence of significant intraoperative hemorrhage was zero in our study of 42 eyes undergoing combined procedures [12]. Bleeding usually stops with gentle pressure applied with a cellulose sponge. The use of intraocular cautery may be dangerous but occasionally is necessary. The fine tips of a "jeweler's" forceps with a bipolar cautery or another type of micro tip cautery are the best instruments for this maneuver.

POSTOPERATIVE COMPLICATIONS

Combined filtration surgery adds to the potential postoperative complications previously

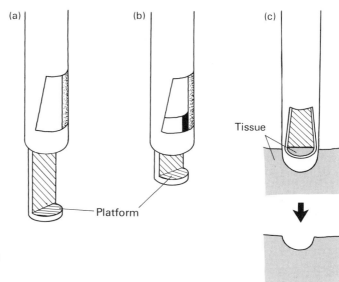

Fig. 15.3 Schematic drawing of the guillotine punch (a). As the shaft advances towards the platform (b), the slot becomes exposed to allow visualization of the tissue resting on the platform (c) before completion of the punch [19].

listed for cataract surgery in the glaucomatous eye. However, visually significant complications unique to combined filtration surgery appear to be minimal.

Hyphema

Postoperative hyphema usually clears without sequelae. However, blood may occlude the sclerostomy opening resulting in an increased IOP (see below). The incidence of postoperative hyphema varies between 5 and 14% [12,13].

Early increase in IOP

Immediate postoperative pressure rises are less common but can still occur following combined procedures. It is important to realize that combined filtration surgery does not prevent this complication. A postoperative IOP greater than 35 mmHg is reported in 5% of combined procedures [13] while an IOP rise greater than 10 mmHg is reported to occur in 14% of eyes 15–18 h following surgery [12]. The etiology for the IOP rise is usually a blocked internal sclerostomy (e.g. blood, fibrin, cortex) or a scleral flap with a tight suture if a trabeculectomy was performed. Argon or Nd:YAG laser treatment to the occluding material through a goniolens can be used to reopen the sclerostomy opening. The argon laser can be used to cut a scleral flap suture which is too tight. External ocular pressure ("massage") and/or medical treatment combined with laser treatment are usually effective in treating this IOP rise. Postoperative monitoring of IOP following combined surgery is important to detect and treat this potentially vision-threatening complication.

Hypotony/choroidal detachment

Hypotony and choroidal detachment are more common in combined (incidence 6–21%) than in cataract only procedures (incidence 4%) in glaucomatous eyes [12,13]. A Seidel test should be performed to detect and treat a conjunctival wound leak which can be the cause for this complication. Hypotony and choroidal detachment can lead to a shallow or flat anterior chamber. In the series by McCartney *et al.* less than 1% of patients undergoing combined surgery required drainage of the choroidal detachment and reformation of the anterior chamber [13]. We manage choroidal detachments medically with frequent topical and occasionally systemic corticosteroids. Surgical intervention is undertaken if there is corneal–lenticular touch and corneal decompensation.

Pupillary block can be a triggering event for a

shallow anterior chamber with subsequent hypotony. Pupillary block can occur in an eye with an intraocular lens implant even with an iridectomy. The iris adheres to the lens implant and causes a localized area of pupillary block. This produces areas of localized shallowing in the anterior chamber depth and regional areas of iris bombé. Laser iridectomy to create multiple openings is the treatment of choice. Occasionally surgery is necessary to create a permanent iridectomy.

LONG-TERM RESULTS

Glaucoma control

Long-term postoperative IOP control following combined surgery is undetermined. It is difficult to separate the positive effects of cataract removal alone from the effects of performing a filtration procedure with the cataract surgery. McCartney *et al.* report IOP control ($\leqslant$21 mmHg) in 92% of eyes undergoing combined surgery at an average follow-up of 16.7 months. No medications were required in 57% of these eyes, and 29% required fewer medications. However, the percentage of eyes controlled on no medications decreased from 67 to 44%, 30 months after surgery [13].

We have recently compared long-term IOP control in eyes with open-angle glaucoma undergoing either ECCE/PCIOL or combined filtration surgery (unpublished data). Eyes undergoing cataract surgery alone had unchanged IOP control over an average 25 months of follow-up. However, there was a significant reduction in the number of medications required to achieve this level of control. Both IOP and the number of medications were reduced at an average of 30.6 months postoperatively in the combined surgery eyes. IOP and the number of medications were significantly reduced in the combined surgery eyes when compared to the cataract only eye. However, only 21% of the combined eyes had a functioning bleb (IOP < 19 mmHg on no medications) at the last follow-up examination. Combined surgery in eyes with open-angle glaucoma provides protection against early postoperative increases in IOP (see above) and improved

long-term IOP control when compared to ECCE/PCIOL alone.

Visual acuity

Visual acuity following combined procedures is similar to that reported after cataract surgery alone. The percentage of eyes with vision better than 6/12 is between 67 and 100% [12,13,20,21].

Staged procedures

FILTRATION SURGERY

The technique for the initial filtration procedure is guided by the surgeon's preference. Filtration surgery is usually performed in the superior-nasal quadrant to allow the subsequent cataract extraction to be performed temporally. This location is not necessary if later cataract removal is to be performed either via a corneal incision anterior to the bleb or at an inferior limbal site. One should consider performing a sector iridectomy at the time of filtration surgery since the enlarged pupil may improve vision and delay the contemplated cataract removal. The sector iridectomy is performed pulling the sphincter out of the anterior chamber using a "hand-over-hand" technique to avoid injury to the lens capsule.

CATARACT REMOVAL

The second stage of cataract removal, if required, is undertaken 4–6 months after the initial filtration procedure. Cataract removal should avoid surgical manipulation of the bleb. The best approach for cataract surgery to maintain functioning of the bleb has not been determined. The incidence of late bleb failure appears to be similar independent of the location of the cataract incision.

Limbal incision

Some surgeons prefer to maintain the limbal anatomy and will perform the incision either to the side of the bleb or at an inferior limbal location. Cataract removal is performed in exactly the same manner as a standard ECCE/PCIOL.

Corneal incision

We prefer a clear corneal incision anterior to the bleb to maintain the usual superior operating position. The anterior location of the incision requires a longer circumferential arc length to achieve the desired chord length needed for delivery of the nucleus. Corneal sutures must be placed radially and at the same uniform tension otherwise significant astigmatism may develop. Wound healing is delayed with a corneal incision and sutures are not removed until 3–6 months postoperatively. Suture induced corneal astigmatism may limit vision during this interval. The long-term degree of astigmatism achieved with this approach is similar to a corneoscleral approach.

Bleb failure

Continued bleb function following cataract surgery is difficult to determine due to the positive effect of cataract removal alone on IOP control. The literature frequently does not differentiate between a preoperatively totally functioning bleb (i.e. IOP < 20 mmHg on no glaucoma medications) and a partially functioning bleb with medications required to control the IOP less than 20 mmHg. Finally, many studies are of relatively short postoperative follow-up.

Studies performed when cataract removal was by intracapsular techniques report continued bleb functioning in 87–100% of cases when a corneal incision was used [22,23]. Duration of follow-up was unspecified in these studies. Baloglou et al. [24] reported the failure rate after intracapsular extraction to be 11% with an inferior approach and 19% with a temporal approach.

Bleb failure following extracapsular techniques appears to be significantly lower than those reported after intracapsular cataract removal. Antonios et al. [25] reported on 29 patients who underwent ECCE/PCIOL via a temporal approach with an average postoperative follow-up of 13 months. No patient required additional surgery, 62% were controlled with no glaucoma medications, and 38% of the patients required medical therapy for IOP control. However, the difference between patients requiring medications before and after cataract surgery was not statistically different. Alpar [26] reported on 85 patients undergoing a temporal approach with either phacoemulsification or ECCE. In all cases the IOP remained controlled; however, there was no mention of the need for additional medications.

We examined the effect of ECCE/PCIOL through a clear corneal incision in 22 patients with a functioning bleb (IOP < 20 mmHg on no medications) (unpublished data). At 1 year of follow-up, 93% of the blebs continued to function with IOP less than 20 mmHg on no medications. Five eyes with extensive glaucomatous damage were also treated with topical β-blockers to achieve a lower IOP. Filtration failure occurred in one eye which required filtration surgery. However, decreased functioning of the blebs with increasing requirement for glaucoma medications occurred over time. Two years after surgery 80% and 3 years after surgery only 60% of eyes were controlled without medications. One eye during these intervals required repeat filtration surgery with IOP in the other eyes controlled less than 20 mmHg with the addition of glaucoma medications. However, it must be remembered that all eyes in this series had a functioning filtration bleb prior to the cataract removal.

Summary

Recent advances in extracapsular cataract removal with a posterior chamber lens implant have improved the visual outcome following cataract removal in glaucomatous eyes. Cataract surgery is more difficult with more frequent operative and postoperative complications in the glaucomatous eye. Long-term IOP control is positively influenced by cataract removal with less medications required postoperatively. The most severe postoperative complication is an acute increase in IOP which may not be tolerated by the glaucomatous optic nerve. Combined cataract and filtration surgery reduces the frequency and magnitude of the postoperative increase in IOP. While combined surgery is associated with a greater incidence of postoperative complications, namely hypotony and choroidal detachment, the long-term IOP control is better than that following cataract removal alone. An alternative approach to the management of cataract in the glaucomatous eye is to do a planned two-staged procedure: filtration surgery followed 4–6 months later with cataract removal. However, bleb failure following cataract removal is a problem.

Continued advances in the field of cataract surgery will continue to have a positive effect in glaucomatous eyes. Improved small incision techniques with reduced surgical manipulation offer the possibility for improved results with combined surgery and for continued functioning of a bleb after cataract removal.

References

1 Shaffer RN, Rosenthal G. Comparison of cataract incidence in normal and glaucomatous population. *Am J Ophthalmol* 1970; **69**: 368.

2 Thomas JV, Simmons RJ, Belcher CD III. Argon laser trabeculoplasty in the pre-surgical glaucoma patient. *Ophthalmology* 1982; **89**: 197.

3 Savage JA, Thomas JV, Belcher CD III, Simmons RJ. Extracapsular cataract extraction and posterior chamber intraocular lens implantation in glaucomatous eyes. *Ophthalmology* 1985; **92**: 1506.

4 Cohen JS, Osher RH, Weber P, Faulkner JD. Complications of extracapsular cataract surgery: The indications and risks of peripheral iridectomy. *Ophthalmology* 1984; **91**: 826.

5 Handa K, Henry C, Krupin T, Keates E. Extracapsular cataract extraction with posterior chamber lens implantation in patients with glaucoma. *Arch Ophthalmol* 1987; **105**: 765.

6 McGuigan LJB, Gottsch J, Stark WJ, Maumenee AE, Quigley HA. Extracapsular cataract extraction and posterior chamber lens implantation in eyes with preexisting glaucoma. *Arch Ophthalmol* 1986; **104**: 1301.

7 Percival SPB. Complications from the use of sodium hyaluronate (Healonid) in anterior segment surgery. *Br J Ophthalmol* 1982; **66**: 714.

8 Passo MS, Ernest TJ, Goldstick TK. Hyaluronate increases intraocular pressure when used in cataract extraction. *Br J Ophthalmol* 1985; **69**: 572.

9 Naeser K, Thim K, Hansen TE, Degn T, Madsen S, Skor J. Intraocular pressure in the first days after implantation of posterior chamber lenses with the use of sodium hyauronate (Healon). *Acta Ophthalmol* 1986; **64**: 330.

10 Ruiz RS, Wilson CA, Musgrove KH, Prager TC. Management of increased intraocular pressure after cataract extraction. *Am J Ophthalmol* 1987; **103**: 487.

11 Barron BA, Busin M, Page C, Bergsma DR, Kaufman HE. Comparison of the effects of Viscoat and Healon on postoperative intraocular pressure. *Am J Ophthalmol* 1985; **100**: 377.

12 Krupin T, Feitl ME, Bishop KI. Postoperative intraocular pressure rise after cataract or combined cataract-filtration surgery in open-angle glaucoma. *Ophthalmology* 1989; **96**: 579.

13 McCartney DL, Memmen JE, Stark WJ et al. The efficacy and safety of combined trabeculectomy, cataract extraction, and intraocular lens implantation. *Ophthalmology* 1988; **95**: 754.

14 Rich WJ, Radtke ND, Cohan BE. Early ocular hypertension after cataract extraction. *Br J Ophthalmol* 1974; **58**: 725.

15 Linn DK, Zimmerman TJ. Effect of intracameral carbachol on intraocular pressure after cataract extraction. *Am J Ophthalmol* 1989; **107**: 133.

16 Cashwell LF, Deok Y. *Effect of cataract extraction on advanced glaucomatous visual field loss*. Presented at the AAO Meeting, New Orleans, October 1989.

17 Taylor DM, Sachs SW, Stern AL. Aphakic cystoid macular edema: Long-term clinical observations. *Surv Ophthalmol* 1984; **28** (suppl): 437.

18 McMahan LB, Monica MI, Zimmerman TJ. Posterior chamber pseudophakes in glaucoma patients. *Ophthal Surg* 1986; **17**: 146.

19 Henry JC, Krupin T, Wax MB, Feitl ME. A modified scleral punch for filtration surgery. *Am J Ophthalmol* 1989; **108**: 740.

20 Ohanesion RV, Kim EW. A prospective study of combined extracapsular extraction, posterior chamber lens implantation and trabeculectomy. *J Am Intraocul Implant Soc* 1985; **11**: 142.

21 Jay JL. Extracapsular lens extraction and posterior chamber lens insertion combined with trabeculectomy. *Br J Ophthalmol* 1985; **69**: 487.

22 Randolph ME, Maumenee AD, Illif CE. Cataract extraction in glaucomatous eyes. *Am J Ophthalmol* 1971; **71**: 331.

23 Kondo T. Cataract extraction after filtering operation. *Glaucoma* 1979; **1**: 265.

24 Baloglou P, Matta C, Asdourian M. Cataract extraction after filtering operations. *Arch Ophthalmol* 1972; **88**: 1.

25 Antonios SR, Traverso CE, Tomey KF. Extracapsular cataract extraction using a temporal limbal approach after filtering operations. *Arch Ophthalmol* 1988; **106**: 608.

26 Alpar JJ. Glaucoma after intraocular lens implantation: Surgery and recommendations. *Glaucoma* 1985; **7**: 241.

16: Conjunctival, Corneal, and Scleral Disease and Cataract Surgery

ROBERT C. ARFFA & RICHARD A. THOFT

Introduction

Patients with cataracts commonly also have diseases of the conjunctiva, cornea, or sclera. Some of these diseases can adversely affect the outcome of surgery, particularly if their presence is not recognized and treatment is not modified. In some cases the standard care is altered by the addition of preoperative medication; in others surgical technique or postoperative care is modified. In addition the risk and types of complications is often different from that in routine cases.

Prospective cataract patients should be examined for the presence of previously unrecognized disease which could affect the course of their surgery. Some diseases can be present in patients with no history of eye problems, and minimal or no symptoms. Probably the most common of these is aqueous tear deficiency, or "dry eyes." Other conditions include impaired lid function, blepharitis, chronic dacryocystitis, and early cicatricial pemphigoid.

Therefore, the following procedures should be included in the routine preoperative evaluation of a surgical candidate:
1 specific questioning about the symptoms of dry eyes, as well as dry mouth and arthritis;
2 evaluation of lid position and function;
3 examination of the lid margins for signs of blepharitis and meibomitis;
4 examination of the tear film; Schirmer testing and rose bengal staining if indicated; and
5 examination of the fornices for evidence of scarring.

Lid and lacrimal disease

Dry eyes

Tear film abnormalities are frequently encountered in cataract patients. Aqueous tear deficiency is the most common of these, but other abnormalities, such as impaired tear surfacing, are also important in cataract surgery.

Aqueous tear deficiency is most often seen in women in their fifth and sixth decades, however, it can develop at any age, and can affect men. It is most often idiopathic, but can be associated with many local and systemic conditions (Table 16.1). Sjögren's syndrome classically consists of dry eyes, dry mouth (xerostomia), and a connective tissue disease, most commonly rheumatoid arthritis [1,2]. The syndrome is often incomplete, and its definition has varied, but it should not be used to refer to cases of isolated dry eyes. The syndrome is divided into two forms: (a) primary: dry eyes and dry mouth; and (b) secondary: dry eyes and/or dry mouth associated with a systemic autoimmune disease [3]. Associated autoimmune diseases include all of those listed in Table 16.1.

The onset usually occurs between 30 and 60 years of age, and women are affected nine times more frequently than men [4]. In addition to the lacrimal and salivary glands, the mucus-secreting glands, respiratory mucosa, and the vagina can also be involved. Many other organ systems can be affected, including the joints, skin, lung, kidneys, peripheral and central nervous systems, blood, and muscle, Impaired

Table 16.1 Conditions associated with aqueous tear deficiency. After [29]

Congenital	*Hematopoietic diseases*
Riley–Day syndrome	Lymphoma
Cri du chat syndrome	Thrombocytopenic purpura
Multiple endocrine neoplasia	Hypergammaglobulinemia
Lacrimal gland hypoplasia	Waldenström's macroglobulinemia
Anhidrotic ectodermal dysplasia	
Holmes–Adie syndrome	*Other systemic conditions*
Paralytic hyposecretion	Celiac disease
	Sarcoidosis
Local conditions	Graft vs. host disease
Dacryoadenitis (viral or bacterial)	Pulmonary fibrosis
Irradiation	Chronic hepatobiliary disease
Trauma	Amyloidosis
Benign lymphoepithelial	
lesion (Mikulicz's disease)	*Medications*
Seventh nerve palsy	Anticholinergic drugs
Blepharitis	Antihistamines
	Tricyclic antidepressants
Autoimmune diseases	Monoamine oxidase inhibitors
Rheumatoid arthritis	β-blockers
Lupus erythematosus	Hydrochlorothiazide
Polyarteritis nodosa	Oral contraceptives(?)
Hashimoto's thyroiditis	Antidiarrheals
Polymyositis	Decongestants
Others	Thiabendazole
	Antiparkinsonian agents
	Antineoplastic agents
	Retinoids (etretinate, isotretinoin)
	Many others [74]

lymphocyte function and lymphoreticular neoplasms also occur [3,5].

CLINICAL FINDINGS

Patient's with dry eyes are prone to sterile corneal ulceration after cataract surgery (Fig. 16.1) [6–8]. Most of the patients who develop ulcers are not severely symptomatic prior to surgery. The precipitating event is not clear, but is probably minor trauma to the corneal epithelium. Healing is impaired, by dryness and superior corneal denervation, and persistence of the epithelial defect leads to stromal loss. Localized drying, related to elevation of the paralimbal conjunctiva or impaired lid function, may contribute. Dry eyes are also more susceptible to infection.

The ulcers tend to be small (2 mm or less in diameter), central or paracentral, and steep walled. Misdiagnosis as bacterial, herpetic, or fungal infection is common. However, in

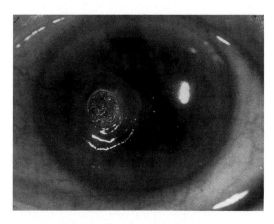

Fig. 16.1 Corneal ulcer occurring after cataract extraction in patient with dry eye. Perforation is sealed with tissue adhesive.

contrast to most infectious ulcers, these are usually not infiltrated or painful, and are often not associated with much conjunctival hyperemia or anterior chamber reaction. The ulcers often deepen rapidly, particularly if topical corticosteroids are being administered, and can perforate if not treated aggressively. Permanent reduction in visual acuity often results from scarring in the visual axis.

PREVENTION AND TREATMENT

Ulceration can usually be prevented by appropriate postoperative treatment. Therefore, it is essential that the dry eye condition be recognized. All candidates for cataract surgery should be questioned about symptoms of dry eyes: burning, foreign-body sensation, dryness grittiness, and mucoid discharge. A history of dry mouth or arthritis should also be elicited. Examination should include the height of the tear meniscus, the presence of excess mucus, and interpalpebral punctate keratopathy. If the diagnosis is suspected Schirmer's testing and rose bengal staining can be performed.

The most important postoperative treatment is tear replacement. Artificial tear solutions and/or ointments should be used frequently, often every 2 h while awake. If the tear deficiency is relatively severe (Schirmer's Type I consistently less than 4 mm) punctal occlusion should be considered. Temporary occlusion can be achieved with silicone plugs (Freeman plugs, Eagle Vision, Memphis), suture closure, or superficial cautery; permanent closure is achieved with deep cautery or extirpation of the canaliculi. It is often convenient to perform these at the time of cataract surgery. In some cases lateral tarsorrhaphy is necessary.

These eyes are also more sensitive to the toxic effects of topical medications. Usage of antibiotics, particularly the more toxic ones, such as gentamicin, tobramycin, and neomycin, and preservatives should be minimized.

Should an epithelial defect or ulcer occur, scrapings and culture should be obtained, to determine whether or not an infection is present. Topical corticosteroids should be avoided if possible; in some cases oral corticosteroids can be administered instead. Occlusive patching or application of a bandage contact lens is used to promote epithelial healing. Sometimes healing is very slow, but steady improvement should be observed. If not, temporary total suture tarsorrhaphy should be considered. If perforation occurs application of tissue adhesive (Fig. 16.1) or lamellar patch grafting is usually necessary.

Impaired lid function

Conditions in which lid function is impaired include: lagophthalmos, seventh nerve paresis, proptosis, infrequent blinking, entropion, ectropion, and localized conjunctival elevations. These conditions interfere with tear surfacing, i.e. the spreading of tears over the surface of the eye by the lid. Even in the presence of normal tear production these can lead to localized drying of the cornea or conjunctiva. Ectropion, entropion, and other lid deformities should be surgically corrected. Sometimes this is also possible with proptosis, lagophthalmos, and conjunctival elevations; in other cases tear replacement or lateral tarsorrhaphy are necessary. Where possible, corrective procedures should be performed prior to or concomitant with cataract surgery. If lagophthalmos is present after surgery ointment should be instilled at bedtime, and either the lids taped closed or occlusive goggles worn. In some cases lateral tarsorrhaphy is necessary.

Blepharitis

Blepharitis is another common condition which can affect the outcome of cataract surgery. It is characterized by the accumulation of material around the base of the lashes and erythema of the anterior lid margin. In staphylococcal blepharitis hard, brittle, fibrinous scales, sometimes forming collarettes, are seen at the base of the lashes (Fig. 16.2) [9–11]. *Staphylococcus aureus* is present on the lids in approximately 50% of patients with staphylococcal blepharitis [12–14]. In the seborrheic form large, yellow, greasy scales are seen loosely attached to the side of the cilia. Patients may be asymptomatic, or may report burning, itching, and irritation, which is frequently worse in the morning. There may be dilated blood vessels on the lid margins, thinning or loss of the lashes (madarosis), white lashes (poliosis), misdirected lashes (trichiasis), broken lashes, or

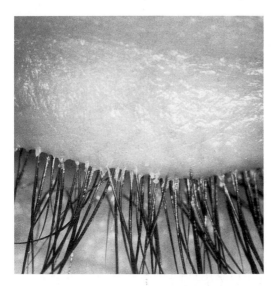

Fig. 16.2 Collarettes along base of lashes in staphylococcal blepharitis.

irregularity of the lid margin (tylosis). Acne rosacea and keratoconjunctivitis sicca are often present. A chronic papillary conjunctivitis is also often present, and this may be accompanied by mucopurulent (predominantly polymorphonuclear) exudate. The conjunctivitis is typically worse in the morning.

Meibomitis is often present. It is seen as dilation of the glands and inspissation of the secretions. Hyperemia, thickening, and tylosis may affect the posterior lid margin. Foamy tears can accumulate in the canthi, or a thick greasy film can be present on the lid margin.

These patients are at a higher risk of postoperative endophthalmitis, conjunctivitis, and corneal ulceration. In addition, patients with blepharitis are prone to hordeola, both external and internal, punctate keratopathy, catarrhal infiltrates, phlyctenules, and pannus formation. The punctate keratopathy predominantly affects the inferior third of the cornea, and consists of fine, flat lesions that stain with rose bengal and sometimes with fluorescein. It can become especially severe when combined with keratoconjunctivitis sicca and/or toxic antibiotic therapy. The corneal epithelium can become diffusely irregular and hazy, markedly reducing vision, and infectious and non-infectious ulceration can occur.

TREATMENT

Blepharitis should be controlled prior to intra-ocular surgery. This can usually be achieved with a combination of lid hygiene and antibiotic application. The lids are scrubbed with a mild detergent, such as baby shampoo, twice daily. Recently, commercially prepared kits (EV Care and EV Lid Cleanser II, Eagle Vision, Memphis; OCuSOFT Lid Scrub, OCuSOFT, Richmond, Texas), became available for this purpose, and they may be superior. Once the blepharitis is under control the frequency can be decreased to once daily, and then continued indefinitely.

Antibiotic ointments also seem to be helpful, erythromycin, bacitracin, or gentamicin should be applied 2–4 times daily. In resistant cases, or cases associated with catarrhal infiltrates or phlyctenulosis, cultures of the lid margin should be performed to direct antibiotic treatment.

If meibomitis is prominent, or acne rosacea is present, oral tetracycline is usually of value. The initial dose is 250 mg q.i.d. for 1 month; if this is effective the dose is reduced to 250 mg b.i.d. for another month, then 250 mg daily. A once or twice daily maintenance dose is necessary in some patients.

If, despite these measures, lid and conjunctival redness or keratitis persist, topical steroids can be used. These can relieve the signs and symptoms of inflammation, but should be used cautiously. Twice daily application of ointment to the lids for 1–2 weeks is usually sufficient.

Dacryocystitis

Chronic dacryocystitis is a cause of recurrent conjunctival inflammation and infection. It is most frequently caused by *Streptococcus pneumoniae* and *Hemophilus influenzae*. There is impairment of tear drainage and frequent shedding of bacteria and purulent material onto the ocular surface. These patients are at higher risk of intraocular and extraocular infection after cataract surgery.

The diagnosis is often unsuspected because the signs can be subtle. Usually there is a complaint of pain, tearing, and discharge from

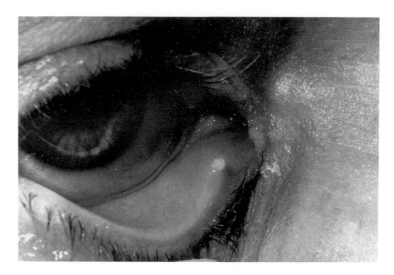

Fig. 16.3 Expression of purulent material from punctum as seen in dacryocystitis.

the eye, and tenderness and swelling is noted in the area of the canaliculi or lacrimal sac. However, in some cases there is only occasional epiphora, and there are no readily evident signs on examination or only pouting of the punctum is present. In these patients the diagnosis is only made when pressure is applied over the canaliculus and lacrimal sac to look for reflux of mucopurulent material (Fig. 16.3). Therefore, this procedure should be performed in all patients with a history of chronic or recurrent conjunctival inflammation.

Patients with dacryocystitis often have an obstruction of the lacrimal outflow system. If possible, material expressed through the punctum should be cultured, to guide antibiotic therapy. Otherwise a penicillinase-resistant penicillin or cephalosporin should be administered, usually orally. Relief of the obstruction is often necessary.

Conjunctival disease

Cicatricial pemphigoid

Cicatricial pemphigoid is an idiopathic scarring disease affecting mainly mucous membranes, especially the conjunctiva. It usually develops after the age of 50, and is more common in women. The main feature is conjunctival inflammation which results in subepithelial

scarring. Cicatricial pemphigoid is nearly always bilateral, although it can be very asymmetric, and only one eye may be active at any given time. It is a chronic and progressive disease, with periods of exacerbation and remission. Over time the scarring can result in symblepharon, trichiasis, entropion, and keratoconjunctivitis sicca. These, in turn, can lead to corneal vascularization and scarring. Similar lesions can be seen in the mouth, nose, larynx, anus, esophagus, and vagina, and, less commonly, the skin [15,16].

Cicatricial pemphigoid appears to be due to an autoimmune reaction against components of the epithelial basement membrane. During active disease immunoglobulins (IgG, and sometimes IgA and IgM) and complement components can be detected along the basement membrane of the conjunctival epithelium [17–20]. In some cases circulating antibasement membrane antibodies have been found [18, 21–23]. The inflammation in the epithelium and substantia propria can lead to subepithelial fibrosis, hyperproliferation of the epithelium cells [24], loss of goblet cells [25,26], and keratinization of the epithelium [27,28].

Cataract surgery in patients with cicatricial pemphigoid can be disastrous; many eyes have progressed to phthisis after an otherwise uncomplicated cataract extraction [29]. The surgery can greatly exacerbate the disease, leading

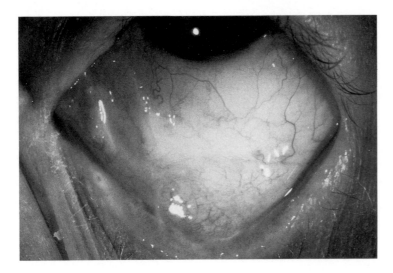

Fig. 16.4 Early forniceal scarring in cicatricial pemphigoid.

to marked inflammation, symblepharon or ankyloblepharon, and eventually corneal opacification.

Therefore, it is essential to recognize the presence of cicatricial pemphigoid prior to surgery. Early in the course of the disease patients can exhibit only recurrent mild bouts of conjunctival inflammation. The first clue to the true nature of the inflammation is usually either slight foreshortening of the inferior conjunctival fornices or gossamer subepithelial scarring (Fig. 16.4). These signs should be sought in surgical candidates, particularly those with a history of chronic or recurrent red eyes.

Once the diagnosis has been made, it is possible to proceed with cataract surgery if proper treatment is given [30]. Patients should be immunosuppressed and quiescent. Immunosuppression is usually achieved with cyclophosphamide, sometimes in conjunction with prednisone [31,32]. This should be performed in cooperation with a physician who routinely administers these drugs, e.g. a hematologist, oncologist, or rheumatologist. It usually requires 2–3 months for sufficient immunosuppression to be achieved. Immunosuppression should probably be continued at least 2 months after surgery.

Dissection of conjunctival adhesions may be necessary at the time of surgery, in order to provide adequate exposure. These often reform despite immunosuppression, symblepharon rings or postoperative lysis. Trichiasis or entropion should be corrected prior to or in conjunction with cataract surgery. If dry eye is also present this must be treated as well, in the manner discussed above.

Atopic dermatitis

Individuals with atopic dermatitis can also exhibit conjunctival inflammation and progressive scarring. During active disease the patients report itching, burning, and mucoid discharge, and the conjunctiva usually appears hyperemic and chemotic. In chronic cases the conjunctiva can be pale and congested, with a papillary response. Medium or giant papillae can be present, usually in the inferior fornix, and gelatinous elevations, thick broad opacifications (usually superior), epithelial cysts, and Trantas' dots can be seen at the limbus. The lids are frequently colonized with staphylococci. Conjunctival scarring (Fig. 16.5) usually develops in patients with relatively severe skin disease. It begins focally, in the centers of the papillae and in the inferior fornix, but can become severe enough to cause symblepharon, entropion, and trichiasis.

A punctate keratitis, marginal ulceration, vascularization, and stromal opacification can occur. Secondary infection with bacteria or herpes simplex is common. Keratoconus is also

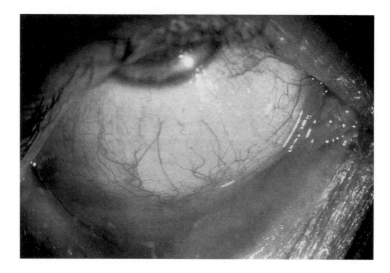

Fig. 16.5 Conjunctival scarring in atopic dermatoconjunctivitis.

more common in these patients [33]. Anterior and posterior subcapsular cataracts occur in approximately 8% of patients [33,34]. The opacities usually begin at 16–18 years of age, and can progress rapidly.

In patients with chronic conjunctival inflammation, particularly those with conjunctival scarring or corneal involvement, cataract surgery may have a higher risk of complications. Healing can be impaired, and there is a higher risk of bacterial and herpetic infection after surgery. Those patients with severe conjunctival involvement may have secondary keratoconjunctivitis sicca, entropion, or trichiasis. There may be risk of progression of the conjunctival or corneal scarring.

It would be prudent to operate on a quiet eye; both the skin and the conjunctiva should not be actively inflamed. In some cases administration of systemic corticosteroids is indicated to achieve a quiescent state and lessen postoperative inflammation and scarring. Entropion or trichiasis should be repaired, and proper dry eye precautions should be taken, as described above.

Erythema multiforme major (Stevens–Johnson syndrome)

This is an acute, self-limited, mucocutaneous inflammatory disease which commonly affects the eye. In some cases a precipitating factor can be identified, such as herpes simplex or other infectious agent, a drug, or carcinoma. Characteristic multiform skin eruptions occur, accompanied by inflammation, bullae and ulcerations of the mucus membranes. The episode tends to resolve after a course of 6–8 weeks, but can recur.

Conjunctival scarring can be extensive enough to result in symblepharon, keratoconjunctivitis sicca, trichiasis, and entropion (Fig. 16.6). However, in nearly all cases the conjunctival disease is stationary after the initial episode; recurrent inflammation is observed only rarely [35]. Corneal scarring and vascularization can occur, usually as a secondary phenomenon, resulting from the effects of conjunctival scarring.

The risks of cataract surgery depend on the extent of ocular surface injury. If lid function and tear production are not very impaired the surgery can be routine. However, if there is extensive injury, with marked drying and secondary corneal scarring, cataract extraction is hazardous. Dry eye precautions, as discussed above, correction of lid function, and removal of trichiatic lashes should be undertaken. There is no evidence concerning the value of immunosuppression.

Chemical burns

Chemical injury is another acute event which can result in severe conjunctival and corneal scarring. Ocular surface function can be

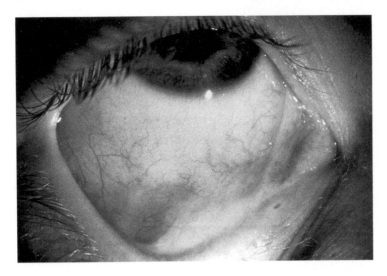

Fig. 16.6 Conjunctival scarring after erythema multiforme major (Stevens–Johnson syndrome).

impaired by dry eye, lid malpositions, and injury to the limbus. Limbal injury appears to reduce the ability of the cornea to heal without vascularization and scarring.

Cataract extraction is sometimes necessary in the acute state; swelling of the lens can cause secondary angle closure. In these cases the injury has been severe, and the prognosis for the eye is poor. Surgery can be difficult, due to excessive bleeding and inflammation, opacification of the cornea, and poor iris dilation. The length of the incision should be minimized, to reduce the risks of impaired healing and melting. Pars plana lensectomy is another alternative.

The risks of late cataract extraction are similar to those in patients who have had erythema multiforme. If tear and lid function are impaired and corneal scarring is present, the risks of poor healing, ulceration, and scarring are substantial.

Corneal and scleral disease

Endothelial disease

Decreased endothelial function places a patient at higher risk for corneal decompensation after cataract surgery. This subject is discussed in more detail in Chapter 24. Most commonly endothelial function is reduced by the loss of cells with aging, and biomicroscopic changes are first noted in the fifth or sixth decades of life. In some cases the endothelial abnormality has an early onset, with frank decompensation developing as early as the fourth decade, and there may be autosomal dominant inheritance. The term Fuchs' dystrophy would seem to apply more appropriately to the latter cases. Endothelial injury can also result from physical or chemical trauma, intraocular inflammation, herpetic keratitis, acute glaucoma, or long-term contact lens wear.

In most cases the manifestations are similar: guttae, stromal edema, and epithelial edema. Guttae are seen as dewdrop-like, wart-like, endothelial excrescences. On specular reflection they are black holes in the endothelial mosaic. They develop first in the central cornea, and gradually spread peripherally and become more numerous. With time Descemet's membrane can develop a beaten-metal appearance. Fine pigment deposition is often seen diffusely on the posterior corneal surface.

If endothelial cell function is insufficient to maintain normal water balance, stromal edema occurs. Stromal edema is more likely with decreased endothelial cell density, but the correlation is not consistent. The number of corneal guttae also does not correlate well; stromal edema can occur in the absence of guttae [36]. When there is early or moderate stromal edema it is difficult to perceive any changes other than a widening of the slit beam. Therefore pachometry is useful to detect its presence.

With further impairment of endothelial function epithelial edema develops. The extent of epithelial edema can depend on the intraocular pressure (higher pressures cause epithelial edema with more normal endothelial function), tear flow, and ambient humidity. Some reduction of vision occurs with marked stromal edema (approximately >0.65 mm), but it is usually not until epithelial edema develops that the patient becomes very symptomatic.

The occurrence of early and permanent corneal decompensation after cataract surgery most likely is mainly determined by two variables: (a) presurgical endothelial status; and (b) surgical trauma. The presence of guttae, endothelial cell density, and endothelial cell morphology are not very helpful in predicting which patients will decompensate [37–39]. Corneal thickness may be a better indicator, but it appears that the extent of surgical trauma is the most significant factor.

The most frequent question is whether or not to combine penetrating keratoplasty with cataract extraction. Currently our approach is to proceed with careful cataract extraction in all patients without evidence of epithelial edema. It appears that the great majority of these patients will not experience corneal decompensation in the first 1–2 years after surgery. Nevertheless, endothelial trauma should be minimized as much as possible during surgery. The technique should be the one with which the surgeon is most comfortable. A viscoelastic agent is recommended, and anterior chamber irrigation should be minimized.

Superior pannus

The growth of vessels onto the corneal surface (pannus) can occur in a wide variety of diseases including: trachoma, phlyctenulosis, acne rosacea, atopic keratoconjunctivitis, contact lens wear, staphylococcal blepharitis, herpes simplex keratitis, inclusion conjunctivitis, superior limbic keratoconjunctivitis, and vernal conjunctivitis.

The increased vascularization at the limbus will increase the amount of bleeding encountered during cataract surgery. More cautery may be required in the region of the incision. It may be preferable to avoid corneal incisions, since they will promote further vascularization after surgery, and local cautery is more difficult. Preoperative laser photocoagulation may be considered to reduce the likelihood of bleeding complications.

If the pannus is gross it can impair visualization of the anterior chamber during surgery. Removal of the pannus and smoothing of the corneal surface may be necessary. Healing of the cataract incision may be accelerated.

Terrien's marginal degeneration

This is an uncommon idiopathic degeneration of the cornea in which there is thinning of the peripheral cornea. It occurs more often in males than females, is most commonly bilateral, and can develop at any age. It is usually asymptomatic, but can be associated with inflammation [40], or decreased vision due to astigmatism.

The characteristic findings on examination are marginal corneal thinning with lipid deposition, and superficial vascularization (Fig. 16.7). The thinning most commonly begins superiorly and extends circumferentially, resulting in an arcuate shape. The epithelium remains intact, and the central edge is gradual rather than steep walled. Marked thinning can lead to a large amount of astigmatism, because of the tilting forward of the central cornea, and perforation.

Cataract extraction can be hampered by the thinning of the superior cornea. The incision should not be placed adjacent to thinned cornea because placement of sutures and achievement of water-tight closure will be impaired. It would be preferable to make a scleral incision, at least 1 mm posterior to the limbus.

If the thinning is so extreme that perforation is threatened, or astigmatism severely reduces vision, a reconstructive full-thickness or lamellar corneoscleral graft can be performed [41,42]. These grafts must be hand-fashioned to fit the defect.

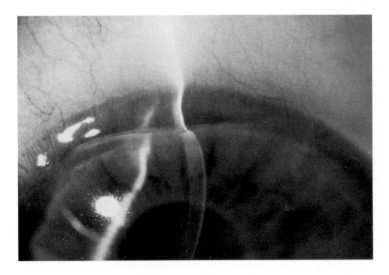

Fig. 16.7 Superior corneal thinning in Terrien's marginal degeneration.

Table 16.2 Causes of decreased corneal sensation. After [29]

Fifty nerve palsy	*Infection*
Surgical	Herpes simplex
Tumors	Herpes zoster
Aneurysms	Leprosy
Others	
	Systemic disease
Congenital	Diabetes [76,77]
Familial dysautonomia (Riley–Day)	
Goldenhar's syndrome	*Medications*
Moebius syndrome	Topical anesthetic abuse
Parry–Romberg syndrome	Atropine [78]
Bassen–Kornzweig syndrome	Timolol (usually temporary)
Isolated congenital trigeminal anesthesia	[79]
	Sulfacetamide 30% [80]
Corneal dystrophies	
Lattice	*Toxic*
Granular (rare)	Chemical burns
	Carbon disulfide exposure
Iatrogenic	Hydrogen sulfide exposure
Contact lens wear [75]	
Trauma to ciliary nerves, by laser,	*Functional*
cryotherapy, scleral buckling, or	Hysteria
diathermy	
Corneal incisions	*Miscellaneous*
Cataract	Any condition with chronic
Keratoplasty	epithelial injury or
Epikeratophakia	stromal inflammation

Neurotrophic keratitis

Whenever corneal sensation is decreased epithelial dysfunction occurs. This can be seen in a wide variety of conditions (Table 16.2). The reason for this is unclear, but it is believed that the corneal nerves normally provide some type of trophic influence on the epithelium. In the absence of innervation epithelial cell vitality is decreased, the ability to heal is markedly reduced, and defects, ulceration, vascularization, and opacification can occur, even in the absence of injury [43]. These eyes are also prone to infection and trauma [44]. Since epithelial integrity is reduced opacification during surgery and development of defects is more likely. Healing of the cataract incision will also be delayed. Prevention of drying of the corneal surface and minimization of trauma are helpful measures. Postoperative lubrication is essential. An ointment (4–8 times daily) is most effective; this can be a non-preserved petrolatum, a relatively non-toxic antibiotic (e.g. sulfacetamide or erythromycin), or a combined antibiotic–corticosteroid medication. Removal of sutures should not be performed until the wound appears well healed.

Epithelial defects most commonly develop in the interpalpebral cornea, and are slow to heal, even with treatment. Patching may be sufficient, but often a bandage contact lens or a tarsorrhaphy is necessary. Bandage contact lens wear is more prone to complications in these patients, particularly sterile hypopyon, which can appear 1–2 days after application of the lens. The use of a cycloplegic agent appears to reduce the risk of hypopyon.

Herpetic keratitis

Patients with recurrent herpes simplex keratitis can have several problems each of which has the potential to affect cataract surgery. They can have superior thinning or pannus, or reduced corneal sensation. The approach to these problems has been discussed above. These patients also tend to have more postoperative inflammation, and surgery can induce viral recurrence.

Postoperative inflammation can be reduced by more intensive corticosteroid use. Usually topical administration (e.g. 1% prednisolone acetate 6–9 times daily) is sufficient, but in some cases 10–14 days of oral corticosteroid (e.g. prednisone 1 mg/kg) is necessary to keep the eye quiet.

There is no data available to indicate the risk of herpetic recurrence after cataract surgery, however, surgical trauma is a known stimulant for recurrence. Information has been accumulated about patients undergoing keratoplasty. Recurrence of herpetic disease after penetrating keratoplasty has occurred in approximately 15% of eyes within 2 years [45–53]. Cor-

ticosteroids do not appear to increase the risk of reactivation [54].

Topical antiviral prophylaxis after keratoplasty does not appear to be beneficial, except during rejection episodes, when recurrence of herpes simplex virus is common [51,55]. However, it may be prudent to administer an antiviral agent (e.g. trifluridine 4 times daily) after cataract extraction, during the early postoperative intensive corticosteroid therapy. If viral keratitis develops during intensive corticosteroid treatment, viral proliferation, and resulting ocular damage, can be enhanced.

Oral acyclovir may be useful in reducing the risk of recurrence. It has been shown to reduce the incidence of genital [56–58] and cutaneous [59] recurrences, as long as the drug is continued. Its effect on ocular occurrences is unclear. The laboratory data is contradictory: in two studies, systemic acyclovir was not able to prevent recurrence of ocular herpes [60,61], but in another it significantly lowered the incidence of ocular viral shedding, geographic ulceration, and stromal keratitis after penetrating keratoplasty [62]. Some clinical experience has suggested that it can reduce ocular recurrences [63], and some surgeons routinely administer oral acyclovir for 10–14 days after keratoplasty [64].

Postkeratoplasty

Any intraocular procedure after keratoplasty poses a risk to the graft, both from endothelial damage and stimulation of rejection. Even with contemporary techniques the risk of graft rejection or failure is approximately 20% [65–67]. Clear corneal grafts more than 12 months after surgery usually have endothelial cell densities of 900–1500, and a thickness of 0.56 mm [68–71]. In our experience there is a high risk of failure after cataract surgery if the preoperative thickness is greater than 0.6 mm, regardless of the endothelial cell density.

Surgical technique is not altered substantially. The use of a viscoelastic substance will help protect the endothelium. Visualization can be hampered by optical distortion caused by an astigmatic surface and opacification at the graft–host interface. Manipulation of the wound can be used to reduce corneal astigmatism; resection of tissue in the flat axis or recession in the steep axis. In our experience up to 4 D of correction can be achieved in some cases, but the overall results are disappointing. Postoperative inflammation should be minimized with topical and/or systemic corticosteroids.

Postkeratotomy

To date few patients who have had radial keratotomy have subsequently undergone cataract extraction, however, in the future this situation will be commonly encountered. In four such cases Koch et al. [72] found that the main problem was in the calculation of the intraocular lens power. After radial keratotomy keratometric measurements do not accurately reflect the functional power of the corneal surface, most commonly overestimating corneal power [73]. Therefore, use of postoperative keratometry in intraocular lens power calculations results in underestimation of the power required [72]. In addition, there appears to be slight postoperative flattening of the corneal surface, averaging 0.4 D.

The authors recommended that the Binkhorst or Holladay lens formula be used, and that the postradial keratotomy corneal curvature be calculated as follows:

preoperative   refractive change
average   – induced by
keratometry   radial keratotomy.

Alternatively, functional corneal curvature could be calculated by overrefracting with a hard contact lens of known power and base curvature. In addition, 0.5 D should be added to the lens power to account for postoperative corneal flattening.

References

1 Sjögren H, Bloch KJ. Keratoconjunctivitis sicca and the Sjögren syndrome. Surv Ophthalmol 1971; 16: 145–59.
2 Bloch KJ, Buchanan WW, Wohl MJ et al. Sjögren's syndrome: A clinical, pathological and serological study of sixty-two cases. Medicine 1965; 44: 187–231.
3 Moustsopoulos HM, Chuset TM, Mann DL et al. Sjögren's syndrome (sicca syndrome): Current issues. Ann Intern Med 1980; 92: 212–26.
4 Tabbara KF, Ostler HB, Daniels TE et al. Sjögren's syndrome: A correlation between ocular findings and labial salivary gland histology. Trans Am Acad Ophthal Otolaryngol 1974; 78: 467–8.
5 Anderson LG, Tala N. The spectrum of benign or malignant lymphoproliferation in Sjögren's syndrome. Clin Exp Immunol 1971; 9: 199–221.
6 Radtke N, Meyers S, Kaufman HF. Sterile corneal ulcers after cataract surgery in keratoconjunctivitis sicca. Arch Ophthalmol 1978; 96: 51–2.
7 Pfister RR, Murphy GE. Corneal ulceration and perforation associated with Sjögren's syndrome. Arch Ophthalmol 1980; 98: 89–94.
8 Insler MS, Boutros G, Boulware DW. Corneal ulceration following cataract surgery in patients with rheumatoid arthritis. J Am Intraocul Implant Soc 1985; 11: 594–7.
9 Smolin G, Okumoto M. Staphylococcal blepharitis. Arch Ophthalmol 1977; 95: 812–16.
10 Thygeson P. The etiology and treatment of blepharitis: Study in military personnel. Milit Surg 1946; 98: 191.
11 Thygeson P. Complications of staphylococcal blepharitis. Am J Ophthalmol 1969; 68: 446–9.
12 Dougherty JM, McCulley JP. Comparative bacteriology of chronic blepharitis. Br J Ophthalmol 1984; 68: 524–8.
13 McCulley JP, Sciallis GF. Meibomian keratoconjunctivitis: Oculodermal correlates. CLAOJ 1983; 9: 130–2.
14 Smolin G, Tabbara K, Whitcher J. Infectious Diseases of the Eyelids. Baltimore: Williams and Wilkins, 1984.
15 Lever WE. Pemphigus and pemphigoid. J Am Acad Dermatol 1979; 1: 2–3.
16 Wright PG. Cicatrizing conjunctivitis. Trans Ophthalmol Soc UK 1986; 105: 1–17.
17 Furney N, West C, Andrews T et al. Immunofluorescent studies of ocular cicatricial pemphigoid. Am J Ophthalmol 1975; 80: 825–31.
18 Griffith MR, Fukuyama K, Tuffanelli D et al. Immunofluorescent studies in mucous membrane pemphigoid. Arch Dermatol 1974; 109: 195–9.
19 Rogers RS, Perry HO, Bean SF et al. Immunopathology of cicatricial pemphigoid: studies of complement deposition. J Invest Dermatol 1977; 68: 39–43.
20 Proia AD, Foulks GN, Sanfilippo FP. Ocular cicatricial pemphigoid with granular IgA and complement deposition. Arch Ophthalmol 1985; 103: 1669–72.
21 Waltman SR, Yarran D. Circulating autoantibodies in ocular pemphigoid. Am J Ophthalmol 1974; 77: 891–4.
22 Dantzig PI. Circulating antibodies in cicatricial pemphigoid. Arch Dermatol 1973; 108: 264–6.
23 Leonard J, Hobday C, Haffenden G et al.

Immunofluorescent studies in ocular cicatricial pemphigoid. *Br J Dermatol* 1988; **118**: 209–17.

24 Thoft RA, Friend J, Kinoshita S *et al.* Ocular cicatricial pemphigoid associated with hyper-proliferation of the conjunctival epithelium. *Am J Ophthalmol* 1984; **98**: 37–42.

25 Ralph RA. Conjunctival goblet cell density in normal subjects and in dry eye syndromes. *Invest Ophthalmol* 1975; **14**: 299–302.

26 Nelson JD, Wright JC. Conjunctival goblet cell densities in ocular surface disease. *Arch Ophthalmol* 1984; **102**: 1049–51.

27 Person JR, Rogers RS. Bullous and cicatricial pemphigoid: Clinical, histopathologic, and immunopathologic correlations. *Mayo Clin Proc* 1977; **52**: 54–66.

28 Anderson SR, Jensen QA, Kristensen EB *et al.* Benign mucous membrane pemphigoid. III. Biopsy. *Acta Ophthalmol* (Copenh) 1974; **52**: 455–63.

29 Grayson M. *Diseases of the Cornea.* St Louis: CV Mosby, 1983.

30 Sainz de la Maza M, Tauber J, Foster CS. Cataract surgery in ocular cicatricial pemphigoid. *Ophthalmology* 1988; **95**: 481–6.

31 Foster CS, Wilson LA, Ekins MB. Immunosuppressive therapy for progressive ocular cicatricial pemphigoid. *Ophthalmology* 1982; **89**: 340–53.

32 Mondino BJ, Brown SI. Immunosuppressive therapy in ocular cicatricial pemphigoid. *Arch Ophthalmol* 1983; **96**: 453–9.

33 Brunsting LA, Reed WB, Bair HL. Occurrence of cataracts and keratoconus with atopic dermatitis. *Arch Dermatol* 1955; **72**: 237–41.

34 Cowan A, Klauder JV. Frequency of occurrence of cataracts in atopic dermatitis. *Arch Ophthalmol* 1950; **43**: 759–68.

35 Foster CS, Fong LP, Azar D, Kenyon KR. Episodic conjunctival inflammation after Stevens–Johnson syndrome. *Ophthalmology* 1988; **95**: 453–62.

36 Abbott RL, Fine BS, Webster RE *et al.* Specular microscopic and histologic observations in non-guttate corneal endothelial degeneration. *Ophthalmology* 1981; **88**: 788–800.

37 Bates AK, Cheng H, Hiorns RW. Pseudophakic bullous keratopathy: Relationship with endothelial cell density and use of a predictive cell loss model. A preliminary report. *Curr Topics Eye Res* 1986; **5**: 363–6.

38 Stur M. Long-term changes of the corneal endothelium following intracapsular cataract extraction with implantation of open-loop anterior chamber lenses. *Acta Ophthalmol* (Copenh) 1988; **66**: 678–86.

39 Bates AK, Cheng H. Bullous keratopathy: A study of endothelial cell morphology in patients undergoing cataract surgery. *Br J Ophthalmol* 1988; **72**: 409–12.

40 Austin P, Brown SI. Inflammatory Terrien's marginal corneal disease. *Am J Ophthalmol* 1981; **98**: 189–92.

41 Brown AC, Rao GN, Aquavella JV. Peripheral corneal grafts in Terrien's marginal degeneration. *Ophthal Surg* 1983; **14**: 931–4.

42 Caldwell DR, Insler MS, Boutros G *et al.* Primary surgical repair of several peripheral marginal ectasias in Terrien's marginal degeneration. *Am J Ophthalmol* 1984; **97**: 332–43.

43 Alper MG. The anesthetic eye: An investigation of changes in the anterior ocular segment of the monkey caused by interrupting the trigeminal nevre at various levels along its course. *Trans Am Ophthalmol Soc* 1976; **72**: 313–65.

44 Schimmelpfennig B, Beuerman R. Sensory deprivation of the rabbit cornea affects epithelial properties. *Exp Neurol* 1980; **69**: 196–201.

45 Langston R, Pavan-Langston D, Dohlman CH. Penetrating keratoplasty for herpetic keratitis. *Trans Am Acad Ophthal Otolaryngol* 1975; **79**: 577–83.

46 Patten JT, Cavanaugh HD, Pavan-Langston D. Penetrating keratoplasty in acute herpetic corneal perforations. *Ann Ophthalmol* 1976; **8**: 287–94.

47 Laibson PR. Surgical approaches to the treatment of active keratitis. *Int Ophthal Clin* 1973; **13**: 65–71.

48 Langston RHS, Pavan-Langston D. Penetrating keratoplasty for herpetic keratitis: Decision making and management. *Int Ophthal Clin* 1975; **15**: 125–40.

49 Pfister RR, Richards JS, Dohlman CH. Recurrence of herpetic keratitis in corneal grafts. *Am J Ophthalmol* 1972; **73**: 192–6.

50 Polack FM, Kaufman HF. Penetrating keratoplasty in herpetic keratitis. *Am J Ophthalmol* 1972; **73**: 908–13.

51 Cobo LM, Coster DJ, Rice NSC, Jones BR. Prognosis and management of corneal transplantation for herpetic keratitis. *Arch Ophthalmol* 1980; **98**: 1755–9.

52 Fine M, Cignetti F. Penetrating keratoplasty in herpes simplex keratitis. *Arch Ophthalmol* 1977; **95**: 613–16.

53 Cohen E, Laibson P, Arentsen J. Corneal transplantation for herpes simplex keratitis. *Am J Ophthalmol* 1983; **95**: 645–50.

54 Kibrick S, Takahashi GH, Liebowitz HM. Local corticosteroid therapy and reactivation of herpetic keratitis. *Arch Ophthalmol* 1971; **86**: 694–8.

55 Ficker LA, Kirkness CM, Rice NSC, Steele ADM. Longterm prognosis for corneal grafting in herpes simplex keratitis. *Eye* 1988; **2**: 400–8.

56 Mindel A, Weller IVD, Faherty A *et al.* Prophylactic oral acyclovir in recurrent genital herpes. *Lancet* 1984; **ii**: 57–8.

57 Straus SE, Takiff HE, Seidlin M *et al.* Suppression of frequently recurring genital herpes. A placebo-controlled double-blind trial of oral acyclovir. *N Engl J Med* 1984; **310**: 1543–50.

58 Douglas JM, Critchlow C, Benedetti J *et al.* A

double-blind study of oral acyclovir for suppression of recurrences of genital herpes simplex virus infection. *N Engl J Med* 1984; **310**: 1551–6.

59 Meyrick Thomas RH, Dodd HJ, Yeo JM *et al*. Oral acyclovir in the suppression of recurrent nongenital herpes simplex virus infection. *Br J Dermatol* 1985; **113**: 731–5.

60 Kaufman HE, Varnell ED, Centifanto-Fitzgerald YM *et al*. Oral antiviral drugs in experimental herpes simplex keratitis. *Antimicrob Agents Chemother* 1983; **24**: 888–91.

61 Nesburn AB, Willey DE, Trousdale MD. Effect of intensive acyclovir therapy during artificial reactivation of latent herpes simplex virus (41563). *Proc Soc Exp Biol Med* 1983; **172**: 316–23.

62 Beyer CF, Arens MQ, Hill GA *et al*. Oral acyclovir reduces the incidence of recurrent herpes simplex keratitis in rabbits after penetrating keratoplasty. *Arch Ophthalmol* 1989; **107**: 1200–5.

63 Schwab I. Oral acyclovir in the management of herpes simplex ocular infections. *Ophthalmology* 1988; **95**: 423–9.

64 Kaufman HE, Rayfield MA. Viral conjunctivitis and keratitis. In: Kaufman HE, Barron BA, McDonald MB, Waltman SR, eds. *The Cornea*. New York: Churchill Livingstone, 1988.

65 Paton RT, Swartz G. Keratoplasty for Fuchs' dystrophy. *Arch Ophthalmol* 1959; **61**: 366–9.

66 Fine M. Therapeutic keratoplasty in Fuchs' dystrophy. *Am J Ophthalmol* 1964; **57**: 371–8.

67 Binder PS. Cataract and lens implant surgery after keratoplasty. Safety and refraction predictability. *Inv Ophthalmol Vis Sci* 1989; **30** (suppl): 276.

68 Matsuda M, Bourne WM. Long-term morphologic changes in the endothelium of transplanted corneas. *Arch Ophthalmol* 1985; **103**: 1343–6.

69 Culbertson WW, Abbott RL, Forster RK. Endo-

thelial cell loss in penetrating keratoplasty. *Ophthalmology* 1982; **89**: 600–4.

70 Bourne WM. Morphologic and functional evaluation of the endothelium of transplanted human corneas. *Trans Am Ophthalmol Soc* 1983; **81**: 403–50.

71 Olsen T. Post-operative changes in the endothelial cell density of corneal grafts. *Acta Ophthalmol* 1981; **59**: 863–70.

72 Koch DD, Liu JF, Hyde LL *et al*. Refractive complications of cataract surgery after radial keratotomy. *Am J Ophthalmol* 1989; **108**: 676–82.

73 Rowsey JJ, Balyeat GD. Preliminary results and complications of radial keratotomy. *Am J Ophthalmol* 1982; **93**: 437–55.

74 Fraunfelder FT. *Drug-Induced Ocular Side Effects and Drug Interactions*. 3rd edn. Philadelphia: Lea & Febiger, 1989.

75 Millodot M. Effect of long-term wear of hard contact lenses on corneal sensitivity. *Arch Ophthalmol* 1978; **96**: 1255–7.

76 Schwartz DE. Corneal sensitivity in diabetics. *Arch Ophthalmol* 1974: **91**: 174–8.

77 Schultz RO, Peters MA, Sobocinski K *et al*. Diabetic keratopathy as a manifestation of peripheral neuropathy. *Am J Ophthalmol* 1983; **96**: 368–71.

78 Von Oer S. Ueber die beziehung des acetylcholine des hornhautepithels zur erregungsu: Bertragung von diesem auf die sensiblen nervenenden. *Pflugers Arch* 1961; **273**: 325–34.

79 Van Buskirk EM. Corneal anesthesia after timolol maleate therapy. *Am J Ophthalmol* 1979; **88**: 739–43.

80 Chang FW, Reinhart S, Fraser NM. Effect of 30% sulfacetamide on corneal sensitivity. *Am J Optom Physiol Opt* 1984; **61**: 318–20.

17: Complications of Cataract Surgery and their Management

MILTON KAHN & STEPHEN A. OBSTBAUM

Introduction

As techniques of cataract surgery have evolved, primarily the conversion from intracapsular to extracapsular surgery, the incidence of many of the complications associated with cataract extraction has declined. This decline has been further augmented by the progress that has been made in intraocular lens (IOL) design and instrumentation. However, a clear understanding of the potential complications that may occur during and after cataract surgery, including their pathogenesis and an approach to their management, is an essential prerequisite for each surgeon every time he or she contemplates operating on a patient, during the surgery itself, and throughout the postoperative period. This understanding will help the surgeon anticipate and prevent many of the complications, and, when they do occur, deal with them in a timely and appropriate manner.

Some of these complications are dealt with in other chapters. In the present chapter, we will review several of the complications that may occur during surgery, emphasizing those that are associated with the extracapsular technique. Although addressed separately, some of these often occur together, such as rupture of the posterior capsule with vitreous loss, and wound leak with hypotony. With each complication, we hope to provide an understanding of its pathogenesis, it clinical presentation, and an approach to its management.

Expulsive hemorrhage

The most dreaded complication of cataract surgery is an expulsive hemorrhage, the incidence being approximately 0.2% [1]. While its precise pathogenesis is unknown, histopathologic studies have shown it to be a consequence of the rupture of one of the posterior ciliary arteries [2]. Factors found to be associated with its occurrence include glaucoma, hypertension, generalized arteriosclerosis, moderate to high myopia, increased blood pressure intraoperatively, and vascular fragility. The etiology is most likely multifactorial.

An expulsive hemorrhage most often occurs intraoperatively. It is postulated that the sudden hypotony secondary to surgical decompression of the globe leads to rupture of the vessel. Clinically, if the process occurs gradually, one may see a dark mass through the pupil. As the intraocular volume increases, the wound gapes, and the intraocular contents (iris, lens, vitreous, retina, and uveal tissue) bulge forward, followed by bright-red blood. An expulsive hemorrhage can also occur after surgery. Some have postulated that an intraoperative choroidal detachment enlarges, leading to stretching of the vessels with eventual rupture [3]. These cases usually occur within the first few days after surgery, the patient complains of severe pain, and one will find a bloody mass extruding through the wound.

Davison [4] has reported on what he termed an acute intraoperative suprachoroidal hemorrhage. The diagnosis is based on clinical suspicion (a "tight," extremely firm eye, with "little room to work") and the observation of a dark choroidal bulge, which he confirmed by indirect ophthalmoscopy. He found a 0.9% incidence in 2839 consecutive cases of extracapsular surgery or phacoemulsification. The only statistically significant risk factors he noted were advanced age and the presence of glaucoma. Through early recognition and prompt treatment, he obtained visual acuity of ≥20/30 in 84% of these cases.

Of further interest is the finding of limited choroidal hemorrhage. Its incidence is much higher: 2.2% with extracapsular surgery [5], and 3.1% with intracapsular surgery [6]. These hemorrhages are, as the name implies, self-limited and do not affect visual acuity.

Unfortunately, it is difficult to predict which patients are predisposed to developing an expulsive hemorrhage. However, if a patient experienced a prior expulsive hemorrhage, one must anticipate its occurrence in the second eye, since bilateral hemorrhages do occur [7]. For these patients, phacoemulsification may be of particular benefit. If an extracapsular technique is used, one should lower the preoperative intraocular pressure to close to zero, use preplaced sutures, deliver the lens slowly, and close the wound with additional sutures. It is also beneficial to lower the patient's systemic blood pressure preoperatively.

For all patients, the key to treating an intraoperative expulsive hemorrhage is its early recognition and immediate treatment. Again, preplaced sutures are invaluable as immediate closure of the wound is of the utmost importance. Fluid may be injected into the anterior chamber through an inferior limbal incision to push back the extruding contents [8]. If one cannot close the wound, a sclerotomy 9 mm posterior to the limbus should be performed [9]. When the bleeding has ceased, one should reopen the wound and remove as much formed vitreous as possible. Postoperatively, intensive topical, periocular, and systemic steroids should be used to lessen the ensuing inflammatory response.

Vitreous loss

Jaffe has stated [10] that operative loss of vitreous is the second most serious complication of cataract surgery. Its incidence has declined over the years, and is less with an extracapsular technique than with an intracapsular technique [11]. Jaffe feels its incidence

should be approximately 3% in experienced hands [10].

In extracapsular cataract surgery, vitreous loss may occur during cortical clean-up, expression of the nucleus, and removal of anterior capsular tags, and results from capsular and/or zonular breaks [12]. The major complication of vitreous loss is cystoid macular edema, although its precise incidence is unknown. Other potential complications include delayed or defective wound healing, corneal edema, retinal detachment, secondary glaucoma, epithelial downgrowth, fibrous ingrowth, vitreous hemorrhage, proliferative vitreoretinopathy, and chronic inflammation.

Unlike an expulsive hemorrhage, the risk factors leading to vitreous loss can often be minimized. Preoperative recognition of an eye with an increased potential for vitreous loss is of great value. Some of these factors include the physical and emotional condition of a patient, such as the presence of chronic obstructive pulmonary disease (COPD), obesity, or excessive agitation, and a past history of loss of vitreous in the fellow eye. One study [12] showed that the only significant risk factor for vitreous loss in patients undergoing an extracapsular cataract extraction was decreasing pupil size. Patients with pupils ≤6.5 mm had twice the incidence, and those with pupils ≤4.5 mm had five times the incidence of vitreous loss. A small pupil makes both expression of the nucleus and cortical clean-up more difficult. Myopia and glaucoma were not found to be risk factors.

Preoperatively, the most important factor to help prevent vitreous loss is to obtain a soft eye. The method of ocular compression depends upon the anesthetic agent that is injected. If a short onset agent is used, we prefer digital pressure for approximately 5 min until the eye feels soft [13]. Its effect is not so much lowering the intraocular pressure as it is a decrease in the vitreous and orbital volume. Other methods used to obtain a soft eye include the use of the mercury bag, super pinkie, or Honan balloon, and are useful when longer onset agents are used, such as bupivicaine. Hyperosmotics administered preoperatively may be used to remove fluid from the vitreous.

It is also beneficial to minimize external pressure on the eye. Adequate lid and globe akinesia is also important since squeezing or eye movements may exert undue pressure on the globe. Intraoperatively, if one experiences gaping of the wound, iris prolapse, forward displacement of the lens and iris, or if one notes horizontal tension lines in the cornea, one should suspect increased posterior pressure and should search for a cause. Releasing the lid speculum and superior rectus suture, and performing a lateral canthotomy may be helpful. The possibility of a suprachoroidal hemorrhage must also be considered.

When vitreous loss has occurred, the management of vitreous removal often determines the long-term outcome of such an eye. The incidence of increased inflammation, cystoid macular edema, and secondary glaucoma are greater in these eyes. Most of the complications of vitreous loss are related to its incarceration within the wound or its contact with the cornea or iris. Modern surgical techniques, especially the use of an automated vitrectomy instrument, have improved the results after vitreous loss. Formed vitreous may be removed from the wound using Weck-cell sponges and scissors. The cyclodialysis spatula sweeps vitreous away from the wound, and a viscoelastic substance may also help push vitreous posteriorly. Several studies have now shown that 75–80% of patients will have a good outcome, with visual acuity ≥20/40 with an anterior or posterior chamber lens [14–16].

Rupture of the posterior capsule

The overall incidence of posterior capsular or zonular disruption is in large part a function of the experience and skills of the surgeon, as it is for the most part an iatrogenic occurrence. The incidence should probably be in the range of ≤5%. Posterior capsular tears occur most often during cortical clean-up [17], but may also occur during expression of the nucleus, removal of anterior capsular flaps, polishing of the posterior capsule, and during phacoemulsification of the nucleus. Tears are unlikely to occur during insertion of the intraocular lens, although zonular dialysis may occur at this

stage of the procedure. One study [12] found that the only significant risk factors for zonular breaks were a small pupil and the presence of pseudoexfoliation, and found no risk factor for capsular breaks. A small incision that does not allow for easy nucleal expression may also increase the risk for disruption of the capsule. The key is avoidance, and thus a meticulous, deliberate, and careful expression and clean-up. Too vigorous an attempt at removing all cortex adherent to the posterior capsule is unwise, given the low incidence of complications from a later Nd:YAG capsulotomy [18].

If a small tear occurs in the capsule whose margins are visible and vitreous is not lost, the IOL may be placed in the capsular bag or in the ciliary sulcus. If, however, there is a small tear with vitreous to the wound, or if there is a disruption of the zonules, the implant should be placed in the sulcus and the vitreous loss must be managed. If a large tear occurs resulting in vitreous loss and its margins are not visible, then anterior chamber lens implantation may be preferable. Recently, there has been interest in iris-sutured or sulcus-fixated posterior chamber lenses in the absence of capsular support [19]. This may be of special benefit for those patients in whom insertion of an anterior chamber IOL may be risky, i.e. in patients with low endothelial cell counts, or those with already compromised angles.

Hypotony

The most common causes of hypotony are a wound leak and a ciliochoroidal detachment, although the two often occur together. Jaffe [10] has provided a useful means of establishing the etiology of postoperative hypotony. If the hypotonous eye has a wound leak which is associated with a normal anterior chamber, then the ciliary body is not detached; if the wound leak is associated with a shallow anterior chamber, then one must suspect an accompanying ciliary body detachment. If the anterior chamber is shallow in the absence of a wound leak, then there is solely a ciliary body detachment.

Wound leaks will be dealt with in a separate section. A ciliary body detachment may be hemorrhagic or serous, and is felt to be a result of the sudden surgical decompression at the beginning of the operation. It may also be a consequence of an accidental cyclodialysis. The prevailing concept is that the hypotony secondary to a detachment of the ciliary body is a result of a decrease in aqueous production [20], although it has been suggested that it is due to an increase in uveoscleral outflow [21].

The majority of patients with hypotony are asymptomatic. However, if it persists, they may show signs of inflammation and may complain of blurred vision. Fundoscopic examination may reveal alternating dark and yellow streaks which are the result of folds in the choroid and retinal pigment epithelium (RPE), and present a characteristic picture by fluorescein angiography [22]. The retina may also be thrown into folds, and some patients have papilledema. Long-standing hypotony is inconsistent with the normal functioning of the eye and will eventually result in phthisis.

Initially, one may observe a hypotonous eye, as long as no danger signs are present. The use of cycloplegics, steroids, and hyperosmotics are usually ineffective [10]. If a wound leak is present and does not respond to pressure patching, it must be surgically corrected. A cyclodialysis cleft can be closed, either with a McCannel suture [23] and cyclocryotherapy, or with the argon laser [24]. Penetrating scleral diathermy [25] has been used in the past to close a cyclodialysis cleft, but is rarely used today.

Choroidal detachment

The mechanism underlying most choroidal detachments is not known and it is unclear whether hypotony causes the detachment or vice versa. Clinically, because of the anatomy of the choroid and its attachments at the optic nerve, ciliary body, and vortex veins, it may take on a multilobular appearance. If extensive, the nasal and temporal portions may come together to form "kissing choroidals."

Some believe that choroidal detachments occurring in the immediate postoperative period are quite common. These usually occur in the inferior quadrants, are asymptomatic, and usually disappear spontaneously. Less common are those which occur 7–21 days postoperatively [10]. While this type may simply be a persistence of the immediate type, it may be a result of a wound leak, and will then be accompanied by a shallow anterior chamber and low intraocular pressure. The patient is often asymptomatic, and the course is usually benign, with resolution within 2 or 3 weeks. Rarely, a choroidal detachment occurs months to year after surgery. While some are associated with a traumatic wound leak, in many the mechanism is unclear. The patient may note sudden onset of decreased vision, the eye will be irritable, and the patient will have a shallow or absent anterior chamber [10].

Prophylaxis involves preoperative softening of the eye and a well-made incision with good closure. Most choroidal detachments require little treatment, since they usually resolve spontaneously within 3 weeks. Medically, cycloplegics and corticosteroids are of some benefit. Should the choroidal detachment be associated with a wound leak with persistent shallowing of the anterior chamber, one should not wait more than a week to repair the leak, since peripheral anterior synechia formation and secondary angle-closure glaucoma can ensue. If one is certain that there is no wound defect, draining the suprachoroidal fluid and filling the anterior chamber with an air bubble often resolves the condition [10].

Wound leak

Shallowing of the anterior chamber may occur with a choroidal detachment, pupillary block, and hypotony, which are discussed elsewhere. The most common cause for shallowing or loss of the anterior chamber is a wound leak, most often occurring in the early postoperative period. Its incidence has declined with newer surgical techniques and suture materials.

The cause of a wound leak is intimately related to problems with the wound. This may include an irregular incision, inadequate closure (too few sutures, poorly spaced sutures, shallow suture depth allowing gaping of the wound, or sutures that are too tight and undergo necrosis), or incarceration of iris, lens fragments, or vitreous in the wound [10]. The wound leak may also be related to accidental trauma.

On examination, the iris may come toward the cornea and wound, the conjunctiva may appear boggy or there may even be a bleb over the wound, and there is usually accompanying hypotony. The fundus should be examined to ascertain whether there is a choroidal detachment. If no obvious leak is noted, use of 2% fluorescein may reveal the leak, i.e. a positive Seidel's test.

Many wound leaks respond to 1–2 days of pressure patching. Untreated, a wound leak may result in hypotony, infection, inflammation, secondary glaucoma, epithelial downgrowth, or fibrous ingrowth. Therefore, if the wound leak does not respond to conservative treatment and persists, or if an anterior chamber IOL is present and is in contact with the cornea, surgical intervention should be considered. Air, viscoelastic, or fluorescein may be injected to help localize the leak.

The key to preventing this complication is careful attention to the incision and its closure. Protection of the eye with an eyeshield during sleep in the early postoperative period is an aid in avoiding inadvertent blunt trauma.

Iris prolapse

Intraoperative prolapse of the iris most often is the result of aqueous trapped in the posterior chamber, and may be solved by simply stroking the iris with the irrigator or iris spatula. It may, however, be the first sign of positive posterior pressure. Any external cause should be searched for and dealt with, such as excessive pressure from the eyelid speculum or bridle suture, or squeezing or Valsalva maneuvering by the patient. If an external cause is not evident, and the prolapse increases, it may be the result of a delayed retrobulbar hemorrhage, or a choroidal hemorrhage. It may also be a result of a beveled cataract incision near the iris root, especially in eyes with shallow anterior chambers.

Postoperative iris prolapse is a rare event [26] which is most often the result of a wound dehiscence. It may be secondary to a poor incision or closure, accidental trauma, or coughing or vomiting by the patient [10]. In the early postoperative period, it is usually accompanied by sudden pain, the appearance of a dark mass underneath the conjunctival flap, and peaking of the pupil. If the prolapse is fresh and the tissue viable, one can attempt to reposit surgically the iris. A straightforward technique uses a small corneal stab incision placed temporally through which acetylcholine is injected. A cyclodialysis spatula is then introduced through this incision to reposit the iris [10]. If the iris appears necrotic, it is best to open the wound, free the iris, excise the necrotic portion, and close the wound tightly. Some use photocoagulation or cryotherapy if the prolapsed iris is covered by the conjunctival flap [10].

Iris prolapse may also occur weeks or months after surgery. This is usually gradual in onset, and if not increasing in size or causing any secondary complications such as increasing astigmatism, and if it is completely covered by conjunctiva, does not require surgical repair. Its progress may be followed with serial keratometry.

While the incidence of postoperative iris prolapse will continue to decrease, especially given the trend toward phacoemulsification, it should not be treated lightly since it may result in poor wound healing, a filtering bleb, excessive astigmatism, secondary glaucoma, and inflammation with subsequent cystoid macular edema (CME) [10].

Iridodialysis

An iridodialysis can be produced when the corneoscleral incision is enlarged, during creation of iridectomies, if the iris becomes incarcerated into the aspiration device, and when instruments are passed into the eye and engage the iris. At times, the same trauma that produces the iridodialysis may also cause a cyclodialysis cleft. Usually an iridodialysis is not a serious long-term problem. If it is small it can be left alone. If large, it should be repaired using the McCannel technique [23] or a modification of the technique [27], since it may present a cosmetic problem, produce optical aberrations, and allow the haptic of a posterior chamber lens to pass through it.

Malposition and dislocation of IOLs

In the past, with the use of iris-fixated and iridocapsular lenses, the rate of subluxation and dislocation was relatively high (1.6% [28], 5% [29]). The present-day use of posterior chamber IOLs has decreased the incidence of malposition significantly to approximately 0.4% [28,30].

Pupillary capture occurs when a portion or all of the optic of a posterior chamber IOL moves anterior to the iris. It has been reported to occur in 0.6% [31] to 2.6% [32] of patients and may be related to pupillary dilation in the early postoperative period. Its incidence has been found to be less with the use of lenses with angulated loops [33]. Patients are usually asymptomatic, and so it is primarily a cosmetic problem. However, in some patients, it may cause a low-grade iritis and lead to lens precipitates and possibly CME. It is therefore best to attempt to correct it early before adhesions have formed. The initial treatment consists of vigorous pupillary dilation with the patient in the supine position to break any synechiaes, followed by mimesis after the optic has repositioned. Lindstrom and Herman [33] advocate the use of two cotton-tipped applicators to exert external pressure over the haptics in the region of the ciliary sulcus to compress the IOL. Steinert and Puliafito [34] have used the Nd:YAG laser to retroplace the optic behind the pupil. It is probably not necessary to intervene surgically since this complication has not been associated with visual loss. If uncorrected, a peripheral iridectomy should be performed as total pupillary capture can result in pupillary block glaucoma.

Decentration of the optic to a minor degree occurs frequently and requires no treatment. However, if the decentration is of such an extent that a positioning hole or the edge of the optic is within the pupillary plane, patients may complain of glare. The incidence of such clinically significant decentration has been reported to be between 0.4% [30] and 3% [35]. The most frequent reason is that one haptic is

in the bag (usually the inferior haptic) while the other is in the ciliary sulcus (usually the superior haptic) [36]. Capsular bag fixation will help prevent this complication. Decentration may also be a consequence of a zonular break with one loop protruding through the break. Many patients are successfully treated with miotics to eliminate the glare. Rarely, surgical intervention is necessary and includes the utilization of McCannel sutures to secure both haptics to the iris and repositioning the optic in the posterior chamber.

The windshield wiper syndrome occurs when the superior portion of the IOL rocks from side to side with head movements. Its incidence is small and results when the diameter of the IOL is too small for the eye. Patients often complain of glare and decreased visual acuity; occasionally it causes diplopia and can lead to a low grade iritis [37]. It is best corrected using the McCannel suture technique [23] or a modification [38].

The sunset syndrome is the most serious form of IOL malposition. This condition occurs when the lens sinks below the visual axis, usually as a result of an inferior zonular dialysis in cases where the implant has been placed vertically outside the capsular bag [30]. The reported incidence is in the range of 1%, but this is probably an overestimate. Patients complain of glare and decreased visual acuity, with problems arising as a result of the aphakic and pseudophakic pupillary zones. Capsular bag fixation and horizontal rotation of the implant both reduce its occurrence. When it occurs, several authors recommend iatrogenically inducing a total pupillary capture [10,27,39]. One may also elect to pull the optic superiorly and secure the superior haptic to the iris with a McCannel suture. A third option is to sclerally fixate the lens. Otherwise, one should remove the lens and insert an anterior chamber IOL.

Complete dislocation of the IOL into the vitreous cavity is a very rare event. It occurs as a result of inadvertent rupture of the posterior capsule or zonules at the time of surgery. If well tolerated, conservative treatment is best, and the eye may be fitted with a contact lens, aphakic spectacle, or implantation of an anterior chamber IOL. However, if there is any evidence of instability of the IOL, or any resultant inflammation, or if the patient cannot be visually rehabilitated, surgical intervention is warranted. A pars plana vitrectomy should be performed and, after the IOL is mobilized, it may be fixated to the iris with a modified McCannel technique, or sclerally fixated [40–42].

Anterior chamber lenses have the least tendency to become severely malpositioned. Their malposition is usually related to inappropriate lens sizing [10]. If the implant is too small, its movement may result in inflammation, iris chafing, and corneal edema. An anterior chamber IOL that is too large may damage angle structures and cause UGH syndrome—a triad of uveitis, glaucoma, and hyphema. The usual remedy for these conditions is lens exchange.

Lindstrom et al. [43] reported a series of cases in which the superior footplate of an anterior chamber lens subluxed through a basal peripheral iridectomy. In some of these patients, the footplate stabilized in the ciliary body–pars plana region and required no intervention. In others, however, the subluxation resulted in instability of the lens, with the inferior haptic contacting the corneal endothelium and causing corneal decompensation, iridocyclitis, and CME. These conditions necessitated lens removal or exchange. To avoid this complication, they recommend performing two midperipheral iridectomies, rather than a single large basal iridectomy.

Pupillary block

Pupillary block was a more frequent occurrence in the past with the use of anterior chamber and iris-fixated IOLs and intracapsular cataract surgery. With the advent of modern extracapsular techniques, the incidence of pupillary block has decreased.

Pupillary or iridovitreal block occurring with intracapsular cataract surgery is a result of a relative or absolute blockage of the iridectomy sites or pupillary aperture by the vitreous face. This disrupts the passage of aqueous from the posterior chamber to the anterior chamber with resultant forward displacement of the iris and

closure of the angle. It may be caused by a wound leak, postoperative inflammation, a large air bubble, inadequate iridectomies, a choroidal detachment, and even by the IOL [10,44].

The mechanism of pupillary block after extracapsular cataract surgery is less clear. Undetected capsular or zonular disruption may allow the vitreous to protrude into the anterior chamber [45]. In eyes which have had excessive postoperative inflammation, posterior synechiae may form between the iris and lens at the pupillary border [46]. Pupillary block after extracapsular surgery occurs within the first 1–2 months postoperatively. Most patients will present with a shallow anterior chamber and iris bombé, resulting in angle closure and increased intraocular pressure. Visual acuity may be reduced because of corneal edema if the intraocular pressure is sufficiently elevated [45]. Pain is variably associated with pupillary block. If untreated for a period of time, it may result in peripheral anterior synechiae, chronic angle-closure glaucoma, and loss of vision.

The occurrence of pupillary block is minimized by adequate wound closure, control of postoperative inflammation, and, in intracapsular surgery, adequate iridectomies. The routine use of iridectomies in extracapsular surgery is a source of much debate. Most surgeons do not perform an iridectomy in an uncomplicated case. Some believe that the potential complications of performing an iridectomy—bleeding, iridodialysis, increased postoperative inflammation, postoperative glare from the exposed edge of the IOL— outweigh the risks associated with pupillary block [47]. Others believe that a peripheral iridectomy should be included if the surgery is complicated in any way [48,49] (a shallow anterior chamber, capsular or zonular disruption, vitreous loss, excessive manipulation, or increased vitreous pressure), or in patients prone to excessive postoperative inflammation [46] (diabetics or patients with pre-existing inflammation).

If pupillary block does occur, the patient should be carefully examined to assess the etiology, paying particular attention to the relationships between the iris, implant, and vitreous. Intraocular pressure should be controlled with β-blockers, carbonic anhydrase inhibitors, and oral hyperosmotics if necessary. Short-acting mydriatics can be used to try to relieve the block if a peripheral iridectomy cannot be performed immediately, but medical therapy is rarely curative [50]. The mainstay of therapy is the laser iridectomy, using either the argon or Nd:YAG laser. Alternatives include laser photomydriasis [51] and, in those cases where the vitreous may be blocking an iridectomy site, Nd:YAG vitrotomy [50]. In selected cases where a laser iridectomy may be difficult in the acute stages of pupillary block, Nd:YAG posterior capsulotomy may be an easier and safer alternative to iridectomy [44]. Finally, after breaking the pupillary block, the angle should be examined and, if synechiae are found, argon iridoplasty may be attempted to pull the synechiae away from the angle [50].

Hyphema

The key to preventing intraoperative bleeding, and thereby many of the instances of postoperative hyphema, is gentle but adequate cauterization of the limbal vessels. Excessive bleeding not only reduces the surgeon's visibility, but also clotted blood in the angle and on the surface of the iris may prevent pupillary miosis after insertion of the IOL, and thus result in pupillary capture. Since scleral flap incisions increase the likelihood of bleeding, one should be meticulous in its creation and suturing [52]. One should also try to avoid the 3 and 9 o'clock positions when making the scleral incisions, and if unavoidable, should make the incision closer to the cornea in these areas. In patients with bleeding diatheses or for patients on anticoagulants which cannot be discontinued prior to surgery, a corneal incision can be considered. During surgery, cautery may also be used to control hemorrhage from the iris secondary to an iridectomy, or from the ciliary body as a result of an iridodialysis [53]. Other methods of controlling intraocular hemorrhage include irrigation of the anterior chamber with buffered saline so-

lution (BSS), and injection of air or viscoelastics to tamponade the bleeding vessels.

Postoperative hyphema usually occurs within the first week. It is most often the result of blood left in the eye at the completion of surgery. Other causes include defective wound healing as a result of inadequate incision and/or closure, a scleral incision, as part of UGH syndrome, secondary to trauma, and from abnormal angle or iris vessels (i.e. rubeosis). Prophylaxis has been discussed above. Since the occurrence of a hyphema is usually a benign and self-limited event in which the blood resorbs within several days, the best initial management is observation. However, if the hyphema does not resorb, or results in prolonged elevation of intraocular pressure, there is a risk of corneal blood staining and surgical intervention is warranted. The simplest method is a wash-out with BSS via two paracentesis tracks. It is not necessary to wash out every last red blood cell. An air bubble can be injected afterwards to prevent a rebleed. Another method employs irrigation and aspiration. One must be cautious and patient however, because the clots are adherent to the iris and IOL [27].

A rare late complication is the "sputtering hyphema syndrome" in which a recurrent hyphema may occur months or years postoperatively [54]. This is related to neovascularization of the wound, may be associated with pain, decreased vision, photophobia, iritis, and increased intraocular pressure, and requires prompt treatment. Gonioscopy should be performed to localize the source, and abnormal blood vessels should be photocoagulated with the argon laser. Transscleral Nd:YAG photocoagulation is also effective [55]. Otherwise, the wound must be reopened and the vessels ablated with diathermy, cauterization, or sutures.

Vitreous hemorrhage

A significant vitreous hemorrhage is an uncommon complication after cataract surgery. Its occurrence should prompt the surgeon to search for a cause, such as a late choroidal hemorrhage, or a retinal detachment. Small vitreous hemorrhages are not as uncommon. According to one study [56], they occur in 36% of intracapsular cases and in 13% of extracapsular cases when specifically looked for, and appear as streaks, a diffuse haze, or beads in the vitreous base. It is most often related to an operative hyphema, with blood then passing from the anterior chamber into the vitreous. It may also be related to zonular traction on peripheral retinal vessels. Most often, the hemorrhage resorbs over time and requires no treatment. However, if it persists for 6 months, or is causing secondary complications such as ghost cell glaucoma [57] or hemolytic glaucoma [58], a pars plana vitrectomy should be performed.

Uveitis

The incidence of postoperative uveitis has decreased sharply over the last few years, in large part as a result of improved surgical techniques, IOL design and manufacture [53]. Most often, inflammation is the result of the accompanying trauma of cataract surgery, is short-lived, and responds to topical corticosteroids. Some patients have a persistent early uveitis which may be the result of breakdown of the blood–aqueous barrier, or perhaps a hypersensitivity to surgical manipulation. The implant itself has been implicated in the etiology of inflammation through several mechanisms, including a hypersensitivity or foreign-body response [59], via materials used in polishing and sterilization of lenses [60], and via iris chafing by the implant [61]. Other foreign matter such as cilia, lint, talc, and impurities in the solutions that are used during surgery may induce a self-limited, well-tolerated inflammatory response [10]. Retained lens material may also initiate a usually benign postoperative inflammation. Uveitis may accompany complications of the surgery, such as incarceration of iris or vitreous into the wound, vitreous loss, and hyphema. Treatment involves the use of corticosteroids and cycloplegics, possibly non-steroidal anti-inflammatory agents [62], as well as removal of the inciting source when appropriate.

Complications associated with phacoemulsification

Many of the complications that occur during conventional cataract extraction occur less frequently during phacoemulsification, in large part, because of the smaller incision. Of those that do occur, most will probably occur during the learning period for any surgeon. The most frequent complications occurring during phacoemulsification include stripping of Descemet's membrane (usually during insertion of the emulsification tip), trauma to the iris by the phacoemulsifier, rupture of the posterior capsule or zonules, and transient corneal edema in the first few postoperative days [63]. Shallowing of the anterior chamber during phacoemulsification is generally a consequence of a wound that is too large, allowing fluid to leak out around the emulsification tip. A potentially serious complication is rupture of the posterior capsule with subsequent loss of fragments of nucleus into the vitreous cavity. This complication is rarely encountered with planned extracapsular techniques. The nuclear fragments can incite an inflammatory response if they remain *in situ*. Definitive treatment of this condition often involves collaborative intervention by a vitreoretinal surgeon.

One of the key means of avoiding complications during phacoemulsification is knowing when to convert to conventional extracapsular surgery, before being forced to. A small pupil or extremely hard nucleus makes phacoemulsification more difficult, as will excessive trauma to the iris resulting in shredded portions being continually aspirated by the phaco tip [10].

Phacoemulsification offers the advantage of cataract extraction in a pressurized environment. Techniques that facilitate safe nucleus removal can be readily learned and mastered. The so-called learning curve does not necessarily include a period of greater complications, but rather the development of a comfort level with a newer technique.

Descemet's detachment

Stripping of Descemet's membrane during surgery is an uncommon event and rarely of much consequence [53]. It may occur when inserting the blades of the scissors to enlarge the wound, when inserting the cystotome for capsulotomy, or during insertion of the irrigation and aspiration tip, phaco tip, or IOL. The diagnosis is not difficult. If it is not noted during surgery, it can be observed post-operatively at the slit-lamp, where there may be overlying corneal edema. If the detachment is small, the corneal edema will usually clear up within several weeks. A large detachment, however, may lead to corneal decompensation requiring a penetrating keratoplasty.

When noted during surgery, one may be able to inject air or a viscoelastic substance into the anterior chamber to uncurl and re-position the detachment. When using a visco-elastic substance, it is injected distal to the point of stromal attachment and allowed to move superiorly in the anterior chamber to compress the loose Descemet's leaf. It should not be allowed to come between Descemet's membrane and stroma or it will prevent re-attachment. Adjunctive means of uncurling the detachment involve the use a cyclodialysis spatula [64] or iris repositor [65]. If the detach-ment is large, it may be necessary to suture the area of stripped membrane to the cornea [27].

Corneal edema

Striate keratopathy and corneal edema are relatively common occurrences after cataract surgery and are usually transient. The inci-dence of persistent corneal edema has de-creased dramatically with the transfer to primarily extracapsular surgery with posterior chamber lens implantation, and with im-provements in IOL design [10,53]. Persistent corneal edema is the hallmark of endothelial cell damage and often results in bullous kera-topathy. There is no effective definitive treat-ment other than a penetrating keratoplasty.

Understanding its cause is the key to its prevention. Patients with pre-existent corneal endothelial disease are at a much higher risk for subsequent corneal decompensation. While some cases are related to a large Descemet's detachment, adherence of vitreous to the back of the cornea, epithelial downgrowth, or fibrous ingrowth, the majority are related to the endothelial trauma that invariably occurs during surgery.

Endothelial trauma may be a particular problem with phacoemulsification, both by a direct effect (secondary to the ultrasound itself) and an indirect effect (via nuclear fragments hitting the endothelium). The large volume of irrigation fluid used may also cause damage, as may the nucleus if it rests against the cornea during anterior chamber phacoemulsification. Jaffe has shown [10] that phacoemulsification resulted in a much greater endothelial cell loss at 6 weeks postoperatively when compared to extracapsular surgery (13.5% vs. 4.8%). However, Kraff et al. [66] have reported that posterior chamber phacoemulsification re-sulted in less cell loss than anterior chamber phacoemulsification (15.2% vs. 27.3%).

The use of viscoelastics to protect the endo-thelium is of great importance in all forms of cataract extraction. In addition, the anterior capsule may help protect the corneal endothe-lium during phacoemulsification. Experimental [67] and clinical [68] studies have shown that the intercapsular technique with phacoemul-sification results in less endothelial cell loss than phacoemulsification with a conventional capsulotomy. Newer techniques of phaco-emulsification using continuous circular cap-sulorhexis, in situ phacoemulsification, low energy phacoemulsification, improved visco-elastic materials, and advanced IOLs should all contribute to further reduction in endothelial cell loss during surgery.

Epithelial downgrowth

Epithelial downgrowth following cataract surgery is a dreaded, but fortunately very rare complication, probably occurring in less than 0.1% of cases. Its pathogenesis is not fully understood, but is usually associated with wound closure problems. Simple implantation of epithelial cells into the anterior chamber will not result in proliferation on the endothelium or iris. It is currently believed that a fistulous wound allows downgrowth of conjunctival epithelium, and that cornea stromal vascularization and contact with uveal tissue provide the nutrition and framework necessary for its proliferation and spread [69]. The most frequent presenting sign is a decrease in visual acuity, and patients may have pain, redness, tearing, and photophobia. On slit-lamp examination there will often be a retrocorneal membrane, painful or painless glaucoma (usually the former), corneal edema, a positive Seidel's test, hypotony, and/or iritis [69]. If the presentation suggests epithelial downgrowth, it may be confirmed by laser photocoagulation of the surface of the iris. If epithelium is present, a white cotton fluff-ball will form immediately. Although not all cases are amenable to surgical intervention, the treatment of epithelial downgrowth involves excising the fistula, involved iris, ciliary body and angle structures, and cryotherapy of the involved cornea with subsequent excision [70]. Unfortunately, most cases are unsuccessful.

Epithelial cysts may also occur postoperatively. They too are related to inadequate wound apposition and implantation of epithelial cells into the anterior chamber. The resultant closed cysts appear translucent or grayish, may distort the pupil, and have a variable growth pattern. If they do grow, they may result in an iridocyclitis, and should then be treated by aspiration and photocoagulation, cryotherapy, or diathermy [10].

Fibrous ingrowth

Fibrous ingrowth is another rare complication related to faulty wound closure. The source of the fibroblasts is unknown, but the tissue can grow over the back of the cornea and throughout the anterior chamber. Clinically, it appears similar to epithelial downgrowth but the retrocorneal membrane has strands of tissue advancing ahead of an irregular border. Little is known about how to treat fibrous ingrowth. Although there may be associated corneal edema and glaucoma, since many eyes do not exhibit the inexorable demise associated with epithelial downgrowth, often no therapy is necessary.

Conclusion

While the incidence of most complications has decreased with the conversion to the extracapsular technique, and may further decline as many surgeon's switch to phacoemulsification, we need to be able to anticipate, recognize and manage complications when they occur, and be constantly aware of the potential for new complications.

We have attempted to provide an understanding of the pathogenesis, presentation, and management of some of the more common and important complications that may occur during and after cataract surgery. While complications are an inevitable part of surgery, it should be apparent from the preceding discussion that many are avoidable if we are attentive at each step of the operation. Furthermore, if we are aware of the potential complication in a particular surgical setting, are able to identify it when it occurs, and understand how to deal with it, these complications may be associated with a satisfactory outcome.

References

1 Taylor DM. Expulsive hemorrhage. *Am J Ophthalmol* 1974; **78**: 961–5.
2 Manschot WA. The pathology of expulsive hemorrhage. *Am J Ophthalmol* 1955; **40**: 15–24.
3 Maumenee AE, Schwartz MF. Acute intraoperative choroidal effusion. *Am J Ophthalmol* 1985; **100**: 147–54.
4 Davison JA. Acute intraoperative suprachoroidal hemorrhage in extracapsular cataract surgery. *J Cataract Refract Surg* 1986; **12**: 606–22.
5 Bukelman A, Hoffman P, Oliver M. Limited choroidal hemorrhage associated with extracapsular cataract extraction. *Arch Ophthalmol* 1987; **105**: 338–41.
6 Hoffman P, Pollack A, Oliver M. Limited choroidal hemorrhage associated with intracapsular cataract extraction. *Arch Ophthalmol* 1984; **102**: 1761–5.
7 Payne JW, Kameen AJ, Jensen AD *et al.* Expulsive hemorrhage: Its incidence in cataract surgery and a report of four bilateral cases. *Trans Am Ophthalmol Soc* 1985: **83**: 181–204.

8 Bair HL. Expulsive hemorrhage at cataract extraction: Report of a case and an additional recommendation for its management. *Am J Ophthalmol* 1966; **61**: 992–4.

9 Shaffer RN. Posterior sclerotomy with scleral cautery in the treatment of expulsive hemorrhage. *Am J Ophthalmol* 1966; **61**: 1307–11.

10 Jaffe NS. *Cataract Surgery and its Complications*. 5th edn. St Louis: CV Mosby, 1989.

11 Acheson JF, McHugh JD, Falcon MG. Changing patterns of early complications in cataract surgery with new techniques: a surgical audit. *Br J Ophthalmol* 1988; **72**: 481–4.

12 Guzek JP, Holm M, Cotter JB *et al*. Risk factors for intraoperative complications in 1000 extracapsular cases. *Ophthalmology* 1987; **94**: 461–6.

13 Obstbaum SA, Robbins R, Best M, Galin MA. Recovery of intraocular pressure and vitreous weight after ocular compression. *Am J Ophthalmol* 1971; **71**: 1059–65.

14 Pearson PA, Owen DG, Maliszewski M *et al*. Anterior chamber lens implantation after vitreous loss. *Br J Ophthalmol* 1989; **73**: 596–9.

15 Balent A, Civerchia LL, Mohamadi P. Visual outcome of cataract extraction and lens implantation complicated by vitreous loss. *J Cataract Refract Surg* 1988; **14**: 158–60.

16 Spigelman AV, Lindstrom RL, Nichols BD *et al*. Visual results following vitreous loss and primary lens implantation. *J Cataract Refract Surg* 1989; **15**: 201–4.

17 O'Donnell FE, Santos B. Posterior capsular–zonular disruption in planned extracapsular surgery. *Arch Ophthalmol* 1985; **103**: 652–3.

18 Shah GR, Gills JP, Durham DG *et al*. Three thousand YAG lasers in posterior capsulotomies: An analysis of complications and comparison to polishing and surgical discission. *Ophthal Surg* 1986; **17**: 473–7.

19 Stark WJ, Goodman G, Goodman D *et al*. Posterior chamber intraocular lens implantation in the absence of posterior capsular support. *Ophthal Surg* 1988; **19**: 240–3.

20 Chandler PA, Maumenee AE. A major cause of hypotony. *Am J Ophthalmol* 1961; **52**: 609–18.

21 Pederson JE, Gaasterland DE, MacLellan HM. Uveoscleral outflow in the rhesus monkey: Importance of uveal reabsorption. *Invest Ophthalmol Vis Sci* 1977; **16**: 1008–17.

22 Gass JDM. The cause of visual loss in hypotony. In: Welsh RC, Welsh J, eds. *The New Report on Cataract Surgery*. Miami, Florida: Miami Educational Press, 1969.

23 McCannel MA. A retrievable suture idea for anterior uveal problems. *Ophthal Surg* 1986; **7**: 98–103.

24 Harbin TS. Treatment of cyclodialysis clefts with argon laser photocoagulation. *Ophthalmology* 1982; **89**: 1082–3.

25 Maumenee AE. Glaucoma: hypotony. *Highlights Ophthalmol* 1966; **9**: 28–53.

26 Kaushik NC, Morgan LH, Morrison AM. Iris prolapse following cataract surgery. *Trans Ophthalmol Soc UK* 1983; **103**: 560.

27 Clayman HM, Jaffe NS, Galin MA. *Intraocular Lens Implantation. Techniques and Complications*. St Louis: CV Mosby, 1983.

28 Worthen DM, Boucher JA, Buxton JN *et al*. Interim FDA report on intraocular lenses. *Ophthalmology* 1980; **87**: 267–71.

29 Poley BJ, Lewin DP. A closed technique for repositioning dislocated iris plane lenses. *Am Intraocul Implant Soc J* 1979; **5**: 316–20.

30 Kratz RP. Complications associated with posterior chamber lenses. *Ophthalmology* 1979; **86**: 659–61.

31 Southwick PC, Olson RJ. Shearing posterior chamber intraocular lenses: Five-year postoperative results. *Am Intraocul Implant Soc J* 1984; **10**: 318–23.

32 Faulkner JD. Advantages and indications for posterior chamber intraocular lens implants. *Contact Intraocul Lens Med J* 1982; **8**: 50–2.

33 Lindstrom RJ, Herman WK. Pupil capture: Prevention and management. *Am Intraocul Implant Soc J* 1983; **9**: 201–4.

34 Steinert P, Puliafito CA. New applications of the Nd:YAG laser. *Am Intraocul Implant Soc J* 1984; **10**: 372–6.

35 Pallin SL, Walman GB. Posterior chamber intraocular lens implant centration: In or out of "the bag." *Am Intraocul Implant Soc J* 1982; **8**: 254–7.

36 Hansen SO, Tetz MR, Solomon KD *et al*. Decentration of flexible loop posterior chamber intraocular lenses in a series of 222 postmortem eyes. *Ophthalmology* 1988; **95**: 344–9.

37 Smith RG, Lindstrom RL. Malpositioned posterior chamber lenses: Etiology, prevention, and management. *Am Intraocul Implant Soc J* 1985; **11**: 584–91.

38 Smith SG, Lindstrom RL. Report and management of the sunrise syndrome. *Am Intraocul Implant Soc J* 1984; **10**: 218–20.

39 Shearing S. Posterior chamber lens implantation. *Int Ophthal Clin* 1982; **221**: 135–53.

40 Sternberg P Jr, Michael RG. Treatment of dislocated posterior chamber intraocular lenses. *Arch Ophthalmol* 1988; **104**: 1391–3.

41 Price FW Jr, Whitson WE. Visual results of suture-fixated posterior chamber lenses during penetrating keratoplasty. *Ophthalmology* 1989; **96**: 1234–40.

42 Apple DJ, Price FW, Gwin T *et al*. Sutured retropupillary posterior chamber intraocular lenses for exchange or secondary implantation. The Twelfth Annual Binkhorst Lecture, 1988. *Ophthalmology* 1989; **96**: 1241–7.

43 Lindstrom RL, Nelson JD, Neist RL. Anterior chamber lens subluxation through a basal peripheral iridectomy. *Am Intraocul Implant Soc J* 1983; **9**: 53–6.

44 Tomey KF, Traverso CE. Neodymium-YAG laser posterior capsulotomy for the treatment of aphakic and pseudophakic pupillary block. *Am J Ophthalmol* 1987; **104**: 502–7.

45 Samples JR, Bellows AR, Rosenquist RC *et al.* Pupillary block with posterior chamber lenses. *Arch Ophthalmol* 1987; **105**: 335–7.

46 Naveh-Floman N, Rosner M, Blumenthal M. Pseudophakic pupillary block glaucoma with posterior-chamber intraocular lens. *Glaucoma* 1985; 7: 262–5.

47 Schulze RR, Copeland JR. Posterior chamber intraocular lens implantation without peripheral iridectomy—a preliminary report. *Ophthal Surg* 1982; **13**: 567.

48 Cohen JS, Osher RH, Weber P *et al.* Complications of extracapsular cataract surgery. The indications and risks of peripheral iridectomy. *Ophthalmology* 1984; **91**: 826–30.

49 Willis DA, Stewart RH, Kimbrough RL. Pupillary block associated with posterior chamber lenses. *Ophthal Surg* 1985; **16**: 108–9.

50 Shrader CE, Belcher CD, Thomas JV *et al.* Pupillary and iridovitreal block in pseudophakic eyes. *Ophthalmology* 1984; **91**: 831–7.

51 Obstbaum SA, Barasch KR, Galin MA, Baras I. Laser photomydriasis in pseudophakic pupillary block. *Am Intraocul Implant Soc J* 1981; **7**: 28–30.

52 Moses L. Postoperative hyphema in cataract surgery with scleral flap technique. *Arch Ophthalmol* 1986; **104**: 793.

53 Goodman DF, Stark WJ, Gottsch JD. Complications of cataract extraction with intraocular lens implantation. *Ophthal Surg* 1989; **20**: 132–40.

54 Swan KC. Hyphema due to wound vascularization after cataract extraction. *Arch Ophthalmol* 1973; **89**: 87–90.

55 Kramer TR, Brown RH, Lynch MG *et al.* Transscleral Nd:YAG photocoagulation for cataract incision vascularization associated with recurrent hyphema. *Am J Ophthalmol* 1989; **107**: 681–2.

56 Littlewood KR, Constable IJ. Vitreous hemorrhage after cataract extraction. *Br J Ophthalmol* 1985; **69**: 911–14.

57 Campbell DG, Simmons RJ, Grant WM. Ghost cells as a cause of glaucoma. *Am J Ophthalmol* 1976; **81**: 441–50.

58 Fenton RH, Zimmerman LE. Hemolytic glaucoma: An unusual case of acute, open-angle secondary glaucoma. *Arch Ophthalmol* 1963; **70**: 236–9.

59 Galin MA, Tuberville AW, Dotson RS. Immunologic aspects of intraocular lenses. *Int Ophthalmol Clin* 1982; **22**: 227–34.

60 Meltzer DW. Sterile hypopyon following intraocular lens surgery. *Arch Ophthalmol* 1980; **98**: 100–4.

61 Ellingson FT. Complications with the Choyce Mark VII anterior chamber lens implant (uveitis–glaucoma–hyphema). *Am Intraocul Implant Soc J* 1983; **9**: 199–205.

62 Kraff MC, Sanders DR, McGuigan L *et al.* Inhibition of blood–aqueous humor barrier breakdown with Diclofenac. A fluorophotometric study. *Arch Ophthalmol* 1990; **108**: 380–3.

63 Emery JM, Wilhelmus KA, Rosenberg S. Complications of phacoemulsification. *Ophthalmology* 1978; **85**: 141–50.

64 Sparks GM. Descemetopexy: surgical reattachment of stripped Descemet's membrane. *Arch Ophthalmol* 1967; **78**: 31–4.

65 Sugar HS. Prognosis in stripping of Descemet's membrane in cataract extraction. *Am J Ophthalmol* 1967; **63**: 140–3.

66 Kraff MC, Sanders DR, Lieberman HL. Specular microscopy in cataract and intraocular lens patients: A report of 564 cases. *Arch Ophthalmol* 1980; **98**: 1782–4.

67 Solomon KD, Gwinn TD, O'Monchoe DJC *et al.* Protective effect of the anterior lens capsule during extracapsular cataract extraction. Part I. Experimental animal study. *Ophthalmology* 1989; **96**: 591–7.

68 Patel J, Apple DJ, Hansen SO *et al.* Protective effect of the anterior lens capsule during extracapsular cataract extraction. Part II. Preliminary results of a clinical study. *Ophthalmology* 1989; **96**: 598–602.

69 Weiner MJ, Trentacoste J, Pon DM *et al.* Epithelial downgrowth: A 30-year clinicopathological review. *Br J Ophthalmol* 1989; **73**: 6–11.

70 Brown SI. Results of excision of advanced epithelial downgrowth. *Ophthalmology* 1979; **86**: 321–8.

18: Complications of Phacoemulsification Surgery

ROBERT J. CIONNI & ROBERT H. OSHER

Introduction

The successful management of intraoperative complications requires a combination of recognition, knowledge, skill, and judgement. The surgeon must respond almost automatically since the intense stress of the moment may impair clear, rapid thinking. Therefore, the best approach to the management of intraoperative complications is preoperative preparation for all possibilities. This chapter will focus upon a constellation of intraoperative complications. Although the majority of these complications will be encountered by every cataract surgeon, a well-prepared, knowledgeable response to these problems will usually result in a successful visual outcome.

Patient movement

The primary drawback of local anesthesia is the patient's ability to move during surgery. Although most movement occurs from talking, coughing, or simply "fidgeting," an occasional patient will abruptly sit up and try to leave the operating room while the surgeon is still working.

Prevention

As always, the best solution to a problem is its prevention. Taping the forehead to the operating table helps decrease small movements by those patients with head tremors or those who lack the concentration to lie still. This is best accomplished before surgery begins so it is better to evaluate the patient's mobility prior to beginning the operation.

Allowing the patient to become over sedated or to fall asleep is also dangerous. The patient may suddenly awaken in a disoriented state and violently thrust the head resulting in severe intraocular damage. It is helpful to remind the somnolent patient periodically the necessity of staying awake. Coughing can also cause sudden head movement as well as significant positive pressure. We ask the patient to warn us if a cough is coming. A box of cough drops located at the microscope has on numerous occasions "saved the day."

To minimize restlessness, it is best to be certain that the patient is comfortable before surgery begins. This includes ample ventilation beneath the drapes, placement of supporting pillows, and proper table tilt.

Management

The anesthesiologist can be of great value in decreasing excessive patient movement by administering appropriate medications when indicated during the procedure. Though the surgeon should always be kind and courteous, it may occasionally become necessary to be stern in order to keep the patient from moving and damaging the eye.

It movement is excessive, the smaller the wound the better. If necessary, the surgeon may quickly close the wound until the patient has settled down. It is often possible to resume surgery once the patient's anxiety or discomfort has been alleviated.

Retrobulbar hemorrhage

Many surgeons cancel surgery in the event of a retrobulbar hemorrhage [1,2]. It is believed that increased orbital or intraocular pressure increases the likelihood of complications which include iris prolapse, posterior capsule rupture, and loss of vitreous.

Management

Although small incision surgery decreases the risks of complications associated with retrobulbar hemorrhage, it does not eliminate complications completely. We have found that in most instances of retrobulbar hemorrhage, phacoemulsification with posterior chamber intraocular lens (IOL) implantation can be performed safely provided that several criteria are met. First, active bleeding must be appropriately managed with direct orbital pressure to facilitate clotication. Once this is accomplished, the surgeon should evaluate the extent of the hemorrhage. Surgery can proceed if the globe is soft, easily retropulsed, the lids are loose and mobile, and not much proptosis exists. If one or more of these parameters are not met, then either digital massage or placement of a mercury bag for 5–10 min may adequately reduce the pressure so that these parameters are fulfilled. Additionally, it may be necessary to perform a lateral canthotomy to reduce lid pressure. If the surgeon remains uncertain about safely proceeding after 30 min, it is probably best to reschedule the surgery.

If the surgery is continued without fulfilling these criteria, then the surgeon should anticipate an extremely difficult case. Iris bombé and prolapse are likely, making every step of the surgery from the insertion of the phacoemulsification tip to wound closure challenging. Positive pressure will be discussed in a subsequent section.

In a recent series of 60 cases of retrobulbar hemorrhage, only three cases failed to satisfy these criteria requiring cancellation [3]. With few exceptions, the eyes undergoing surgery did not encounter a higher incidence of intraocular complications and the postoperative visual results were similar to a control group of patients who had not developed a retrobulbar hemorrhage.

Tight lids

Extensive pressure from tight lids is a common occurrence during cataract surgery. Tight lids, associated with narrow palpebral fissures or resulting from a relative proptosis, may lead to a multitude of intraoperative difficulties and potential intraoperative complications. It is in the surgeon's best interest to do everything that is possible to reduce the pressure that the lids exert upon the globe.

Evaluation

There are several clues that indicate excessive lid pressure. When the eyelids are opened after the retrobulbar or peribulbar anesthetic, the surgeon may observe narrowed fissures with little visible sclera. There may also be a blunted lateral canthal angle restricting the width of the fissure. Another sign of potential lid pressure is indentation of the conjunctiva by either the lid margin or the speculum. A final indication of tight lids may be resistance of the globe to rotation as the bridal suture is being placed.

Management

The first step is to select a lid speculum that lifts the lids off the globe (e.g. Osher–Cionni Lid Speculum, Storz Ophthalmics Inc., St Louis, Missouri). It may be necessary to perform a lateral canthotomy in some cases. This is accomplished after the speculum has been inserted by clamping a few millimeters of the lateral canthal angle with a hemostat for a minute or two. After releasing the hemostat, the canthus is incised with scissors and little if any bleeding results. This procedure should allow easy globe rotation with a reduction in lid pressure.

Incision

The incision has always been important to the surgeon as its closure is his or her signature. In phacoemulsification, however, its importance goes well beyond appearance. A poorly con-structed incision will make a routine case dif-ficult. Likewise, a carefully planned and precise incision may convert an extremely difficult case into an enjoyable and successful procedure. This important point must be firmly engraved into every cataract surgeon's mind lest he or she be reminded by iris prolapse, hemorrhage, wound leak, and astigmatism.

Placement

The surgeon must first decide at which axis to center the wound. This decision usually depends upon pre-existing astigmatism and occasionally upon anatomic landmarks (i.e. vessels, peripheral anterior synechiae, corneal opacity, etc.). Of even greater importance is where best to gain comfortable access to the globe so that a prominent supraorbital rim will not interfere. The distance the incision is placed from the cornea must also be determined and several factors must be considered. The closer the incision is to the cornea, the greater the tendency for induced cylinder at that axis [4]. This wound, however, is also more difficult to close as there is less surface area of the flap for appositional closure. On the other hand, a more posterior incision affords a more water-tight closure with less induction of astigma-tism. Yet a more posterior incision requires careful construction to avoid premature entry. A greater number of vessels will be encoun-tered with more bleeding and a more difficult "uphill" procedure may ensue. Other factors must be considered before placing the incision. A very deep anterior chamber warrants a more anterior incision in order to gain access to the superior aspect of the capsular bag for cortical removal. Similarly, a very shallow anterior chamber must be entered more anteriorly to avoid iris prolapse. A young patient will tend to form a wound gape due to "molding" around the phacoemulsifier shaft. Therefore, a more posterior incision with a larger bed of apposition is desirable and will be more likely to allow a water-tight closure. If a posterior lip sclerectomy is planned with a combined procedure, a more posterior wound is con-ducive to better filtration.

Size

The length of the incision must allow entry of the handpiece and the IOL and must be tapered to these dimensions. A larger wound will allow "against-the-rule" slide and may be used to decrease "with-the-rule" astigmatism [5,6]. Yet too large an incision may also result in a leaky incision with constant chamber shallowing throughout the operation requiring a tem-porary suture. An undersized wound will not permit sufficient sliding of the phacoemulsifier shaft causing excessive eye rotation during the emulsification. In addition, too small an in-cision is more likely to result in trauma to Descemet's membrane, a wound gape and a difficult lens implantation. A certain amount of "snugness" is desirable but if excessively tight, the wound should be extended. Proper sizing of the wound can be assured by using an internal caliper to measure the actual length of the incision prior to the IOL implantation (e.g. Osher Internal Caliper, Storz Ophthalmics Inc., St Louis, Missouri).

Depth

Too deep an incision may result in entry into the suprachoroidal space or premature entry into the chamber angle. The former may be associated with bleeding and hypotony while the latter is associated with iris prolapse. A guarded knife for performing the incision is helpful and we prefer a depth of one-half to two-thirds scleral thickness.

Descemet's tear

A tear of Descemet's membrane at the anterior chamber entry site can be caused by improper insertion of an instrument through the incision. It is important to direct the leading tip pos-teriorly whenever inserting an instrument to avoid this occurrence. The ability to do so is compromised in eyes with shallow chambers where a posteriorly directed passage would engage the iris. The use of a viscoelastic agent to deepen the chamber prior to entry with a keratome or a phaco tip will aid the surgeon in preventing this complication. As mentioned, an adequate incision size will also minimize the likelihood of a Descemet's tear.

The most important step in managing a tear in Descemet's membrane is recognizing its presence. If unnoticed, continued instrument manipulation may increase the extent of the detachment. Inadvertent injection of a viscoelastic agent into the separation can also extend the detachment. Once recognized, Descemet's membrane can usually be reattached by one or two simple maneuvers. Placing pressure on the posterior lip of the wound at the site of the tear will generate an egress of fluid which will reposit a small Descemet's flap in most instances. Alternatively, a small air bubble or a viscoelastic agent can be used to tamponade a Descemet's flap into position during suturing of the wound.

A more extensive tear may require suturing. The needle should pass through clear cornea central to the "hinge" of the tear and is then directed peripherally to splint Descemet's membrane into position.

Iris prolapse

Prolapse of the iris is not only an aggravating event for the surgeon but it may also lead to an irregular pupil, peripheral anterior synechiae, or incarceration into the wound. Prostaglandin release may cause a constriction of the pupil while rupture of vessels from the minor iris circle may cause intraocular bleeding. Iris prolapse is less common with the newer types of incisions yet the surgeon should know how to properly manage it.

Prevention

As mentioned previously, a well-placed incision, scleral flap, and entry will help to prevent iris prolapse, while a posterior entry will ensure its occurrence. Efforts of both minimizing iris trauma and reducing positive pressure will decrease the likelihood of iris prolapse. Care should be taken to avoid excessive injection of fluid or viscoelastics into the eye which may also cause iris prolapse.

Management

The surgeon should try to identify the etiology of the iris prolapse in order to properly manage it. Excessive intraocular pressure can be reduced by eliminating sources of external pressure such as proper speculum positioning and release of the bridal suture. The intraocular pressure can be further lowered by aspirating fluid or viscoelastic material from the anterior chamber, preferably via the second incision site. The iris can be gently reposited in most cases by the cannula on the viscoelastic syringe leaving some viscoelastic agent on the iris surface. If these attempts fail, the surgeon should not hesitate to perform a small peripheral iridectomy to neutralize the pressure gradient between the anterior and posterior chambers. Repeated iris manipulation should be avoided since the iris becomes increasingly more frayed and flaccid. A few drops of intracameral miotic, judicious use of viscoelastics, iridotomy, and deeply placed sutures will reduce the possibility of iris incarceration in the wound.

Intraocular hemorrhage

Hemorrhage from the wound may compromise visibility and obscure the surgical events within the eye. Blood may also accumulate behind an IOL and prove difficult to remove. Although, intraocular hemorrhage will invariably absorb, it may acutely reduce vision, stimulate inflammation, accelerate capsular opacification, and prevent pupillary movement by clot formation. For these reasons we attempt to discontinue anticoagulants prior to surgery with the approval of the patient's internist.

We have found that intraocular hemorrhage occurs more commonly when the incision is placed either more temporal, more posterior, or deeper than usual. In these locations, larger blood vessels are encountered and bleeding is often more brisk. Viscoelastic material, because of its space-occupying properties will often limit the amount of intraocular bleeding and may serve to tamponade the bleeding site. Elevating the intraocular pressure by overfilling the chamber with adrenalized balanced salt solution is also an advantage with small incision surgery. Point cautery to the feeder vessel away from the wound itself is often helpful. It is best for the surgeon to evacuate intraocular blood before clot formation occurs by simply depressing the posterior lip of the wound with a cannula at the site where blood has entered the eye. However, if there is a tendency for anterior chamber collapse, intraocular blood should be ignored until the chamber is controlled by suturing the wound. Blood can then be aspirated and exchanged for balanced salt solution either through the side stab incision or between sutures. There are cannulas available for simultaneous aspiration and infusion, yet we use a miniature irrigation and aspiration (I&A) tip that will slip between sutures aspirating the clot in a closed system at the end of the case.

Anterior capsulectomy

Can opener vs. continuous tear

Many surgeons have recently adopted capsulorhexis as their preferred anterior capsulectomy technique. This type of capsulectomy is much stronger and resistant to peripheral extension during nucleus manipulation, cortical removal, and IOL implantation [7]. We have found that our incidence of posterior capsular tears has been reduced (0.2%) since incorporating capsulorhexis into our surgical technique [8]. Moreover, if a tear in the posterior capsule should occur, there is a greater likelihood of being able to place a posterior chamber IOL into the capsular bag. Our comments on the complications encountered during capsulectomy will be directed toward capsulorhexis.

Peripheral extension

The surgeon just learning capsulorhexis will encounter this problem more often than one who is more experienced with this technique. Certain conditions predispose to this event. Anterior bowing of the lens–iris diaphragm will always encourage peripheral extension. This condition is more common in patients

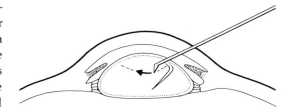

Fig. 18.1 Anterior bowing causing the capsulorhexis to run peripherally.

with shallow anterior chambers and in those patients with positive pressure. The effect is that a "hill" is formed and the capsule will always pursue the downhill course resisting any attempted redirection uphill (Fig. 18.1).

In young patients the leading edge of the anterior capsular tear tends to run peripherally which is possibly due to the elastic forces of the zonules, intralenticular pressure, and the chamber shallowing tendencies secondary to reduced scleral rigidity. The widely dilated pupil may also lend itself to a larger capsulectomy and if the zonular insertions are encountered, the tear will have a strong tendency to follow the radial course of the zonule rather than the desired circumferential course. Therefore, we make a conscientious effort to perform a slightly smaller capsulectomy in the young patient, but not so small as to compromise nuclear manipulation or superior cortical aspiration.

The best management of a complication is its prevention. In young patients and those with either shallow anterior chambers or positive pressure, it is imperative to push the lens–iris diaphragm posterior with a generous amount of viscoelastic material. If the viscoelastic material is extruded, additional amounts may be required to prevent peripheral extension. This may be accomplished by attaching a bent needle or cystotome to the viscoelastic syringe thereby eliminating the tendency for viscoelastic escape as one enters and exits the anterior chamber. Once the chamber deepens, the capsulorhexis will be easier to guide in the desired direction (Fig. 18.2).

Occasionally, the anterior capsular tear will extend too far peripherally to be recovered. Persistent attempts to force the tear centrally may cause it to further extend around the

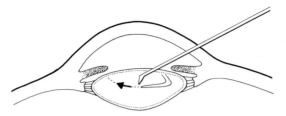

Fig. 18.2 After placing viscoelastic substance to flatten the lens–iris diaphragm, the tear runs as desired.

equator into the posterior capsule. An experienced surgeon will know when the tear is too far peripheral by the feel of resistance to effort to redirect the tear. The surgeon should return to the starting point and proceed with either a second continuous tear or a can opener technique until the capsulectomy is completed.

If the anterior capsular tear has extended peripherally or if a notch is present in the anterior capsular ring, phacoemulsification must be performed with extreme care in order to avoid stress to the capsular bag. The second instrument is used to manipulate the nucleus away from the area of peripheral extension without generating forces that may extend the tear further. A low aspiration–infusion system allows phacoemulsification to occur slowly without sudden chamber shallowing or excessive fluid movement through compromised zonules. Aspiration of cortex is also performed gently in the area of the peripheral extension. The IOL should be inserted and oriented away from the tear in the weakened capsular bag.

Small capsulectomy

A capsulectomy that is too small makes manipulation of the superior nucleus more difficult. Often it is virtually impossible to use a tipping or prolapsing technique if the anterior capsule is holding the nucleus back. The surgeon may select a number of maneuvers that will facilitate the emulsification even when the capsulectomy is too small. One technique involves rotation and emulsification of the nucleus within the capsular bag. Another technique depends upon the dividing or sectioning of the nucleus within the capsular bag [9]. Debulking the

nucleus and using a second instrument to lift its malleable rim away from the posterior capsule is a third effective technique.

A small capsulectomy also makes cortical aspiration difficult at the superior pole. It may be necessary to nearly verticalize the I&A tip while rotating the eye superiorly to reach the superior cortex. This, however, causes cornea and wound distortion. An alternative method is to use a manual aspiration system with a curved cannula introduced through either the superior or the side stab incision.

It may occasionally be necessary to enlarge a capsulectomy. If a "tag" with an edge is present, it can be grasped and the tear can be guided with either forceps or with the I&A tip. If there is not a tag present, Vanass scissors can be used to create a tear orienting the cut in the desired direction and then proceeding with a capsule forceps. This is most safe when performed under the protection of a viscoelastic agent after the IOL has been implanted.

Phacoemulsification

A variety of complications can occur during phacoemulsification.

Insertion

Insertion of the phacoemulsification tip can cause stripping of Descemet's membrane, iris stromal chafing, and even disinsertion of the iris. These complications are more likely to occur in eyes with shallow chambers where there is little room between the iris and the cornea. If the incision is made properly, and the instruments are carefully angled toward the pupil, these complications can be minimized. An effective technique in decreasing iris chafing is to introduce the phacoemulsification tip beveled down and then rotating the bevel upward while either irrigation is on or while passing through a viscoelastic agent without irrigation. Another technique is to "reverse" aspiration in which the footswitch is activated causing infusion from the tip to displace the iris posteriorly.

If there is iris prolapse plugging the incision

prior to or during the phacoemulsification entry then the technique must be modified. The prolapsed iris is reposited as described earlier. A viscoelastic agent is then instilled onto the adjacent iris. If an attempt is made to insert the phaco tip with irrigation on, prolapse will inevitably recur. Instead the irrigation line should be pinched off until the phaco tip is well within the anterior chamber.

Excessive globe movement

This problem is usually due to either too tight an incision, too long a scleral tunnel, or improper manipulation of the phaco handpiece. If the surgeon's movements are adjusted so that the wound site acts as a fulcrum for the handpiece, excessive movement of the globe should not occur. If the problem persists, then the incision should be enlarged slightly.

Shallow anterior chamber

The presence of a shallow anterior chamber makes phacoemulsification extremely difficult. Descemet's detachments and difficulty reaching superior cortex are more likely to occur as the surgeon tends to direct his wound more anteriorly to avoid the iris upon entry into the anterior chamber. Whenever iris bombé is present, peripheral anterior capsular extensions are more likely to occur. Iris prolapse and damage to both the iris and the corneal endothelium may occur during insertion of the phacoemulsifier. The possibility of spontaneous prolapse of the nucleus can be minimized by avoiding hydrodissection in these cases. Fortunately, the anterior chamber will usually deepen significantly upon completion of the emulsification.

CAUSES

Footswitch inattentiveness

The anterior chamber will routinely shallow if the surgeon is so preoccupied with intraocular maneuvering that control of the footswitch is forgotten. Continuous irrigation is necessary to maintain the anterior chamber depth.

Insufficient inflow

As a general rule, the irrigation stream should be just enough to maintain the depth of the anterior chamber, since trauma to the endothelium secondary to excessive irrigation should be avoided. If the infusion is insufficient, however, shallowing of the chamber will occur. When prompt elevation of the bottle height fails to increase the infusion, an air block, venting problem, faulty tubing, or even an error in preparation is probably responsible. A wound of insufficient size might compress the collapsible sleeve that accompanies some systems. Kinking of this sleeve may compromise infusion, resulting in chamber shallowing.

Excessive outflow

In contrast to a tight incision, an excessive incision allows fluid to escape. A more subtle problem is a tendency for the surgeon to elevate the instrument, which causes the wound to gape and the chamber to empty. This error tends to occur in patients with deep orbits since it is quite easy to inadvertently distort the wound by lifting the handpiece.

External globe compression

Compression against the sclera from any source may shallow the anterior chamber. Possible causes include retrobulbar hemorrhage, excessive retrobulbar anesthetic, tight lids, pressure from the lid speculum, and traction from the superior fixation suture. If the shaft of an instrument is inadvertently pressed against the sclera while the surgeon is working (for example during a two-handed phacoemulsification), problems maintaining the chamber will occur.

Intraocular factors

Several specific circumstances that originate within the eye cause chamber shallowing. If the posterior capsule has been ruptured or a zonular dialysis has occurred, persistent irrigation will hydrate the vitreous which may result in anterior displacement of the capsule and iris. Air may also shallow the chamber by getting behind the iris and by producing air-induced pupillary block. Scleral collapse can produce chamber shallowing either in young patients or in eyes that have been "over-softened." Finally, a choroidal hemorrhage or effusion will shallow or flatten the anterior chamber.

MANAGEMENT

Except in cases of scleral collapse, an eye that is not firm will invariably act on the surgeon's behalf regardless of which causes are present. Familiarity with and careful preparation of the irrigating system along with footswitch dexterity will minimize the mechanical potential for chamber loss. Rarely, a defective bottle or tubing will require replacement. Careful attention to the wound is mandatory, and if the wound appears too large, the surgeon should not hesitate to pass a temporary suture reducing its length. Intermittent shallowing should cause the surgeon to question whether the shaft of an intraocular instrument being used is compressing the sclera, separating the wound, or whether there is kinking of the sleeve. An awareness of excessive tension from the speculum, lids, or traction suture should develop with experience. A well-designed speculum is crucial and careful attention to the patient's head position will reduce or even eliminate the force exerted by a fixation suture in most cases.

If the surgeon has exhausted his mental check-list, the use of a viscoelastic agent should aid in deepening the chamber. This is particularly valuable during the anterior capsulectomy and implantation of the IOL. During the emulsification, it may be necessary to hold the nucleus back with a second instrument until sufficient sculpting has been accomplished at which time the chamber may deepen.

Rarely, IOL implantation will be jeopardized by persistent chamber collapse despite the use of a viscoelastic substance. Under these circumstances, several emergency maneuvers can be extremely helpful. First, if the implant can be introduced into the anterior chamber without jeopardizing the cornea, the wound can

be sutured quickly to allow the insertion procedure to resume within a closed system. If this is not possible and implantation is necessary, the chamber can be deepened by aspirating fluid vitreous using a syringe and 25 gauge needle via an external approach at the pars plana. Because these maneuvers carry risk, they should be reserved as emergency measures. Of course, if the chamber shallowing is progressive and if the surgeon suspects suprachoroidal hemorrhage, rapid closure of the eye followed by indirect ophthalmoscopy is essential. The case can always be resumed at a later time when the intraocular environment is more favorable.

Fortunately, deepening of the anterior chamber is generally a matter of elevating the infusion bottle. Nevertheless, a thorough understanding of the causes and the corresponding management of chamber shallowing will prove useful to the surgeon.

Positive pressure

The presence of positive pressure makes phacoemulsification a more difficult procedure with a higher incidence of complications. The chamber will tend to shallow leaving little room for phacoemulsification. Iris prolapse and progressive miosis are more likely. The nucleus will often spontaneously prolapse and it may be difficult to reposition, forcing the surgeon to perform emulsification in the anterior chamber. The posterior capsule assumes a convex configuration which is easier to tear. Moreover, the capsular bag closes making cortical aspiration and IOL placement very challenging. If positive pressure is encountered, the surgeon must take all steps necessary to decrease it. Proper design and placement of the lid speculum, lateral canthotomy, and other techniques for minimizing lid pressure have already been discussed. Excessive traction of a fixation suture may increase the intraocular pressure by either excessive downward rotation of the globe or by actually lifting the globe from the orbit. Therefore, if a traction suture is used, an effort should be made to maintain the globe in its primary position. The intraocular pressure may also increase if the patient is straining with a full bladder, attempting to suppress a cough, or is generally apprehensive or uncomfortable leading to a Valsalva. Giving the patient a cough drop, repositioning until comfortable or allowing the patient to urinate will often help decrease the pressure. Another overlooked cause of positive pressure is body habitus. Patients with large, heavy abdomens, when laying flat will have a tendency toward an increased intraocular pressure. By placing the patient in a Trendelenburg position, the positive pressure can be significantly diminished.

Phacoemulsification in the face of positive pressure can be difficult and several factors may decrease the risks of complications. Capsulorhexis and phaco insertion techniques in the face of positive pressure have already been described. An anterior entry in to the anterior chamber as in the "no-stitch" wound construction is helpful. Hydrodissection is not recommended in order to avoid spontaneous prolapse of the nucleus. The aspiration level should be kept to a minimum so as not to accelerate chamber collapse. Even so, the chamber may tend to collapse with each attempt at emulsification. It is then necessary to elevate the bottle increasing infusion and emulsifying in short bursts. The latter technique allows the chamber to reform between each burst of ultrasound. It may also be necessary to use a second instrument to either hold the nucleus posteriorly or to restrain the posterior capsule with this instrument while performing the emulsification immediately over its protection. It may be helpful to "play" with the phacoemulsification shaft position in an attempt to decrease its tendency to scleral depress, gape, or twist the wound. The surgeon should suppress the reflex to request intravenous hypertonic solutions which may cause shrinkage of the vitreous and enhance scleral collapse thereby worsening chamber shallowing.

Iris trauma

Damage to the iris during phacoemulsification can be caused by either iris prolapse or by direct injury from the tip of the phacoemulsifier. Iris prolapse or injury may cause loss of pigment, flaccidity, bleeding, pupillary irregularity, or late cystoid macular edema.

Direct trauma to the iris from the phacoemulsification tip can be prevented in most if not all cases. Insertion techniques to decrease iris chafing have already been presented. By utilizing low aspiration rates during phacoemulsification, events occur more slowly and the iris is much less likely to jump into the phaco port. It is imperative to be overly cautious once the iris has been injured as it will become much more flaccid and susceptible to additional damage. It may be necessary to restrain a flaccid miotic iris with a second instrument, maneuver it with a viscoelastic agent, or cut it with scissors to reduce the pressure gradient between the anterior and posterior chamber.

Often overlooked is the damage caused by the exposed metal at the neck of the titanium tip. If this metal touches the iris during emulsification, it will cause damage. For this reason, it is best to leave minimal metal showing when performing phacoemulsification in eyes with small pupils.

Miosis

Any trauma to the iris may stimulate the iris sphincter to contract during the procedure. Additionally, volatile chambers with multiple collapses will also result in pupillary constriction. Preoperative topical non-steroidal anti-inflammatory agents in combination with intraoperative adrenaline added to the buffered saline solution (BSS) infusion may help to maintain pupillary dilatation [10]. Several small pupil phacoemulsification techniques are discussed in a later section yet the surgeon must feel comfortable and capable of utilizing these techniques. If miosis prevents safe emulsification and the surgeon becomes uncomfortable proceeding, he or she should not hesitate to either perform a radial iridotomy, sphincterotomies, or convert to an extracapsular technique.

Posterior capsule tears

The torn posterior capsule is probably the most frequent significant complication encountered by the surgeon learning phacoemulsification and continues to occur, albeit rarely, in even the expert's hands. It is well recognized that an open posterior capsule increases the risk of cystoid macular edema and retinal detachment [11]. In most instances, posterior capsule rupture can be prevented. However, if a tear does occur, proper management can allow for a successful procedure with safe implantation of a posterior chamber IOL.

Prevention

The incidence of a torn posterior capsule decreases with increasing experience of the surgeon. There is mounting evidence that capsulorhexis can greatly diminish this complication [7]. The stability of a continuous, strong anterior capsular edge prevents peripheral extension into the posterior capsule that may occur during nucleus manipulation. The use of low aspiration phacoemulsification will also reduce the likelihood of a torn posterior capsule since chamber volatility is decreased and the tendency toward sudden shallowing or collapse is minimized. Moreover, when the emulsification is performed at a lower phaco power, there is less chance of piercing through the nucleus into the posterior capsule.

The most severe posterior capsule tears occur during attempted emulsification of the nucleus. Two-handed phacoemulsification permits the most precise control of the nucleus for most surgeons. We prefer a specially designed dull-fingered nucleus manipulating hood which is utilized through a second stab incision site (Osher Nucleus Manipulator, Storz Ophthalmics Inc., St Louis, Missouri). The majority of the nucleus is sculpted *in situ* until it is thin and malleable. When the pupil dilates well, the nucleus manipulator retracts the superior anterior capsular edge until the superior pole of the nucleus is visualized, and engaged, and lifted away from the posterior capsule where it can be emulsified with minimal risks of a tear. Since there is no inferior counterpressure with another instrument, there is no chance of inadvertently passing through the nucleus and rupturing the posterior capsule. As the emulsification pro-

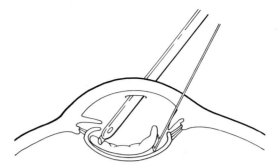

Fig. 18.3 Two-handed direct-lift technique. A second instrument pulls the superior anterior edge back to slide under the nucleus and prolapse its superior pole.

gresses, a second instrument should be used to avoid an inadvertent posterior capsular tear by placing it behind the remaining nucleus in order to physically prevent the posterior capsule from contacting the phacoemulsification tip. This is especially useful in eyes with an anterior chamber shallowing tendency.

If the pupil fails to dilate well, we prefer two techniques that have a high level of capsular safety. The first technique involves sculpting the central core in the nucleus followed by decentering the nucleus bowl inferiorly and posteriorly with the phacoemulsification tip which has a broader surface area than the second instrument so that nuclear penetration with injury to the posterior capsule cannot occur. A dull-fingered second instrument retracts the superior iris and anterior capsular ring embedding itself in the superior pole which is lifted away from the posterior capsule as in the technique used for the dilated pupil (Fig. 18.3). The emulsification is completed in the plane of the iris affording maximal protection to the posterior capsule. A second technique is a variation of the "divide and conquer" technique introduced by Howard Gimbel MD [11]. A large central furrow is sculpted through the nucleus which is emulsified after being divided into halves by creating a crack using the opposing forces of the phaco tip and second instrument pressed against the nucleus. Each half of the fetal nucleus is removed followed by the bimanual removal of the adult and epinuclear layers. This technique is safe to the posterior capsule if a continuous tear capsulectomy has been accomplished.

Several types of cataracts deserve special mention since they may be associated with a higher risk of posterior capsular tear. The brunescent cataract should not be hydrodissected since it is very large and can disinsert zonules if mobile. Moreover, its hardness can traumatize all ocular structures. We patiently perform an *in situ* emulsification without nuclear loosening until only a thin peripheral shell is remaining which can then be safely loosened by either hydrodissection or the second instrument.

By contrast, the young patient with a very soft cataract is at greater risk of a torn posterior capsule since the second instrument or a phacoemulsification tip will readily penetrate this cataract. A low scleral rigidity results in a strong tendency for anterior chamber shallowing so minimal aspiration and low phaco power is very helpful.

A morgagnian cataract is associated with an escape of liquefied cortex from the capsule bag when an initial puncture into the anterior lens capsule is made. The anterior and posterior capsular leaves will approach each other and the later is at risk of being torn during the anterior capsulectomy. Therefore, a viscoelastic agent is injected through this puncture site refilling the capsular bag before proceeding.

Management

Knowledgeable and skillful management of a posterior capsular tear is essential to the successful outcome of the procedure. At whatever stage the tear is discovered, establishment of a semi-closed pressurized system is advantageous. Allowing the anterior chamber to collapse will promote forward movement of the vitreous with possible extension of the tear.

If a tear is discovered during phacoemulsification, residual nuclear material must be removed by either emulsification or by converting to an extracapsular technique. If most of the nucleus has already been emulsified, the surgeon may use the second instrument to manuever the remaining nucleus away from the tear in order to complete the emulsification.

Alternating the second instrument may be placed over a smaller rent to prevent loss of nuclear material. Short bursts of low energy ultrasound with low aspiration and irrigation settings will decrease the risk of nuclear loss, chamber shallowing, and vitreous prolapse. When a nucleus has been emulsified, a phaco handpiece should not be removed without simultaneously injecting a viscoelastic through the second stab site to prevent a vitreous prolapse with extension of the tear. This is a critical maneuver and may make the difference between the necessity of a vitrectomy and successful lens implantation into the capsular bag.

Cortical removal can be safely accomplished without extending the tear by following several surgical principles. "Low flow" irrigation will not excessively hydrate vitreous and will therefore minimize the likelihood of vitreous prolapse through the tear. The cortex remote from the tear should be removed initially so that the majority of cortex will have been removed before manipulating cortex near the rent. Cortex should be stripped toward the rent since any force generated away from it will certainly cause its extension. The removal of as much cortex as possible is desirable, yet efforts to remove all cortex should be avoided as these might extend the tear and further compromise the integrity of the capsular bag. The same warning applies to vacuuming the central posterior capsule when the tear is peripheral since the YAG laser can be safely used postoperatively. Cortical removal by a "dry" technique may also be accomplished by injecting a viscoelastic agent and aspirating cortex with a syringe and 25 gauge cannula. As with the phacoemulsification handpiece, the withdrawal of the I&A handpiece should be accompanied by a simultaneous injection of air or viscoelastic agent into the eye in order to maintain the anterior chamber depth.

If vitreous is encountered at any point in the procedure, a "low flow" two-handed vitrectomy is performed. This is best accomplished by using a dripping cannula for infusion at the second stab site in combination with a separate thin-board automated vitrector which is passed through the rent where an anterior vitrectomy is performed. An alternative technique is a "dry" vitrectomy which utilizes a viscoelastic agent to maintain the anterior segment while the vitrectomy is performed through an opening in the torn capsule without using infusion. Recently, other techniques have been reported such as converting a linear tear in the posterior capsule to a continuous round capsulorhexis. Another technique involves the use of the sheets' glide to tamponade the opening in the posterior capsule [14,15].

IOL placement

The key to successful placement of an IOL in the face of a posterior capsule tear is clear visualization of the capsular–zonular anatomy. Only by determining the exact anatomy of the tear can the extent of capsular support be understood. We instill viscoelastic and generally retract the iris with a rounded instrument (Osher Iris Retractor, Storz Ophthalmics Inc., St Louis, Missouri). The optimal lens selection, technique of lens implantation, desired location, and orientation of the lens will become evident to the surgeon. It is better not to implant the posterior chamber lens than for a surgeon who is unsure of the anatomy to rely on "chance."

Several guidelines have proven to be helpful in implanting the posterior chamber IOL. If the tear is small with well-defined borders, the bag can be inflated with viscoelastic and the lens inserted using a technique relying on superior loop compression. By contrast, a dialing technique may cause extension of the tear. If the tear is large with peripheral extension and poorly defined borders, a viscoelastic agent is placed over the anterior capsular rim to collapse the bag and allow implantation into the ciliary sulcus. The IOL power for the ciliary sulcus should be decreased 0.5 D from the capsular bag calculation as presented at the Welsh Cataract Congress in 1986 [12]. Whether the lens is placed into the bag or into the ciliary sulcus, it should be positioned with the haptics oriented for best support which is usually 90° away from the axis of the tear. Once the lens is centered, its fixation should be evaluated by slightly decentering the lens toward each haptic

and releasing it to see if it will spontaneously recenter (bounce-back test). If it does not recenter, the haptic should then be rotated to a different axis. If the lens shows signs of poor fixation and will not center, it can either be repositioned in the ciliary sulcus, sutured into the ciliary sulcus, or removed and exchanged for an anterior chamber IOL providing this latter alternative is suitable for the patient. Once the lens is well-centered and its stability has been confirmed acetylcholine should be instilled onto the iris sphincter for pupillary constriction followed by the injection of either air or a viscoelastic agent to establish a formed, pressurized chamber.

Once the wound has been closed, a miniature I&A tip can be inserted between or under a suture for the removal of viscoelastic material. Air should be injected simultaneously with tip withdrawal in order to prevent vitreous prolapse. The air is then removed in small aliquots and exchanged for BSS so that the anterior chamber depth is maintained.

Zonular dialysis

Zonular dialysis may be present prior to surgery as a result of pre-existing trauma or conditions where the lens may be dislocated such as Marfan's syndrome or Marchesani's syndrome. Phacodonesis, iridodonesis, vitreous in the anterior chamber, visibility of the lens equator or a slit view of the nucleus which appears off-center may provide clues to this diagnosis. Pseudoexfoliation syndrome is another condition that has a propensity for zonular dehiscence. Surgical management of these cases is beyond the scope of this chapter yet may be reviewed elsewhere [13].

Acquired zonular dialysis may result from a traumatic capsulectomy, excessive maneuvering of the nucleus, or aspiration of the anterior or posterior capsule with the I&A tip. Prompt recognition and the avoidance of further trauma is the best initial response. Similar principles to the torn posterior capsule exists in that all forces generated within the eye should be directed toward rather than away from the zonular dialysis to avoid additional "unzipping" of the zonules. If the phacoemulsification is being performed when the zonular dialysis is discovered, we use very low vacuum aspiration and ultrasound power in addition to a second instrument to accomplish a lamellar dissection lifting layer by layer toward the dialysis as the lens is emulsified.

Both nuclear and cortical removal may be very difficult when countertraction is absent from a loose capsular bag. Occasionally, nuclear or cortical visco dissection is necessary to loosen these structures. Cortical stripping may require frequent foot pedal reflux if the capsule is drawn into the aspiration port. The last cortex to be removed should be that in proximity to the zonular dialysis. It should not be stripped radially but rather parallel to the dialysis. Heroic perseverance is to be avoided. If vitreous presents, the surgical principle of either low infusion or dry anterior vitrectomy should apply as discussed in the preceding section on posterior capsular tears. The IOL can be implanted into the capsular bag as long as the anterior capsular ring is intact and the zonular dialysis is not in excess of the four or five hours. A larger holeless optic is recommended since a slight decentration may occur as postoperative forces generated by the remaining zonules come into play. If the zonular dialysis is extremely large, the surgeon who wishes to implant an IOL has several choices. Alpha-chymotrypsin may be instilled allowing delivery of the entire capsular bag and its contents followed by either a sutured posterior chamber lens or an anterior chamber lens. If the surgeon has been successful at removing nuclear and cortical material, the remaining capsule may be left since it probably does have some stabilizing effect and occasionally the suturing of one haptic will be sufficient if there is some adequate capsular–zonular support. As in the case of the torn posterior capsule, the IOL decision must be based upon direct inspection of the anatomy which offers the highest chances of a successful outcome.

Dropped nucleus

Losing a partially emulsified nucleus into the vitreous cavity is a complication dreaded by every phaco surgeon. If the surgeon keeps a clear sensorium, this situation can often be safely managed at the time of the complication. The first step is to remove any residual nucleus in the anterior segment by whatever technique the surgeon chooses.

Next, a generous two-handed anterior vitrectomy is performed. If the nucleus does not present during vitrectomy, the surgeon may attempt to float it forward by directing a gentle stream of irrigation fluid through a 22 gauge cannula posteriorly into the vitreous cavity. When the nucleus becomes visible, it can then be recovered by sliding a loop beneath it. Delivery of the nucleus from the eye is facilitated by an incision size exceeding the diameter of the remaining nucleus. If the nucleus fails to present, additional vitrectomy is recommended. If still unsuccessful, the surgeon should remove as much cortex as is possible and the patient should be referred to a vitreoretinal specialist. Whether or not the original surgeon elects to implant an IOL or leave the task to the vitreoretinal specialist must be considered on an individual basis.

Expulsive hemorrhage

This catastrophic complication is more likely to occur in older patients with pre-existing uveitis, glaucoma, and high myopia. Hypertension and anticoagulation therapy are also risk factors. Early recognition is the key to successful management. An eye that is becoming firm with chamber shallowing may be developing an expulsive hemorrhage. The surgeon may notice a loss of red reflex and the patient may be complaining of pain despite adequate anesthesia. If the process is gradual, indirect ophthalmoscopy may be performed to determine if a choroidal hemorrhage is occurring. If abrupt, however, immediate closure of the eye is mandatory. If the surgeon is unable to close the wound due to extensive pressure, proceed by tamponading the incision with a finger while mannitol is given [16]. 7/0 or 8/0 sutures are best selected since they are less likely to break or "cheese-wire" through tissues when challenged by positive pressure. Once the eye is closed, tissue which has prolapsed can be repositioned and the anterior chamber can be deepened with air, BSS, or a viscoelastic material. If the anterior chamber fails to deepen or if closure of the incision is unsuccessful, the surgeon should attempt to drain the choroidal hemorrhage via a posterior sclerotomy 3.5–4 mm posterior to the limbus. The importance of cortical removal or IOL implantation pales in relation to the crisis at hand since the goal is to save the eye. A secondary procedure can always be performed at a later date if the vital structures within the globe are preserved. Fortunately, this complication is extraordinarily rare in phacoemulsification surgery since the small wound is protective against this disastrous event.

Summary

Phacoemulsification is an elegant and safe procedure rewarding to both the patient and the surgeon. Complications will occasionally be encountered by every cataract surgeon and the management will depend upon experience, skill, and sound judgement. We have presented a spectrum of common complications and offered our perspective in handling these situations. There are yet many surgical alternatives that could not be discussed given the scope of this chapter so the reader should be encouraged to expand these principles and do what ever it takes to achieve a successful outcome.

References

1 Reibel R. Current concepts in retrobulbar anesthesia. *Surv Ophthalmol* 1985; **30**: 102–10.
2 Ellis P. Retrobulbar injection. *Surv Ophthalmol* 1974; **18**: 425–30.
3 Cionni R, Osher R. *Cataract surgery in the face of retrobulbar hemorrhage. Ophthalmol* 1991; **98**: 1153–1155.
4 Jaffe N, Claymann H. The pathophysiology of corneal astigmatism after cataract extraction. *Trans Am Acad Ophthal Otolaryngol* 1975; **79**: 615–30.
5 Jaffe N. *Cataract Surgery and its Complications*, 3rd edn. St Louis: CV Mosby, 1981: 92–110.
6 Masket S. Nonkeratometric control of postoperative astigmatism. *J Am Intraocular Implant Soc* 1985; **11**: 134–47.
7 Neuhann T, Utrata P, Brint S, Osher R. Special focus on continuous capsulectomy. *Audio Video J Cataract Implant Surg* 1989 (Issue II) **5**.
8 Osher R, Cionni R. The torn posterior capsule: Its intraoperative behavior, surgical management and long term consequences. *J Cataract Refract Surg* (Issue 4) 1990; **16**: 490–4.
9 Gimbel H. Divide and conquer. *Audio Video J Cataract Implant Surg* 1990 (Issue II) **6**.
10 Keates R, McGowan K. Clinical trial of flurbiprofen to maintain pupillary dilation during cataract surgery. *Ann Ophthalmol* 1984; **16**: 919–21.
11 Jaffe N. *Cataract Surgery and its Complications*, 3rd edn. St Louis: CV Mosby, 1981: 368, 576–9.
12 Osher R, Corcoran K. *Modification of the IOL power: ciliary sulcus versus capsular bag.* Welsh Cataract Congress, Houston, 1986.
13 Osher R. Surgical approach to the traumatic cataract. *Audio Video J Cataract Implant Surg* (Issue II) 1987; **3**.
14 Michelson M. The Sheets' glide. *Audio J Cataract Implant Surg* 1991; **7**.
15 Gimbel H. Posterior capsulorhesis. *Audio J Cataract Implant Surg* 1991; **7**.
16 Osher M. Emergency treatment of vitreous bulge and wound gaping complicating cataract surgery. *Am J Ophthalmol* 1957; **44**: 409–11.

19: Intraocular Lens Removal

MICHAEL COBO

Introduction

The decision to remove an intraocular lens (IOL) from a patient's eye may be amongst the most difficult an ophthalmologist can make. It is doubtful that there is any other elective surgical procedure which is more likely to leave the patient with a poor or unimproved visual result after surgery as elective implant removal. By definition, IOL removal is occurring in a sick eye, where a problematic implant is contributing to one or more specific clinical problems. Adding the necessary surgical trauma to the pre-existing iatrogenic problem compounds the stress on ocular tissues, increasing the risk for corneal decompensation, protracted glaucoma, or recalcitrant cystoid macular edema.

To complicate matters further, the guidelines for removing a lens that is presumed to be problematic are not well established, and so the indications for implant removal may vary greatly amongst practitioners, as well as in different communities.

Alternatives to implant removal can and should be attempted, including the use of topical anti-inflammatory agents when indicated, antiglaucoma therapy for secondary glaucoma, and cycloplegia when chafing of the implant against the iris contributes to the clinical problem. Ultimately the clinician must determine a threshold suitable for a given patient based on the potential for visual rehabilitation of the eye, the status of the fellow eye, the ease of implant removal, and the patient's visual needs. These are balanced against the severity and chronicity of the observed complication, i.e. a single event such as a hyphema may not mandate removal of the implant, however a chronic process such as uveitis or secondary glaucoma unresponsive to medical therapy may induce early removal. On occasion, non-invasive surgical maneuvers such as laser photoablation of bleeding vessels in the iris or angle may be utilized to delay or avoid surgery. However, once the eye has become symptomatic, a patient is faced with the prospect of further visual loss or complicated rehabilitative maneuvers. Given the extreme variability in ease of implant removal, surgical outcome, and baseline vision, the patient must have a thorough understanding of the nature of the problem and the potential risk for further complication.

The technique of implant removal is predicated by the design of the implant present in the eye. The myriad of designs introduced over the years create a variety of surgical challenges for the explanting surgeon. It is important, therefore, that the surgeon thoroughly analyzes the preoperative state of the eye so as to determine the best surgical approach and any unusual surgical maneuvers that may be necessary. Additionally, secondary problems such as glaucoma or inflammation should be under maximum medical treatment prior to surgical intervention to reduce the potential for compounding postoperative complications. This review will include a summary based on the author's experience of the relative indications for implant removal, therapies that may be attempted, preoperative evaluation of the eye due to undergo explantation, and a summary of varied techniques for removal of different styles of implants.

Indications for IOL removal

The threshold for implant removal varies with the individual surgeon, the ease with which a given implant can be removed, and the severity or chronicity of the complication observed. The complications of IOLs range from trivial problems to debilitating or vision-threatening problems.

In the evaluation of any patient with post-operative complications felt to be related to a given implant, one must rule out other potential etiologies related primarily to surgery such as cystoid macular edema or corneal edema. With this perspective, this brief list of varied intraocular implant complications is presented.

Recurrent hyphema

The highly vascularized tissues which support an implant will on occasion sustain either erosive trauma or chronic inflammation leading to recurrent hyphema. This may be associated with secondary elevation in intraocular pressure and iritis. One should seek alternative etiologies including bleeding diathesis, the presence of wound neovascularization (Swan's syndrome), and on rare occasion, a retinal tear with a bridging vessel resulting in a vitreous hemorrhage with blood presenting in the anterior chamber. Excluding these possibilities, one should then observe the implant with respect to its relationship to the iris to determine if malposition or dislocation of the implant has occurred resulting in chafing of the iris. If such a site can be identified, cycloplegia or focal photocoagulation may ameliorate bleeding and lessen the contact between iris and implant.

Uveitis

The etiologies of implant-related uveitis remain highly speculative. Varied lens materials, improper sizing of implants, excessive contact of implant with uveal tissues, and malpositioning of an implant have all been implicated. Patients may concurrently exhibit symptoms of discomfort, photophobia, or tenderness to touch. A key differential point is the exclusion of chronic endophthalmitis caused by an organism of low pathogenicity, for example, fungus, *Staphylococcus epidermitis*, or *Propionibacterium acnes*. Alternatively, in the patient with underlying vasculitis or collagen vascular disease, aggravation of an underlying uveitis secondary to systemic inflammatory disease should be considered.

Cystoid macular edema

This well-established complication of cataract surgery has been reduced in incidence as mechanized extracapsular surgical techniques have evolved. Nonetheless, this may be associated with or aggravated by a lens implant especially in the setting of a primary procedure complicated by vitreous loss. The empiric use of topical or systemic anti-inflammatory agents is advocated by some in the treatment of cystoid edema. Removal of the implant may not substantially improve the visual status of the macula in these patients. The presence of coexisting intraocular inflammation may perhaps be a stronger indication for implant removal.

More ominously, cystoid edema may serve as a sentinel of more serious ocular complications. It is not uncommon to see an eye that has first developed cystoid macular edema progress to corneal decompensation months or years later. Whereas cystoid macular edema is a symptomatically binary process that is either present or not, it may indicate ongoing intraocular inflammation that may contribute to chronic attrition of corneal endothelial cells.

Corneal endothelial compromise

Pseudoaphakic bullous keratopathy is amongst the more serious complications of a problematic lens implant. The development of diffuse corneal edema indicates that maximal endothelial damage has occurred, and simple removal of an implant in this setting is of no value. Rehabilitation of an eye with pseudophakic bullous keratopathy ultimately requires penetrating keratoplasty with implant removal or replacement. A more sensitive indicator of corneal compromise is specular microscopy. While this technique is not readily available to every ophthalmologist, it is often available in referral centers or where resources are pooled. This technique allows quantification of corneal endothelial cells as well as analysis of cell morphology. Marked diminution of the cell count with 400–600 cells/mm^2 indicates advanced compromise of the cornea. The surgical manipulation involved in implant removal, particularly if traumatic, is almost certain to result in diffuse corneal edema. A low cell number may encourage a conservative approach of non-intervention anticipating future keratoplasty combined with implant removal. At the other extreme, a healthy endothelial cell count provides a baseline against which endothelial cell counts can be compared at 6–12 month intervals. One is more interested here in the general trend of cell counts over time rather than in one absolute cell count as counts may vary 10% from reading to reading. For example, an eye that has gone from a cell count of 2200 to 1800 cells/mm^2 and then 1500 demonstrates definite loss of cells over a period of time strengthening the indications for removal before the cornea is more severely compromised.

If specular microscopy is not readily available, an estimate can be undertaken in the office with the slit-lamp using high magnification to obtain a specular reflection from the posterior corneal surface. The presence of peripheral edema is a useful indicator of central endothelial viability. If edema involves one-quarter to one-third of the peripheral cornea, it is almost always associated with marked central attrition of endothelial cells even in the setting of a clinically normal appearing central cornea and good visual acuity.

Glaucoma

Elevated intraocular pressure is another known postoperative complication of cataract surgery, and an implant may play a contributory role either through mechanical obstruction when positioned in the angle or through contact with the iris resulting either in inflammation or dispersion of pigment. Alternative etiologies to be considered include corticosteroid-induced glaucoma, primary open-angle glaucoma,

and chronic angle closure due to pupillary block. Angle closure may present both acutely or chronically in patients when there is no iridectomy present or the iridectomy has been obstructed. Gonioscopy confirms this diagnosis and allows one to proceed with laser iridotomy.

Miscellaneous problems

Varied problems can arise due either to the size, power, or location of the implant. These include improper sizing leading either to a mobile lens often with direct corneal endothelial contact, or an oversized lens that may result in marked tenderness to touch. Similarly, dislocation or malpositioning of the lens, often after blunt trauma, can result in a lens with excessive uveal contact. Improper power selection either as a result of manufacturing error or miscalculation of the implant power can occur. Finally, edge glare may present as a debilitating complication, unresponsive to topical miotics.

Medical therapy

Medical therapy of implant-related complications are predicated by the specific complication. In the setting of chronic inflammatory disease such as uveitis with or without cystoid macular edema, the use of variable doses of topical corticosteroids may be in order. This likewise has been advocated in patients with early endothelial compromise. Topical corticosteroid use on a chronic basis, however, can be complicated by secondarily elevated intraocular pressure.

In the setting of direct contact between implant and iris resulting either in chafing of the anterior iris surface or dispersion of pigment from the posterior iris surface, the use of long-acting chronic cycloplegia may be in order. Finally, in the setting where the patient is known to rub the affected eye excessively, the use of a shield, particularly at bedtime, can be helpful.

Preoperative evaluation

Specific aspects of the comprehensive preoperative eye examination merit emphasis. In the setting of anterior chamber lens removal, gonioscopy is a key maneuver. This allows one to enter surgery with full knowledge of the state of the implant haptics within the angle, reducing the risk that inadvertent traumatic removal of the implant may result in cyclodialysis or iridodialysis. Evaluation of the corneal endothelium is once again important, even if it serves only to give the patient a better sense of the prognosis relative to a late corneal decompensation. Finally, treatable problems should be addressed prior to surgical intervention. In particular, the diagnosis of iritis or glaucoma should result in the institution of appropriate topical therapies.

Technique of IOL removal

Basic principles

The technique of removal varies with the type of lens to be removed as well as the anatomic abnormalities induced by the implant. Given the proximity of the implant to the cornea, one major goal of explantation is to minimize corneal damage with the generous use of viscoelastic materials. Adhesions which are evident at the slit-lamp by gonioscopy are often obscure at the time of surgery. Visualization into the angle is achieved by intraoperative gonioscopy, or by direct viewing through an air-filled anterior chamber for synechiolysis. The risk in this maneuver, however, is that sudden loss of air from the anterior chamber may result in collapse of the cornea onto the implant optic.

Closed loop implant removal is achieved by cutting IOL haptics and then rotating the haptics through the synechial tunnels rather than attempting to tear or disrupt the synechial tunnels. The cutting of a haptic, especially if rather coarse or blunt scissors are used on prolene, may result in barbs protruding from the prolene which may tear angle structures as they are rotated out of the eye, much as a fish hook will tear tissue upon removal. Therefore, an instrument designed specifically for cutting implant haptics or a pair of sharp intraocular scissors should be used.

Typically, the implant is removed through a limbal incision. Presence of an alternative stab incision at a limbal site may be of value. Attempting to perform maneuvers through the larger limbal wound may result in loss of the chamber or insufficient access to extremes of the implant.

It should also be recognized that concurrent vitreous loss often occurs in these cases. The performance of an adequate anterior vitrectomy is critical if visual results are to be optimized. While some advocate performing a vitrectomy prior to the removal of the implant, the author shares the opinion that this potentially increases the chances of collapse of the anterior chamber and contact of iris with optic. The author's preference is to perform a very limited vitrectomy at the start of surgery if there is marked pathology such as vitreous incarceration in the wound, with subsequent removal of the implant and finally more complete vitrectomy if required.

A final concern is that at times remnants of an amputated implant may not be easily removed. While no large experience is available to inform us of the true fate of these remnants, anecdotal reports indicate but they may be tolerated. This, however, presents a problem if one feels that contact of implant material with uveal tissue is contributing to a chronic inflammatory process since this process may continue after the partial extirpation of the lens. Thus, every attempt should be made to remove the implant completely at the time of explantation balancing this against the trauma of additional complicated surgery.

In the following pages, the techniques of removal, and various general styles of lens implant are reviewed. The techniques outlined here should be adaptable to the removal of a specific implant.

Surgical techniques of IOL explantation

Given the varied IOL designs and materials, the surgical description of lens explantation cannot be stereotyped beyond the general principles previously outlined. Similarly, the technique of explantation varies not only with lens design but additionally with the specific anatomic puzzle that intraocular inflammation or fibrosis has produced about the fixation points of the implant. Therefore, rather than adopt an encyclopedic approach for all lens designs, the focus is on more common or generic implant styles, emphasizing general principles adaptable to specific clinical situations.

One-piece rigid polymethylmetacrylate (PMMA) lenses

These are amongst the earliest type of lens design and are also the easiest to remove. The rigid configuration with large feet without and closed loop configuration (as demonstrated in the Choyce style lens) generally results in insignificant angle fibrosis with respect to entrapment of the implant. The one exception is the setting where the implant feet have been modified with positioning holes or unusual angulation of the PMMA. In this setting, the lens should be treated as a closed loop lens with a high probability of macroscopic or microscopic fibrotic attachment through the positioning holes or feet. In general this implant style provides the opportunity to emphasize the basic points of removing an easily mobilized implant from the anterior chamber. With other lens styles where more complicated maneuvering may be required, the goal is to free the implant of adhesions and effectively convert it to an anteriorly located lens which can then be linearly extracted from the anterior chamber through a limbal incision.

A limbal groove is created overlying the axis of orientation of the implant, of a length sufficient to remove the implant. A groove incision is recommended to minimize the distortion of the wound that may occur upon opening the wound with scissors, perhaps increasing the risk of loss of anterior chamber loss and corneal implant contact. If the previous wound has healed well and tissue does not appear extremely attenuated or irregular, one can proceed with removal through the same limbal incision that was used for primary implantation. Alternatively, if the previous wound is irregular, one could go either more corneal or scleral, in the latter case dissecting up to the limbus. A limbal wound is ideal for providing access to the ante-

rior chamber and reducing the need for more gross distortion of the implant during the process of explantation. Prior to entering the anterior chamber, a stab incision is recommended which is separate from the wound, ideally through clear cornea. This incision may not necessarily be used during the procedure but it provides a port through which the anterior chamber can be formed with viscoelastic material, where a second instrument can be placed for intraocular manipulation if unexpected problems arise; and it creates a port for infusion during postexplantation vitrectomy. The manipulation of this stab incision would probably be less prone to cause collapse of the anterior chamber than the limbal wound.

Having prepared the surgical entry site, the surgeon must decide whether vitrectomy prior to implant removal is necessary. In the absence of gross vitreous pathology such as broad incarceration enveloping the implant and going up to the wound, it is preferable to perform the vitrectomy after the implant is removed. This reduces the risk of inadvertent collapse of the anterior chamber. If it is necessary to proceed with vitrectomy prior to lens explantation, one can consider the stab incision for infusion and then through a limited incision in the previous groove, one can insert an appropriate vitrectomy instrument. The infusion needle can minimize implant contact with the cornea if it is held over the anterior chamber implant gently pressing it posteriorly to minimize any forward movement of the IOL.

Subsequently, going through the clear corneal incision, the anterior chamber is well formed with viscoelastic material taking care not to put this behind the implant. An alternative is the use of air although the risk of air creeping behind the implant and propelling it forward is significant. Having formed the chamber, the groove incision previously formed is entered and opened to its full extent. The superior footplates can then be mobilized into the wound in stepwise manner, grasped with platform forceps, linearly extracting the implant from the eye.

At this point, a more complete vitrectomy can be undertaken. Because viscoelastic material is generally removed and may be mistaken for vitreous, it is recommended that the viscoelastic material be removed with a mechanized vitrectomy instrument. An anterior vitrectomy can then be performed with careful inspection of the wound at the end of the procedure to ensure that no vitreous remains incarcerated.

Closed-loop all-PMMA large haptic lenses

The Pannu-style lens serves as the classic prototype with a relatively large diameter haptic broadly in contact with angle structures, with a large closed loop at the end of the haptic that prevents simple rotation of the haptic through a synechial tunnel. The large diameter of the haptic may serve as a mechanical block to explantation through a synechial tunnel. Nonetheless, preoperative gonioscopy is critical for careful inspection of the angle since, in general, these synechiae need to be directly dissected. This results in part from the fact that the cutting of solid PMMA haptics can be difficult with scissors and, additionally, the haptics frequently have a gradually increasing taper toward the optic which may preclude simple rotation through the synechial tunnel.

Thus, the major challenge presented by this implant is the intraoperative dissection of synechiae. Not only are synechiae difficult to visualize directly, but also intraoperative hemorrhage further obscures the view. The latter problem may be ameliorated by ensuring that appropriate intraocular diathermy instrumentation is available, remembering that lesser degrees of cauterization are required inside the eye. Ideally one may use intraocular cautery instrumentation such as that typically used by posterior segment surgeons.

To cut synechiae directly, the haptics within the angle can be visualized in one of two ways. First, the angle may be viewed directly with the aid of gonioscopic lenses such as those used in congenital glaucoma surgery. The initial technique is identical to that previously described for rigid all-PMMA lenses with respect to formation of a limbal groove as well as a clear corneal stab incision. In preparation for gonioscopy, the anterior chamber is filled with viscoelastic material and the haptic is approached with a sharp steel blade, e.g. Ziegler knife. The principle difficulty experienced by the surgeon unaccustomed to gonioscopic imaging intraoperatively is the reversed image. The use of a viscoelastic material minimizes the risk of anterior chamber collapse and the view provided should allow one to mobilize the haptic.

A second alternative for visualization of the angle consists of taking advantage of the change in refractive index of the anterior segment when the anterior chamber is filled with air. Using the previously mentioned stab incision, air is carefully injected in front of the optic taking care to limit the amount of air injected, therefore minimizing the risk of it moving behind the implant. This allows one to look directly into the angle with the operating microscope and using a very small limbal stab incision, one can dissect synechiae within the angle. A major risk of this maneuver is the inadvertent and rapid loss of air from the anterior chamber resulting in IOL/corneal endothelial contact. Visualization of the superior angle can be accomplished by the use of a dental mirror held in the inferior fornix, again with the difficulties of reversed imaging. An alternative is to directly visualize the haptic superiorly through the limbal stab wound and lyse synechiae under direct visualization.

Once the surgeon has lysed synechiae, it is then recommended that an attempt be made to move the implant slightly with a right-angle hook so as to ensure its ready mobility prior to the time that the limbal incision is completely open. Once this is accomplished, the implant is removed linearly through the limbal incision as previously described.

Open-loop flexible IOL

The prototype of this implant is the Dubroff lens. The open-loop configuration results in rather facile removal of the implant. Groove and stab incisions are created as previously described and the anterior chamber is formed with a viscoelastic material. The limbal wound is opened, the superior haptic (in this case of a three-pronged implant) is rotated slightly and mobilized out of the wound. Linear extraction is not advocated as much as a gentle rotation of the implant with a right-angle hook utilizing a limbal stab incision and wound with either one or two instruments to spin the lens out of the anterior chamber.

Flexible closed-loop IOLs

This large class of IOLs, amongst the more commonly implanted in the early and middle part of the 1980s, has been recently reported as contributing to postoperative inflammatory problems. Implant removal is complicated by the narrow caliber of the implant haptic, typically prolene, which is often associated with synechial entrapment either as the result of the relatively small diameter of the haptic in association with chronic inflammation. Three principles are stressed:

1 if synechial entrapment of the haptic is present, cut the haptics rather than attempt direct dissection;

2 cut the haptics relatively close to the optic. This recommendation is contrary to intuition which suggests that cutting the haptic more closely to the angle minimizes the amount of haptic material needing removal from the eye. However, this eliminates a level that can be used to distort the haptic, so as to elongate it, making it easier to slide it through the synechial tunnel while utilizing a second instrument. The additional 2 or 3 mm of haptic that needs to be rotated from the eye is not as great a problem as is the removal of an irregular-shaped haptic with various acute angles which can only be removed by distorting the haptic material with a second instrument. Thus, one should always start surgery with a game plan with respect to where one wishes to cut the haptic so as to allow for ease of mobilization or distortion of the haptic as required; and

3 use your best scissors. Again, this is counter-intuitive in the sense that one does not wish to use fine, expensive scissors. However, in particular with the cutting of the 4/0 or 5/0 prolene used in these haptics, the compression of the prolene by a relatively blunt pair of scissors creates small hooks or barbs which

radiate out from the haptic material. These microscopic barbs may not be appreciated intraoperatively but as one begins to rotate the haptic through the synechial tunnel within the angle, these will tear angle structures and often create considerable bleeding or make it difficult if not impossible to remove the haptic from the eye. Thus, either a specialized pair of scissors for cutting haptics such as the Raposso scissors, specialized disposable scissors, or a fine pair of Vannas scissors are requried. My personal preference is intraocular vitrectomy scissors (angled Southerland).

In the process of cutting the haptics, if one does not use specialized scissors with a notch to stabilize the haptic, the haptic may slide out of the scissors making cutting more complicated. For this reason, a second instrument can be introduced through the limbal stab incision such as a Jaffe–Bechert nucleus manipulator with its Y-shaped end prong which allows one to stabilize the haptic while cutting it with an instrument such as Vannas scissors brought in through the limbal wound. Having amputated the haptic material from the optic superiorly, one can amputate a single arm of the inferior haptic and then grasp the optic as a means of sliding the implant and inferior haptic out of the eye. With implants where the inferior haptic is rounded or obtuse such as the Azar lens, this can be linearly extracted since the haptic will flex in the process of removal. The superior haptic, having been completely amputated from the optic, is subsequently removed by rotating and distorting the haptic material, utilizing two platform forceps and adequate amounts of viscoelastic material. Throughout these maneuvers, closely observe the iris tissue adjacent to the angle for any signs of distortion suggesting that there is residual synechial adhesion which if dealt with too brusquely, may result in cyclodialysis, irido-dialysis, or bleeding.

Acutely angled multiple closed-loop haptics

Removal of these implants through a limbal incision can be very difficult. The acute angles make it difficult to maneuver the lens through the synechial tunnel and additionally some configurations, in this case the most representative being the ORC Stableflex lens, are effectively double looped so that synechiae occur not only around the outer part of the haptic but also in the inner part of the haptic. In the setting of advanced corneal compromise, e.g. peripheral corneal edema with central corneal clarity retained, one may propose to the patient deferring surgery since the manipulation of this lens may hasten the decompensation of the cornea. This lens is far more easily removed through a penetrating keratoplasty wound. Nonetheless, if implant removal is required, the maneuver is not unlike that described for closed loop haptics with the additional caveat of dealing with synechiae enclosing both outer and inner haptic loops. The maneuver here consists of again amputating haptics from the optic, in the case of the Stableflex, at all four haptic insertion sites. One then proceeds with a wishbone type of maneuver, using a Jaffe–Bechert manipulator to push the outer haptic against the angle while using a platform forceps to grasp the inner haptic while splaying this toward the center, thus breaking the synechiae which encompass the inner portion of the haptic, leaving those that encompass the outer portion of the haptic intact. One can, at this point, distort and rotate the haptic through the synechial tunnel recognizing that, in the case of the Stableflex lens, this will need to be performed four times in view of the four closed loops present. Optionally one can snare the inner loop of the haptic with right-angle hooks.

Consideration of removal of this implant style raises the question of whether haptics need to be removed. No convincing study exists to suggest the appropriateness of this intraoperative decision. However, in some cases, the trauma of removing an implant haptic may be greater than the limited risk of leaving the haptic behind. The problem that arises consists of leaving residual material in an eye which is prone to inflammation where the question will persist as to whether the implant remnant is contributing to postexplantation inflammatory disease or cystoid macular edema.

Iris plane lenses

If these lenses are not fixed within the capsular bag, as was done during the evolution of contemporary extracapsular surgery, removal of the implant is generally quite facile. In principle, one wishes to mobilize the iris plane lens into the anterior chamber, facilitating removal. With regard to removal of the planar Copeland lens, where no haptic loops are present, this is relatively straightforward, as one haptic is mobilized at a time. If there are closed loops as with a Binkhorst-style lens, one may need to either individually lyse iris adhesions with a Ziegler knife or cut haptics and rotate through a synechial tunnel. If the haptic is enmeshed in the capsular remnant, this likewise may need to be gently dissected. Be aware that many of these lenses were stabilized within the eye with an iris fixation suture often through the superior iridectomy and one must be certain to inspect these eyes for this. Failure to note this pre-existing condition may result in a major iris tear as the lens is explanted. Once the implant is mobilized into the anterior chamber, it may then we removed linearly through a limbal incision as previously described.

Posterior chamber lens and posterior chamber IOL

The key to removing the lens is to convert it to an anterior chamber lens. This is done by first using two peripheral corneal stab incisions and then using a closed eye system to mobilize the IOL, prior to creating a limbal 7 mm entry site. The stab incisions are used to loosen and manipulate the implant in a closed eye system. Either the positioning holes or the crotch where the haptic enters the optic are used. The two instruments can be used to spin or rotate the implant anteriorly twisting it from either the ciliary sulcus or the capsular bag. If the pupil is adequately dilated the IOL can then be mobilized into the anterior chamber and extracted linearly. In the setting of the encasement of the haptics either within the sulcus or within the capsular bag, it may be necessary to amputate haptics and leave them behind. This is less problematic than with anteriorly fixated implants inasmuch as the capsular fixation of the haptic generally precludes major contact with iris tissue; there is certainly less of a risk than tearing the posterior capsule and the process of traumatically removing a haptic remnant. This is particularly true with posterior chamber lens designs which include double closed loop haptics or notched haptics with maneuvering holes.

In the setting of an entrapped haptic where one has chosen to leave the haptic remnant, enter the eye through the limbal incision, cut the haptic with appropriate intraocular scissors, mobilize the optic and residual haptic material, and then elect to leave the remaining haptic if this is not problematic. One question that arises in the setting of repositioning a posterior chamber lens rather than removing it is whether the implant needs to be replaced or simply repositioned. If the implant has been fixed within the capsular bag, there is frequently distortion of the haptic material which may have lost its resilience or memory thus deforming the lens to a smaller effective diameter. In an attempt to mobilize this lens in the ciliary sulcus, one may be left with a smaller diameter haptic than required for implant fixation in the sulcus. Thus, it should be determined if, after mobilizing the IOL, the IOL is loose, so that it can then be pulled up into the anterior chamber, removed, and replaced with another implant rather than risking a loose implant postoperatively.

Conclusion

The removal of an implant may be either an extremely facile procedure or a highly complicated one depending on the type of implant and the relative experience of the surgeon. Remember the caution stated at the beginning of this chapter that this procedure may in principle leave the eye seeing more poorly than it did preoperatively and may in fact require subsequent surgical maneuvering. It is encouraging to discuss the risk:benefit ratio at length with the patient using ancillary tests such as fluorescein angiography or specular microscopy to better inform the patient about

long-term prognosis. Additionally, given the complicated nature of these cases, a second opinion from a respected colleague may often help to reassure both the patient and provide the surgeon with an additional perspective on technique and potential problems. The decision to remove the implant is often coupled with the request for implant replacement by the patient. The decision to replace an implant rather than simply remove one is complicated and must be individualized to the patient, taking into consideration the status of the fellow eye, the potential for visual rehabilitation of the involved eye, the indication for implant removal (since the alternative implant style might cause similar inflammatory problems), and the relative state of the eye with respect to the replacement with an alternative lens such as a posterior chamber lens, that is, if there is sufficient residual posterior capsule remaining. More recently, empiric clinical experience has led to an interest in transclerally fixated posterior chamber lenses in the absence of capsular support. One should appreciate that this technique has not been extensively studied and the results may vary widely in the hands of different surgeons depending on their previous experience. Significant complications do exist with respect to persistent hypotony or endophthalmitis. An alternative to implant replacement is either the use of a contact lens postoperatively or an epikeratophakia procedure.

Finally, it must be recognized that observation of an adverse effect from an implant is important and reportable information. The primary implanting surgeon should carry out appropriate reporting to the company that has produced this implant in keeping with the guidelines of the Food and Drug Administration, USA.

Further reading

Anderson WB, Cobo LM, Foulks GF, Mitchell C. *Atlas of Ophthalmic Surgery*, vol I. *Surgery of the Anterior Segment*. St Louis: CV Mosby, 1991.
Apple DJ, Mamilis H, Loftield K *et al.* Complications of intraocular lenses. A historical and histopathological review. *Surv Ophthalmol* 1984; **29**: 1–54.

Cobo LM. Intraocular lens removal: indications and techniques. COVE Videotape No. 025104, AAO, 1988.

Ellingson FT. The uveitis–glaucoma–hyphema syndrome associated with the Mark VIII anterior chamber lens implant. *J Am Intraocul Implant Soc* 1978; **4**: 50–3.

Hagan JC. Complications while removing the Iolab 91Z lens for the UGH-UGH+ syndrome. *J Am Intraocul Implant Soc* 1984; **10**: 209–13.

20: Postcataract Inflammation and Endophthalmitis: Diagnosis, Prevention, and Management

NICK MAMALIS

There are many different causes of inflammation following cataract surgery with intraocular lens (IOL) implantation. A generalized, infectious endophthalmitis following cataract surgery is a rare, but potentially devastating complication of cataract surgery. In addition, postoperative endophthalmitis may be localized or have a more chronic indolent course. There are also many causes of postoperative inflammation which are sterile, or noninfectious forms of endophthalmitis. These may be caused by problems with the IOL itself, sterilizing agents or polishing compounds, toxic effects from intraocular fluids, and finally, inflammation caused by residual lens cortex. The diagnosis, prevention, and management of these various forms of inflammation following cataract surgery is of utmost importance to the clinician in order to insure optimum postoperative results for the patient.

Infectious endophthalmitis

Generalized endophthalmitis

A generalized, infectious endophthalmitis is a rare complication following cataract surgery with or without IOL implantation. Overall, the incidence of postoperative bacterial endophthalmitis has decreased markedly over the last 40 years. The rate of postoperative bacterial endophthalmitis has dropped from approximately 1% in 1950 to 0.35% in the early 1970s [1,2]. The more recent Food and Drug Administration (FDA) report on IOLs found the incidence of pseudophakic bacterial endophthalmitis to be 0.06% [3]. Thus, it

appears that the present incident rate is extremely low, at approximately 0.05%. The fact that postoperative endophthalmitis is seen so infrequently increases the need for the clinician to be aware of the presenting signs, symptoms, and diagnosis.

Although the implantation of a foreign material such as an IOL into the eye may cause one to expect a higher incidence of endophthalmitis associated with pseudophakia, this has not been the case. Newer surgical techniques such as extracapsular cataract extraction (ECCE) and phacoemulsification may actually help lower the incidence of infectious endophthalmitis with an intact posterior lens capsule creating a protective barrier effect which may help prevent the posterior extension of bacteria [4,5].

Driebe et al. [6] reported one of the largest series of pseudophakic endophthalmitis. Of 83 patients reported, cultures were positive for a bacterial source in 57 cases. Gram-positive bacteria accounted for 76% of the isolates. Staphylococcus epidermidis accounted for one-half of all the Gram-positive infections (38% overall). This was followed by Staphylococcus aureus (21%) and various streptococcal species (11%). Gram-negative bacteria accounted for only 16% of the isolates, of which Proteus was the most common. The remaining five culture-positive cases were secondary to fungal endophthalmitis.

The overall incidence of fungal endophthalmitis is very low with Mosier et al. [7] estimating fungal endophthalmitis occurring in 0.062% of postoperative cases at most. The present incidence may be even less. Driebe et al. [6] found a fungal etiology for endoph-

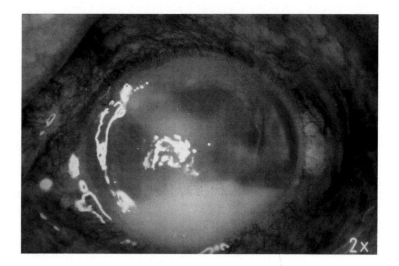

Fig. 20.1 Clinical photograph of a patient following extracapsular cataract extraction with posterior chamber intraocular lens implantation who developed a severe postoperative bacterial endophthalmitis. The conjunctiva is markedly hyperemic and the cornea is edematous. A large hypopyon is present.

thalmitis in only 8% of their reported cases of pseudophakic endophthalmitis.

Although fungal endophthalmitis is a rare complication of intraocular surgery, there have been two major outbreaks which occurred secondary to contamination of solutions used during surgery. The first major outbreak consisted of 13 cases of *Paecilomyces lilacinus* secondary to a contaminated lot of sodium bicarbonate neutralizing solution in which the sterilized IOLs had been rinsed [7,8]. The fungus was isolated from the eye in 11 of 13 cases and also from three different vials of neutralizing solution from the same production lot. Visual results of patients from this outbreak were very poor with eight eyes eventually requiring enucleation and only two eyes recovering useful vision. A second outbreak of postsurgical fungal endophthalmitis was reported by Stern *et al.* [9]. Fifteen patients developed postoperative *Candida parapsilosis* endophthalmitis secondary to a contaminated lot of intraocular irrigating solution. Results of this outbreak were not nearly as serious in that eight of 15 patients achieved a final visual acuity of 20/60 or better.

Isolated incidences of fungal contaminated intraocular solutions are still being reported. Isenberg *et al.* [10] reported an incidence of an unopened bottle of balanced salt solution which was noted to have a small black spot inside. Cultures determined the isolate to be a species of *Ulocladium* fungus. Although fungal contamination is rare, cases such as this stress the importance of a surgical team member inspecting all solutions prior to use in cataract surgery.

Adequate diagnosis and treatment of patients with endophthalmitis requires prompt recognition of signs and symptoms of endophthalmitis. Patients with postoperative bacterial endophthalmitis will often present with a history of severe pain, ocular tenderness, ad decreased vision in the operated eye occurring 2–4 days after surgery. External examination reveals marked lid swelling or edema, as well as a possible discharge. Slit-lamp examination will often reveal severe conjunctival hyperemia, chemosis, and diffuse corneal edema. Examination of the anterior chamber shows a marked inflammatory reaction with aqueous flare, cells, and usually the presence of a hypopyon (Fig. 20.1). The vitreous may be hazy which can markedly reduce the red reflex.

In general, patients with fungal endophthalmitis tend to have a later onset of symptoms than those with postoperative bacterial endophthalmitis. In addition, the course seems to be more indolent in fungal endophthalmitis with relatively mild symptoms. Examination of the anterior chamber may reveal a fibrino-purulent exudate, and examination of the vitreous can show various opacities such as snowballs or puff balls [9].

Patients who present with postoperative pain, swelling, chemosis, and hypopyon should immediately undergo anterior chamber and vitreous taps with aspiration of fluid for cultures, as simply tapping and culturing fluid from the anterior chamber is often not adequate for establishing the proper diagnosis [11]. Driebe *et al.* [6] stressed the importance of sampling the vitreous to establish the diagnosis of endophthalmitis in that sampling the aqueous fluid alone would have missed the organisms in half of their cases.

The method for obtaining cultures is also very important. The patient should be taken to the operating room and intraocular samples taken under sterile conditions. Sterile tapping of the anterior chamber is achieved using a 25 gauge needle attached to a tuberculin syringe with aspiration of 0.1–0.2 ml of fluid [11]. A vitreous sample may be obtained by using a 22 gauge needle on a tuberculin syringe. In patients who are aphakic or have an anterior chamber IOL, the needle may be placed through the limbus into the vitreous. In patients who are phakic or have a posterior chamber lens, the vitreous may be obtained via a sclerotomy through the pars plana or during the time of vitrectomy if this is being performed [6,11,12]. Once the fluid is aspirated, it should immediately be inoculated onto blood agar, chocolate agar, Sabouraud's agar, and thioglycolate broth.

The treatment of presumed infectious endophthalmitis requires immediate antibiotic therapy, with later adjustment of the medication depending on culture results. Intravitreal injection of antibiotics has now become the preferred route of antibiotic administration for the treatment of endophthalmitis. Current recommendations for intravitreal antibiotics in postoperative endophthalmitis include gentamicin 0.1 mg for coverage of Gram-negative organisms and cefazolin 2.25 mg for coverage of Gram-positive organisms [6]. Most recently, vancomycin 1 mg has been suggested for coverage of Gram-positive organisms. [12]. Patients with suspected fungal endophthalmitis are treated in a similar fashion with an intravitreal injection of amphotericin B 0.005–0.01 mg [9,13].

In addition to intravitreal antibiotic injections, most clinicians are still using periocular, topical, and systemic antibiotics. Topical or systemic steroids may be added to the therapeutic regimen 24–48 h following the beginning of antibiotic therapy [6,12]. Subconjunctival antibiotics consisting of gentamicin 40 mg and cefazolin 100 mg are often used. In addition, fortified topical antibiotic drops consisting of gentamicin 15 mg/ml and cefazolin 50 mg/ml may be used. Systemic antibiotics may also be added to the treatment regimen with cefazolin given intravenously 1 g every 6 h and gentamicin intravenously 1 mg/kg of body weight every 8 h, with adequate monitoring of renal function [14].

The question of the need for repeat intravitreal injection of antibiotics has been raised. It is recommended that if the cultures are negative after 48 h, that the intravitreal antibiotics do not need to be repeated [11]. In their study on postoperative endophthalmitis, Stern *et al.* [12] found that all culture-negative patients were successfully treated with a single intravitreal injection of antibiotics. However, they found that five of seven culture-positive patients who were treated with only a single intravitreal injection of antibiotics and no vitrectomy were either incompletely treated or failed to respond. They felt that the culture-positive patients responded best to an aggressive approach that included the use of repeat intravitreal injection of antibiotics and/or vitrectomy.

In cases of more severe endophthalmitis, vitrectomy has become a frequent therapeutic modality. Some of the reasons given for the use of vitrectomy to manage postoperative endophthalmitis include: (a) removing infectious material; (b) obtaining an adequate specimen for culture; (c) allowing better distribution of intraocular antibiotics; and (d) removing opaque debris from the visual axis [15]. Olk and Bohigian [13] stated that vitrectomy should be given strong consideration in any of the following situations: (a) profound visual loss to a level of light perception with a history of rapid deterioration; (b) deterioration despite appropriate therapy; (c) lack of visualization of the fundus or marked vitreous involvement on ultrasound; (d) a virulent organism on culture; and (e) suspected fungal endophthalmitis.

The removal of an IOL is usually unnecessary for adequate treatment of postoperative endophthalmitis. Zaidman and Mondino [16] found that in cases of infective endophthalmitis, the response to treatment and final visual outcome were unrelated to removal or retention of the IOL. Driebe et al. [6] in their study of pseudophakic endophthalmitis found that only one of the 57 eyes that were infected with bacteria required removal of the IOL for subsequent sterilization. Hopen et al. [17] developed an experimental rabbit model and found that there was no difference between aphakic eyes and pseudophakic eyes in terms of clinical response or onset of negative cultures after inducing endophthalmitis. Thus in most instances, the IOL can be left in place unless the vitreous surgeon requires removal of the lens to perform surgery or if there is a suspected fungal endophthalmitis [13].

One of the most important factors in the final visual outcome in patients with infectious endophthalmitis is the specific infecting organism. Organisms with low virulence have a better visual prognosis than organisms with a high degree of virulence. Patients with *Staphylococcus epidermidis* infections had the best prognosis in a large series of pseudophakic endophthalmitis patients studied by Driebe *et al.* [6]. Of these patients 78% achieved vision of 20/400 or better with 33% seeing 20/40 or better. Overall, 19% of their patients with culture-positive endophthalmitis lost all vision. Other studies have shown similar results with patients having *Staphylococcus epidermidis* endophthalmitis having the best visual prognosis [12,15]. Patients who were culture-negative were also found to have a better visual prognosis than patients with positive cultures [12,15]. Driebe et al. [6] found that 94% of their patients with negative cultures achieved a vision of 20/400 or better with 44% seeing 20/40 or better.

One factor that is very important in preventing postoperative endophthalmitis is a carefully controlled aseptic surgical technique. Care should be taken to prevent placing the sterile IOL on the external aspect of the eye before implantation in order to prevent contamination [18]. Preoperative preparation of the eye may also be an important factor in the prevention of endophthalmitis. Isenberg et al. [19] found that using a combination of topical Neosporin ophthalmic solution three times daily for 3 days prior to surgery along with irrigating the eye preoperatively with dilute, half-strength (5%) povidone–iodine solution was successful in sterilizing the conjunctiva in 83% of the cases. Methods of preventing intraocular contamination include micropore filtration of ocular irrigating solution [20], as well as the use of intraocular dilute antibiotics [21].

Intraoperative complications may also be a factor in the development of postoperative endophthalmitis. Driebe et al. [6] found a very high incidence of associated wound complications in patients with endophthalmitis. More than one in five of the patients who developed endophthalmitis had a problem with the cataract wound which was felt to directly contribute to the development of endophthalmitis. These authors stressed the importance of a well-closed wound as well as careful technique in removing sutures postoperatively. Another factor that was associated with the development of endophthalmitis was vitreous loss at the time of cataract surgery. They found that vitreous loss occurred in 11% of their patients with endophthalmitis. This fact stresses the importance of carefully removing all vitreous from the area of the wound and anterior chamber at the time of surgery in order to prevent this complication.

Although postoperative endophthalmitis following cataract surgery is very rare and most often occurs sporadically, it is important for a hospital or surgical center to have a specific endophthalmitis protocol to try to ascertain the cause of the endophthalmitis, as well as to prevent or minimize recurrences. We have developed a specific protocol at the Intermountain Ocular Research Center, Utah to help identify potential sources of postoperative endophthalmitis.

The first step is to carefully review the

patient's preoperative data. Potential sources of postoperative endophthalmitis, such as blepharitis, poor lid hygiene, or concurrent infections, must be assessed. In addition, patient adherence to postoperative care must be evaluated. A discussion of any irregularities in postoperative medications use and patient hygiene must be carefully assessed.

All operative data must be evaluated to look for possible deviations from the surgical protocol. The surgeon, assistants, and nursing staff should be identified. Any changes in nursing staff or surgical assistants should also be noted. Careful attention should be paid to any preoperative medications administered to the patient and who administered them. The preparation of the operating room, as well as the patient preoperatively, must then be evaluated. Then, instrument preparation and sterilization techniques employed should be assessed with special attention to handpieces, canulas, and tubing. Proper sterilization of the instrument tray must be established by reviewing the time, temperature, and pressure that was used in the sterilization. All intraocular solutions and medications used in the case should be noted, and lot numbers and manufacturers for each one checked off. If possible, all intraocular or irrigating solutions used during the procedure should be cultured. If the specific solutions used during the surgery have been discarded, samples should be obtained from similar lot numbers and sent for culture. The solutions should also be checked for clarity, precipitates, or signs of any growth inside the container.

The type of equipment and handpieces used in the surgery should be noted. Cultures need to be taken from phacoemulsification or irrigation/aspiration handpieces and tips. Methods of cleaning the instruments prior to surgery need to be reviewed. In addition, notation of the style, as well as the manufacturer of an IOL if it was used in the surgery, should also be recorded.

It is important to check the report of the operative procedure for any signs of intraoperative complications which may predispose the patient to endophthalmitis. As mentioned previously, patients who develop endophthalmitis often have problems with the catar-

act wound. In addition, such complications as vitreous loss or vitreous strands to the wounds may contribute to the etiology of postoperative endophthalmitis.

Any patients who underwent surgery at the hospital or surgery center the same day as the endophthalmitis patient should be carefully evaluated postoperatively for any signs of endophthalmitis or unusual postoperative intraocular inflammation.

Following this extensive evaluation, deviations from the normal surgical protocol, from preoperative sterilization to postoperative instruction on use of medications to the patient, should be corrected immediately. If any specific causes for postoperative endophthalmitis are found, it is important to correct these immediately, prior to proceeding with further surgery. Fortunately, most cases of postoperative endophthalmitis are sporadic and not related to a specific break in technique. In fact, most bacteria causing endophthalmitis are felt to be from the patient's endogenous ocular flora. Nonetheless, it is important for the hospital or surgical center to investigate each case of postoperative endophthalmitis, using a specific protocol as outlined here to rule out all possible sources of preventable contamination.

Chronic or localized endophthalmitis

Occasionally following cataract surgery, there can be a low grade or late onset of endophthalmitis caused by bacteria of low virulence. Ficker *et al.* [22] have termed these cases of indolent postoperative endophthalmitis "chronic bacterial endophthalmitis." Pathogens of low virulence such as coagulase-negative *Staphylococcus epidermidis* are a common cause of this entity. In contrast to the usual course of postoperative bacterial endophthalmitis, these patients typically complain of redness, photophobia, and visual impairment rather than severe pain, decrease in vision, and tissue swelling with purulent discharge [22]. These signs can appear anywhere from 4 days to 12 weeks postoperatively and are often followed by a chronic uveitis picture which is often suppressed by administration of topical or systemic steroids. Schanzlin *et al.* [23] describe the case of a patient following cataract surgery who developed a hypopyon that cleared with topical corticosteroid therapy but recurred whenever the steroid therapy was reduced. The persistence of the inflammation and the recurrence of the hypopyon whenever the corticosteroids were decreased suggested an endophthalmitis due to an organism of low virulence and cultures of the anterior vitreous confirmed the presence of Staphylococcus epidermidis. These authors felt that the corticosteroids may completely mask an endophthalmitis from an organism of low virulence such as Staphylococcus epidermidis. Other authors also believe that the steroids mask or suppress the signs and symptoms of chronic bacterial endophthalmitis [22].

Cases of chronic, low-grade, postoperative inflammation which show an incomplete clinical response to corticosteroids or recurrence of inflammation following decrease of steroid therapy, should raise the question of a chronic bacterial endophthalmitis. In this situation, it is important to obtain cultures of the vitreous as well as the aqueous, as aqueous taps are often unreliable. The treatment is similar to that of a routine postoperative endophthalmitis. As in other cases of endophthalmitis, it appears as though IOL removal is not required for successful treatment of the infection [22].

A recently described cause for chronic postoperative inflammation after cataract surgery and IOL implantation is chronic Propionibacterium acnes endophthalmitis. Meisler et al. [24] described a series of six patients with chronic Propionibacterium endophthalmitis in 1986. These patients all had undergone uncomplicated ECCE with implantation of a posterior chamber IOL. The interval between cataract surgery and the onset of postoperative inflammation ranged from 2 to 6 months in these patients. The inflammation was characterized by an indolent course and appeared clinically as a chronic granulomatous iridocyclitis. Of interest, five of these six patients had accumulation of a white exudative material on the posterior capsule or the IOL. In all these patients, the inflammation improved transiently with corticosteroid therapy. The diagnosis of Propionibacterium endophthalmitis

was made following anaerobic cultures of vitrectomy specimens, although the interval between the onset of the inflammation and the diagnosis ranged from 5 to 15 months. The delay in onset and chronic indolent nature of the inflammation observed in patients with P. acnes is very similar to that seen with chronic Staphylococcus epidermidis endophthalmitis, although the course in these patients with Propionibacterium acnes seems to be even more delayed in onset and prolonged [24,25].

Meisler and Mandelbaum [26] have recently updated their original paper and reviewed 16 reported cases of Propionibacterium associated endophthalmitis after ECCE. The inflammation was observed anywhere from 2 to 10 months following cataract surgery and occurred after laser posterior capsulotomy in four patients. Clinically, this entity was characterized by a chronic iridocyclitis which had hypopyon in 10 cases and granulomatous-appearing keratic precipitates in five cases. A white plaque was noted on the posterior capsule or IOL in half of the cases. These patients all had a transient response to corticosteroid treatment.

There is a subset of patients with chronic postoperative inflammation in which the microorganisms may be localized to the capsular bag following cataract surgery, thus creating a localized smoldering infection. This entity has been termed "localized endophthalmitis," and seven patients with this condition have been reviewed [27,28]. Pathologic evaluation of materials extracted from these cases showed Gram-positive organisms sequestered within the residual lens capsule (Fig. 20.2a). It was thought that this sequestration by the lens capsule prevented a more widespread infection. Of interest, Tetz et al. [29] reported a case of a patient who developed a generalized endophthalmitis secondary to P. acnes following an Nd:YAG capsulotomy. It appears that the organisms were initially confined within the capsular bag and were released into the vitreous following the Nd:YAG laser capsulotomy.

Propionibacterium acnes is a Gram-positive, anaerobic pleomorphic bacillus (Fig. 20.2b). It is a relatively ubiquitous organism which is commonly found in the normal anaerobic flora

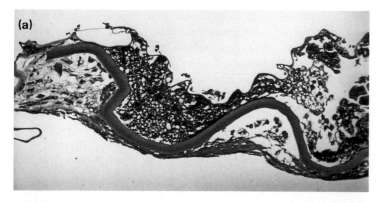

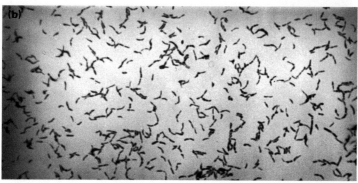

Fig. 20.2 (a) Photomicrograph of the capsular sac removed from a patient with *Propionibacterium acnes* endophthalmitis. The lens capsule is seen in the center of the photograph with a small amount of anterior fibrous metaplasia of the lens epithelium. Note the deeply staining material next to the capsular bag which is composed of a large mass of Gram-positive organisms. (PAS stain; original magnification ×100.) (b) Gram-positive, pleomorphic bacilli from a culture of *Propionibacterium acnes*. (Gram stain; original magnification ×700.)

of the conjunctiva [24]. In addition, this bacterium may originate from several other sources, including the patient's own skin, as well as the skin of the surgeon or other operating room personnel [28,30].

Microbiologic diagnosis of *P. acnes* endophthalmitis can be difficult due to the fact that this is a relatively fastidious organism which may be difficult to culture [24]. Ormerod *et al*. [31] describe a technique of obtaining a vitreous specimen under relatively anaerobic conditions with immediate culturing of the specimen. The organism may be dismissed by a microbiologic laboratory as a contaminant; therefore, it is imperative to inform the laboratory of a suspected diagnosis of *P. acnes* endophthalmitis. In addition, many laboratories routinely discard anaerobic cultures 48 h after incubation, and *P. acnes* may take 5–7 days to grow in culture [24,26]. Cultures of suspected *P. acnes* bacterium should be held for at least 1 week, in order not to miss the diagnosis.

Meisler *et al*. [24] have also postulated that *P. acnes* and residual lens cortex may form a synergistic reaction that may produce or exacerbate postoperative inflammation. *Propionibacterium acnes* has some of the properties of an adjuvant, and this could play a role in promoting sensitization to lens proteins following ECCE. *Propionibacterium acnes* may persist for extended periods in the eye postoperatively, precipitating prolonged or delayed postoperative infection and inflammation [25].

Therapy for patients with *P. acnes* endophthalmitis consists of a combination of surgical intervention and antibiotics [24,31,32]. Zambrano *et al*. [32] have devised a management approach for the treatment of *P. acnes* endophthalmitis. For cases with a mild initial presentation, vitreous cultures are performed, followed by injection of intravitreal vancomycin (1 mg). Vancomycin has been shown to be effective against *P. acnes* as well as coagulase-negative *Staphylococcus epidermidis* which can cause a similar chronic endophthalmitis [33]. Anaerobic bacteria such as *Propionibacterium acnes* are relatively resistant to aminoglycosides, and these antibodies are not recommended for management of this entity. In more advanced cases with a more severe initial presentation, a pars plana vitrectomy with a central capsulectomy is performed in addition to intravitreal vancomycin. If this approach fails to eliminate the infection, these authors suggest that an attempt should be made to remove the IOL and all lens capsular remnants.

In their recent review of 16 cases of *Propionibacterium* endophthalmitis, Meisler and Mandelbaum [26], noted that treatment consisted of surgical intervention in all cases. Seven patients had removal of the posterior chamber IOL and capsular bag from the limbal approach. The remaining nine patients underwent a pars plana vitrectomy, some of which had a partial capsulectomy. Twelve of 16 patients were treated with intravitreal antibiotics at the time of surgery. Visual results in these patients were very good, with 11 of 16 patients achieving a visual acuity of 20/40 or better.

Sterile (non-infectious) endophthalmitis

Inflammation following cataract extraction with IOL implantation is caused by many different factors. These factors include trauma from the surgical procedure, infectious agents (discussed earlier), mechanical irritation from the IOL itself, problems with lens design or finish, toxic effects from lens sterilizing agents or polishing compounds, toxic effects from intraocular fluids, and inflammation caused by residual lens cortex. Any one of these factors causing postoperative inflammation may lead to a breakdown of the blood–aqueous barrier [34], as well as activation of various inflammatory mediators. An in-depth overview of the inflammatory process is beyond the scope of this chapter but has been thoroughly summarized by Apple *et al.* [35].

Inflammation caused by the IOL

Postoperative inflammation may be directly caused by the IOL itself. Several mechanical factors may be involved relating to specific lens design or type of lens. Other important mechanical factors are related to lens finishing and manufacturing defects, as well as bio-

compatibility of lens components. A final important factor in inflammation caused directly by the IOL is related to the fixation of the IOL with subsequent uveal contact, breakdown of the blood–aqueous barrier, and release of inflammatory mediators.

Anterior segment inflammation following cataract surgery with IOL implantation may be directly related to mechanical factors such as IOL manufacturing, finish, and design. Ellingson [36] and others [37] recognized a group of postoperative patients who had a triad of uveitis, glaucoma, and hyphema, and coined the descriptive term "UGH syndrome." This syndrome was initially seen in patients with poorly made copies of the Choyce Mark VIII style anterior chamber lenses. Ellingson felt that this inflammation was due to warping of the IOL footplates. However, examination of lenses removed from patients with UGH syndrome by Keates found that the lenses were poorly finished with sharp, irregular edges [37]. Scanning electron microscopic study of explanted Choyce lens copies demonstrated that sharp edges rather than warped footplates were most likely the causative factor of UGH syndrome in these patients [38].

Problems with lens design and finish became especially apparent in the early 1980s with a high incidence of anterior segment inflammation and UGH syndrome associated with various closed looped, poor quality, anterior chamber IOLs (Fig. 20.3). One lens which was frequently associated with UGH syndrome was the Azar 91Z lens. Beehler [39] reported on the UGH syndrome association with the Azar 91Z. Hagen [40] also reported multiple patients who developed UGH syndrome following implantation of the Azar 91Z lens. Some of these patients also had an associated vitreous hemorrhage for which he coined the term UGH+ syndrome. An extensive study in our laboratory of explanted Azar 91Z IOLs by scanning electron microscopy revealed multiple areas of poorly finished, sharp edges on the lens optic [41] (Fig. 20.4). In addition, several flaws were found in the lens design relating to the closed loops with subsequent vaulting and uveal erosion.

Analysis of other closed loop, anterior chamber IOLs has shown similar problems.

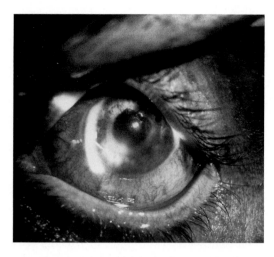

Fig. 20.3 Clinical photograph of a patient with the UGH syndrome associated with an anterior chamber intraocular lens. (Courtesy Dr Alan S. Crandall.)

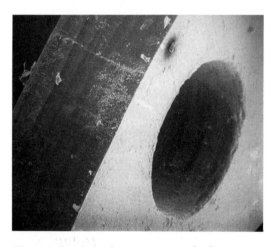

Fig. 20.4 Scanning electron micrograph of an Azar 91Z style anterior chamber intraocular lens removed secondary to the UGH syndrome. Note the sharp edge of the optic as well as the poorly finished edge of the positioning hole. In addition, the edge of the optic is irregular. (Original magnification ×100.)

Reidy *et al.* [42] reported on extensive inflammatory problems and UGH syndrome in patients with a semiflexible closed loop, Leiske-style, anterior chamber IOL. In addition, Isenberg *et al.* [43] documented the association of UGH syndrome with the Stableflex-style, anterior chamber IOL. Findings such as these

led to the removal of closed loop, anterior chamber lenses from the market [44].

These findings illustrate the problems caused by poorly finished IOLs with sharp edges as well as other mechanical problems such as lens design. This stresses the importance of good quality control and lens finishing in the manufacturing process as well as good lens design. This is especially true for anterior chamber IOLs with the potential for direct uveal contact.

UGH syndrome is very rare in patients with posterior chamber IOLs due to the fact that these lenses are positioned behind the iris and have less chance of direct uveal contact. However, it is still possible to have posterior iris chafing with these lenses. Johnson *et al.* [45] reported a series of patients with iris transillumination defects and microhyphemas thought to be secondary to posterior iris chafing. Masket [46], and Samples and Van Buskirk [47] have described similar posterior iris chafing in patients with posterior chamber IOLs with some associated pigmentary glaucoma. Iris chafing may also lead to episodes of decreased vision with both white cells and red cells leaking into the anterior chamber. This was called the "intermittent visual white-out" syndrome by Lieppman in 1982 [48] in patients with iris plane IOLs. The incidence of this complication in patients with posterior chamber lenses is fortunately extremely rare.

A very rare cause of inflammation secondary to an IOL is that of ciliary body erosion of a lens loop causing anterior segment ischemia. Apple *et al.* [49] reported a patient with marked anterior segment ischemia resulting from deep erosion of a posterior chamber lens loop into the ciliary sulcus with pressure on the major arterial circle of the iris. This created a picture similar to that of an anterior uveitis.

Much has been written about the biocompatibility of IOL components [50,51]. Fortunately, both of the most commonly used polymers in present-day IOLs, polymethylmetacrylate (PMMA) and polypropylene appear to be relatively biocompatible within the eye and are felt to have a minimal chance of causing postoperative inflammation.

Different varieties of nylon were initially used in the manufacture of IOL haptics as well

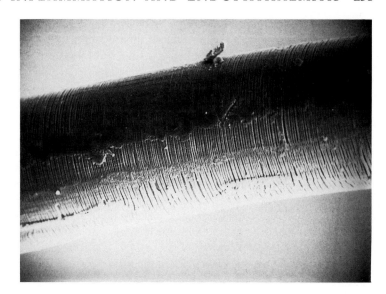

Fig. 20.5 Scanning electron micrograph of a polypropylene intraocular lens loop. The loop shows multiple, parallel transverse fissures in the outer layers of the polymer. (Original magnification ×100.)

as sutures. Drews *et al.* [52] found signs of degradation of IOL loops manufactured with nylon, especially in areas of iris touch. Studies in our laboratory confirmed the intraocular degradation of nylon IOL loops [50]. This was not shown to directly cause intraocular inflammation, but at present nylon is no longer used as an IOL material.

Although an ideal polymer for the manufacture of an IOL does not exist, PMMA has shown excellent long-term biocompatibility within the human eye [51]. There is no evidence of PMMA degradation within the eye and it has not been shown to cause directly severe postoperative inflammation [35].

Polypropylene (prolene) is the most frequently used biopolymer in IOL loops. Clayman [53] reviewed polypropylene extensively and noted that it was relatively biologically inert. An extensive review from our laboratory [50] found signs of superficial degradation of polypropylene loops. Superficial cracking and fissuring was noted in cases where the polypropylene loops had been in contact with uveal tissue for more than 2 years (Fig. 20.5). Although there is a possibility this degradation may contribute to postoperative inflammation, this has not been conclusively shown. If an IOL with polypropylene loops is used, any possible effects or degradation would be minimized if the loops are placed in the capsular bag, thereby sequestering the polymer from uveal tissue.

Sterile hypopyon—"toxic lens syndrome"

IOL implantation may be associated with a sterile postoperative inflammation with a hypopyon and/or anterior vitreous reaction. This condition was initially called the "toxic lens syndrome" [54,55]. Although earlier cases of direct ocular toxicity caused by polishing compounds or lens sterilization techniques have been reported, inflammation in this syndrome is often unrelated to the IOL itself. Thus, at present, the term "toxic lens syndrome" is probably inappropriate and sterile endophthalmitis or sterile hypopyon is used to describe this syndrome.

A potential source of postoperative inflammation is the method used for sterilization of the IOL. Worst [56] presented a history of the sterilization of IOLs and subsequent difficulties with sterile hypopyons. He reviewed the history of the original sterilizing agents used which were quaternary ammonium compounds such as cetrimide. These were found to cause postoperative inflammatory reactions such as sterile hypopyons, intense inflammation, and fibrosis. Because of these problems, a technique of "wet-pack" sterilization with caustic soda or sodium bicarbonate was developed

[57]. Binkhorst advocated using ultraviolet radiation to sterilize IOLs, but it was soon discovered that this may possibly damage the PMMA, so this was abandoned [58].

Sodium hydroxide (wet-pack) sterilization of IOLs was used successfully until the late 1970s. These lenses were then rinsed in a sodium bicarbonate neutralizing solution. Unfortunately, two major outbreaks of contamination of this neutralizing solution were reported involving *Paecilomices lilacinus* fungus [8] and *Pseudomonas aeruginosa* [59]. Following these outbreaks, the FDA banned wet-pack sterilization and a method of dry sterilization using ethylene oxide gas was adopted.

Worst [56] felt that increased inflammatory episodes would occur using ethylene oxide to sterilize the implant. Initially, increased inflammation was reported with the dry-pack sterilization [60]. Stark *et al.* [61] found that the incidence of postoperative inflammatory reactions in the group using ethylene oxide sterilization was 7% as compared to a 1.5% incidence of hypopyon in the sodium hydroxide or wet-pack sterilization group. At the present time, using proper aeration and the ethylene oxide technique, reactions due to sterilization techniques of IOLs are extremely rare.

Residual polishing compounds on the surface of the IOL optic or loop are another potential source of intraocular inflammation. Meltzer [62] reported several patients with sterile hypopyons following IOL implantation. Analysis of the IOLs using energy dispersive X-ray techniques found residual polishing compound on the lenses. He found that the residual polishing compound was apparently fused to the surface of the lens and could not be removed. Ratner [63] also analyzed the surface of several IOLs using energy-dispersive X-ray analysis. Gross particulate contaminants and surface films on the IOL were found. Due to better manufacturing techniques of IOLs, this condition is also very rare today.

Talc is a possible source of postoperative inflammation or sterile hypopyon. Bene and Kranias [64] reported a patient with a severe postoperative iritis who was noted to have deposits on the surface of the IOL optic felt to be secondary to contamination by surgical glove powder. Other possible sources of sterile endophthalmitis include contaminated intraocular fluids or viscoelastic substances used during surgery. Finally, Richburg *et al.* [65] reported several cases of a sterile hypopyon occurring 24 h after an uncomplicated cataract surgery with posterior chamber IOL implantation. While all cases responded to steroid treatment, a direct cause for the inflammation was not immediately found. It was eventually determined that instruments placed in older ultrasound cleaning solution caused the hypopyon. Further analysis of these instruments found that they were contaminated by heat-stable endotoxin that remained on the instruments through the autoclaving process. Daily changing of the solution in the ultrasonic instrument cleaner was felt to alleviate this problem.

On occasion, there is an acute intraocular inflammation following uncomplicated cataract extraction with implantation of a posterior chamber IOL in which no etiology can be found. We have found three unrelated cases of this condition at our center which we have named the "toxic anterior segment syndrome" (TASS) (Monson, in press). The hallmark of this entity is an acute toxic reaction occurring in the anterior segment typified by a fixed, or almost fixed, dilated pupil with diffuse corneal endothelial damage and widespread corneal edema. Marked inflammation is seen on the first postoperative day, and a severe secondary glaucoma often develops. No etiology has been found for this syndrome despite extensive testing.

The most important factor in postoperative patients who present with a sterile hypopyon or sterile endophthalmitis is differentiating these patients from those who have a true infectious endophthalmitis. Although these patients may present with reduced visual acuity, hypopyon, and vitreous opacity, the most important factors are that these patients have no pain, no lid edema, and little or no conjunctival injection or chemosis [54,66]. If there is any question of an infectious etiology, aqueous and vitreous taps must be performed to rule out endophthalmitis. Patients with a sterile inflammatory reaction postoperatively may be treated with a course of intense topical corticosteroids and followed closely. The hypopyon or other anterior inflammatory changes should clear rapidly following this treatment. Patients who show signs of recurrence of inflammation after tapering off corticosteroids raise the suspicion of a chronic bacterial endophthalmitis [22], *Propionibacterium acnes* endophthalmitis [26], or possibly phacoanaphylactic endophthalmitis [67]. These entities usually have a much more delayed onset and prolonged course than a sterile uveitis.

Inflammation related to residual lens cortex—phacoanaphylactic endophthalmitis

On rare occasions, a successful ECCE with posterior chamber IOL implantation can be complicated by a chronic, sterile inflammatory process in which other causes of sterile hypopyon or the "toxic lens syndrome" (previously discussed) have been ruled out. In these instances, the inflammation is caused not by the IOL itself or other factors, but rather by a hypersensitivity reaction to the patient's own lens protein. This inflammation has been termed phacoanaphylactic endophthalmitis.

Verhoeff and Lemoine [68] originally called this entity endophthalmitis phacoanaphylactica and postulated that this reaction was a hypersensitivity to the patient's lens protein which is liberated after capsular rupture. The entity of phacoanaphylactic endophthalmitis was described at length by Irvine and Irvine [69] in 1952 as a sterile granulomatous inflammatory reaction to retained lens cortex. Rahi and Garner [70] have stated that the term "phacoanaphylaxis" is probably not accurate since there is no evidence of IgE involvement in this entity. Normally, an intact lens capsular membrane provides a protective barrier around the lens that prevents a cell-mediated autosensitization to the patient's own lens protein [71,72]. Disruption of the normally intact lens capsule due to trauma or surgery will expose the lens proteins which are normally sequestered to the immune system which may lead to a chronic inflammation [67].

The exact incidence of phacoanaphylactic endophthalmitis is presently unknown. Following some of the earliest reports of this entity, phacoanaphylaxis was not seen in the era of intracapsular cataract extraction (ICCE). With ophthalmologists making the transition from ICCE to ECCE, it was felt that there would be a resurgence of lens cortex-induced uveitis. However, with modern techniques of ECCE and meticulous cortical removal, this entity is still relatively rare. Several reports of complications in large series of ECCEs done in the early 1980s reported no distinct cases of phacoanaphylactic endophthalmitis [3,73]. In fact, very few reports of phacoanaphylactic endophthalmitis following ECCE were noted. Smith and Weiner [74] reported an isolated case of phacoanaphylactic endophthalmitis which followed phacoemulsification with no IOL implantation. The diagnosis in this case was confirmed by an anterior chamber paracentesis which showed foamy macrophages present. Ishikawa et al. [75] subsequently reported three cases of phacoanaphylactic endophthalmitis— all following ECCE. These cases were not confirmed histologically; however, clinically they fit the pattern of this disease entity. It is difficult to tell if the entity of phacoanaphylactic endophthalmitis is indeed extremely rare, or if this entity is simply being diagnosed as a chronic uveitis.

Smith [25] states that phacoanaphylactic endophthalmitis, "an old enemy," is making a come-back. He prefers the term "phacoantigenic" endophthalmitis for this entity. Several recent reports have documented cases of phacoanaphylactic endophthalmitis following cataract extraction with IOL implantation [67,76,77]. We initially reported a case of a patient with a severe intractable uveitis that was shown to be consistent with phacoanaphylactic endophthalmitis on histopathologic examination in 1984 [67]. Since that time, several other cases of presumed phacoanaphylactic endophthalmitis have been reported [76].

Clinically, the onset of inflammation in phacoanaphylactic endophthalmitis occurs between 1 and 14 days after traumatic or surgical disruption of the lens capsule [70,72]. However, there have been unusual cases

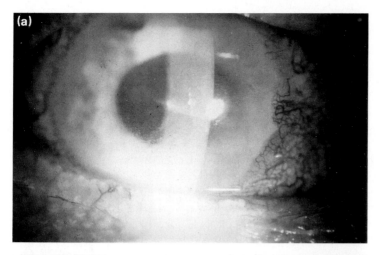

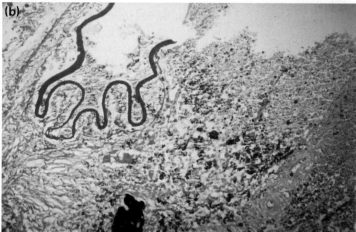

Fig. 20.6 (a) Clinical photograph of a patient who developed a low-grade anterior uveitis 1 month following cataract surgery with implantation of a posterior chamber IOL. The patient was subsequently found to have phacoanaphylactic endophthalmitis on histopathologic examination of removed lens cortical material. (b) Photomicrograph from a patient with phacoanaphylactic endophthalmitis. A small piece of residual lens capsule is surrounded by a chronic inflammatory cell infiltrate with extensive necrosis and disruption of tissue. (PAS stain; original magnification ×40.)

reported where the reaction as early as several hours or as late as several months following capsular rupture [74]. These patients usually present with blurred vision and an anterior uveitis without severe pain, chemosis, or eyelid edema (Fig. 20.6a).

Histopathologically, the entity of phacoanaphylactic endophthalmitis is characterized by a zonal granulomatous inflammatory reaction around the lens or lens remnant [67,71, 78] (Fig. 20.6b). The central part of the reaction consists predominantly of polymorphonuclear cells which are in turn surrounded by concentric layers of epithelioid and giant cells, and finally lymphocytes and plasma cells. Foamy macrophages have also been seen associated with this entity [67]. The entire inflammatory

mass may become surrounded by dense fibrous or granulation tissue. The iris and ciliary body adjacent to the inflammation typically show an infiltrate of mononuclear plasma cells and lymphocytes.

The most important factor in the management of phacoanaphylactic endophthalmitis is early recognition and diagnosis. If left untreated, phacoanaphylactic endophthalmitis may lead to severe sequelae of chronic uveitis including synechia formation, cyclitic membranes, retinal detachment, and phthisis bulbi [79]. This entity should be considered in any patient who presents with a sterile uveitis that improves initially with cortical steroid treatment but recurs when the steroids are tapered. Chronic infectious etiologies such as

Staphylococcus epidermidis and *Propionibacterium acnes* may be ruled out using appropriate taps.

Once infectious etiologies have been ruled out and the diagnosis of phacoanaphylactic endophthalmitis is likely, the treatment is surgical removal of the IOL and any remaining lens cortex and capsule. The inflammation may continue or even worsen if only the IOL is removed. Wohl *et al.* [77] have described a technique of removing the IOL through a limbal incision. This is followed by removal of the entire remnant lens capsule using α-chymotrypsin. Surgical removal of the lens and capsule remnants along with aggressive cortical steroid therapy should quiet the inflammation.

Recently, the question has arisen as to whether phacoanaphylactic endophthalmitis is actually a hypersensitivity response to lens protein or a disease of infectious origin [35]. Meisler *et al.* [24] have raised the question of a possible synergy between bacteria and residual lens proteins exacerbating the inflammation in *P. acnes* endophthalmitis. In addition, Piest *et al.* [27] also raise the question that perhaps the entity of phacoanaphylactic endophthalmitis is actually a disease of infectious origin. Further research is necessary in this area to address these questions.

References

1 Allen HF, Mangiaracine AB. Bacterial endophthalmitis after cataract extraction. *Arch Ophthalmol* 1964; **72**: 454–62.

2 Jaffe NS. *Cataract Surgery and Its Complications*. 4th edn. St Louis: CV Mosby, 1984; 497–529.

3 Stark WJ, Worthen DM, Holladay JT *et al.* The FDA report on intraocular lenses. *Ophthalmology* 1983; **90**: 311–17.

4 Beyer TL, Vogler G, Sharma D, O'Donnell FE Jr. Protective barrier effect of the posterior lens capsule in exogenous bacterial endophthalmitis: An experimental pseudophakic primate study. *J Am Intraocul Implant Soc* 1983; **9**: 293–6.

5 Gross KA, Pearce JL. Protective barrier effect of the posterior lens capsule in exogenous bacterial endophthalmitis: A case report. *J Cataract Refract Surg* 1986; **12**: 413–14.

6 Driebe WT Jr, Mandelbaum S, Forster RK *et al.* Pseudophakic endophthalmitis: Diagnosis and management. *Ophthalmology* 1986; **93**: 442–8.

7 Mosier MA, Lusk B, Pettit TH *et al.* Fungal endophthalmitis following intraocular lens implantation. *Am J Ophthalmol* 1977; **83**: 1–8.

8 Pettit TH, Olson RJ, Foos RY, Martin WJ. Fungal endophthalmitis following intraocular lens implantation: A surgical epidemic. *Arch Ophthalmol* 1980; **98**: 1025–39.

9 Stern WH, Tamura E, Jacobs RA *et al.* Epidemic postsurgical *Candida parapsilosis* endophthalmitis: Clinical findings and management of 15 consecutive cases. *Ophthalmology* 1985; **92**: 1701–9.

10 Isenberg RA, Weiss RL, Apple DJ, Lowrey DB. Fungal contamination of balanced salt solution. *J Am Intraocul Implant Soc* 1985; **11**: 485–586.

11 Forster RK, Abbott RL, Gelender H. Management of infectious endophthalmitis. *Ophthalmology* 1980; **87**: 313–19.

12 Stern GA, Engel HM, Driebe WT Jr. The treatment of postoperative endophthalmitis: The results of differing approaches to treatment. *Ophthalmology* 1989; **96**: 62–7.

13 Olk RJ, Bohigian GM. The management of endophthalmitis: Diagnostic and therapeutic guidelines including the use of vitrectomy. *Ophthal Surg* 1987; **18**: 262–7.

14 Smith SG, Lindstrom RL. *Intraocular Lens Complications and Their Management*. Thorofare, New Jersey: Slack Inc., 1988: 58–62.

15 Olson JC, Flynn HW Jr, Forster RK, Culbertson WW. Results in the treatment of postoperative endophthalmitis. *Ophthalmology* 1983; **90**: 692–9.

16 Zaidman GW, Mondino BJ. Postoperative pseudophakic bacterial endophthalmitis. *Am J Ophthalmol* 1982; **93**: 218–23.

17 Hopen G, Mondino BJ, Kozy D, Lipkowitz J. Intraocular lenses and experimental bacterial endophthalmitis. *Am J Ophthalmol* 1982; **94**: 402–7.

18 Vafidis GC, Marsh RJ, Stacey AR. Bacterial contamination of intraocular lens surgery. *Br J Ophthalmol* 1984; **68**: 520–3.

19 Isenberg SJ, Apt L, Yoshimori R, Khwarg S. Chemical preparation of the eye in ophthalmic surgery. IV. Comparison of povidone–iodine on the conjunctiva with a prophylactic antibiotic. *Arch Ophthalmol* 1985; **103**: 1340–2.

20 Neumann AC. Particulate and microbial contamination of intraocular irrigating solutions. *J Cataract Refract Surg* 1986; **12**: 485–8.

21 Gills JP. Prevention of endophthalmitis by intraocular solution filtration and antibiotics. *J Am Intraocul Implant Soc* 1985; **11**: 185–6.

22 Ficker L, Meredith TA, Wilson LA *et al.* Chronic bacterial endophthalmitis. *Am J Ophthalmol* 1987; **103**: 745–8.

23 Schanzlin DJ, Goldberg DB, Brown SI. *Staphylococcus epidermidis* endophthalmitis following intraocular lens implantation. *Br J Ophthalmol* 1980; **64**: 684–6.

24 Meisler DM, Palestine AG, Vastine DW *et al.* Chronic propionibacterium endophthalmitis after extracapsular cataract extraction and intraocular lens implantation. *Am J Ophthalmol* 1986; **102**: 733–9.

25 Smith RE. Inflammation after cataract surgery (Editorial). *Am J Opthalmol* 1986; **102**: 788–90.

26 Meisler DM, Mandelbaum S. *Propionibacterium-*associated endophthalmitis after extracapsular cataract extraction: Review of reported cases. *Ophthalmology* 1989; **96**: 54–61.

27 Piest KL, Kincaid MC, Tetz MR *et al.* Localized endophthalmitis: A newly documented cause of toxic lens syndrome. *J Cataract Refract Surg* 1987; **13**: 498–510.

28 Tetz MR, Apple DJ, Hansen SO *et al.* "Localized endophthalmitis": A complication of extracapsular cataract extraction. *Implant Ophthalmol* 1987; **1**: 93–7.

29 Tetz MR, Apple DJ, Price FW Jr *et al.* A newly described complication of Nd:YAG laser capsulotomy: Exacerbation of an intraocular inflammation. *Arch Ophthalmol* 1987; **105**: 1324–5.

30 McNatt J, Allen SD, Wilson LA, Dowell VR Jr. Anaerobic flora of the normal human conjunctival sac. *Arch Ophthalmol* 1978; **96**: 1448–50.

31 Ormerod LD, Paton BG, Haaf J *et al.* Anaerobic bacterial endophthalmitis. *Ophthalmology* 1987; **94**: 799–808.

32 Zambrano W, Flynn HW, Pflugfelder SC *et al.* Management options for *Propionibacterium acnes* endophthalmitis. *Ophthalmology* 1989; **96**: 1100–5.

33 Davis JL, Koidou-Tsiligianni A, Pflugfelder SC *et al.* Coagulase-negative staphylococcal endophthalmitis: Increase in antimicrobial resistance. *Ophthalmology* 1988; **95**: 1404–10.

34 Cunha-Vaz JG: The blood–ocular barriers. *Surv Ophthalmol* 1979; **23**: 279–96.

35 Apple DJ, Mamalis N, Olson RJ, Kincaid MC. *Intraocular Lenses: Evolution, Designs, Complications, and Pathology.* Baltimore: Williams & Wilkins, 1989: 225–54.

36 Ellingson FT. Complications with the Choyce Mark VIII anterior chamber lens implant (uveitis–glaucoma–hyphema). *J Am Intraocul Implant Soc* 1977; **3**: 199–201.

37 Keates RH, Ehrlich DR. "Lenses of chance": Complications of anterior chamber implants. *Ophthalmology* 1978; **85**: 408–14.

38 Apple DJ, Brems RN, Park RB *et al.* Anterior chamber lenses. Part I: Complications and pathology and a review of designs. *J Cataract Refract Surg* 1987; **13**: 157–74.

39 Beehler CC. UGH syndrome with the 91Z lens. *J Am Intraocul Implant Soc* 1983; **9**: 459 (letter).

40 Hagen JC III. A comparative study of the 91Z and other anterior chamber intraocular lenses. *J Am Intraocul Implant Soc* 1984; **10**: 324–8.

41 Mamalis N, Apple DJ, Brady SE *et al.* Pathological and scanning electron microscopic evaluation of the 91Z intraocular lens. *J Am Intraocul Implant Soc* 1984; **10**: 191–9.

42 Reidy JJ, Apple DJ, Googe JM *et al.* An analysis of semi-flexible, closed-loop anterior chamber intraocular lenses. *J Am Intraocul Implant Soc* 1985; **11**: 344–52.

43 Isenberg RA, Apple DJ, Reidy JJ *et al.* Histopathologic and scanning electron miscroscopic study of one type of intraocular lens. *Arch Ophthalmol* 1986; **104**: 683–6.

44 Apple DJ, Olson RJ. Closed-loop anterior chamber intraocular lenses. *Arch Ophthalmol* 1987; **105**: 19–20 (letter).

45 Johnson SH, Kratz RP, Olson PF. Iris transillumination defects and microhyphema syndrome. *Am Intraocul Implant Soc J* 1984; **10**: 425–8.

46 Masket S. Pseudophakic posterior iris chaffing syndrome. *J Cataract Refract Surg* 1986; **12**: 252–6.

47 Samples JR, Van Buskirk EM. Pigmentary glaucoma associated with posterior chamber intraocular lenses. *Am J Ophthalmol* 1985; **100**: 385–8.

48 Lieppman ME. Intermittent visual "white-out": A new intraocular lens complication. *Ophthalmology* 1982; **89**: 109–12.

49 Apple DJ, Craythorn JM, Olson RJ *et al.* Anterior segment complications and neovascular glaucoma following implantation of a posterior chamber intraocular lens. *Ophthalmology* 1984; **91**: 403–19.

50 Apple DJ, Mamalis N, Brady SC *et al.* Biocompatibility of implant materials: A review and scanning electron microscopic study. *J Am Intraocul Implant Soc* 1984; **10**: 53–66.

51 Apple DJ, Mamalis N, Loftfield K *et al.* Complications of intraocular lenses: A historical and histopathological review. *Surv Ophthalmol* 1984; **29**: 1–54.

52 Drews RC, Smith ME, Okun N. Scanning electron microscopy of intraocular lenses. *Ophthalmology* 1978; **85**: 415–24.

53 Clayman HM. Polypropylene. *Ophthalmology* 1981; **88**: 959–64.

54 Alpar JJ. Toxic lens syndrome. *J Ocul Ther Surg* 1982; **1**: 306–8.

55 Shepherd DD. The "toxic lens" syndrome. *Contact Intraocul Lens Med J* 1980; **6**: 158–61.

56 Worst JGF. A retrospective view on the sterilization of intraocular lenses and the incidence of sterile hypopyon (Editorial). *J Am Intraocul Implant Soc* 1980; **6**: 10–12.

57 Ridley F. Safety requirements for acrylic implants. *Br J Ophthalmol* 1957; **41**: 359–67.

58 Binkhorst CD, Flu FP. Sterilization of intraocular acrylic lens prostheses with ultralviolet rays. *Br J Ophthalmol* 1956; **40**: 665–8.

59 Gerding DN, Poley BJ, Hall WH *et al.* Treatment of pseudomonas endophthalmitis associated with prosthetic intraocular lens implant. *Am J Ophthalmol* 1979; **88**: 902–8.

60 Boyaner D, Solomon LD. Ocular reaction to the use of wet-pack versus dry-pack intraocular lenses. *J Am Intraocul Implant Soc* 1980; **6**: 252–4.

61 Stark WJ, Rosenblum P, Maumenee AE, Cowan CL. Postoperative inflammatory reactions to

intraocular lenses sterilized with ethylene-oxide. *Ophthalmology* 1980; **87**: 385–9.

62 Meltzer DW. Sterile hypopyon following intraocular lens surgery. *Arch Ophthalmol* 1980; **98**: 100–4.

63 Ratner BD. Analysis of surface contaminants on intraocular lenses. *Arch Ophthalmol* 1983; **101**: 1434–8.

64 Bene C, Kranias G. Possible intraocular lens contamination by surgical glove powder. *Ophthal Surg* 1986; **17**: 290–1.

65 Richburg FA, Reidy JJ, Apple DJ, Olson RJ. Sterile hypopyon secondary to ultrasonic cleaning solution. *J Cataract Refract Surg* 1986; **12**: 248–51.

66 Parelman AG. Sterile uveitis and intraocular lens implantation. *J Am Intraocul Implant Soc* 1979; **5**: 301–6.

67 Apple DJ, Mamalis N, Steinmetz RL *et al.* Phaco-anaphylactic endophthalmitis associated with extracapsular cataract extraction and posterior chamber lens implantation. *Arch Ophthalmol* 1984; **102**: 1528–32.

68 Verhoeff FH, Lemoine AN. Endophthalmitis phaco-anaphylactica. *Am J Ophthalmol* 1922; **5**: 737–45.

69 Irvine SR, Irvine AR Jr. Lens-induced uveitis and glaucoma. Part I. Endophthalmitis phaco-anaphylactica. *Am J Ophthalmol* 1952; **35**: 177–86.

70 Rahi AHS, Garner A. The lens. In: Rahi AHS, Garner A, eds. *Immunopathology of the Eye*. Oxford: Blackwell Scientific Publications, 1976: 204–20.

71 Apple DJ, Rabb MF. *Ocular Pathology: Clinical Applications and Self-assessment*, 3rd edn. St Louis: CV Mosby, 1985: 138.

72 Schlaegel TF Jr. Uveitis following cataract surgery. In: Bellows JG, ed. *Cataract and Abnormalities of the Lens*. New York: Grune & Stratton, 1975; 429–34.

73 Emery JM, McIntyre DJ. *Extracapsular Cataract Surgery*. St Louis: CV Mosby, 1983: 337–58.

74 Smith RE, Weiner P. Unusual presentation of phaco-anaphylaxis following phacoemulsification. *Ophthal Surg* 1976; **7**: 65–8.

75 Ishikawa Y, Kawata K, Ishikawa Y. Three cases of endophthalmitis phaco-anaphylactica in the fellow eye after extracapsular lens extraction. *J Japan Contact Lens Soc* 1977; **23**: 1260–5.

76 Apple DJ, Mamalis N, Steinmetz RL *et al.* Phaco-anaphylactic endophthalmitis following ECCE and IOL implantation (Guest editorial). *J Am Intraocul Implant Soc* 1984; **10**: 423–4.

77 Wohl LG, Klein OR Jr, Lucier AC, Galman BD. Pseudophakic phacoanaphylactic endophthalmitis. *Ophthal Surg* 1986; **17**: 234–7.

78 Yanoff M, Fine BS. *Ocular Pathology: A Text and Atlas*, 3rd edn. Philadelphia: JB Lippincott, 1989: 71–4.

79 Riise P. Endophthalmitis phaco-anaphylactica and clinical ophthalmology. *Am J Ophthalmol* 1965; **60**: 911–15.

21: The Realities of Endophthalmitis

MICHAEL A. NOVAK & THOMAS A. RICE

Introduction

Infectious endophthalmitis is a dreaded and potentially catastrophic complication of intraocular surgery. It can occur following cataract extraction, glaucoma filtering procedures, penetrating keratoplasty, scleral buckling procedures, vitrectomy, pneumatic retinopexy, and repair of an eye sustaining penetrating trauma. Because cataract removal with intraocular lens implantation is by far the most common intraocular surgery performed, most cases of infectious endophthalmitis occur after this procedure. Advances in the treatment of endophthalmitis, including the use of diagnostic vitreous aspiration, intraocular antibiotics, and vitrectomy, usually eliminate the infection and sterilize the eye. Many eyes, however, have poor vision from the damage of the infection or the associated inflammation. Some aspects of the treatment of patients with endophthalmitis are controversial, including the choice of antibiotics and their route of administration; the use, timing, and route of administration of steroids; and the role of vitrectomy. This chapter presents an overview of these controversies and our guidelines for the management of postoperative endophthalmitis.

Incidence

The true incidence of endophthalmitis occurring after cataract surgery is difficult to determine from the series reported. In earlier series, cases were included in which endophthalmitis was diagnosed clinically but was not proven by culture of intraocular fluids. Such series tend to overestimate the true incidence of endophthalmitis because sterile inflammation can mimic infectious endophthalmitis. In contrast, other errors tend to underestimate the true incidence. If only intraocular culture-positive cases are included, some cases of endophthalmitis may be missed because of false-negative cultures, in part because some organisms are fastidious and difficult to culture. For example, the anaerobic bacteria *Propionibacterium acnes* does not grow unless anaerobic culture media are used. *Propionibacterium acnes* endophthalmitis may be misdiagnosed as presumed aseptic postoperative uveitis, iridocyclitis, or presumed lens-induced uveitis [1]. Another difficulty in accurately determining the incidence of endophthalmitis is that the incidence of endophthalmitis is so low that a large number of cataract extractions are necessary in a series to determine the incidence accurately.

In the past several decades, the incidence of postoperative infectious endophthalmitis has decreased. This has been attributed to improved sterile techniques, widespread use of the operating microscope for cataract extraction with the use of smaller synthetic sutures, better instrumentation for intraocular manipulation and wound closure, and the prophylactic and possibly therapeutic role of preoperative, intraoperative, and postoperative antibiotics.

The incidence of endophthalmitis occurring after cataract extraction has been reported to be in the range of 0.05 to 0.5% (or from 1 in 2000 to 1 in 200 cataract surgeries), but most series in developed countries seem to show an incidence of about 1 in 1000 cataract surgeries

Table 21.1 Incidence of endophthalmitis following cataract extraction

Period	Number of operations	Number of infections	Incidence of endophthalmitis (%)	Intraocular culture proven	Reference
1950–64	20 000	22	0.11	No	[4]
1964–73	16 000	9	0.056	Yes (4/9)	[5]
1957–72	77 093	382	0.5	No	[2]
1979–85	77 015	80	0.1	No	[3]
1965–75	3 864	8	0.21	No	[8]
1969–79	10 032	7	0.07	Yes	[6]
1976–82	12 800 (est.)	16	0.125	Yes	[7]

(Table 21.1). The largest series of postoperative endophthalmitis cases was reported by Christy and Lall [2]. Of 77 093 cataract extractions performed in Pakistan, 382 cases of endophthalmitis developed postoperatively, for an incidence of 0.5%. The high incidence of endophthalmitis in this report may be attributed to a number of factors, including poor nutrition and physical health of the patients, and a no-touch, gloveless surgical technique. Thirteen years later, Christy and Lall [3] reported a marked decrease in the incidence of endophthalmitis. In 77 015 cataract extractions, only 80 eyes (0.1%) developed postoperative endophthalmitis. This decline in the incidence of postoperative endophthalmitis was attributed to the use of either subconjunctival or retrobulbar prophylactic antibiotics.

Allen and Mangiaracine identified 22 cases of endophthalmitis in their first series [4] of 20 000 cataract extractions (0.11%), whereas they reported only nine cases in their second series [5] of 16 000 operations (0.056%). The cases of endophthalmitis were not culture-proven in the first series, and four of nine cases were culture-proven in the second series.

Berler [6] reported a similar incidence of 0.07%. In a series of 10 032 cataract extractions, seven patients developed culture-proven postoperative endophthalmitis. Bohigian and Olk [7] found 16 cases of culture-proven endophthalmitis in an estimated 12 800 cataract extractions, resulting in an incidence of 0.125%. Cameron and Forster [8] reported an incidence of postoperative endophthalmitis of 0.21% (eight cases of endophthalmitis following 3864 cataract extractions). However, no intraocular cultures were taken to confirm the diagnosis.

It is not fully known why the incidence of postoperative infectious endophthalmitis is not greater. The eye and ocular adnexa cannot be completely sterilized, and bacteria enter the eye during cataract surgery. The incidence of postoperative infection is lower after cataract surgery than after surgery on most other organs or other parts of the body. The anterior chamber resists an infectious microorganism although the vitreous is less resistant [9].

Etiology and microbiology

Infectious microorganisms can enter the eye during surgery when the eye is open, or postoperatively by passage of organisms through the unhealed cataract wound or other tract into the eye. Allen and Mangiaracine [4] have identified four potential sources of infection after cataract extraction:

1 from the skin in the operating field, lids, and lid margins; from the lacrimal sac, conjunctiva, and preocular tear film; or from the surgeon's gloves;

2 surgical instruments, intraocular lenses, and sutures;

3 solutions and medications, such as intraocular irrigating solutions; or

4 airborne contaminants, such as respiratory flora of the surgeon, assistants, or patient.

The most common source of infection is contamination from the patient's skin, preocular tear film, and ocular adnexa. Bacteria from the patient's lid margins, lashes, and lacrimal system, if the lacrimal system is partially

Table 21.2 Microbiology of endophthalmitis following cataract extraction

| | Organisms | | | | | | | | | | | | | | | | | |
| | Gram-positive | | | | | Gram-negative | | | | | | | | | | | | |
Period	Staph. epiderm.	Staph. aureus	Strep. spp.	Bacillus spp.	Prop. acnes	Proteus	Pseudo- monas	Serratia	H. influ- enzae	Entero- bacter	Other Gram(−)	Fungi	Other	Mixed	No growth	Total	Total culture positive	Reference
1969–75	4	1	1	0	1	3	1	0	1	0	0	0	0	0	0	12	12	[18]
1974–83	24	13	7	0	3	4	2	1	2	0	1	5	1	0	0	63	63	[21]
1976–81	11	8	0	0	0	0	2	2	0	2	0	0	6	3	3	37	34	[30]
1976–82	12	5	7	1	0	1	1	1	1	0	0	1	0	0	19	49	30	[7]
1977–80	10	2	0	0	0	1	1	1	0	0	0	0	2	0	0	17	17	[54]
1979–81	10	6	7	0	0	1	0	0	0	1	0	0	1	0	10	36	26	[49]
1981–84	16	8	2	0	0	1	0	0	0	0	0	0	0	3	0	30	30	[22]
Number of eyes	87	43	24	1	4	11	7	5	4	3	1	6	10	6	32	244	212	
% culture- positive eyes	41	20	11	0.5	2	5	3	2	2	1	0.5	3	5	3	—	—	100	

or completely obstructed, are an important source of infection. The normal preocular tear film has indigenous flora, and *Staphylococcus epidermidis* (*Staphylococcus* coagulase-negative), *Staphylococcus aureus* (*Staphylococcus* coagulase-positive), and *Streptococcus* spp. are commonly found. Gram-negative rods may be found in the preocular tear film of up to 10% of normal adults [10]. Prophylactic topical antibiotics can reduce the number of bacteria in the preocular tear film but can rarely sterilize it. Occasionally, medical personnel carrying pathogenic bacteria may be responsible for an epidemic of postoperative infectious endophthalmitis. Airborne pathogens from the surgeon's nose [4], operating room air, or the air-conditioning system may be a source of bacterial contamination. Other important sources of contamination are the solutions and medications irrigated into the anterior segment during surgery [11]. Endophthalmitis from contamination of the neutralizing solution (sodium bicarbonate), in which intraocular lens implants were once stored, has been eliminated by ethylene oxide sterilization of intraocular lenses [12]. Fungal endophthalmitis rarely develops in the early postoperative course, but when it does develop, it is usually a result of contaminated intraocular solutions, medications, or intraocular lenses.

The microorganism most commonly responsible for postoperative endophthalmitis is *Staphylococcus epidermidis* (Table 21.2). In the studies listed in Table 21.2, *Staph. epidermidis* was isolated in 41% of eyes. *Staphylococcus aureus* was the second most common isolate found in 20% of eyes. *Streptococcus* spp. were isolated in 11% of eyes. *Bacillus* spp. were cultured in 0.5% of eyes. *Propionibacterium*, a group of anaerobic Gram-positive bacilli commonly found in the flora of the conjunctiva, was cultured in 2%. Therefore, in the studies listed in Table 21.2, Gram-positive organisms were cultured from 75% of eyes with postoperative culture-positive endophthalmitis.

Gram-negative bacteria were responsible for 15% of the cases of endophthalmitis from the studies in Table 21.2. The most common Gram-negative bacteria was *Proteus* spp., which was cultured in 35% of cases of Gram-negative bacterial endophthalmitis, or 5% of all cases. *Pseudomonas* spp. were isolated in 22% of cases of Gram-negative bacterial endophthalmitis, or 3% of all cases. Other Gram-negative bacteria that were cultured include *Serratia* spp. and *Haemophilus influenzae*.

Fungi, which usually produce signs of infectious endophthalmitis that is delayed by weeks or months, accounted for only 3% of all cases of postoperative endophthalmitis (Table 21.2).

Late postoperative endophthalmitis can result from less virulent organisms or delayed inoculation. If less virulent organisms are introduced into the eye at the time of cataract extraction, a smoldering, indolent course of endophthalmitis may result. Such less virulent organisms include *Propionibacterium acnes*, *Corynebacterium* spp., *Actinomycetes* spp., and some fungi.

Delayed inoculation can result from:
1 dehiscence of the cataract wound [13];
2 suture abscess, which may communicate with the anterior chamber;
3 suture removal [13] in which the suture drags microorganisms through the suture tract and into the anterior chamber;
4 conjunctival filtering blebs, whether intentional (following glaucoma filtering procedures) or unintentional [14];
5 Nd:YAG laser posterior capsulotomy [15, 16], which may release into the vitreous low virulent bacteria, such as *Propionibacterium acnes*, that were sequestered in the capsular bag and inactive; and
6 vitreous wick syndrome [17] with direct communication between an exposed vitreous wick and the inside of the eye.

The microorganisms responsible for delayed inoculation are similar to those that are responsible for early postoperative endophthalmitis—*Staphylococcus* and *Streptococcus* spp., and, infrequently, Gram-negative rods. Postoperative endophthalmitis associated with an intentional or unintentional conjunctival filtering bleb may develop months or years after the initial surgery. In a series of 30 culture-proven cases, Mandelbaum *et al.* [14] isolated *Streptococcus* spp. in 57%, *Haemophilus influenzae* in 23%, and *Staphylococcus aureus* in 7% of cases.

In the studies listed in Table 21.2, 13% of all eyes had no microorganisms recovered from cultures. There are a number of possible explanations for negative culture results in patients with presumed infectious endophthalmitis. Prior topical, periocular, or systemic antibiotic treatment may prevent the growth of microorganisms from intraocular cultures. The intraocular specimen may be inadequate because of small sample volume, sampling of a sterile area of vitreous after infection has loculated to other areas, or failure to obtain a vitreous specimen. If the specimen is improperly handled, a negative culture may result. Transport media should not be used; rather, the culture media must be inoculated immediately. The appropriate culture media should be selected and must be maintained in the correct environment. As mentioned, anaerobic media are necessary to culture organisms such as *Propionibacterium acnes* [18]. Certain organisms are fastidious and difficult to grow despite proper media and techniques.

Signs and symptoms of endophthalmitis

The classic clinical features of a patient with endophthalmitis are a hypopyon (Fig. 21.1) and a significant vitreous inflammatory cellular response (Fig. 21.2) that often precludes a view of the retina. However, the appearance may range from a mild iritis or anterior uveitis to a fulminant suppurative process. The clinical presentation of endophthalmitis is determined by a variety of factors: (a) the infecting organism; (b) the relative severity of the infection; (c) duration of the infection before examination; (d) anatomic factors; (e) host immune status; and (f) previous antibiotic treatment.

The characteristic clinical features of postoperative infectious endophthalmitis typically appear within 24–72 h after surgery. However, these signs and symptoms may be delayed if the infecting organism is less virulent, or if postoperative antibiotics and/or steroids were administered. Although pain and decreasing vision are the most prominent initial symptoms, painless, culture-proven bacterial endophthalmitis is not rare [19]. Pain is especially

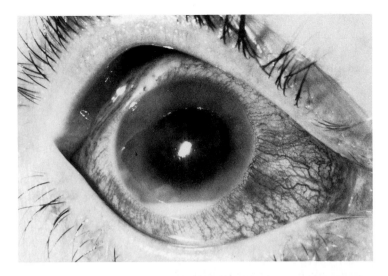

Fig. 21.1 Postoperative endophthalmitis due to *Staphylococcus epidermidis* following a phaco-emulsification procedure 2 days earlier. There is intense episcleral and conjunctival hyperemia, corneal edema, and a small hypopyon.

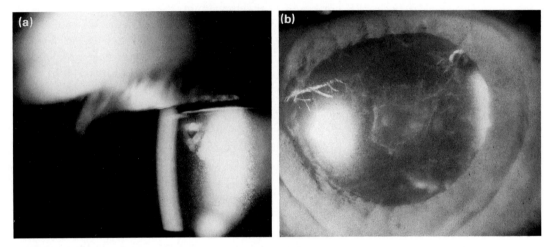

Fig. 21.2 Endophthalmitis due to *Staphylococcus epidermidis* following an uncomplicated extracapsular cataract extraction and posterior chamber intraocular lens implantation 6 days earlier. (a) There is intense vitreous inflammation with numerous inflammatory cells in the anterior vitreous, behind the intraocular lens.
(b) Moderate anterior chamber inflammation is present with fibrinous exudate on the anterior surface of the intraocular lens.

significant if it occurs after the usual postoperative pain has subsided and there has been a pain-free period. Other frequent findings are lid edema and erythema, episcleral and conjunctival hyperemia with chemosis, purulent discharge from the cataract wound, epithelial and/or stromal corneal edema, inflammatory anterior chamber reaction with fibrin (Fig. 21.2) and usually a hypopyon, and inflammatory cellular reaction in the vitreous, which may result in loss of the red fundus reflex. In a series of 28 cases of coagulase-negative staphylococcal endophthalmitis, there was an average delay of 7 days between surgery and the diagnosis [20]. Such organisms may produce a smoldering inflammatory reaction that may be difficult to differentiate initially from a sterile inflammatory reaction. The administration of postoperative subconjunctival and/or topical antibiotics and steroids may suppress the inflammatory component of the infection and temporarily reduce the severity of the signs and symptoms.

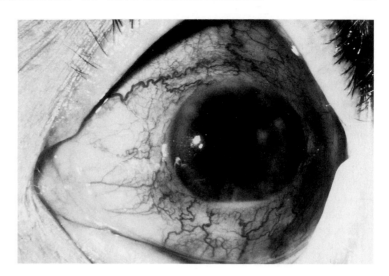

Fig. 21.3 Endophthalmitis due to *Candida parapsilosis* after an uncomplicated extracapsular cataract extraction and posterior chamber intraocular lens implantation 4 months earlier. There is mild conjunctival infection, a hypopyon, and white infiltrates adjacent to the iris and in the anterior vitreous.

In fungal endophthalmitis, the early postoperative course may be uneventful until 2 or more weeks after surgery. Fungal endophthalmitis is an indolent process with a quiet external ocular appearance compared with that of most types of bacterial endophthalmitis [12]. Characteristically, there is a smoldering inflammatory process with minimal pain, minimal or mild conjunctival hyperemia, transient hypopyon, and progressive iridocyclitis and vitritis, especially at the iris–pupillary border or in the anterior vitreous (Fig. 21.3). There may be progressive white infiltrates in the anterior vitreous or adherent to the iris or lens capsule that may produce only a reduction in vision. Delayed onset fungal endophthalmitis caused by intraocular irrigating solution contaminated by *Candida parapsilosis* has been reported in a series of 15 patients [11].

When postoperative endophthalmitis is identified weeks or months after surgery, the possibility of cataract wound dehiscence [13], conjunctival bleb formation [14], or cataract suture microabscess [13] must be considered. Driebe *et al.* [21] identified cataract wound abnormalities in 22% of 83 eyes with infectious endophthalmitis that developed after cataract extraction and intraocular lens implantation. These wound abnormalities consisted of (a) vitreous wicks; (b) wound leaks; (c) wound ruptures; (d) premature suture removal; (e) absorbable sutures that degraded more rapidly

than the wound healed, leading to wound dehiscence; (f) infected necrotic wound margins; and (g) inadvertent filtering bleb. In these patients, loose, untied, or broken sutures were common and may have contributed to endophthalmitis. In delayed onset endophthalmitis with a cataract wound abnormality, the organism presumably enters the eye sometime following surgery. If a wound abnormality is absent, a less pathogenic or virulent organism may have entered and inoculated the eye at the time of the initial operation.

Endophthalmitis in patients with an intentional or unintentional conjunctival bleb often is a virulent infection that produces sudden ocular pain and hyperemia of the conjunctiva and episclera. In a series of 36 patients with late onset endophthalmitis in patients with filtering blebs, endophthalmitis developed 4 months to 60 years after bleb formation [14]. The conjunctiva over these blebs appeared intact, although purulent exudate was visible in the blebs. Presumed conjunctivitis (five patients), upper respiratory infection (two patients), and contact lens wear (four patients) were associated with these late onset cases of endophthalmitis. Patients with a conjunctival filtering bleb who develop symptoms of ocular irritation or conjunctivitis must be examined immediately. If intraocular inflammation is not present, and if bacterial conjunctivitis is suspected, conjunctival cultures must be taken and treatment with topical antibiotics should be started. Four of five such patients developed endophthalmitis in spite of topical antibiotic treatment for presumed bacterial conjunctivitis [14].

Another cause of delayed onset postoperative endophthalmitis is the vitreous wick syndrome. Ruiz and Teeters [23] reported six cases of endophthalmitis occurring 2–4 weeks following cataract surgery with a fornix-based conjunctival flap. The endophthalmitis was believed to be caused by microscopic cataract wound breakdown resulting from overly tight corneoscleral sutures. Following the wound breakdown, there was vitreous prolapse onto the external surface of the eye. This vitreous wick permitted the bacteria from the conjunctiva to pass into the eye and produce endophthalmitis. Although in this series the cases presented with features of typical bacterial endophthalmitis, no intraocular cultures were obtained to confirm the diagnosis. Lindstrom and Doughman [17] described a case of culture-proven bacterial endophthalmitis, caused by a *Streptococcus* sp. and a coagulase-negative *Staphylococcus* sp., that developed 26 days after cataract extraction. When a careful examination of the anterior hyaloid and corneoscleral wound demonstrates a vitreous wick communicating with the external ocular surface, prompt surgical repair is needed before the onset of endophthalmitis [17,23].

Propionibacterium acnes, a Gram-positive, anaerobic bacillus found on conjunctiva and skin, is another cause of delayed onset postoperative endophthalmitis [1]. It may develop 2–10 months following extracapsular cataract extraction. In a compilation of 16 previously reported cases, Meisler and Mandelbaum [1] found the characteristic clinical presentation to include a chronic iridocyclitis with large granulomatous-appearing precipitates on the corneal endothelium and intraocular lens implant surfaces (five cases), hypopyon (10 cases), and a white plaque on the posterior capsule or intraocular lens implant (eight cases). Other characteristic features that may be found are vitritis, non-granulomatous uveitis, beaded fibrin strands in the anterior chamber, and diffuse intraretinal hemorrhages. The chronic and indolent intraocular inflammation usually intensified slowly over many months, even slower than the days or weeks found with most aerobic bacterial and fungal infectious endophthalmitis. *Propionibacterium acnes* endophthalmitis usually shows an improvement with corticosteroid treatment, especially in the early phases of inflammation. Some cases diagnosed previously as phacoanaphylactic endophthalmitis may actually have been *P. acnes* infections [1]. The tendency of the *P. acnes* organism to loculate within the capsular bag may alter the host response. Iridocyclitis or uveitis may flare up if there is intermittent release of sequestered bacteria either spontaneously or due to Nd:YAG laser posterior capsulotomy [15]. *Propionibacterium*-associated endophthalmitis should be considered in any eye with chronic uveitis following intraocular surgery.

Differential diagnosis

If the intraocular inflammation following cataract extraction is more severe than the usual mild or minimal inflammation seen, then infectious endophthalmitis must be suspected. The differential diagnosis of infectious endophthalmitis must include other causes of intraocular inflammation including vitreous loss, manipulation of vitreous, retained lens material, non-infectious toxic foreign matter introduced at the time of surgery, and incarceration of vitreous, iris, or lens material in the corneoscleral wound. Loose red blood cells or ghost red blood cells in the vitreous may also simulate inflammatory cells in the vitreous.

Sterile postoperative iridocyclitis is common. There is generally less hyperemia, swelling of the lids, and conjunctiva than in cases of infectious endophthalmitis. Also, there is usually no hypopyon or cellular reaction in the vitreous. Some eyes with severe sterile inflammation can develop hypopyon; however, endophthalmitis must always be ruled out by cultures of the aqueous and vitreous.

When there is significant retained cortical or nuclear lens material following cataract extraction, postoperative uveitis may develop and mimic endophthalmitis.

Phacoanaphylactic endophthalmitis is a

chronic, zonal granulomatous inflammation centered around lens material. It occurs after lens trauma or surgery as a result of auto-sensitization to lens proteins that previously were sequestered from the immune system [24]. Phacoanaphylactic endophthalmitis usually occurs within 2 weeks of cataract surgery or rupture of the lens capsule, but it can also develop several months after extracapsular cataract extraction [24]. The intraocular inflammation may range from a mild iritis with or without hypopyon to fulminant endophthalmitis. The duration of the latent period and the severity of the intraocular inflammation may have no relationship to the amount of residual lens material [24]. In contrast to bacterial endophthalmitis, chemosis, lid edema, and pain are usually not associated with phaco-anaphylactic endophthalmitis. Whereas treatment with steroids usually does not improve the signs and symptoms in acute bacterial endophthalmitis, such treatment usually improves the inflammation associated with phacoanaphylactic endophthalmitis.

Diagnostic technique

If infectious endophthalmitis is suspected, then aspiration of aqueous and vitreous specimens is necessary to establish fully the diagnosis, isolate the infecting microorganism, and perform sensitivity studies to allow the most effective antibiotic treatment. A vitreous specimen gives a higher proportion of positive culture results than does an anterior chamber specimen [25]. Animal models show that the anterior chamber is better able than the vitreous to resist infection, and this may explain this finding. In one study [26], 500 000 or more *Staphylococcus epidermidis* organisms or 2000 or more *Staphylococcus aureus* organisms injected into the anterior chamber of the rabbit produced endophthalmitis, but fewer organisms did not. In a study by Maylath and Leopold [9], only 700 *Staphylococcus aureus* organisms injected into the vitreous produced endophthalmitis. In contrast, in another study, Meredith *et al.* [27] injected up to 460 000 *Staphylococcus epidermidis* organisms into the vitreous cavity of rabbits. Although these less

virulent bacteria multiplied rapidly on the first day, it was unusual to recover bacteria after the third day, and the vitreous cavity became spontaneously sterilized without any antibiotic treatment. Although cultures of an aqueous specimen may not be positive as frequently as cultures of the vitreous, an aqueous culture may occasionally be positive when the vitreous culture is negative. In 51 cases of culture-proven endophthalmitis, Bohigian and Olk [7] identified two in which cultures of the aqueous were positive, but cultures of the vitreous were negative. Therefore, an aqueous specimen should be obtained in addition to the vitreous specimen unless the anterior chamber and vitreous cavity freely communicate.

Patients with suspected infectious endophthalmitis usually have intraocular specimens taken in the operating room, and this is mandatory if a cataract wound leak must be repaired or a vitrectomy is planned. Occasionally cultures of the anterior chamber and vitreous can be taken outside the operating room, at the slit-lamp, if only simple aspiration is required. This is followed by injection of intravitreal antibiotics immediately thereafter. If there are signs of external ocular infection, cultures of the eyelid and conjunctiva are taken before administration of an anesthetic and preparation of the eye for surgery. Usually the procedures are performed under local anesthesia with a retrobulbar block whether they are done in the clinic or in the operating room. General anesthesia is usually required only if there is a significant wound leak that must be repaired and there is a risk that retrobulbar hemorrhage from retrobulbar injection might cause expulsion of the intraocular contents through the open wound. If the cataract or corneoscleral wound demonstrates leakage, dehiscence, or a positive Seidel test preoperatively, the corneoscleral wound must be cultured, cleaned, and closed with interrupted monofilament nylon sutures before intraocular specimens are obtained. A 25, 26, or 27 gauge needle attached to a tuberculin syringe is inserted into the clear cornea near the limbus with the needle directed so it passes between the iris and the back of the cornea (Fig. 21.4). The authors prefer a 27 gauge needle to the larger diameter needles

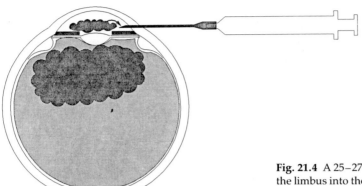

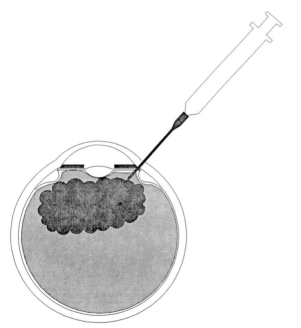

Fig. 21.4 A 25–27 gauge needle is inserted through the limbus into the anterior chamber and used to aspirate a fluid specimen into a tuberculin syringe.

Fig. 21.5 A 22–27 gauge needle is inserted through the limbus, through an iridectomy, and around an intraocular lens into the vitreous cavity. It is used to aspirate a fluid vitreous specimen into a tuberculin syringe.

ness keratotomy may allow easier insertion of the needle. Approximately 0.1 ml of aqueous is aspirated. Aspiration of more than 0.1 ml of aqueous should be avoided to prevent collapse of the anterior chamber, particularly in an eye in which this would result in touch of an intraocular lens to the corneal endothelium.

To obtain a vitreous specimen in an aphakic and in certain pseudophakic eyes, a 22–27 gauge needle attached to a tuberculin syringe is placed through the cornea at the limbus and through the pupil, going around the intraocular lens, or through the iridectomy into the vitreous (Fig. 21.5). Again, the authors prefer the smaller diameter needle. With only minimal manipulation of the needle and mild suction, 0.2–0.3 ml of liquid vitreous is aspirated into the syringe. Excessive suction is not used, because it may cause traction on the vitreous gel and creation of retinal breaks and detachment.

An alternative approach is to pass the needle through the pars plana (Fig. 21.6). A 22–27 gauge needle is placed through the pars plana, 3 mm posterior to the limbus, into the anterior vitreous. A partial-thickness pars plana sclerotomy may aid in placement of the needle through the sclera and pars plana. With careful manipulation of the needle, 0.2–0.3 ml of liquid vitreous is aspirated into the syringe. If resistance is met on application of mild suction, and an adequate vitreous specimen cannot be obtained, then the suction is released and the needle is carefully withdrawn from the eye.

A third technique, using a vitrectomy instrument, can be used in the operating room to

because there is less chance after removal of the needle of persistent leakage from the anterior chamber along the needle tract. An even smaller 30 gauge needle might be considered; however, this small size may be too small to allow aspiration of even the loose portions of a hypopyon. The bevel of the needle is directed anteriorly toward the cornea. A partial thick-

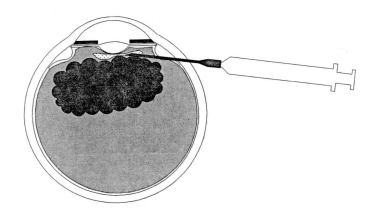

Fig. 21.6 A 22–27 gauge needle is inserted through the pars plana into the vitreous cavity and used to aspirate a fluid vitreous specimen into a tuberculin syringe.

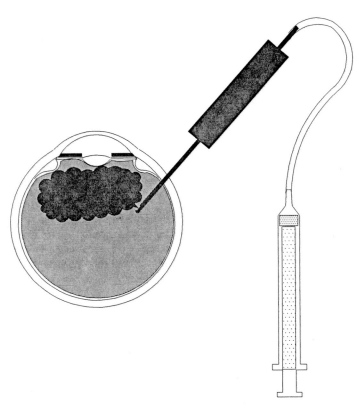

Fig. 21.7 A 20 gauge vitrectomy instrument is inserted through the pars plana into the vitreous. A tuberculin syringe is used to aspirate vitreous gel through tubing attached to the vitrectomy probe. The vitrectomy instrument is used to cut and aspirate the specimen.

obtain a vitreous specimen (Fig. 21.7). This can be done without first resorting to attempted aspiration of liquid vitreous with a needle, or it can be used if simple aspiration is tried and fails. A full-thickness pars plana sclerotomy is made 3 mm posterior to the limbus to accommodate a 20 gauge vitrectomy instrument. If a pars plana sclerotomy was performed earlier, the previous entry site can be enlarged to permit introduction of a 20 gauge vitrectomy cutter instrument. The collection tubing coming from the vitrectomy probe is cut approximately 5 cm (2 in) from the vitrectomy instrument, and the free end is attached to a blunt needle on a tuberculin syringe. The vitreous cutter is inserted through the pars plana sclerotomy and into the anterior vitreous. Using mild suction on the tuberculin syringe, and a rapid cutting rate (more than 400 cuts/min), the vitreous cutter is used to cut and aspirate 0.2–0.3 ml of vitreous gel into the syringe and tubing. While the vitrectomy instrument is in the anterior vitreous, vigorous suction and traction on the vitreous gel is avoided so as to minimize the risk of creating a retinal break. An infusion port and endoilluminator are not needed if vitreous surgery is not planned. This third technique can safely remove vitreous gel when liquid vitreous is unaccessible by simple aspiration.

A sterile plug is placed over the tip of each specimen-containing syringe, and the syringe is labeled. Once adequate specimens have been obtained, a more complete pars plana vitrectomy can be done if desired. After the specimens have been obtained and whatever vitreous surgery has been completed, broad-spectrum antibiotics are injected into the anterior vitreous, and the keratotomy and sclerotomy incisions are closed.

Within 30 min of being removed from the eye, the aqueous and vitreous specimens are inoculated onto fresh culture media: chocolate agar, liquid thioglycolate or other anaerobic media, and Sabouraud's agar. If adequate material is available, blood agar can also be inoculated. Ideally, the material to be cultured is plated on the media in the operating room. The chocolate agar, and blood agar if used, is kept at 37°C in carbon-dioxide-containing atmosphere. Anaerobic cultures are kept at 37°C in an anaerobic atmosphere. Sabouraud's agar is kept at 25°C. In cases of endophthalmitis that develop during the night or during the weekend when the proper culture media are not available, the aqueous and vitreous specimens can be injected into aerobic and anaerobic blood culture bottles [28]. For fungal isolation, Sabouraud's agar, or blood agar if Sabouraud's agar is unavailable, is inoculated and incubated at 25°C. Several drops of each specimen are placed on glass slides for Gram, Giemsa, and Grocott's methenamine silver stains. If the amount of specimen is inadequate to inoculate all required media, the first medium inoculated should be chocolate agar; the second, thioglycolate; and the third, Sabouraud's. All plates are observed daily and maintained for 10 days to rule out the presence of a slow-growing or fastidious organism.

Forster [29] defined a positive culture as growth of the same organism on two or more culture media, or semiconfluent growth on one or more solid media at the inoculation site. When there is growth only in one liquid culture medium, or scant growth on one solid medium, it was considered an equivocal positive culture [29]. Inoculation onto solid media is also desirable because a single contaminating bacteria can cause a positive culture in liquid media. In contrast, a contaminant on solid media may be a single colony, sometimes not even at the inoculation site.

Examination of the endophthalmitis patient

A careful measurement of visual acuity is important because it has been shown to be a prognostic factor in endophthalmitis cases. Bohigian and Olk [7] found that, when preoperative visual acuity was light perception, only 21% of eyes developed 20/400 or better vision. However, when initial visual acuity was 20/400 or better, 88% of eyes had final vision of 20/400 or better.

The anterior segment examination should be performed with a slit-lamp. The conjunctiva is evaluated to determine whether a bleb is present, and the cornea is carefully examined for stitch abscess or ring infiltrate. If the cornea is opacified, it will not be possible to perform vitrectomy, and the eye will have to be cultured by simple aspiration of fluid from the anterior chamber and vitreous. The cataract wound is examined to identify any wound dehiscence, wound leak, or vitreous wick, and to determine whether the corneoscleral wound is completely covered by conjunctiva. If an obvious wound dehiscence or wound leak is present clinically, then a Seidel test is not needed. Otherwise, a Seidel test is performed using either sterile 2% fluorescein or a sterile fluorescein strip. This is performed with and without light pressure, using a fingertip to apply pressure on the globe through the upper lid. The height of any hypopyon is determined. The examiner should also note whether iris details are visible. The presence and type of intraocular lens and the status of the posterior capsule is determined, and the intraocular pressure is measured in both eyes. Indirect ophthalmoscopy is performed to assess the presence of a red reflex and to determine the overall view of the fundus and vitreous, including both the posterior pole and the peripheral retina. Any vitreous opacification is noted. When ocular media opacities preclude ophthalmoscopic evaluation of the retina, then B-scan ultrasonography is performed to determine whether choroidal detachment and/or retinal detachment is present. If large choroidal detachments or retinal detachment is present, it may not be possible to perform vitreous surgery, and simple aspiration of the anterior chamber and vitreous is performed instead.

Treatment with antibiotics

Successful management of postoperative infectious endophthalmitis requires elimination of the infecting organism and control of the host inflammatory response before significant ocular tissue damage occurs. There is disagreement regarding the means to these goals. The indications for therapeutic vitrectomy and the use, timing, and route of administration of steroids remain controversial. However, the use of intravitreal antibiotics is now generally agreed to be essential to proper management.

Before the advent of intravitreal antibiotic treatment, the conventional routes of antibiotic administration were topical, subconjunctival, and intravenous. Most experimental animal and clinical studies have concluded that any regimen of antibiotic treatment that does not include intravitreal antibiotics is markedly less successful in sterilizing eyes with endophthalmitis. These routes of administration often do not produce sufficient levels of antibiotics in the vitreous to treat most infections adequately. From 1944 to 1966, nine reviews of 103 cases of endophthalmitis treated with intravenous, topical, and/or subconjunctival antibiotics without intravitreal antibiotics reported a final visual acuity of less than counting fingers in 73% of eyes [30]. In a study by Cameron and Forster [8], six of eight eyes (75%) with postoperative endophthalmitis had final visual acuity of hand motions or worse, and two of the eight eyes (25%) were eviscerated.

Better results were found by O'Day et al. [31] who used combined systemic antibiotic and steroid therapy to treat 18 consecutive cases of postoperative endophthalmitis caused by Staphylococcus epidermidis. Fourteen (78%) eyes achieved final visual acuity of 20/50 or better without intravitreal antibiotics or vitrectomy. These improved results can be attributed to the low virulence of the organism.

Because of the poor results with conventional antibiotic treatment, and the inability of the antibiotics to penetrate into the vitreous, some ophthalmic surgeons began direct injection of dilute concentrations of antibiotics into the vitreous. However, it was not until 1982 that there was a consensus that injection of intravitreal antibiotics was essential in the treatment of patients with bacterial endophthalmitis [32]. Such treatment produces immediate bactericidal intraocular levels of antibiotic to sensitive organisms. Experimental animal studies helped determine the maximal, nontoxic doses of intravitreal antibiotics and their clearance. From those studies doses for human use were established. The safe dose for intravitreal injection of gentamicin is 100–200 μg [33]; of cefazolin, 2.25 mg [34]; of vancomycin, 1 mg [35]; of tobramycin, 100 μg [36]; and of amikacin, 400 μg [37].

Generally, two different intravitreal antibiotic injections have been given in each case, one covering predominantly Gram-positive bacteria and one predominantly Gram-negative bacteria. Although cefazolin and gentamicin were the two intravitreal antibiotics most commonly used in recent years, there have been reports of endophthalmitis due to Streptococcus faecalis [14] and Staphylococcus epidermidis [38] resistant to these antibiotics. Antibiotics with an even broader spectrum of activity have been recommended. Intravitreal vancomycin given as a 1 mg dose is non-toxic and effective against many Gram-positive bacteria [35]. Intravitreal vancomycin combined with an aminoglycoside is now preferred (Table 21.3) [38]. Amikacin is active against certain Gram-negative bacilli that are resistant to other aminoglycosides [39]. It is one-fourth as toxic as gentamicin, and studies have shown no other aminoglycoside to be superior to amikacin, especially with

Table 21.3 Initial treatment of postoperative infectious endophthalmitis [65]

Antibiotics

Intravitreal antibiotics. Administer once only, unless clinical course or culture results dictate otherwise:
    Amikacin 0.4 mg/0.1 ml
    Vancomycin 1 mg/0.1 ml

Topical antibiotic drops. Alternate one drop of each every 4 h if no evidence of wound infection, stitch abscess, or corneal infection. If such an infection is present, alternate drops of each every hour:
    Amikacin 20 mg/ml
    Vancomycin 50 mg/ml

Subconjunctival antibiotics. Administer once only, unless clinical course or culture results dictate otherwise:
    Ceftazidime 100 mg/0.5 ml
    Vancomycin 25 mg/0.5 ml

Intravenous antibiotics. Administer for 5–14 days, unless clinical course or culture results dictate otherwise:
    Amikacin 7.5 mg/kg initial dose, followed by 6 mg/kg every 12 h (total 12 mg/kg per day) if renal function normal
    Ceftazidime 2 g initial dose, then every 8 h (1.5 g every 8 h if patient weighs less than 50 kg)

Steroids

Topical steroids. Administer 1 drop every 1–4 h for 5–21 days, unless clinical course or culture results dictate otherwise:
    Prednisolone acetate 1%

Subconjunctival steroids. Administer once only, unless clinical course or culture results dictate otherwise:
    Dexamethasone 6 mg

Oral steroids. Begin 1 day after surgery and administer for 5–14 days, unless clinical course or culture results dictate otherwise:
    Prednisone 30 mg twice a day

Others

Topical cycloplegics. Administer 1 drop 2–4 times daily:
    Atropine 1% or scopolamine 0.25%

Intravitreal antifungal agent. Administer if fungal endophthalmitis is strongly suspected clinically or from the results of fungal stains of the aqueous or vitreous. If clinical course and/or culture results confirm diagnosis, then topical, subconjunctival, and intravenous antibiotics may need to be changed:
    Amphotericin B 5 µg/0.1 ml

Consultation with infectious disease specialist

---

gentamicin-resistant organisms [40]. Therefore, vancomycin 1 mg and amikacin 400 µg, each in a volume of 0.1 ml and injected separately, are the initial intravitreal antibiotics of choice in postoperative bacterial endophthalmitis (Table 21.3) [41]. The antibiotics are injected into the anterior vitreous after diagnostic aspiration of the aqueous and vitreous and completion of any vitreous surgery.

Antibiotics for intravitreal administration should be prepared by the hospital pharmacist just prior to their use. This reduces the risk of dilutional errors that commonly occur if the antibiotics are mixed by non-pharmacists [42]. The intravitreal antibiotics are diluted with sterile normal saline without preservatives.

It is important to check that the antibiotics that are being injected are those diluted antibiotics prepared by the pharmacist. Inadvertent injection of undiluted antibiotics results in blindness. Each diluted antibiotic is then drawn into a labeled tuberculin syringe, and a new, 30 gauge needle is placed on the end of the syringe. The needle is then inserted through the pars plana, 3 mm posterior to the limbus, into the anterior vitreous cavity. Once the needle is visualized, and the bevel is directed away from the retina, the 0.1 ml volume of the antibiotic solution is slowly injected, and then the needle is withdrawn. Slow injection will minimize the jet-stream effect and prevent direct toxic or mechanical retinal damage. This is performed separately for the amikacin and the vancomycin, and these antibiotics are not mixed together before injection.

Although periocular antibiotic injections penetrate poorly into the vitreous, some produce high concentrations of antibiotic in the anterior segment. Subconjunctival antibiotics therefore may be of benefit, especially if there is cataract wound infection, cataract suture abscess, conjunctival bleb infection, or vitreous wick syndrome. Because of the high frequency with which coagulase-negative staphylococci are identified as the infectious organism, the use of subconjunctival vancomycin seems reasonable. Although 100 mg of vancomycin administered subconjunctivally was quite irritating in rabbit eyes [43], 25 mg of vancomycin given subconjunctivally is well tolerated in human eyes (Table 21.3), although it penetrates poorly into the vitreous.

Of the antibiotics with activity against Gram-negative bacteria, aminoglycosides and cephalosporins can be considered for subconjunctival injection. The third-generation cephalosporins, like ceftazidime, have been found to produce higher aqueous and vitreous concentrations than do the aminoglycosides [44]. Ceftazidime is more effective against Gram-negative bacteria, including *Pseudomonas aeruginosa*, than are other third-generation cephalosporins. Ceftazidime and vancomycin are therefore recommended for subconjunctival administration as part of the treatment for postoperative endophthalmitis (Table 21.3).

Although it is common to administer intravenous antibiotics as part of the treatment of endophthalmitis, Pavan and Brinser [45] reported excellent visual outcome in 16 eyes with culture-proven exogenous bacterial endophthalmitis treated with intravitreal and subconjunctival antibiotics alone. Fifteen eyes recovered a visual acuity of 20/400 or better, and 12 eyes achieved 20/80 or better vision. A National Institutes of Health study, the Endophthalmitis Vitrectomy Study, is examining whether intravenous antibiotics are necessary in the treatment of postoperative infectious endophthalmitis.

Although the vitreous concentration of antibiotics administered intravenously is far lower than the concentration produced by intravitreal injection, the use of intravenous antibiotics can still be considered. There is some intraocular penetration of intravenous antibiotics, and their use is part of the standard of care for the treatment of infectious endophthalmitis. In a study of inflamed rabbit eyes, cefazolin administered intravenously exceeded the minimum inhibitory concentration in the rabbit vitreous for cefazolin-sensitive bacteria [46]. Because of their spectrum of activity and their penetration into the vitreous, the third-generation cephalosporins are a useful adjunct to systemically administered amikacin. Ceftazidime penetrates the meninges of humans quite readily and is employed for periocular injection [47]. Ceftazidime and amikacin can be considered for intravenous administration for at least 5 days and up to 14 days as part of the treatment of postoperative bacterial endophthalmitis (Table 21.3). It is often possible to discontinue one of these antibiotics after the culture results and sensitivities are known.

It is also common to administer an aminoglycoside systemically. Amikacin is currently recommended because it has a broader spectrum of activity than does gentamicin. The systemic toxicity of amikacin is no greater than that of gentamicin or tobramycin. Careful monitoring of renal function, with measurements of serum creatinine every day or two and measurement of peak and trough serum aminoglycoside levels twice a week, is necessary to reduce the risk of toxicity. Consultation with an infectious disease specialist may also be helpful in avoiding toxicity and dealing with allergic reactions.

The value of topical antibiotics in the absence of corneal infection is uncertain. Topically applied antibiotics are unlikely to penetrate well into the vitreous. However, some penetration into the anterior chamber occurs. If there are signs of cataract wound infection, stitch abscess, or corneal infection, then "fortified" or concentrated topical antibiotics are more likely to be useful and should be administered every hour. If there is no evidence of such an infection, then the antibiotic drop should be given every 4 h. Because of their activity against Gram-positive cocci and Gram-negative rods, vancomycin and amikacin are the recommended topically applied antibiotics (Table 21.3).

If the culture result is positive and the organism is sensitive to both of the antibiotics used intravenously or topically, then one of two antibiotics, the one thought to be least effective, may be discontinued. If the bacteria is a virulent variety, such as *Pseudomonas aeruginosa* or *Streptococcus faecalis*, or the eye is not improving, then both antibiotics can be continued. If the organism is sensitive to only one antibiotic, then that one is continued and the other is stopped. If the organism is sensitive to neither antibiotic, then another antibiotic can be chosen based on bacterial antibiotic sensitivity testing.

Table 21.4 Results of treatment of postoperative culture-positive endophthalmitis via intraocular antibiotics alone

	Number of eyes	20/400 or better final vision % (no. of eyes)	20/20–20/40 final vision % (no. of eyes)	20/50–20/100 final vision % (no. of eyes)	20/200–20/400 final vision % (no. of eyes)	Reference
	14	57 (8)	14 (2)	14 (2)	29 (4)	[25]
	12	83 (10)	25 (3)	50 (6)	8 (1)	[48]
	10	80 (8)	50 (5)	10 (1)	20 (2)	[49]
	16	94 (15)	31 (5)	38 (6)	25 (4)	[21]
Total	52	79 (41)	29 (15)	29 (15)	21 (11)	

In addition to the above topically administered medications, a topical cycloplegic and steroid are recommended (Table 21.3). Either atropine 1% or scopolamine 0.25% may be employed as a topical cycloplegic. Prednisolone acetate 1% can be administered every 1–2 h.

The role of systemic or intravitreal steroids in the management of patients with postoperative infectious endophthalmitis is controversial. Although some ophthalmologists do not use steroids at all, many use systemic steroids to control the inflammatory damage produced by infection, and some even inject steroids into the vitreous following intravitreal antibiotic injection. Intravitreal injection of steroids may be dangerous, however, because commercially available preparations contain toxic preservatives. Because systemic use is probably beneficial, we begin oral prednisone, 30 mg twice per day, on the day after surgery and continue it for at least 5 days following surgery. Because of possible gastric upset or peptic ulceration from oral steroids, antacids or histamine H_2-receptor antagonists may be given concomitantly. If fungal endophthalmitis is suspected, then steroids by any route should be avoided.

Results of intraocular antibiotic treatment

The visual results following treatment of postoperative infectious endophthalmitis with intravitreal antibiotics are superior to those achieved without their use. In a study of eyes given conventional treatment, 73% had final visual acuity of less than counting fingers [30]. In contrast, of eyes treated with intraocular antibiotics, 79% had a final visual acuity of 20/400 or better (Table 21.4). Despite the fact that these were different studies, the large difference in results suggests that treatment with intravitreal antibiotics is beneficial.

Forster et al. [25] reported a series of 140 eyes with suspected infectious endophthalmitis following ocular surgery, penetrating trauma, or associated with conjunctival bleb or a metastatic endogenous source. Of those 140 eyes, 78 (56%) yielded positive cultures from aqueous or vitreous specimens. Fourteen of those culture-positive eyes were treated with intraocular antibiotics without vitrectomy. Eight of 14 eyes (57%) recovered 20/400 or better final visual acuity. Of those eight eyes, two had 20/20 to 20/40 vision, and two had 20/50 to 20/100 vision.

Diamond [48] studied 26 eyes with culture-positive endophthalmitis. Twelve of those eyes had prior ocular surgery, and endophthalmitis had been diagnosed less than 72 h after the onset of infection. These eyes received intravitreal antibiotics but did not have vitrectomy. Ten of the 12 eyes (83%) had final visual acuity of 20/400 or better. The other two eyes had central retinal vein occlusion and inoperable retinal detachment.

In a retrospective study by Olsen et al. [49] of 40 cases of postoperative endophthalmitis, cultures were positive in 29 eyes (72%). Ten of these eyes were treated with intraocular antibiotics with no vitrectomy. Of these 10 eyes, eight (80%) had final visual acuity of 20/400 or better. Six of these eyes (75%) had 20/50 or better final vision. Thirteen of the 29 eyes had what was judged to be a poor clinical response to initial treatment. These eyes had a repeat intraocular culture taken at the same time as a repeat intraocular antibiotic injection was given, between 24 and 72 h after initial aspiration of aqueous and vitreous and intraocular antibiotic injection. The choice of the antibiotic injected was determined by the sensitivity of the organism isolated. All 13 repeat cultures had no growth, indicating that the initial intravitreal injection had probably sterilized the eye and that the poor clinical response was probably from persistent sterile inflammation.

Driebe et al. [21] reported a series of 62 eyes with culture-positive endophthalmitis following cataract extraction with intraocular lens implantation. Sixteen of those eyes were treated with intraocular antibiotics alone. Fifteen of 16 eyes (94%) had final visual acuity of 20/400 or better.

In a retrospective study of 26 patients with postoperative bacterial endophthalmitis, Stern et al. [50] identified seven culture-positive cases in which a single injection of intravitreal antibiotics had been given. Five of the seven patients (71%) developed recurrence of the infection or failed to respond to treatment. Two of four patients infected with Staphylococcus epidermidis and treated initially with a single intravitreal injection of antibiotics without vitrectomy were not cured. However, all six patients infected with Staphylococcus epidermidis and treated with multiple antibiotic intravitreal injections and/or vitrectomy were successfully managed and recovered useful vision. Similar results were affirmed when patients were infected with other organisms. Recurrent infections developed in four of nine patients infected with other organisms. Of these four, three were treated with a single intravitreal antibiotic injection without vitrectomy. Four of five patients receiving multiple intravitreal injections of antibiotics and/or vitrectomy were successfully treated. This study suggested that more aggressive management, such as multiple intravitreal injections of antibiotics and/or vitrectomy, must be considered, especially when the causative organism is highly virulent. The high frequency of persistent infection after

one intravitreal antibiotic injection is at odds, however, with the experience of most clinicians treating endophthalmitis, although it is not uncommon to see signs such as increasing hypopyon height from sterile inflammation. Furthermore, repeated intravitreal antibiotic injections may substantially increase the risk of toxic effects of the antibiotics [41]. When there are clinical signs of worsening, the ophthalmic surgeon can consider repeating the cultures from the anterior chamber and vitreous and reinjecting antibiotics only if the cultures are positive. Unfortunately, this method of management would delay retreatment, and it is not fully known whether such a delay is advisable. This depends mainly on what percentage of eyes that show signs of worsening, such as increased hypopyon, truly continue to be infected.

Although there are no studies establishing the safety of multiple intravitreal antibiotic injections, Forster et al. [25] recommend that, for culture-positive eyes, repeat intravitreal antibiotic injections be considered at 48 and 96 h after the initial injection. Gentamicin could not be consistently found, 48 h after intravitreal injection, in the vitreous of patients with endophthalmitis [51]. Based on these studies, Cobo and Forster [51] have suggested that, when clinically indicated, intravitreal antibiotics be reinjected between 36 and 48 h after the initial intravitreal injection. Repeat intravitreal antibiotic injections in an eye with culture-positive endophthalmitis may be indicated at 48 and/or 96 h following initial antibiotic injection if there are signs of worsening such as increasing hypopyon height, increasing opacity of the vitreous, or development of corneal ring infiltrate. If bacterial sensitivity studies have shown resistance to the antibiotics previously used and the eye is not improving, a different appropriate intravitreal antibiotic should be injected to treat the offending organism. The choice of the intravitreal antibiotic should be based on the bacterial antibiotic sensitivity studies of the organisms. Repeat reinjection probably should not be given just because a virulent organism has been isolated from the original culture(s) unless there are clinical signs of worsening. Repeat intravitreal antibiotic injections may be performed, with topical anesthesia, at the bedside, in the minor surgery room, at the slit-lamp, or in the operating room, depending on the cooperation of the patient.

Treatment with antibiotics and vitrectomy

The role of vitrectomy in the management of patients with postoperative infectious endophthalmitis is controversial. There are several theoretic advantages to its use in patients with endophthalmitis. Vitrectomy may be analogous to drainage of an abscess elsewhere in the body. Vitreous surgery permits bulk removal of the offending organisms and their toxins, inflammatory debris, and vitreous opacities. It might allow for better dispersion of intravitreal antibiotics in a fluid space. However, there is no evidence that antibiotics injected into an eye that has not had vitrectomy fail to disperse. Finally, in eyes in which an adequate vitreous specimen cannot be obtained with vitreous aspiration, vitrectomy allows a means of obtaining an adequate specimen for culture, which is a crucial step in properly managing endophthalmitis. Vitreous surgery, however, is more complex and potentially more hazardous than is simple aspiration or biopsy of fluid from the eye.

Although the timing and role of vitrectomy in the management of patients with endophthalmitis are not fully proven, one study advocates that vitrectomy should be considered in the following situations [52]:

1 severe cases, in which initial examination demonstrates profound visual loss to light perception or no light perception, presence of an afferent pupillary defect, corneal ring infiltrate, or loss of red reflex;

2 eyes with severe vitreous opacities that are sufficiently dense to preclude visualization of retinal vessels by indirect ophthalmoscopy, or eyes with moderately dense vitreous opacities on ultrasound examination;

3 eyes from which Gram-negative rods are cultured or from which virulent organisms are cultured from the aqueous or vitreous aspirate, when the clinical status of the patient is not improving;

4 eyes in which fungal endophthalmitis is suspected; and

5 patients whose clinical condition is deteriorating despite the use of appropriate topical, periocular, intravitreal, and intravenous antibiotics.

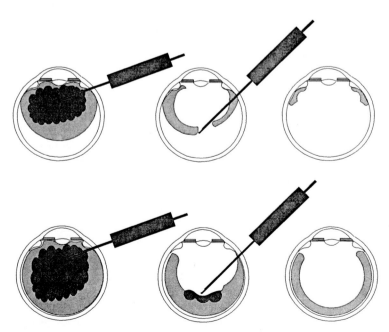

Fig. 21.8 A vitrectomy is performed with a 20 gauge vitrectomy instrument to remove infected vitreous gel in an eye with endophthalmitis. Top row: all the vitreous gel except the peripheral anterior vitreous is removed in an eye with a pre-existing posterior vitreous separation. Bottom row: only the core vitreous is removed in an eye with no posterior vitreous separation.

Table 21.5 Results of treatment of postoperative culture-positive endophthalmitis with intraocular antibiotics and vitrectomy

	Number of eyes	20/400 or better final vision % (no. of eyes)	20/20–20/40 final vision % (no. of eyes)	20/50–20/100 final vision % (no. of eyes)	20/200–20/400 final vision % (no. of eyes)	Reference
	14*	64 (9)	29 (4)	21 (3)	14 (2)	[48]
	11	36 (4)	0 (0)	18 (2)	18 (2)	[54]
	34	50 (17)	9 (3)	21 (7)	21 (7)	[21]
Total	59	51 (30)	12 (7)	20 (12)	19 (11)	

* Includes cases of endophthalmitis following ocular trauma.

The authors recommend vitrectomy in eyes suspected of having fungal endophthalmitis and eyes that are worsening that have only had a vitreous tap or biopsy previously. Vitreous surgery or tap can be considered in the other suggested situations as enumerated above, although there is no evidence that it is superior to a simple tap. Biopsy or tap rather than vitrectomy should be done in eyes with severe corneal opacity that precludes vitreous surgery. Vitrectomy for eyes with endophthalmitis has been performed through a limbal route in aphakic eyes, but this is difficult in eyes with intraocular lenses. We recommend a pars plana approach for all eyes suspected of having endophthalmitis (Fig. 21.8). The main objectives are to excise the central vitreous gel, remove inflammatory debris, and create a fluid space. No effort is made to separate the posterior cortical vitreous from the retina if a posterior vitreous separation is not present. Inflammatory debris may create adhesions between the posterior vitreous surface and the inner retina. Since the retina may be weakened by damage from bacterial toxins and lysosomes from inflammatory cells, separation of the vitreous from the retina may result in retinal tears or bleeding.

Vitrectomy is performed only after specimens from the anterior chamber and the vitreous have been taken for culture and staining. In many cases it is also necessary to first remove opacities from the anterior chamber before vitrectomy can be done. Following the vitrectomy, antibiotics are injected slowly into the anterior vitreous cavity, with the bevel of the needle directed away from the posterior retina, as described earlier.

Most studies of eyes with postoperative infectious endophthalmitis report that the response to treatment and the final visual acuity are not dependent on the removal or retention of an intraocular lens [53]. In the series reported by Driebe et al. [21], only one of 57 eyes with bacterial endophthalmitis could not be sterilized while the intraocular lens was retained. Therefore, the intraocular lens may be left in place in most cases.

Results of treatment with intraocular antibiotics and vitrectomy (Table 21.5)

In reviewing the reports of visual results in patients who had vitrectomy in addition to the injection of antibiotics into the vitreous for the management of infectious endophthalmitis, it is important to remember that most eyes selected for vitrectomy, as compared with those managed with a tap, are those with a worse clinical presentation. Therefore, in these non-randomized retrospective studies, the final visual results from eyes receiving a tap and injection of intraocular antibiotics alone cannot be compared with those from eyes that underwent vitrectomy and intraocular injection of antibiotics. There is a selection bias, with the worst cases undergoing vitrectomy. The Endophthalmitis Vitrectomy Study is the first randomized, controlled clinical trial that will determine the role of vitrectomy in the management of patients with postoperative infectious endophthalmitis.

Of Diamond's 26 patients with culture-positive endophthalmitis, 14 had pars plana vitrectomy [48]. The eyes undergoing vitrectomy had the worst prognosis, with late diagnosis, trauma-related endophthalmitis, and/or organized vitreous opacities on ultrasound examination. In the eyes receiving intraocular antibiotics alone, the diagnosis was confirmed within 72 h from the onset of the infection, endophthalmitis was the result of surgery, and it was caused by less virulent organisms. Final visual acuity of 20/400 or better was found in 64% of the eyes undergoing vitrectomy.

In a retrospective series by Puliafito et al. [54] of 36 patients with infectious endophthalmitis, one-half of the patients were treated with both vitrectomy and intraocular antibiotics. Of these 18 patients, 11 developed endophthalmitis after cataract extraction. Of these 11 eyes, 36% had no light perception, 36% had visual acuity of 20/400 or better, and 18% had visual acuity of 20/100 or better. When the vitrectomy was performed within 24 h of the clinical appearance of endophthalmitis, 25% of eyes had no light perception. However, when vitrectomy was not done until after the first 24 h, 70% of eyes had no light perception.

Driebe et al. [21] reviewed 83 cases of pseudophakic endophthalmitis and a therapeutic vitrectomy was performed in 46 eyes (55%). Vitrectomy was performed in those eyes with more aggressive infections and severe, rapidly progressive intraocular inflammation. Of the 34 culture-positive eyes that underwent vitrectomy without removal of the intraocular lens, 29% of the eyes had no light perception, 50% had 20/400 or better vision, and 29% had 20/100 or better vision.

There are risks associated with pars plana vitrectomy, and these must be balanced against the potential benefits in each patient. Vitrectomy may be a difficult procedure in an eye with a hazy or edematous cornea, or with fibrin in the anterior chamber or on the iris or intraocular lens. Olsen et al. [49] reported rhegmatogenous retinal detachments in three of 22 eyes (14%) that had undergone vitrectomy and one of 18 eyes (6%) that had received intraocular antibiotic injection alone

for postoperative infectious endophthalmitis. Nelsen et al. [55] confirmed these findings. They reviewed the case histories of 55 consecutive patients with a clinical diagnosis of bacterial endophthalmitis. However, in only 30 patients were the cultures positive. All patients had received systemic, periocular, topical, and intravitreal antibiotics. Of the 55 patients, 33 also underwent pars plana vitrectomy. Of the 55 patients, nine (16%) developed rhegmatogenous retinal detachments within 6 months of the initial diagnosis. Nelsen et al. [55] hyopthesized that the higher frequency of retinal detachment in the patients undergoing vitrectomy (21%) as compared with those not receiving vitrectomy (9%) could be explained by the surgical complications and the increased severity of the endophthalmitis in the vitrectomy group. Two patients developed retinal detachments during the vitrectomy procedure, and these eyes rapidly progressed to no light preception. Furthermore, simple aspirations of fluid and injections of intravitreal antibiotics in certain instances can be done sooner than vitreous surgery, and therefore treatment for this rapidly progressive infection can sometimes be initiated more quickly than vitreous surgery.

In a retrospective study of 82 eyes with endophthalmitis, Bohigian and Olk [7] identified three prognostic factors associated with a poor final visual result, defined as a visual acuity of less than 20/400. These factors were (a) poor initial visual acuity of less than 20/400; (b) a positive intraocular culture; and (c) identification by intraocular culture of a virulent organism, which was defined as any organism other than *Staphylococcus epidermidis*. However, two of the 16 patients with *Staphylococcus epidermidis* endophthalmitis had poor final visual acuity, one with light perception vision and the other with count-fingers vision.

Prophylaxis (Table 21.6)

Because infectious endophthalmitis can produce severe visual loss in spite of adequate treatment, all possible means of prevention must be considered. These include careful preoperative examination, preoperative cul-

Table 21.6 Antibiotics in the treatment of infectious endophthalmitis

Antibiotic	Topical	Subconjunctival	Intravitreal (per 0.1 ml)	Systemic (intravenous)*
Amikacin	20 mg/ml	20 mg	0.4 mg	7.5 mg/kg initially, 6 mg/kg every 12 h
Amphotericin B	2–5 mg/ml	0.5–2 mg	0.005–0.01 mg	0.25–0.6 mg/kg per day in 1 dose
Ampicillin	—	100 mg	0.5 mg	2 g every 4 h (200 mg/kg per day)
Bacitracin	10 000 U/ml	10 000 U	—	—
Carbenicillin	4 mg/ml	100 mg	0.25–2 mg	2–6 g every 4 h
Cefazolin	50 mg/ml	100–125 mg	2.25 mg	1–1.5 g every 6 h
Ceftazidime	—	100 mg	—	2 g every 8 h (1.5 g every 8 h if <50 kg)
Cephalothin	50 mg/ml	50–100 mg	—	1–2 g every 4 h
Chloramphenicol	5 mg/ml	1–2 mg	2 mg	50 mg/kg per day in 4 doses
Clindamycin	50 mg/ml	75 mg	1 mg	0.3–1.2 g every 6 h (40 mg/kg per day)
Colistin	5–10 mg/ml	15–37.5 mg	—	5 mg/kg per day in 4 doses
Erythromycin	50 mg/ml	100 mg	0.5 mg	1 g every 6 h
Flucytosine	10 mg/ml	—	—	oral: 50–150 mg/kg per day in 4 doses
Gentamicin	8–15 mg/ml	20–40 mg	0.1–0.2 mg	1–1.7 mg/kg every 8 h (3–5 mg/kg per day)
Ketoconazole	—	—	—	oral: 200–400 mg per day in 1 dose
Lincomycin	—	150 mg	1.5 mg	600 mg every 8 h
Methicillin	—	20–100 mg	2 mg	1–2 g every 4 h (200 mg/kg per day)
Miconazole	10 mg/ml	5 mg	0.025 mg	200–1200 mg every 8 h (20–40 mg/kg per day)
Natamycin	50 mg/ml	—	0.025 mg	—
Neomycin	5–8 mg/ml	250–500 mg	—	—
Nystatin	100 000 U/g (ointment)	50 000 U	—	—
Penicillin G	100 000 U/ml	500 000 U	—	2–6 M u every 4 h
Polymyxin B	16 250 U/ml	10 mg	—	—
Streptomycin	—	50–100 mg	—	0.5–1 g every 12 h (20–30 mg/kg per day)
Sulfacetamide	100–300 mg/ml	—	—	—
Tobramycin	14 mg/ml	20 mg	0.1–0.2 mg	3–5 mg/kg per day in 3 doses
Vancomycin	50 mg/ml	25 mg	1 mg	1 g every 12 h

* Dosage in adults with normal renal function
The authors have made every effort to ensure that the drug dosage schedules are accurate and in accord with the standards accepted at the time of publication. Readers are advised to check the product information sheet included in the package of each drug they plan to administer to be certain that changes have not been made in the recommended dose or in the contraindications for administration. This is of particular importance in regard to new or infrequently used drugs.

tures, preoperative topical antibiotics, chemical and mechanical preparation of the eye prior to surgery, and subconjunctival antibiotics at the time of surgery.

The most important step in the prevention of infectious postoperative endophthalmitis is careful preoperative examination. The patient must be in the best possible physical condition. Diabetes should be well controlled, and respiratory and skin infections must be eliminated. Patients with diabetes and/or peripheral vascular disease should be carefully examined for infected or gangrenous toes and feet. The facial skin, ocular adnexae including lids and lacrimal apparatus, and ocular surface should be examined carefully to avoid operating in the presence of chronic blepharitis, bacterial conjunctivitis, or dacryocystitis.

Routine preoperative cultures are probably of no value unless there are signs of infection of the lids, conjunctiva, or lacrimal apparatus. Allansmith et al. [56] obtained weekly cultures of the conjunctiva and lid margins of normal high school students to study the natural history of the ocular flora, especially Staphylococcus aureus. There was a 21% chance that Staphylococcus aureus would be present on the lid margin at any given time, regardless of previous negative cultures. Likewise, routine cultures taken several days before cataract surgery do not indicate the type or quantity of bacteria present at the time of the surgery. In another study, Allansmith et al. [56] found that, if a culture was taken 7 days before surgery and was positive for *Staphylococcus aureus*, the untreated patient had a 43% chance of having the bacteria on the lids on the day of surgery. If the culture was negative, there was a 24% chance of having the organism on the lids on the day of surgery. If the culture was negative for *Staphylococcus aureus* on the day before surgery, there was a 20% chance that the bacteria would be present on the lids on the day of surgery. The routine use of preoperative cultures of the conjunctiva or lids is therefore not practical or cost effective.

Preoperative cultures, however, should be performed if there are clinical signs of a conjunctival, skin, or ocular adnexal infection, if the patient wears an extended wear contact lens, if the fellow eye is phthisical, or if an ocular prosthesis is present in the fellow orbit [57]. A cotton applicator moistened with a nutrient liquid medium, such as trypsinase soy broth, should be rubbed on the conjunctiva and lid margins. A blood agar plate can be inoculated and maintained at 37°C. The culture will identify and quantitate the organisms present and permit selection of appropriate antibiotics. If there are symptoms or signs of nasolacrimal duct obstruction, then pressure should be applied over the lacrimal sac to obtain reflux of mucopurulent material through the punctum. Any reflux should be cultured, and appropriate systemic antibiotics should be started. Further treatment, including nasolacrimal duct probing or dacryocystorhinostomy, may be needed.

Topical antibiotics given preoperatively for a short period of time reduce the number of lid and conjunctival bacteria, compared with untreated controls. Burns *et al.* [58] have reported several randomized, controlled, double-blind clinical studies in which patients were randomly allocated to different treatment groups. In one study, preoperative bacterial cultures of the lower palpebral conjunctiva, lower lid, and inner canthus were obtained from 66 patients who were to undergo cataract extraction. Following surgery, the control eyes received lubricating ointment, while the treated patients received either neomycin ointment 0.5% or gentamicin ointment 0.3% for 5 days at the time of the daily dressing change. Cultures were taken again on the fifth postoperative day. Of the 18 control eyes, two (11%) eyes showed a decrease in the bacterial count, while the remaining eyes showed an increase. The eyes treated with neomycin or gentamicin ointment showed a reduction of bacterial count to 48% and 86%, respectively. This study demonstrated the effectiveness of both antibiotics over the control, and the superiority of gentamicin over neomycin.

In a similar study, Burns and Oden [59] found gentamicin 0.3% drops to be more effective than chloramphenicol 0.5% drops in reducing bacterial counts of *Staphylococcus epidermidis*, which is the most common cause of postoperative infectious endophthalmitis (see Table 21.2).

In another study, Burns [60] compared the effects of gentamicin 0.3% drops, gentamicin 0.3% ointment, sulfacetamide 30% drops, neomycin–polymixin B–gramicidin drops, and chloramphenicol 1% ointment on the preoperative and postoperative bacterial counts from cultures of the lower palpebral conjunctiva, lower lid margin, and the inner canthus. Gentamicin was found to be the most effective in reducing the bacterial count postoperatively.

Fahmy [61] studied the effectiveness of six different antibiotics in eradicating bacteria on the conjunctiva in 60 patients before cataract extraction. The antibiotics evaluated were chloramphenicol 0.5% drops; gentamicin 0.3% drops; oxytetracycline 3%–polymixin B 0.1% ointment; sulfamethizole 4% drops; bacitracin 1%–neomycin 0.5% drops; and ristocetin 0.5%–polymixin B 0.25% drops. Each drug was applied five times beginning shortly after admission, or 18 h before cataract surgery, and stopping at bedtime. Gentamicin 0.3% drops eliminated 21 of 22 bacteria isolated prior to surgery in nine of 10 eyes and was the most effective antibiotic.

Topical antibiotics administered for a short period prior to cataract surgery reduced the number of lid and conjunctival bacteria compared with untreated controls. The degree to which the bacterial flora will be reduced depends on the antibiotic and on the frequency and duration of its administration. An antibiotic with a broad-spectrum of activity is preferred, and gentamicin has been found to be most effective in reducing bacterial counts in these studies.

Allen and Mangiaracine [4,5] reported the efficacy of topical antibiotics in the prevention of endophthalmitis in an uncontrolled retrospective study. In their initial series of 660 patients undergoing cataract extraction without the use of preoperative topical antibiotics, endophthalmitis developed in five eyes (0.76%) [4]. Among 19 340 patients who received a variety of topical antibiotics hourly for 5 h, and an ointment at bedtime, prior to cataract extraction, only 12 developed endophthalmitis (0.062%). This suggests that the use of prophylactic antibiotics reduces the incidence of endophthalmitis. In their second series, two combinations of antibiotics were evaluated, neomycin 0.5%–polymixin B 0.1% drops, and chloramphenicol 0.4%–polymixin B 0.1% drops. These were administered hourly during the afternoon and evening before cataract surgery. Erythromycin ointment 0.5% was applied to all eyes at bedtime prior to surgery. Of the 1000 patients receiving the neomycin treatment, six cases of endophthalmitis (0.6%) developed during the postoperative period. However, in the 15 000 patients receiving chloramphenicol, presumed infectious endophthalmitis developed in three eyes (0.02%).

Currently, the recommended treatment is gentamicin sulfate 3 mg/ml or tobramycin 3 mg/ml at hourly intervals for 5–6 h the evening before and the morning of the cataract surgery. Gentamicin ointment 3 mg/g or tobramycin ointment 3 mg/g may be given at bedtime, the night before surgery. In eyes with blepharoconjunctivitis or blepharitis, lid and conjunctival cultures should be obtained from both eyes. Antibiotic selection is determined by the results of the cultures, and the topical antibiotics should be continued for 5–7 days in both eyes. Lid scrubs with an antibiotic ointment may also be valuable in such cases.

Most cases of endophthalmitis probably originate from contamination of the anterior chamber and/or vitreous with organisms of sufficient quantity to overcome the natural resistance of the host to infection. Therefore, the critical time to establish bactericidal levels of prophylactic antibiotics is either during or at the completion of cataract surgery. The purpose of subconjunctival antibiotics given immediately at the conclusion of cataract surgery is to inhibit the growth of bacteria inadvertently introduced into the eye or on the wound margin during the operation. To inhibit bacterial growth, subconjunctival antibiotics must produce bactericidal levels in the early postoperative period.

Christy and Sommer [62] studied 6618 patients who underwent cataract extraction and were randomized in a masked trial to either preoperative topical antibiotics alone or topical antibiotics and subconjunctival antibiotics at the time of surgery. The topical antibiotics were chloramphenicol and sulfadimidine. Penicillin (500 000 U) was given subconjunctivally at the time of surgery to the treatment group. Of the 3309 patients receiving topical antibiotics alone, 0.5% developed postoperative endophthalmitis, which was not culture-proven. Of the 3309 patients receiving both topical and subconjunctival antibiotics, 0.15% developed postoperative endophthalmitis. Another group of 21 829 patients received both preoperative topical antibiotics and subconjunctival antibiotics at the time of cataract surgery. The incidence of endophthalmitis in this group was 0.14%. Another group of 2071 patients received subconjunctival antibiotics alone at the time of cataract surgery. In this group, the incidence of postoperative endophthalmitis was 0.43%. Combined topical and subconjunctival prophylactic antibiotic treatment was more effective in preventing postoperative endophthalmitis than either topical or subconjunctival antibiotics alone.

Because the prophylactic use of subconjunctival antibiotics appears beneficial, the use of broader spectrum antibiotics injected subconjunctivally is advisable. Gentamicin 20 mg, tobramycin 20 mg, or vancomycin 25 mg with or without a cephalosporin, such as cefazolin 50 to 100 mg or ceftazidime 100 mg, can be used. The aminoglycosides and vancomycin have a broader spectrum of activity than penicillin, but their activity against streptococci and coagulase-negative staphylococci is variable.

Therefore, by including a cephalosporin with gentamicin, tobramycin, or vancomycin, there will be better coverage of the bacteria most commonly found to cause postoperative endophthalmitis.

The antibiotics should be administered adjacent to the limbus, in the bulbar conjunctiva. A study by Forster [57] measured the gentamicin level in the anterior chamber at the beginning of cataract surgery after injection of 20 mg of gentamicin at one of three sites: (a) adjacent to the limbus in the bulbar conjunctiva; (b) subconjunctivally in the cul de sac adjacent to the orbital rim; and (c) infraorbitally through the lower lid. Therapeutic levels of the gentamicin were demonstrated when the antibiotic was administered subconjunctivally in the bulbar conjunctiva, adjacent to the limbus. Negligible levels of gentamicin were found when the other two routes were used.

The use of antibiotic prophylaxis should not minimize the importance of a preoperative preparation of the eye, including mechanical cleansing of the lids and adnexae and the use of antiseptic solutions in the operating room. The goal of antibiotic prophylaxis and the chemical and mechanical preparation of the eye is to reduce the bacterial count in the operative field to the lowest possible level.

Apt *et al.* [63] studied half-strength (5%) povidone–iodine (Betadine) solution used topically as part of the preoperative chemical preparation of the eye in 30 patients undergoing ophthalmic surgery. In each patient, both eyes underwent identical preoperative chemical preparation, except one randomly chosen eye received one or two drops of half-strength povidone–iodine solution, filling the upper and lower fornices. The control eye did not receive povidone–iodine, and neither eye was irrigated. Aerobic and anaerobic cultures were taken before and after preparation of the eye. In the povidone–iodine treated eyes, the bacterial count decreased by 91%, and the number of species decreased by 50%.

Isenberg *et al.* [64] compared the antibacterial effect of the topical antibiotic combination containing polymixin B, neomycin, and gramicidin given three times daily for 3 days preoperatively with half-strength povidone–iodine solution

administered with the preoperative preparation. Bacterial conjunctival cultures were taken before and after the preoperative preparation of both eyes of 35 patients undergoing ocular surgery. When used individually, the topical antibiotic and povidone–iodine caused a similar and substantial decrease in the bacterial count and species of bacteria cultured. When both were used together, the decrease was greater, with 83% of the conjunctival cultures negative.

A povidone–iodine preparation of the periocular skin and face should include careful cleansing of the lid margins with povidone–iodine moistened cotton applicators. Several drops of half-strength povidone–iodine should be instilled to fill the upper and lower conjunctival fornices while the lid is manipulated. The povidone–iodine should not be removed from the skin or initially irrigated from the eye. The patient should be draped with either disposable or laundered–sterilized head drape and split sheets. Adhesive plastic drapes over the lids, lashes, and periorbital skin will isolate the eye and conjunctiva from the surrounding facial skin, hold down and cover the lashes, and cover the lid margins when the lid speculum is properly positioned. Once the lid speculum is positioned, the eye then should be irrigated to remove the povidone–iodine solution before surgery is begun. Also, an attempt should be made to reduce the pooling of irrigating solutions in the conjunctival cul de sac.

Summary

Although infectious endophthalmitis is a dire complication of intraocular surgery, advances have been made in its management. Through the use of cultures of aqueous and vitreous specimens, intravitreal antibiotics, systemic steroids, and/or vitrectomy, most eyes have the infection controlled and some recover useful vision. Successful treatment of infectious endophthalmitis depends on early detection and treatment and therefore requires a keen awareness of the signs and symptoms. Even when treated promptly, however, the damage from infection and the associated inflammation may result in a blind eye.

References

1 Meisler DM, Mandelbaum S. *Propionibacterium*-associated endophthalmitis after extracapsular cataract extraction. Review of reported cases. *Ophthalmology* 1989; **96**: 54–61.

2 Christy NE, Lall P. Postoperative endophthalmitis following cataract surgery. Effects of subconjunctival antibiotics and other factors. *Arch Ophthalmol* 1973; **90**: 361–6.

3 Christy NE, Lall P. A randomized, controlled comparison of anterior and posterior periocular injection of antibiotic in the prevention of postoperative endophthalmitis. *Ophthalmic Surg* 1986; **17**: 715–18.

4 Allen HF, Mangiaracine AB. Bacterial endophthalmitis aftre cataract extraction. A study of 22 infections in 20,000 operations. *Arch Ophthalmol* 1964; **72**: 454–62.

5 Allen HF, Mangiaracine AB. Bacterial endophthalmitis after cataract extraction. II. Incidence in 36,000 consecutive operations with special reference to preoperative topical antibiotics. *Arch Ophthalmol* 1974; **91**: 3–7.

6 Berler DK. Endophthalmitis in 10,032 cataract operations. *J Ocul Ther Surg* 1982; **1**: 159–62.

7 Bohigian GM, Olk RJ. Factors associated with a poor visual result in endophthalmitis. *Am J Ophthalmol* 1986; **101**: 332–4.

8 Cameron ME, Forster TDC. Endophthalmitis occurring during hospitalization following cataract surgery. *Ophthal Surg* 1978; **9**: 52–7.

9 Maylath FR, Leopold IH. Study of experimental intraocular infection. *Am J Ophthalmol* 1955; **40**: 86–101.

10 Allansmith MR, Ostler HB, Butterworth M. Concomitance of bacteria in various areas of the eye. *Arch Ophthalmol* 1969; **82**: 37–42.

11 Stern WH, Tamura E, Jacobs RA *et al.* Epidemic postsurgical *Candida parapsilosis* endophthalmitis. *Ophthalmology* 1985; **92**: 1701–9.

12 Theodore FH. Symposium: Postoperative endophthalmitis. Etiology and diagnosis of fungal postoperative endophthalmitis. *Trans Am Acad Ophthalmol* 1978; **85**: 327–40.

13 Gelender H. Bacterial endophthalmitis following cutting of sutures after cataract surgery. *Am J Ophthalmol* 1982; **94**: 528–33.

14 Mandelbaum S, Forster RK, Gelender H, Culbertson W. Late onset endophthalmitis associated with filtering blebs. *Ophthalmology* 1985; **92**: 964–72.

15 Carlson AN, Koch DD. Endophthalmitis following Nd:YAG laser posterior capsulotomy. *Ophthalmic Surg* 1988; **19**: 168–70.

16 Neuteboom GHG, Vries-Knoppert WAEJ. Endophthalmitis after Nd:YAG laser capsulotomy. *Doc Ophthal* 1988; **70**: 175–8.

17 Lindstrom RL, Doughman DJ. Bacterial endophthalmitis associated with vitreous wick. *Ann Ophthalmol* 1979; **11**: 1775–8.

18 Forster RK, Zachary IG, Cottingham AJ Jr, Norton EWD. Further observations on the diagnosis, etiology, and treatment of endophthalmitis. *Trans Am Ophthalmol Soc* 1975; **73**: 221–30.

19 Deutsch TA, Goldberg MF. Painless endophthalmitis after cataract surgery. *Ophthalmic Surg* 1984; **15**: 837–40.

20 Bode DD Jr, Gelender H, Forster RK. A retrospective review of endophthalmitis due to coagulase-negative staphylococci. *Br J Ophthalmol* 1985; **69**: 915–9.

21 Driebe WT Jr, Mandelbaum S, Forster RK, Schwartz LK, Culbertson WW. Pseudophakic endophthalmitis. Diagnosis and management. *Ophthalmology* 1986; **93**: 442–8.

22 Weber DJ, Hoffman KL, Thoft RA, Baker AS. Endophthalmitis following intraocular lens implantation. Report of 30 cases and review of the literature. *Rev Infect Dis* 1986; **8**: 12–20.

23 Ruiz RS, Teeters VW. Vitreous wick syndrome. A late complication following cataract extraction. *Am J Ophthalmol* 1970; **70**: 483–90.

24 Apple DJ, Mamalis N, Steinmetz RL, Loftfield K, Crandall AS, Olson RJ. Phacoanaphylactic endophthalmitis associated with extracapsular cataract extraction and posterior chamber intraocular lens. *Arch Ophthalmol* 1984; **102**: 1528–32.

25 Forster RK, Abbott RL, Gelender H. Management of infectious endophthalmitis. *Ophthalmology* 1980; **87**: 313–9.

26 Tucher DN, Forster RK. Experimental bacterial endophthalmitis. *Arch Ophthalmol* 1972; **88**: 647–9.

27 Meredith TA, Trabelsi A, Miller MJ, Aguilar E, Wilson LA. Spontaneous sterilization in experimental *Staphylococcus epidermidis* endophthalmitis. *Invest Ophthalmol Vis Sci* 1990; **31**: 181–6.

28 Joondeph BC, Flynn HW Jr, Miller D, Joondeph HC. A new culture method for infectious endophthalmitis. *Arch Ophthalmol* 1989; **107**: 1334–7.

29 Forster RK. Symposium: Postoperative endophthalmitis. Etiology and diagnosis of bacterial postoperative endophthalmitis. *Ophthalmology* 1978; **85**: 320–6.

30 Rowsey JJ, Newsome DL, Sexton DJ, Harms WK. Endophthalmitis. Current approaches. *Ophthalmology* 1982; **89**: 1055–66.

31 O'Day DM, Jones DB, Patrinely J, Elliott JH. *Staphylococcus epidermidis* endophthalmitis. Visual outcome following noninvasive therapy. *Ophthalmology* 1982; **89**: 354–60.

32 Baum J, Peyman GA, Barza M. Intravitreal administration of antibiotic in the treatment of bacterial endophthalmitis. III. Consensus. *Surv Ophthalmol* 1982; **26**: 204–6.

33 Zachary IG, Forster RK. Experimental intravitreal gentamicin. *Am J Ophthalmol* 1976; **82**: 604.

34 Fisher JP, Civiletto SE, Forster RK. Toxicity, efficacy, and clearance of intravitreally injected

cefazolin. *Arch Ophthalmol* 1982; **100**: 650–2.

35 Pflugfelder SC, Hernandez E, Fliesler SJ, Alvarez J, Pflugfelder ME, Forster RK. Intravitreal vancomycin. Retinal toxicity, clearance, and interaction with gentamicin. *Arch Ophthalmol* 1987; **105**: 831–7.

36 Mandelbaum S, Forster RK. Endophthalmitis associated with filtering blebs. *Int Ophthalmol Clin* 1987; **27**: 107–11.

37 Talamo JH, D'Amico DJ, Kenyon KR. Intravitreal amikacin in the treatment of bacterial endophthalmitis. *Arch Ophthalmol* 1986; **104**: 1483–5.

38 Davis JL, Koidou-Tsiligianni A, Pflugfelder SC, Miller D, Flynn HW, Forster RK. Coagulase-negative staphylococcal endophthalmitis. *Ophthalmology* 1988; **95**: 1404–10.

39 Gammon JA, Schwab I, Joseph P. Gentamicin resistant *Serratia marcescens* endophthalmitis. *Arch Ophthalmol* 1980; **98**: 1221–3.

40 Edson RS, Terrell CL. The aminoglycosides: streptomycin, kanamycin, gentamicin, tobramycin, amikacin, netilmicin, and sisomicin. *Mayo Clin Proc* 1987; **62**: 916–20.

41 Oum BS, D'Amico DJ, Wong KW. Intravitreal antibiotic therapy with vancomycin and aminoglycoside. An experimental study of combination and repetitive injections. *Arch Ophthalmol* 1989; **107**: 1055–60.

42 Jeglum EL, Rosenberg SB, Benson WE. Preparation of intravitreal drug doses. *Ophthal Surg* 1981; **12**: 355–9.

43 Barza M, Baum JL, Slikowski M. Ocular pharmacokinetics of LY146032 (LY), teicoplanin, and vancomycin in a rabbit model. Program and abstracts of the 27th Interscience Conference on Antimicrobial Agents and Chemotherapy, 4–7 October, 1987, American Society for Microbiology (Abstract 152, p. 123).

44 Shockley RK, Fishman P, Aziz M, Yannis RA, Jay WM. Subconjunctival administration of ceftazidime in pigmented rabbit eyes. *Arch Ophthalmol* 1986; **104**: 266–8.

45 Pavan PR, Brinser JH. Exogenous bacterial endophthalmitis treated without systemic antibiotics. *Am J Ophthalmol* 1987; **104**: 121–6.

46 Martin DF, Ficker LA, Aguilar HA *et al*. Vitreous cefazolin levels after intravenous injection. Effects of inflammation, repeated antibiotic doses, and surgery. *Arch Ophthalmol* 1990; **108**: 411–14.

47 Thea D, Barza M. Use of antibacterial agents in infections of the central nervous system. *Infect Dis Clin N Am* 1989; **3**: 553–70.

48 Diamond JG. Intraocular management of endophthalmitis. A systematic approach. *Arch Ophthalmol* 1981; **99**: 96–9.

49 Olson JC, Flynn HW Jr, Forster RK, Culbertson WW. Results in the treatment of postoperative endophthalmitis. *Ophthalmology* 1983; **90**: 692–9.

50 Stern GA, Engel HM, Driebe WT Jr. The treatment of postoperative endophthalmitis. Results of differing approaches to treatment. *Ophthalmology* 1989; **96**: 62–7.

51 Cobo LM, Forster RK. The clearance of intravitreal gentamicin. *Am J Ophthalmol* 1981; **92**: 59–62.

52 Olk RJ, Bohigian GM. The management of endophthalmitis. Diagnostic and therapeutic guidelines including the use of vitrectomy. *Ophthal Surg* 1987; **18**: 262–7.

53 Zaidman GW, Mondino BJ. Postoperative pseudophakic bacterial endophthalmitis. *Am J Ophthalmol* 1982; **93**: 218–23.

54 Puliafito CA, Baker AS, Haaf J, Foster CS. Infectious endophthalmitis. Review of 36 cases. *Ophthalmology* 1982; **89**: 921–9.

55 Nelsen PT, Marcus DA, Bovino JA. Retinal detachment following endophthalmitis. *Ophthalmology* 1985; **92**: 1112–17.

56 Allansmith MR, Anderson RP, Butterworth M. The meaning of preoperative cultures in ophthalmology. *Trans Am Acad Ophthal Otolaryngol* 1969; **73**: 683–90.

57 Forster RK. Antibiotics and asepsis. In: Sears M, Tarkkanen A, eds. *Surgical Pharmacology of the Eye*. New York: Raven Press, 1985; 57–80.

58 Burns RP, Hansen T, Fraunfelder FT, Klass AM, Allen A. An experimental model for evaluation of human conjunctivitis and topical antibiotic therapy: Comparison of gentamicin and neomycin. *Canad J Ophthalmol* 1968; **3**: 132–7.

59 Burns RP, Oden M. Antibiotic prophylaxis in cataract surgery. *Trans Am Ophthalmol Soc* 1972; **70**: 43–57.

60 Burns RP. Effectiveness study of antibiotics. *Symp Ocul Ther* 1972; **5**: 105–12.

61 Fahmy JA. Bacterial flora in relation to cataract extraction. V. Effects of topical antibiotics on the preoperative conjunctival flora. *Acta Ophthalmol* (Copenh) 1980; **58**: 567–75.

62 Christy NE, Sommer A. Antibiotic prophylaxis of postoperative endophthalmitis. *Ann Ophthalmol* 1979; **11**: 1261–5.

63 Apt L, Isenberg S, Yoshimori R, Paez JH. Chemical preparation of the eye in ophthalmic surgery. III. Effect of povidone–iodine on the conjunctiva. *Arch Ophthalmol* 1984; **102**: 728–9.

64 Isenberg SJ, Apt L, Yoshimori R, Khwarg S. Chemical preparation of the eye in ophthalmic surgery. IV. Comparison of povidone–iodine on the conjunctiva with a prophylactic antibiotic. *Arch Ophthalmol* 1985; **103**: 1340–2.

65 *Endophthalmitis Vitrectomy Study Manual of Operations*, 1990.

22: Prevention of Postoperative Astigmatism and its Management

SPENCER P. THORNTON

One should always attempt to prevent the induction of astigmatism with one's cataract surgical technique, but the possibility of induced astigmatism is still present, even in the best of hands. Fortunately, high postoperative astigmatism after cataract surgery is very uncommon but it is best prevented than corrected. The surgeon should attempt to modify his or her surgical technique to compensate for those factors which predispose to astigmatism. Techniques which minimize changes in corneal curvature should be used.

Basic concepts

Surgical definition of astigmatism

One can define astigmatism by the cylindrical lens that is used to neutralize the refractive error. This neutralizes both corneal and lenticular astigmatism. It should be noted however that astigmatism measured by keratometry does not exactly equal the refractive astigmatism. In general, 3 D of astigmatism measured by keratometry will usually produce about 2 D of manifest astigmatism. This relationship is a progressive one with both higher hyperopic and higher myopic refractive errors.

When a patient has significant steepness in the vertical meridian, it is described as "with-the-rule" astigmatism. Conversely, significant astigmatism produced by the steep corneal curvature in the horizontal meridian is termed "against-the-rule" astigmatism.

Wound compression and wound relaxation

Multiple sutures, sutures that are tight, sutures that pass through long distances of corneal tissue, and deeper sutures compress the wound, shortening its cord length and creating a steeper corneal meridian. All of these produce wound compression and secondary steepening (Table 22.1).

Wound relaxation is produced by too few sutures, widely spaced sutures, sutures with a short and shallow course through tissue, posteriorly or sclerally placed sutures, sutures that are removed early (or absorbable sutures), or wounds treated with significant corticosteroids (Table 22.2). These produce a lengthening of the cord length of that meridian with resultant relaxation and flattening. Wound compression thus induces plus cylinder or a steeper meridian whereas wound gape and relaxation induces flattening in that meridian and a plus cylinder in the meridian 90° away.

Surgical planning

To retain low degrees of pre-existing astigmatism one should use techniques which minimize change in corneal curvature. With phacoemulsification posterior scleral pocket incisions should be used, and with planned extracapsular cataract extractions incisions should be made in the sclera 1–2 mm posterior

Table 22.1 Factors which produce corneal steepening

Multiple sutures
Tight sutures
Long bites
Sutures deep on the scleral side

Table 22.2 Factors which produce corneal flattening

Too few sutures
Posteriorly or sclerally placed sutures
Suture removal
Prolonged steroid treatment

to the cornea with an extension of the incision into the clear cornea before entering the anterior chamber. Suture bites should be in the sclera, not in the cornea, with deep, even bites tied for apposition without compression.

To correct with-the-rule astigmatism of higher amounts the 90° axis should be flattened with a more posterior incision, non-tight sutures, and postoperative steroid drops. Some with-the-rule astigmatism should be retained.

For against-the-rule astigmatism the vertical axis should be steepened with a more anterior incision with midlimbal 10/0 nylon sutures with deep bites tied slightly tighter. Another method of reducing against-the-rule astigmatism is to make the incision temporal, using non-tight, non-absorbable sutures and a shelving incision to flatten the horizontal axis. It is generally easier to induce permanent flattening than to induce permanent steepening.

For oblique astigmatism the incision should be centered over the steep axis using a flattening technique.

For larger amounts of preoperative astigmatism (3.5 D or greater) transverse astigmatic keratotomy may be considered either at the time of surgery or postoperatively.

Alignment of the wound margins is an important determinant of the amount of astigmatism remaining when the eye is fully healed. Non-radial interrupted suture bites or the shift of single running sutures produces a significant horizontal misalignment resulting in irregular steep and flat areas. On the other hand, by vertically mismatching the wound margins one can produce a regular and predictable cylindric modification. A mnemonic proposed by John Corboy helps one to remember the technique: "Shallow to deep will make it steep; the reverse of that will make it flat." By making the first corneal bite shallow and the opposing scleral bite deep one can steepen that meridian of the

cornea. By making the first corneal bite deep and the scleral bite shallow, the cornea tends to flatten in that area. In general the rules of astigmatism control and modification are these:

1 wound gape or "relaxation" flattens the cornea;

2 wound compression (and wedge resection) steepens the cornea;

3 deep to shallow placement flattens the cornea; and

4 shallow to deep suture placement steepens the cornea.

The problems of astigmatism control must not be compounded by placing long compressing tight sutures. The immediate result may look good but with decay of tight sutures, the patient is frequently left with against-the-rule astigmatism. One must be precise in wound alignment and suture for apposition of tissue without compression.

When operative precautions fail

Despite best efforts on the part of the surgeon, biologic and technical variables continue to conspire to produce unwanted astigmatism following cataract surgery. A number of approaches for postcataract astigmatism correction have been tried including radial corneal relaxing incisions, transverse corneal relaxing incisions, trapezoidal (Ruiz) relaxing incisions of "ladder" configuration, and wedge resections. The non-intersecting transverse incisions advocated by this author have been shown to be effective and predictable. In some respects postcataract astigmatism can be treated like idiopathic astigmatism but there are some significant differences.

Principles of postcataract astigmatism correction

1 Not all astigmatism needs to be corrected surgically;

2 be aware of the correction of the fellow eye and correct only if there is a significant difference between the two;

3 there is a wide range of results for any and all astigmatism procedures;

4 both the effect and the variability of the result increases with age;

5 try selective cutting of sutures before considering any other method of astigmatism correction;

6 cut no sutures before 8 weeks after cataract surgery. The best time to modify postoperative astigmatism with suture cutting is from 2 to 4 months after the operation but the technique may be effective even at 6 months;

7 wait a minimum of 6 months after cataract surgery (the longer the better) before astigmatic keratotomy;

8 use astigmatic keratotomy only if the patient is symptomatic;

9 attempt to leave some with-the-rule astigmatism; and

10 remember that postoperative keratometry readings do not coincide with postoperative refraction.

Candidates for postcataract astigmatic keratotomy

1 Against-the-rule astigmatism which is more than 2.5 D;

2 against-the-rule astigmatism more than 1 D if the patient is symptomatic and the preoperative cylinder was with-the-rule; or

3 with-the-rule astigmatism of over 2.5 D when there is a significant difference between the two eyes.

Wound decay

The concept of leaving about 2 D steepening in the area of cataract wound closure is because of the known decay effect of cataract wounds (Fig. 22.1). This is more pronounced with elastic or absorbable sutures but occurs to a lesser degree with non-absorbable sutures. One should not be in a hurry to correct postcataract astigmatism. To do so may compound the problem.

When surgical modification is necessary the approach must be indicated by the result desired. Relaxing incisions (astigmatic keratotomy) tend to flatten the cornea and reduce the dioptric power whereas wedge resections tend to steepen the cornea and increase the dioptric power.

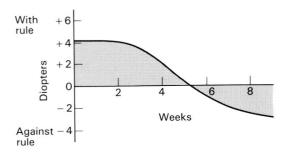

Fig. 22.1 Usual postcataract wound decay.

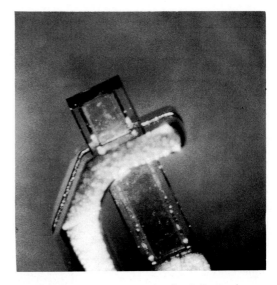

Fig. 22.2 Square-tipped, triple-edged diamond blade.

The effect of relaxing incisions is more predictable and longer lasting than tightening procedures, therefore astigmatic keratotomy has been recommended as the procedure of choice for correcting postcataract astigmatism.

Astigmatic keratotomy

Astigmatic keratotomy procedures are performed much as radial keratotomy procedures in that an appropriate axis is determined and marked, ultrasonic pachymetry is used to determine the depth of the incisions, an appropriate optical zone is determined, and then properly patterned incisions are made, preferably with a square-tipped, triple-edged diamond blade (Fig. 22.2; Tables 22.3 and 22.4).

Table 22.3 Transverse incision guide. Cylinder corrected by transverse incisions placed on each side of the cornea

Length (segment)	Correction (D)
1/2	0.75–1.25
2/3	1.25–1.5
3/4	1.5–1.75
1	1.75–2.25
Two 1/2	2–2.5
Two 2/3	2.5–2.75
Two 3/4	2.75–3
Two 1	3.25–3.5

Improved instrumentation has improved the predictability of the procedure and led to earlier stability of the correction. The square-tipped triple-edged diamond blade provides an assured full depth cut throughout the length of the incision and when specific lengths are needed for transverse incisions at any given otpical zone, a press-on corneal ruler is available which, when pressed on the cornea at the desired optical zone, leaves a very precise ruler marked on the cornea which can be easily seen by the surgeon with a cutting instrument in place (Fig. 22.3).

RESULTS OF POSTCATARACT ASTIGMATIC KERATOTOMY

In postcataract refractive surgery as in primary refractive surgery for myopia and astigmatism, the surgical approach is aimed at reduction of astigmatism and bringing the operated eye to a correction similar to the fellow eye. The amount of correction is determined by the number, length, and placement of the transverse incisions on the cornea. The relative length of transverse incisions is based on degrees of arc (Fig. 22.4). Basic to this concept is the awareness that one segment, the distance between two of eight radials, is equal to 45° of arc (Fig. 22.5). The effective central corneal curvature change is essentially the same whether the incision is placed at a 5 mm optical zone or an 8 mm optical zone if the cord length of the incision is the same measured in degrees of arc (Fig. 22.6).

The length and placement of the transverse incisions is important. The longer the transverse incision and the closer it is to the optical zone the greater is the effect. However the closer one comes to the optical center of the

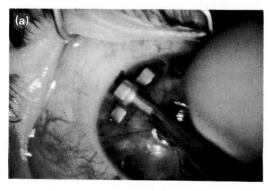
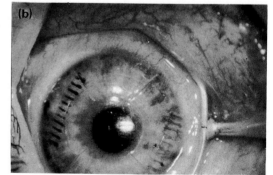

Fig. 22.3 Press-on corneal ruler.

Table 22.4 Incision lengths at varying optical zones (OZ)

Length (segment)	At 5 mm OZ (mm)	At 6 mm OZ (mm)	At 7 mm OZ (mm)	At 8 mm OZ (mm)
1/2	1.1	1.3	1.5	1.7
2/3	1.4	1.7	2	2.3
3/4	1.6	1.9	2.3	2.6
1	2.1	2.5	3	3.4

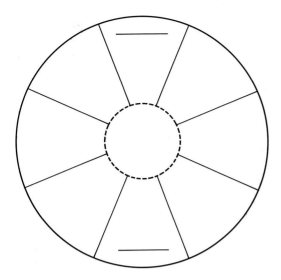

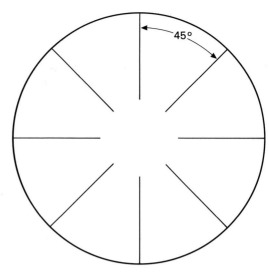

Fig. 22.4 The relative length of transverse incisions is based on degrees of arc.

Fig. 22.5 One segment is equal to 45° of arc.

cornea, the greater is the amount of glare and the greater the potential for inducing irregular astigmatism. Table 22.3 shows the amount of cylinder corrected by varying lengths of incisions and Table 22.4 shows the incision lengths at varying optical zones.

Coupling

In analyzing the effect of postcataract transverse incisions it becomes apparent that incisions that relax and flatten the steeper (primary) meridian also tend to steepen the flatter (secondary) meridian. The total amount of astigmatism corrected is equal to the sum of the change which takes place between the primary and secondary meridians. This ratio of change is termed coupling (Fig. 22.7).

The amount of astigmatism corrected and the amount of coupling induced is a function of the size of the central optical zone and the length of the incisions, modified by the presence or absence of radials alongside the transverse incisions (Fig. 22.8). It becomes apparent that transverse incisions may be used in combination with radial incisons (which enhance their effect in the primary meridian) to alter predictably the curvature of the cornea and reduce virtually any type of astigmatism.

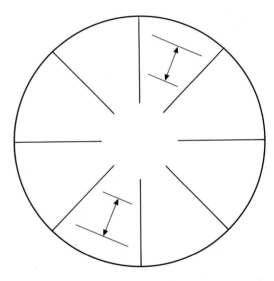

Fig. 22.6 Incisions at a 5 mm or 8 mm optical zone have the same effective central corneal curvature change.

By determining the spherical equivalent of a postcataract astigmatic error, theoretically one can determine the postoperative refractive power. The living human eye, however, does not behave as the theoretic eye and there is a great deal of variability in the results obtained by different surgeons. Because of this variability it is advisable to avoid or minimize overcorrection by careful preoperative planning.

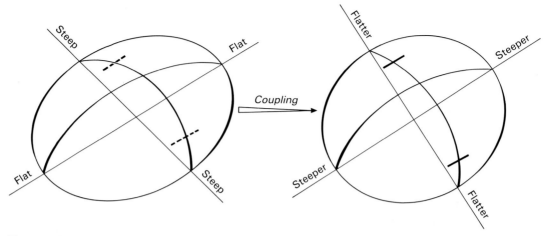

Fig. 22.7 Coupling: steepening of the cornea 90° away from transverse relaxing incisions.

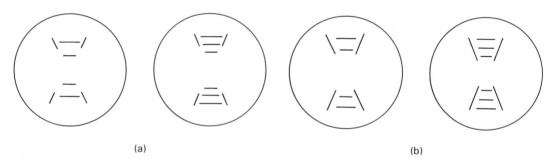

(a)   (b)

Fig. 22.8 (a) Short radials outsize "T" optical zone reduce coupling from 30 to 60% (depending on length) and add to meridional flattening. (b) Long radials at or inside "T" optical zone isolate and increase meridional flattening and reduce coupling from 80 to 90%.

Summary

Modification of postcataract astigmatism by refractive surgery has provided a means of restoring a quality of vision not achieved by cataract and lens implant surgery alone. Although improved instrumentation such as diamond blades, smaller corneal needles, better suture material, and surgical keratometry have reduced the incidence of higher degrees of postoperative astigmatism, both pre-existing and postoperative astigmatism remain a problem.

Low degrees of postcataract astigmatism can be corrected by single pairs of transverse incisions across the axis of steeper curvature and by adding a second pair of transverse incisions increasing amounts of astigmatism can be corrected. By increasing the number of transverse incisions and adding radials to either side as in the Ruiz procedure even higher degrees of astigmatism are correctable. By utilizing the effect of coupling it is possible, by lengthening the transverse incisions and adjusting the optical zone, to steepen predictably one meridian while flattening the other. As these techniques evolve the authors believe that by combining transverse incisions with other incision patterns, astigmatism correction will develop into a more predictable and effective procedure.

23: Accommodation after Intraocular Lens Implantation

SPENCER P. THORNTON

Introduction

This chapter deals with the potential for restoration of accommodation concurrently with the implantation of an intraocular lens (IOL). Basic to dealing with this concept is an understanding of both optical principles and physical characteristics of the eye which bring about the ability to focus at both distance and near. Beginning with a historic look at our understanding of how the eye focuses, we look at applications of this knowledge to the restoration of accommodation with an artificial lens. Our discussion begins with considerations of pupil size, astigmatism, and residual myopia which can produce an apparent or "pseudo-accommodation." The second area of discussion is bifocal IOLs, multifocal, and defractive IOL designs. Finally, we shall discuss the potential for restoration of accommodation with "moveable" in-the-bag IOL which are dependent on lens position, shape of the lens, haptic support, and potential vitreous movement on accommodative effort.

How the eye focuses

The physical characteristics of the eye which determine its focal power include the length of the eye, the curvature of the cornea, and the effective focal power of the lens.

The cornea, aqueous, and vitreous each have a fixed refractive power. Though the lens tissue has a fixed refractive power, this power is changed in accommodation. In order for an image to come into focus on the retina, light must be bent so that the rays converge at the fovea. The nearer an object is to the eye, the more the light must be bent for the object to be seen in focus. In accommodation, the lens curvature can be steepened and the lens itself may be moved forward, thereby increasing its focal power. Donders [1] in his treatise *On The Anomalies of Accommodation and Refraction of the Eye*, credits Heinrich Mueller with the anatomic investigations of the action of the ciliary muscle in accommodation in which he saw, in the action of the most external layers of the ciliary muscle, a means of augmenting the pressure of the vitreous humor and pushing the lens forward. In addition, he noted the advance of the surface of the pupil and the retrogression of the periphery of the iris in accommodation for near objects. In his treatise on physiologic optics, Helmholtz noted that the lens is suspended by zonular filaments projecting from the ciliary muscle which he described as non-elastic filaments holding the lens taut with the ciliary muscle in its relaxed state, and relaxed when the ciliary muscle is contracted. He described a slight anterior movement of the ciliary body on contraction, reducing the stress on the zonules and thereupon allowing the lens to undergo elastic recovery. He described the lens becoming thicker from front to back and its surfaces becoming more sharply curved as the lens focused on progressively closer objects. Thus the lens is maximally accommodated—most steeply curved and most refractive—when it is under the least stress and the ciliary muscle fully contracted. The idea of multiple factors affecting accommodation is therefore not new.

Microscopic studies of the structural organization of the lens have shown that because of the interlocking nature of cortical fibers, that these fibers do not stretch and cannot slide past one another, and so the only way that the shape of the lens can be changed is for the fibers to alter their curvature by compression. Recent studies with computer models have indicated that the forces acting on the surface of the accommodating lens are approximately equal, and are in a direction approximately perpendicular to the lens surface providing a uniform compressive force against the entire surface of the lens. The zonules exert a force that has both a stretching (parallel) component, and a compressive (perpendicular) one. The capsular fibers, however, resist stretching, and so the main force transmitted to the lens is perpendicular [2].

Most but not all of the shape change seen in the lens during the elastic recovery of accommodation can be accounted for by relaxation of the zonules. Another component suggested in the focusing process is the vitreous humor which acts by its support in the relaxed state and possible forward movement during ciliary contraction on accommodative effort.

The gradual reduction of focal power of the lens with age is not fully understood. We know that the lens continues to grow throughout life with increasing steepness in both anterior and posterior surfaces with age. Despite the increased curvature of both anterior and posterior surfaces the refractive power decreases with age, thereby producing a paradox. Why is it that an older lens has to be curved more than a younger one to focus on the same object? One suggested possibility is that the nature of the cytoplasm in the lens fibers changes chemically in a way that decreases the refractive index of the lens with age. It is clear that a number of mechanisms are involved in age-related changes of the lens. The decrease in the refractive index of the lens is partly compensated for by increasing steepness in curvature of the anterior and posterior surfaces as well as increasing zones of discontinuity within the lens.

The gradual overall decrease in the index of refraction and reduced elastic recovery of the lens with age explains the phenomenon of presbyopia. The problem of restoration of accomodation in pseudophakia then becomes one of the manipulation of factors exclusive of an elastic lens. There are several alternatives: (a) pseudoaccommodation; (b) bifocal IOLs; (c) multifocal or defractive lenses; and (d) "moveable" in-the-bag IOLs.

Pseudoaccommodation

Some aphakic patients have been noted to have good near vision while wearing only their correction for emmetropia at distance [3]. With improved control of postoperative refractive power and the deliberate induction of a small amount of with-the-rule myopic astigmatism, an increasing number of patients have been provided a means of apparent accommodation without corrective lenses. Nakazawa and Ohtsuki [4] measured apparent accommodation in a number of pseudophakic eyes after implantation of posterior chamber IOLs. They found that the primary factor producing increased depth of field and apparent accommodation was the ability of the pupil to constrict on accommodative effort. There appeared to be no correlation between apparent accommodation and corrected visual acuity, refractive error, corneal astigmatism, or axial length. The apparent accommodation appeared to be inversely related to the anterior chamber depth. In essence, the diameter of the pupil appeared to be the most important factor in apparent accommodation, with accommodation being greater the smaller the pupil.

Another factor which appears to contribute to apparent accommodation or increased depth of field is the posterior placement of the pseudophakos. The greater the distance of the posterior pseudophakos surface from the cornea, the greater the focal power and the less anterior movement necessary for increasing that focal power [5] (Fig. 23.1).

Patients with an implanted IOL have been shown to be capable of near spectacle independence by increasing the depth of focus of the uncorrected implanted eye by careful preoperative planning and surgical technique. With simple myopic astigmatism the visual acuity can be brought to 20/50 or better from

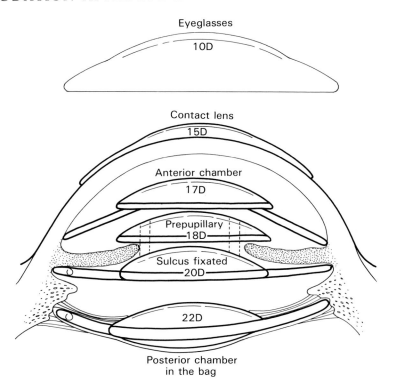

Fig. 23.1 Focal power for emmetropia with various lens positions.

far to near because the size of the blurred retinal image changes less than its shape as the object of fixation approaches the eye. For simple myopic astigmatism the change in corneal power must be included in the calculation of IOL power. The postoperative shape of the cornea can be predicted and the IOL power then calculated to make the flatter meridian emmetropic and the stronger meridian of the cornea myopic from −1.5D to −2.5D. With simple myopic astigmatism of −1.5D an uncorrected distance acuity of about 20/40 is possible [6]. The increase in the depth of focus is achieved at the cost of a slight reduction in the uncorrected visual acuity compared to the emmetropic eye for distance vision.

Astigmatism can be predictably produced by using non-absorbable sutures and adjusted suture tension. Huber [6] described a technique in which he did not adjust the amount of astigmatism during surgery, but controlled the amount of surgical ametropia by cutting the corneoscleral nylon sutures in the steeper meridian during the postoperative period. With this technique the postoperative shape of the cornea can be predicted and adjusted. If the flatter meridian is calculated for emmetropia then the steeper corneal meridian produces a simple myopic astigmatism. Best acuities and depth of focus have been found in subjects with about −0.75D to −3D of simple myopic astigmatism.

Bifocal, multifocal, and diffractive IOLs

The specifications of IOLs have tended to follow the lead of the contact lens industry using the same principles of optics. The most common type of bifocal IOL uses the simultaneous vision principle and has two concentric optical zones. The concentric bifocal has the distance portion in the center of the lens and the add portion in the periphery of the lens. The lens is manufactured in such a way that the bifocal or reading portion is seen at near simultaneously with the distance portion. As the wearer fixates on the near object, the image focused by the stronger lens becomes appreciated and the distance image is ignored. This requires a learning process but patients apparently adapt to it with little difficulty.

Bifocal IOL design requires an add involving about one-half of the area of the lens and uses the alternating vision principle of the traditional bifocal design. The add can be varied in power just as in eyeglasses or contact lenses. Theoretically one can have any power at distance and near while maintaining 20/20 vision with full appreciation of the bifocal effect. The difficulty with these designs is that decentration of such a lens may produce problems such as monocular dyplopia, binocular dyplopia, constant blurring of images, and change of focal power or loss of bifocal power with myosis. Despite these difficulties a number of patients have had bifocal IOLs implanted and the results have appeared encouraging.

Diffractive optics

A recent innovation in IOLs is a lens utilizing diffractive optics providing simultaneous bifocal imaging using the effects of diffraction rather than relying on conventional refractive optics. The apparent advantage of this diffractive design is that it provides a constant intensity of the two foci independent of pupil aperture size. The diffractive microstructure of the lens is composed of 20 to 30 concentric optical zones of minute steps of a few microns at the zone boundaries. Thus the lens utilizes both the conventional ray as well as the wave nature of light, resulting in a true multifocal lens [7]. At the time of this writing it is yet undetermined whether the quality of vision will equal that of monofocal lenses. Short-term results appear quite good and there is optimism for the long term. With a base power calculated for emmetropia at distance, and an add power of 3 D for near, the diffractive lens has two powers. When focusing at distance, the higher power focuses anterior to the retina. When its share of light reaches the retina, it is highly defocused and has no informational structure. The intensity of the focused light from distance overwhelms the defocused light from near, resulting in a clear image of the distant object. The brain apparently receives one image clearly

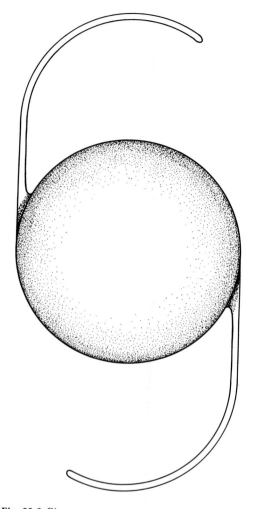

Fig. 23.2 Biconvex optic, shorter haptic diameter assures better in-the-bag placement and potential anterior movement on accommodative effort.

in focus with some blurred light that has no structure. There appears to be a slight reduction in contrast compared with monovision, but only one focused image.

In near vision, the incoming light is divergent from a near object so the two foci move posteriorly and the 3 D add power is at the retina and the distance foci moves beyond the retina, again producing a clear single image accompanied by a structureless defocused one. This focusing ability appears to function independently of pupil aperture and is tolerant of moderate decentration. Because of the reduction in light intensity some patients have noted

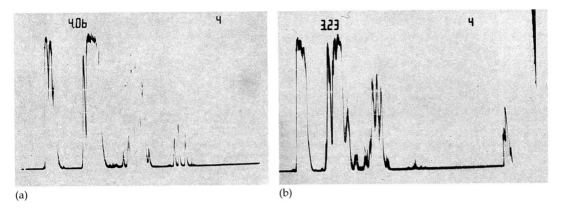

(a)   (b)

Fig. 23.3 Real time A-scan of 70-year-old female, right eye, 2 D power change on accommodative effort. (a) Fixing at distance AC depth 4.06 mm. (b) Fixing at near AC depth 3.23 mm.

a deficit in their reading ability, particularly in low illumination.

Potential for restored accommodation with in-the-bag implantation of an IOL

The potential for restored accommodation with a monofocal IOL appears possible with lenses designed with biconvex optics for implantation in the bag with the posterior convexity firmly held against the posterior capsule so that the capsule is slightly on stretch, and the lens positioned so that there is no pseudophakodonesis (Fig. 23.2). Such a lens has been designed and studied from the standpoint of apparent accommodation produced by change in pupil size, posterior positioning of the lens allowing greater depth of focus, and movement of the lens produced by anterior vitreous movement on ciliary contraction with accommodative effort [8]. A-scan ultrasound measurements of changes in the anterior chamber depth in pseudophakic accommodation tend to confirm Mueller's theory of vitreous pressure pushing the lens forward with ciliary contraction on accommodation (Fig. 23.3).

Any refractive change based on movement of the lens is dependent both on the shape and position of the lens (Fig. 23.4). The more posterior the lens, the more significant the change in refraction with any given anterior movement. Any movement of an IOL implanted posteriorly in the bag will result in a significant

change in refraction when compared to movement of a lens positioned just behind or just anterior to the iris plane. A lens implanted in the bag with the convexity against the posterior capsule will produce approximately twice the change in near focal power compared with a lens with convexity forward.

It is not uncommon on slit-lamp examination of aphakic patients to see the vitreous face bulging forward through the pupil on accommodative effort. Studies have shown that following extracapsular cataract surgery and sulcus fixation of an IOL the posterior capsule goes from a preoperative average of 7.6 mm from the cornea to 4.68 mm, a change of 2.92 mm. The approximately 3 mm forward movement of the capsule appears to be due to its tendency to tighten in its zonular support. This leaves a space that is filled by forward movement of the vitreous face, or an accumulation of a fluid interface between the capsule and the vitreous face [9].

A solid polymethylmetacrylic (PMMA) lens with an optic size of 6.5 mm and a total haptic diameter of 12.5 or 13 mm with biconvex optics and slight posterior angulation of the haptics allows for in-the-bag placement with posterior convexity against the posterior capsule. With the lens properly placed within the capsular bag, accommodative effort produces ciliary body contraction and an apparent pulling forward of the vitreous. If the posterior convexity of the lens optic is positioned against the posterior capsule, any forward movement of

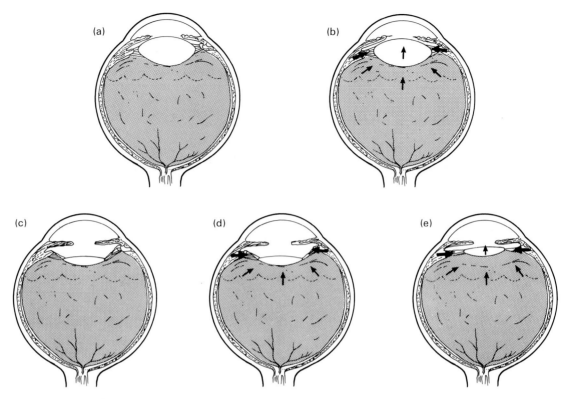

Fig. 23.4 Accommodation of pseudophakia. (a) The natural lens at rest. (b) On accommodation, the vitreous is forced forward. (c) With intraocular lens implanted in the bag. (d) On accommodative effort the vitreous is forced (pulled) forward. (e) Anterior movement of intraocular lens produces increased focal power.

the vitreous will push the lens forward. Thus on accommodative effort, if the lens moves even 0.25–0.5 mm, a significant effect is produced in the effective focal power increase. Clinically this has been demonstrated by reduction of the power of bifocal adds for patients who wear glasses and a number of patients who are quite comfortable without further lens correction.

With a biconvex monofocal IOL implanted posteriorly the apparent accommodative potential is enhanced by preoperatively planning a postoperative focal power of −0.5 to −0.75 and a surgical technique which results in simple myopic astigmatism of about −1.5 D.

References

1 Donders FC. *On the Anomalies of Accommodation and Refraction of the Eye.* London: New Sydenham Society, 1864.

2 Koretz J, Handleman G. How the human eye focuses. *Sci Am* 1988; July; **32**: 92–9.

3 Bettman JS. Apparent accommodation in aphakic eyes. *Am J Ophthalmol* 1950; **33**: 921.

4 Nakazawa M, Ohtsuki K. Apparent accommodation in pseudophakic eyes after implantation of posterior chamber intraocular lenses. *Am J Ophthalmol* 1983; **96**: 435–8.

5 Holladay JT, Koch DD, Green MT *et al.* Determining intraocular lens power within the eye. *Am Intraocul Implant Soc J* 1985; **11**: 353–63.

6 Huber C. Planned myopic astigmatism as a substitute for accommodation in pseudophakia. *Am Intraocul Implant Soc J* 1981; **7**: 244–9.

7 Sanders DR, ed. *Symposium on Innovations on Multifocal Lens Design.* Copenhagen, Denmark: *Ocul Surg News* 1988; (suppl) September.

8 Thornton S. Lens implantation with restored accommodation. *Curr Canad Ophthal Pract* 1986; **4**: 60–82.

9 Hoffer KJ. The effect of axial length on posterior chamber lens and posterior capsule position. *Curr Concept Ophthal Surg* 1985; **1**: 20–2.

24: Corneal Decompensation following Cataract Surgery: Prevention and Management

PETER C. DONSHIK & WILLIAM H. EHLERS

Introduction

Cataract surgery is one of the safest and most effective operations in modern medicine. When complications do occur, they are generally responsive to therapeutic modalities. Patient expectations have kept pace with the improvement in microsurgical techniques and instrumentation, and thus even the best informed consent has little power to satisfy the patient with poor vision after a postoperative complication. Corneal edema following cataract extraction can have a disastrous effect on the patient's acuity and comfort. Corneal edema may occur in the early postoperative period or years after successful cataract surgery, resulting in painful bullous keratopathy or irreversible stromal scarring and neovascularization. It is important to note at the outset that corneal edema may have two components: (a) stromal edema; and (b) epithelial edema. This distinction allows the surgeon to note the differences in pathophysiology, effect on vision, and treatment dictated by these entities. The modern cataract surgeon has the responsibility to anticipate this potential problem and respond in the appropriate manner should it arise.

Corneal structure and physiology

The cornea's function as the major refractive surface of the human ocular system is dependent on the maintenance of a smooth epithelial surface and stromal transparency. An understanding of the structure and physiology involved in maintaining corneal transparency is essential to the anticipation and treatment of postoperative corneal edema.

Traditionally the cornea is said to be composed of five layers: (a) the epithelium; (b) Bowman's layer; (c) corneal stroma; (d) Descemet's membrane; and (e) the endothelium (Fig. 24.1). These layers have special properties that contribute to corneal clarity: they are avascular and devoid of pigment. The epithelium forms a barrier to the external environment and provides a scaffold upon which the tear film is evenly distributed. When epithelial edema occurs, it has a greater effect on visual acuity than stromal edema. Epithelial edema, however, is rare if the intraocular pressure is in the normal range until corneal thickness reaches 0.65–0.75 mm, compared to 0.5 mm for normal corneas [1]. The stroma is composed of collagen fibrils embedded in a glycosaminoglycan (GAG) matrix. The collagen fibers of the cornea are small with a diameter of 190–340 Å and highly regular spacing. The spatial separation of these small fibrils is less than half of the wavelength of visible light, and therefore little scattering of light occurs as it passes through the cornea [2]. In stromal corneal edema the space between the fibrils is increased, resulting in increased scattering of incident light (Fig. 24.2). The endothelium is the site of the active pump mechanism which plays an essential role in the maintenance of corneal deturgescence.

The corneal stroma normally contains 78% water by weight. This is a relative state of dehydration compared to other connective tissue structures in the body. The cornea,

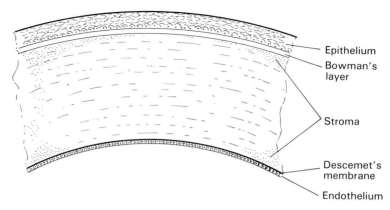

Fig. 24.1 The cornea is composed of five layers. The epithelium is the non-keratinized surface composed of four to six cell layers. Bowman's layer is in contact with the basement membrane of the basal epithelial cells and continuous with the corneal stroma posteriorly. The stroma is composed of lamellar layers of collagen in a glycosaminoglycan matrix. Descemet's membrane is the basement membrane of the endothelial cells. The endothelium is a single cell layer which does not display mitotic activity in adults.

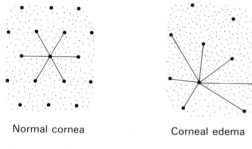

Normal cornea   Corneal edema

Fig. 24.2 In the normal cornea, small diameter collagen fibrils have a highly regular arrangement. The distance between the fibrils is less than half the wavelength of visible light so little scattering occurs. With stromal edema, the regular pattern is disrupted and the space between the collagen fibrils increases with increased scattering of light rays.

in the corneal stroma. Because the bundles of fibrils extend from limbus to limbus, the swelling of the stroma affects only the thickness of the cornea. It follows that corneal thickness and hydration are directly related. The concept of stromal hydration (H) has been helpful in defining this relationship. It is defined as the weight of water in the stroma divided by the dry weight of the stroma. The result is an "index" that has a value of about 3.5 in humans, and increases in a linear fashion with increases in corneal thickness. For example, if a cornea doubles in thickness, it's water content has only increased to 87% (normally 78%). Corneal hydration, however, has doubled, increasing to 6.8 from 3.4 [3].

Epithelium

The epithelium performs several vital functions in the maintenance of corneal clarity. It is composed of four to six cell layers with three distinct cell types: (a) superficial cells; (b) wing cells; and (c) basal cells. The barrier function of the epithelium is enhanced by the presence of "tight junctions" (zonula occludens) between adjacent surface cells, creating a hydrophobic barrier to the influx of water. When the integrity of the ocular surface is lost through

therefore, has a natural tendency to imbibe water and swell. A dynamic equilibrium exists between this tendency and the various elements that maintain the relative dehydration of the cornea (Fig. 24.3). If the barrier function of the epithelium or the pump function of the endothelium is lost, this tendency of the stroma is unchecked and the stromal thickness can increase to several times its normal thickness. This ability to swell is also unusual for a connective tissue and is felt to be due to the relative paucity of interweaving of the collagen fibrils

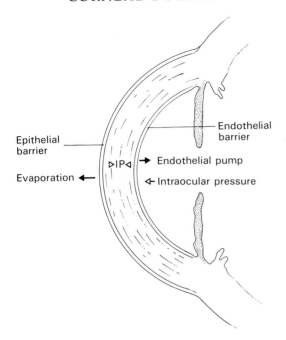

Epithelial barrier

Evaporation ←

▷IP◁ →

Endothelial barrier

→ Endothelial pump

← Intraocular pressure

Fig. 24.3 A dynamic equilibrium exists between factors which tend to increase corneal hydration and factors that tend to keep the cornea in a relative state of dehydration. The imbibition pressure (IP) of the stroma and the intraocular pressure tend to increase stromal hydration. The endothelial pump, along with evaporation and the endothelial and epithelial barriers tend to maintain dehydration.

injury, the epithelium acts quickly with mitotic activity and sliding of cells to cover the defect. Surface studies of the superficial epithelial cells show polygonal cells with an abundance of microvilli. The muscin layer of the tear film is adsorbed onto this surface and provides a hydrophilic interface allowing the even distribution of the tear film over the ocular surface, thus providing a smooth refractive surface. The wing cells are joined to each other and to the basal layer by desmosomes. The basal cells are columnar cells with an apically displaced nucleus. This is the mitotically active layer of the epithelium. Cells produced in this layer have a 3–5 day lifespan, becoming wing cells and finally superficial cells as they migrate to the ocular surface where they are desquamated. The basal cell layer is attached to the basal lamina by hemidesmosomes and the basal lamina is attached to Bowman's layer with anchoring fibrils. Sensory nerve fibers penetrate the basal lamina and reach the upper third of the epithelium before terminating as free nerve endings. The epithelium also contains an energy dependent ion pump mechanism but it is felt this pump contributes little to stromal deturgesence.

Basal lamina/Bowman's layer

The basal lamina of the epithelium merges imperceptibly with Bowman's layer. This layer is 8–16 µm in thickness and is composed of collagen fibrils that are smaller in diameter and less densely packed than those of the stroma. Bowman's layer fuses with the stromal fibrils posteriorly.

Corneal stroma

The stroma accounts for 90% of the thickness of the cornea. It is composed of bundles of collagen fibrils in a GAG matrix (primarily chondroitin and keratin sulfate). These bundles are arranged in a highly regular series of lamellae. The fibrils of adjacent lamellae are oriented nearly perpendicularly in the posterior cornea but intersect at angles less than 90° in the anterior portion of the cornea. The negative charges of GAG create repulsive electrostatic forces, which tend to separate the fibrils, and are felt to be responsible for the tendency of the stroma to imbibe water and swell [4]. These negative charges are also responsible for the higher concentration of positive ions in the stroma. The endothelium and epithelium provide a barrier to the passage of ions, resulting in an osmotic pressure that favors the flow of water into the cornea, contributing a small amount to the overall swelling pressure. This tendency normally results in a swelling pressure exerted against the epithelium and endothelium that measures 50–60 mmHg [5]. It is helpful to note that intraocular pressure tends to counterbalance the swelling pressure (SP) and the difference between these two values is termed the imbibition pressure (IP). Imbibition pressure is approximately 30–40 mmHg under normal conditions [6].

The SP of the stroma decreases as its thickness increases. When the intraocular pressure exceeds the SP of the cornea there is a net flux of water moving into the cornea. When the epithelium is intact, it forms a barrier to the passage of fluid. Pockets of fluid may therefore collect beneath the epithelium, forming bullae. Epithelial edema with bullae formation causes a marked reduction in visual acuity with significant pain if the bullae rupture. This has particular importance for the prognosis of marginally functioning corneas in the postoperative period. If a cornea has modest thickening with the attendant decrease in SP, postoperative pressure spikes (or even normal pressure) may tip the dynamic balance and decompensation can occur.

Descemet's membrane

Descemet's membrane is secreted by the endothelial cells as fine fibrils of collagen in a glycoprotein matrix, and forms the basement membrane of the endothelium. A banded anterior segment is formed in fetal development but deposition of the non-banded posterior layers continues throughout life. If excess amounts of basal lamina are produced, the excrescences are apparent clinically as corneal guttata centrally or Hassall–Henle warts peripherally. When corneal swelling occurs, the elastic properties of Descemet's membrane cause it to be thrown into folds. These folds do not effect vision to the degree that surface irregularities reduce visual acuity because the relative difference between the indices of refraction is much greater at the air–cornea interface than at the cornea–aqueous interface.

Endothelium

The endothelium is a single layer of cells on the posterior surface of the cornea that contains the pump mechanism primarily responsible for corneal dehydration. The cell apices face the anterior chamber and appear primarily hexagonal near the surface, but show marked interdigitation with adjacent cells below the surface. Junctional complexes located near the apical borders are the primary site of the endothelial barrier. The barrier function of the endothelium is felt to be less important than the barrier function of the epithelium, and the fact that it is a single cell layer makes it a "leakier" barrier with a permeability approximately 15 times greater than the epithelium. The integrity of the junctional complexes is dependent on calcium ions and is subject to damage when anterior chamber irrigation is performed with a calcium-free solution.

At birth, the endothelial cell density is approximately 3500–4000 cells/mm^2. Endothelial cells do not display mitotic activity after birth. When cells are lost through normal attrition in aging, surgical trauma, inflammation, and other insults, the remaining cells restore the integrity of the endothelial surface by sliding and enlarging to cover the defect. This results in a variable decrease in endothelial cell density in the older population, and variability in size and shape termed polymegathism. The average endothelial cell density has been shown to be 2400 cell/mm^2 for patients between 40 and 90 years of age [7]. Marked individual variation exists, and although the average cell density appears to be relatively stable in this age group, the range increases with increasing age. The minimum cell density required to maintain corneal deturgescence appears to vary from person to person, but cell counts of 400–700 cells/mm^2 appear to be the lower limit tolerated. Some patients with cell counts in this range do, however, maintain clear corneas. Loss of barrier function of the endothelium as occurs with corneal guttata results in leakage of fluid and ions that may exceed the pump capacity of the remaining cells. Some studies have suggested that the degree of polymegathism is a better predictor of postoperative corneal decompensation than actual cell counts [8].

The existence of intact epithelial and endothelial barriers do not completely prevent ions or water from gaining access to the corneal stroma. The existence of an active pumping mechanism is therefore necessary to maintain corneal fluid balance. The endothelial pump is located in the lateral cell membrane of the endothelial cells. A series of membrane-bound enzymes controls the movement of ions between the stroma and aqueous, and water follows the osmotic gradient created, maintaining corneal fluid balance. Glucose from the aqueous is metabolized via the tricarboxylic acid (TCA) cycle and the hexose monophosphate shunt (HMS) by mitochondria in the cytoplasm to provide the adenosine triphosphate (ATP) required for this energy-dependent pump. The required oxygen is obtained primarily from the tears and aqueous humor, although a small amount is obtained from the limbal circulation. The details of ionic transportation and the movement of fluids are exceedingly complex and some of the mechanisms remain unknown. The endothelial cells contain carbonic anhydrase and recent work suggests that bicarbonate ions and sodium are transported from the stroma to the aqueous, and water passively follows the osmotic gradient, maintaining the dynamic balance of corneal hydration.

Intraocular pressure

Intraocular pressure normally has little effect on corneal hydration until it exceeds the corneal SP [9]. This explains the ability of normal corneas to tolerate chronic elevation of intraocular pressures to 50–60 mmHg without developing corneal edema. As discussed above, the corneal SP decreases significantly as corneal thickness increases. This decreases the differential between the stromal SP and the intraocular pressure. Therefore, a cornea already compromised and thickened by mechanical trauma during surgery is more susceptible to the pressure increases that can occur in the postoperative period.

Evaporation

Evaporation of water from the tear film occurs at a variable rate which is dependent on the integrity of the various layers of the tear film, area of corneal exposure, relative humidity, temperature, and air movement (average approximately $3\,\mu l/h$ at 30% relative humidity) [10]. The importance of this variable is evident in the fact that normal corneas show a 5% thinning through the day (visual acuity is not affected) and in the visual difficulties experienced by patients with marginal corneal

function upon awakening. As corneal evaporation occurs, the tonicity of the tear film increases, drawing fluid from the epithelium, much the same as the application of hypertonic solutions.

Preoperative considerations and evaluation

Pre-existing disease states

A number of pre-existing ocular conditions can compromise the health of the corneal endothelium and increase the possibility of postoperative decompensation. These include uveitis, Fuchs' endothelial dystrophy, previous trauma or surgery, and glaucoma.

CHRONIC INFLAMMATION

The history of chronic inflammation may be associated with generalized or localized decreases in endothelial cell density, although the degree of cell loss is usually not severe. Long-standing inflammatory conditions such as herpes simplex keratitis or iridocyclitis secondary to sarcoidosis are frequently associated with long-term use of steroids and cataract formation. Active inflammation can compromise endothelial cell function by decreased pump rate or loss of endothelial barrier function. It is therefore desirable to suppress chronic inflammation before undertaking cataract surgery and to reduce inflammation as rapidly as possible after surgery. Many clinicians feel intraocular lenses (IOLs), especially anterior chamber lenses, are contraindicated in patients with a history of chronic inflammation, although anecdotal accounts of successful implantation abound. A controlled clinical evaluation of the safety of posterior chamber lens implantation in patients with uveitis is currently underway.

TRAUMA (PENETRATING, NON-PENETRATING, RETAINED FOREIGN BODIES)

An eye that has sustained significant trauma may have endothelial cell loss. Blunt trauma has been shown to be associated with endothelial cell loss which may be mild to severe [11]

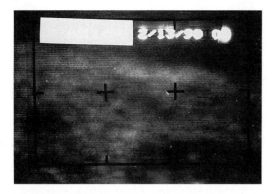

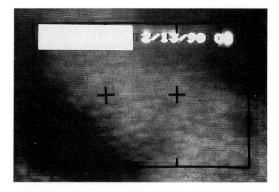

Fig. 24.4 A 15-year-old male sustained significant blunt trauma in the right eye resulting in angle recession, hyphema, and traumatic cataract. Specular microscopy 4 weeks after the injury show a 30% decrease in endothelial cell density and increased polymegathism compared to the uninjured left eye (Fig. 24.5).

Fig. 24.5 Specular microscopy of uninjured left eye of patient in Fig. 24.4.

(Figs 24.4 and 24.5). Penetrating injuries will result in variable loss of endothelial cells depending on the extent of the injury, repair, and accompanying infection or inflammation. A retained foreign body in the anterior chamber can cause corneal edema by mechanical or toxic damage to the endothelium. Copper, iron, and organic matter may induce marked anterior chamber inflammation and endothelial toxicity. If the retained foreign body is inert (i.e. glass or plastic), it will usually settle in the inferior angle and the resulting corneal decompensation begins inferiorly [12]. The cornea may recover if the offending object is removed and the remaining endothelial cells are able to restore normal corneal hydration. The reduction in endothelial cell density, however, may place these patients at risk for decompensation with additional surgical insult.

FUCHS' DYSTROPHY

Fuchs' corneal dystrophy is a slowly progressive, degenerative condition of unknown etiology. The majority of the studies favor an autosomal dominant mode of inheritance, but females are affected 2–4 times as often as males. The condition is bilateral but involvement and progression are frequently asym-

metric. Individuals with early involvement are asymptomatic with slow progression over a 10–20 year period. Early symptoms include blurred vision, glare, and colored halos around lights. Symptoms may be worse early in the day, with vision improving as water is drawn out of the cornea by evaporation and hypertonicity of the tear film. Central corneal guttata are the first sign of the disease and may progress to involve the entire cornea. The presence of fine pigment granules gives the endothelium a characteristic "beaten metal" appearance (Plate 24.1). Corneal sensitivity is reduced. Endothelial dysfunction leads to increasing stromal edema, striate keratopathy, and epithelial involvement with painful bullous keratopathy, fibrosis, and vascularization (Plate 24.2). Histologically, the endothelium is thinned and the nuclei appear widely separated. Vacuoles and clumps of pigment may be present, and late in the disease a fibrillar layer may be seen between Descemet's membrane and the endothelium. Descemet's membrane is thickened with localized excrescences (guttata) [13].

The fact that patients with Fuchs' dystrophy frequently first experience symptoms of their disease at the same age that cataracts are becoming significant makes this entity of particular interest to the cataract surgeon. Although advanced disease is not likely to be overlooked, early signs of the disease may be missed at the slit-lamp during a busy office schedule.

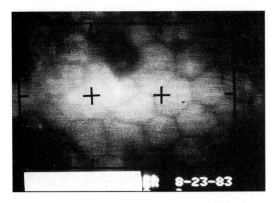

Fig. 24.6 Specular microscopy demonstrating decreased endothelial cell count, polymegathism, and polymorphism. Endothelial guttata displace the endothelial cells creating dark areas in the specular pattern.

Cataract surgery may lead to corneal decompensation. A retrospective study by Lugo *et al.* [14] reported that 67% of the patients with pseudophakic bullous keratopathy and posterior chamber IOLs showed signs of endothelial dystrophy, but only 12% of patients with anterior chamber IOLs showed similar changes. This suggests unrecognized endothelial dystrophy may be a significant factor in corneal decompensation cases that are not associated with anterior chamber lenses.

Patients with slit-lamp findings suggestive of endothelial dystrophy may be evaluated by specular microscopy, pachymetry, or fluorophotometry. Specular findings consist of increased polymegathism and polymorphism. Because guttata push the endothelial cells out of the plane of focus, they appear as dark, acellular areas (Fig. 24.6). Variable stromal thickening (up to 1 mm in severe cases) is found by pachymetry. Although it is generally agreed that the endothelium in Fuchs' dystrophy allows greater aqueous penetration of the stroma, the exact nature of the abnormality remains an area of debate. Burns *et al.* [15] reported significantly increased endothelial permeability in patients with Fuchs' dystrophy, but Wilson *et al.* [16] found no significant difference in permeability compared to normals and concluded that the endothelial pump rate was lower in Fuchs' patients.

RUPTURE OF DESCEMET'S MEMBRANE

Rupture of Descemet's membrane is seen in several conditions, including birth trauma, congenital glaucoma, and keratoconus. Ruptures associated with birth trauma are usually associated with the use of forceps in delivery. The pressure exerted on the head and eye causes a rupture which tends to be oriented vertically. Localized edema may be seen but the endothelium migrates to cover the defect and Descemet's membrane is regenerated with restoration of corneal clarity. Slit-lamp examination in later years reveals vertically oriented striae with a scroll-like, double contour appearance (Plate 24.3). This condition was more common with the use of midposition forceps in the past. In congenital glaucoma the increased intraocular pressure can result in rupture of Descemet's membane. If the pressure is reduced, restoration of endothelial integrity can occur as described above. In both situations, a variable localized decrease in endothelial cell density can occur. The cornea may remain clear for years, but late decompensation can occur and a suggestive history or slit-lamp examination should alert the cataract surgeon to this possibility [17].

Rupture of Descemet's membrane also occurs in keratoconus, and usually presents as an acute event later in life with the sudden development of marked corneal edema, usually accompanied by severe pain and visual loss. The corneal edema usually resolves over a period of months but severe scarring may result. The scarring associated with this condition is a common indication for penetrating keratoplasty.

GLAUCOMA

Long-standing modest elevation of the intraocular pressure appears to have little effect on normal corneal endothelium. On the other hand, the extreme pressure elevations that occur with angle closure episodes are very poorly tolerated and can result in an average 23–40% reduction of endothelial cell density when cell counts from the affected eye are compared to counts from the unaffected fellow eye [18,19]. The history of such an episode or the presence of a surgical or laser iridectomy should alert the surgeon to the possibility of endothelial compromise requiring additional preoperative evaluation.

PREVIOUS EYE SURGERY

A history of previous eye surgery obviously means the eye has had prior exposure to at least some of the many potentially harmful agents discussed in this chapter. It should also be noted that laser surgery of the anterior or posterior segment may be associated with injury to the cornea. Mechanical injury or laser burns to the epithelium during treatment usually heal without consequence. Endothelial laser burns may occur with a very shallow anterior chamber or a poorly focused laser. These burns may result in localized corneal edema that clears relatively rapidly, but endothelial cell loss of 12–19% has been reported after argon laser iridotomy or trabeculoplasty [20]. Laser procedures are frequently associated with a period of inflammation which may also contribute to corneal decompensation. With a history of ocular surgery of any kind, careful preoperative evaluation with special attention to the endothelium is essential. The surgical approach may require modification based on slit-lamp examination, specular evaluation of the endothelium, the presence of a functional filter, or other factors. The surgeon may wish to consider a combined procedure or give special attention to the possibility of late corneal decompensation in obtaining informed consent.

DRY EYE SYNDROME/EYE MEDICATIONS

The frequent use of topical medications and lubricants is the cornerstone of treatment of many ocular diseases, including keratoconjunctivitis sicca, glaucoma, and various inflammatory diseases. The use of preservatives in these preparations has been associated with epithelial and endothelial toxicity [21,22]. Benzalkonium chloride, the most common preservative used in ophthalmic preparations, has been associated with progressive endothelial damage requiring corneal transplantation [23].

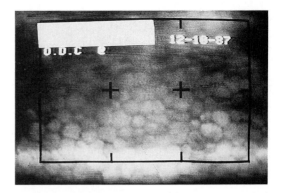

Fig. 24.7 Specular microscopy in a long-term contact lens wearer demonstrates increased polymegathism. Polymegathism has been documented in wearers of polymethylmetacrylate, hydrogel, and rigid gas permeable lens.

A history of any condition requiring the long-term use of topical preparations may be associated with compromise of the endothelium. Preservative-free solutions should be considered for patients requiring chronic use of topical medications.

CONTACT LENS USE

It has been well documented that contact lens wearers experience changes in their endothelium after long-term lens wear. Various investigators have documented polymegathism with daily wear PMMA (polymethylmetacrylate) lenses, rigid gas-permeable lenses, and hydrogel lenses [24,25] (Fig 24.7). The coefficient of variation and the ratio of smallest cell size to largest cell size is increased in these patients, but no evidence exists that the endothelial cell counts are actually decreased. It is felt that the endothelial changes seen in these patients may be the result of hypoxic stress induced by lens wear. Relatively few studies have examined endothelial function in these patients. One study showed that corneas with polymegathism have a decreased deswelling rate compared to normals [26]. Lass *et al.* [25] found increased endothelial permeability by fluorophotometric analysis in long-term wearers of both PMMA and daily wear hydrogel lenses. Because they found no increase in corneal thickness, they concluded a compensatory increase in the endothelial pump rate had occured. Other investigators reported no increase in endothelial permeability. The long-term significance of endothelial changes associated with contact lens use is unknown, but research continues, and more data will be available as increasing numbers of long-term contact lens wearers develop cataracts and undergo surgery.

Evaluation

ENDOTHELIAL CELL COUNTS

A variety of methods are available to study the endothelial mosaic and obtain cell counts. A number of variables affect the accuracy of these counts and the relative density of endothelial cells throughout life. Many studies have been performed with sometimes contradictory results. Debate continues regarding the importance of endothelial cell counts in predicting corneal clarity.

Endothelial cell counts may be evaluated at the slit-lamp utilizing the specular reflection from the endothelium. The illuminating beam and the microscope are positioned to form an angle of approximately 30° with the visual axis. High magnification is required (25× oculars), as well as considerable patience and practice. Careful observers can make a qualitative estimation of the endothelial pattern. The use of comparators or a grid in the slit-lamp oculars can enhance the accuracy of specular observations, and are available from commercial sources.

The specular microscope is designed to study the endothelium in the specular reflection of a narrow slit-beam. A very small area of the central cornea is studied in high magnification. An electronic flash is used to obtain a clear mosaic pattern. Contact and non-contact specular microscopes are available, and some models allow study of the peripheral cornea. A variation using a video recorder allows the tape of the study to be reviewed to select the clearest image for counting. Cell counts are performed on the images obtained in a specified area and multiplied by the appropriate number

to give the cell count per square milliliter. In addition to providing cell density, the mosaic may be studied for variation in cell size and shape (polymegathism). The significance of these various factors is an area of ongoing research and debate. As discussed above, cell counts generally decrease with age, and most clinicians feel a minimum of three separate counts should be made and averaged; if the cell count is low, 9–12 counts should be made because greater variation exists in these corneas.

There are a number of variables which can affect the accuracy of the endothelial cell counts, such as age of the patient, operator skill, and the area of the cornea where the measurement is taken. This last factor is of particular importance in cases where surgical or other trauma has resulted in localized loss of endothelial cells. In patients who have had previous cataract surgery, there is frequently a decreased endothelial cell density superiorly as this area sustains the greatest surgical trauma. Central endothelial cell counts in these patients may be falsely reassuring. This has been termed "vertical cell disparity" by Hoffer [27]. Additional surgical insult may cause local decompensation although the cell count centrally or inferiorly suggests a margin of safety. The surgeon contemplating lens removal or exchange by the superior approach should attempt to determine the cell count in the superior cornea, and modify the approach or consider a combined procedure if the cell density in that area is dangerously low. For eyes that have not had prior surgery, the central endothelial cell count is believed to reflect accurately the overall cell density.

PACHYMETRY

Many investigators and clinicians consider measurement of corneal thickness (pachymetry) to be the single most useful measure of endothelial cell function. It is a functional study, and many patients with clear corneas of normal thickness but marginal endothelial cell counts have undergone successful cataract surgery. The importance of this measurement in prediction of postoperative corneal decompensation is related to the fact that marked thickening of the stroma can occur with little effect on visual acuity until epithelial edema occurs [1]. Serial measurements can provide evidence of progressive endothelial dysfunction preoperatively, or a measure of endothelial recovery in the postoperative period.

The normal cornea measures 0.52 ± 0.02 mm centrally and approximately 0.65 mm in the periphery, although peripheral readings up to 1 mm are considered normal [28]. Clinically, corneal thickness can be measured by an optical pachymeter at the slit-lamp, by the contact specular microscope, or by ultrasonic means. All these methods give accurate results in skilled hands, but ultrasonic pachymetry is most commonly employed at this time. If significant corneal edema is present with striate keratopathy, accurate pachymetry readings are difficult. Preoperative pachymetry measurements greater than 0.65 mm usually indicate a poorer prognosis for postoperative corneal clarity.

FLUOROPHOTOMETRY

Fluorophotometry is a dynamic study of the integrity of the endothelial barrier as measured by its permeability to fluorescein. For the purposes of this study the movement of fluorescein is assumed to be proportional to the movement of water. The patient receives 5 mg/kg fluorescein, either in 10% solution taken orally or by intravenous injection. The dye enters the aqueous humor and crosses the endothelial barrier to enter the corneal stroma. The fluorophotometer measures the concentration of fluorescein in the cornea and aqueous humor. The endothelial barrier is compromised by disease states and surgical trauma. Fluorophotometry can be used to assess the health of the endothelium in corneas with uveitis, Fuchs' dystrophy, or previous surgery. Serial studies can be used to monitor disease progress or endothelial recovery postoperatively. However, this is not a practical clinical tool.

Summary

In conclusion, careful preoperative evaluation including ocular history, complete ocular exam-

ination, and special studies, when indicated, will allow each surgeon to tailor his or her approach to the individual patient. The approach we use in planning surgery in patients with visually significant cataracts is summarized in Fig. 24.8.

Intraoperative factors

Surgical technique

Each step in the preparation and execution of cataract surgery involves choices which affect the degree of surgical trauma to the cornea and attention to potential pitfalls will reward the careful surgeon with fewer postoperative complications. By far the most common cause of postoperative corneal edema is injury to the endothelium. Protection of this vital and fragile cell layer should be of paramount importance at every step in the surgical procedure. Selection of surgical technique, irrigating fluids, viscoelastics, and lens style all affect the degree of endothelial cell loss secondary to surgical trauma. It should be noted that damage to the epithelium or Descemet's membrane are potential causes of corneal decompensation and these will be considered prior to discussion of endothelial problems.

Preparation for intraocular surgery involves a number of steps which are potentially damaging to the corneal epithelium and can result in loss of the epithelial barrier. Digital or mechanical ocular massage can traumatize the epithelium, particularly if they are inadvertently applied with the lid open. The various solutions used in the surgical preparation can be irritating or toxic to the epithelium if prolonged contact is allowed. MacRae *et al.* [29] studied various solutions commonly used in surgical skin preparation to determine their effect on the corneal epithelium of rabbits. They reported marked epithelial toxicity 5 min after application of the following solutions studied: tincture of iodine, Hibiclens, pHisohex, 70% ethanol, povidone—iodine with detergent, and povidone—iodine without detergent. At 3 h, all groups except the group receiving povidone—iodine without detergent showed evidence of epithelial injury. All groups returned to normal

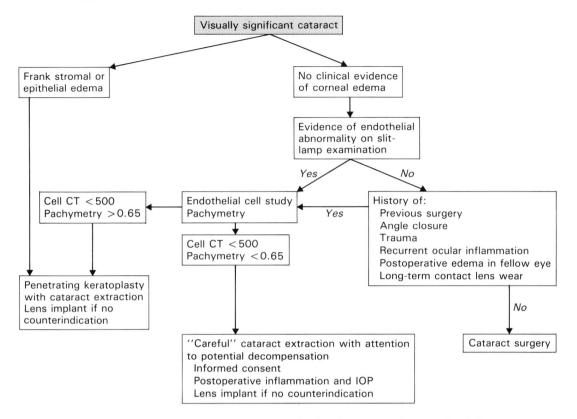

Fig. 24.8 Preoperative evaluation of cataract patients emphasizes the status of the corneal endothelium.

within 1 week [29]. It is wise to irrigate the ocular surface and fornices at the conclusion of the surgical preparation. In addition to protecting the ocular surface, the chance of these solutions entering the eye after the incision is made is likewise decreased by this step. The epithelium is susceptible to drying, and care must be taken to keep the ocular surface moist with a physiologic solution while the lids are restrained by the speculum. It is also possible for the epithelium to be damaged by surgical instruments during the procedure. Careful attention on the part of the surgeon and assistants can minimize these inadvertant injuries.

An unusual cause of corneal edema following cataract surgery is detachment of Descemet's membrane during surgery. If the instrument used to enter the anterior chamber is dull or misdirected, Descemet's membrane and the endothelium may be stripped from the posterior corneal surface (Plate 24.4). If the surgeon

proceeds without recognizing this event, the detachment can be enlarged by injection of a viscoelastic agent or insertion of another instrument. A small detachment will usually not cause significant problems and the viscoelastics or an air bubble may be used to reapproximate the membrane. If a large detachment is noted, it should be repaired at the time of surgery. The membrane may be reattached with double-armed 10/0 nylon suture passed through the membrane and stroma and tied with the knot on the epithelium. Another approach is to purposely incarcerate the membrane in the wound as it is sutured. Care must be used when handling the membrane as it is very friable. A small peripheral detachment may cause a period of localized edema, but this is seldom significant because of the superior location far outside the visual axis.

The popularity of phacoemulsification continues to grow, and it is predicted that it will bypass extracapsular cataract extraction in the near future [30]. Many studies have been completed comparing various methods of cataract extraction and lens implantation with results that are frequently contradictory. It should also be noted that analysis of cell loss can take several forms and may be reported as a "mean percentage decrease" in endothelial cell density, or as a percentage of eyes experiencing a specified level of loss. The coefficient of variation of endothelial cell size and percentage of hexagonal cells are parameters that tend to reflect endothelial cell loss and have been analyzed by some investigators.

Some authors have reported a greater decrease in endothelial cell density postoperatively following phacoemulsification compared to extracapsular and intracapsular cataract extractions (ECCE and ICCE) [31–35]. Other authors have found no significant difference in cell loss comparing posterior chamber phacoemulsification and ECCE or ICCE [36,37]. Levy and Pisacano [38] compared endothelial cell loss in four types of cataract procedures with the following results: ICCE (10.8%), ECCE (10.7%), anterior chamber phacoemulsification (19.2%), and posterior chamber phacoemulsification (17.2%). It is generally agreed that "difficult" cases are associated with much higher endothelial cell loss regardless of the technique used. Complications associated with increased endothelial cell loss include vitreous loss, hypopyon, uveitis, subluxation, shallow anterior chamber, and cystoid macular edema [39]. Several authors have reported that endothelial cell loss and morphologic alterations tend to stabilize 3 months after uncomplicated surgery [40,41]. Persistent inflammation, vitreous touch, and problems associated with IOL design, placement, and stability can lead to progressive cell loss for years after surgery [39].

The importance of maintaining a soft globe and deep anterior chamber to minimize the possibility of vitreous loss or instrument contact with the endothelium was emphasized by leading implant surgeons in a panel discussion at the American Implant Society Meeting in 1981 (N.S. Jaffe, personal communication). The use of adequate anesthesia, speculum, traction sutures, ocular massage, and pharmacologic agents to achieve this goal was encouraged.

IOLs

The ophthalmic literature has devoted a great deal of attention in recent years to the effects of IOL implantation on the corneal endothelium. Cell loss may occur with endothelial contact during or after lens insertion, persistent inflammation, lens defects, or rarely, with toxic lens syndrome associated with IOL materials [42]. Published reports of cell loss following IOL implantation reflect dramatic improvement in lens design, quality control, and surgical technique. The average period of time between lens implantation and the onset of pseudophakic corneal edema is approximately 24 months. There is, therefore, a delay in the appearance of lens-related problems in the literature. It should also be noted that regional variations in lens marketing and distribution may distort the clinical observations of the practicing ophthalmologist.

The early reports comparing endothelial cell loss following cataract extraction with lens implantation to lens extraction alone found significantly higher cell loss with implantation. These reports were based on the use of iris-supported lenses (i.e. Binkhorst, Copeland, and Worst Medallion lenses) with average cell loss of approximately 40% [43]. It is likely that some patients with excessive iridodonesis and chronic low grade inflammation sustained continued damage to the endothelium postoperatively. The use of iris-fixated lenses with metal haptics was associated with persistent inflammation and continued endothelial cell loss.

Average endothelial cell loss with anterior chamber lenses are comparable to losses with iris clip lenses, although less individual variation was seen. Semiflexible, closed loop anterior chamber lenses in particular have been documented to cause continued endothelial cell loss through intermittent touch syndrome, persistent inflammation, and the triad of uveitis, glaucoma, and hyphema (UGH) syndrome (Plates 24.5 to 24.7). These lenses include Azar 91Z, Leiske, Stableflex, and others [44–47].

Reports on IOL explantation have underscored the problems associated with this lens design. Additional reports also indicate a significant visual loss with these lenses secondary to chronic cystoid macular edema [46]. This is a significant factor limiting the vision of patients undergoing penetrating keratoplasty for pseudophakic corneal edema. On the other hand, one-piece all-PMMA open loop anterior chamber lenses such as the Kelman Multiflex and model 120 Feaster are designed to maintain the proper vault yet have sufficient flexibility to avoid problems with sizing. In addition, their open loop design allows for easier explantation should it become necessary [47]. The endothelial cell loss associated with these lenses in uncomplicated cases is probably comparable to posterior chamber lenses (PCLs).

Posterior chamber lenses now represent 94% of lenses being implanted in the USA [30]. Endothelial cell loss associated with these lenses is believed to be about 10% in uncomplicated cases. Most reports of pseudophakic bullous keratopathy associated with PCLs implicate pre-existing endothelial dystrophy as the cause of decompensation [48]. It should be remembered that reports of lens-associated problems lag behind their use, and familiarity with the current literature is important as trends in lens usage change.

Lens materials and insertion technique can be a factor in endothelial cell loss as documented by Levy and Pisacano [49]. They compared the endothelial cell loss with insertion of silicone versus PMMA PCLs following posterior chamber phacoemulsification. They found endothelial cell losses greater than 1200 cells/mm^2 in 12% of the patients receiving PMMA lenses. This degree of cell loss was seen in 7.7% of patients when a silicone lens was inserted flat, but increased to 14.3% and 16.9% with folded and syringe style insertion respectively [49].

Recently, the manufacturers of IOLs have developed surface modifications which may decrease postoperative inflammation and improve visual results. Three types of surface modification are currently under investigation: (a) heparin-grafted modification; (b) surface passification; and (c) polyvinylpyrrolidone-grafted modification (PVP). Approval of some models is expected in the near future.

Fluids and viscoelastics

The use of viscoelastic substances has dramatically changed the nature of intraocular surgery and greatly improved the protection of the endothelium during surgery. The protective effect of these agents has been well documented. Reported endothelial cell losses after cataract extraction with the use of viscoelastics vary widely but are felt to average 10–12% at 2–3 months after surgery and remain relatively stable in uncomplicated cases [38,50,51]. It must be noted that the use of viscoelastics has been associated with postoperative intraocular pressure increases.

Complicated and lengthy intraocular procedures are associated with prolonged endothelial exposure to irrigating solutions. Use of solutions with a composition that closely resembles aqueous humor will minimize trauma to the endothelium. Calcium ions are essential to maintaining the integrity of the endothelial barrier and therefore an essential component of irrigating solutions. Epinephrine is commonly used in irrigating solutions to maintain pupillary dilatation. Endothelial toxicity has been associated with commercial epinephrine solutions containing 0.1% sodium bisulfate as a preservative. Non-preserved epinephrine solutions are recommended or dilution of 1:1000 preserved solution to 1:5000 also dilutes the preservative to a non-toxic level [52].

Postoperative considerations

In the immediate postoperative period the epithelium may be compromised by a variety of insults. Persistent surgical anesthesia, coupled with facial nerve block, render the cornea at risk if the dressing is applied improperly. Various topical medications applied before and after surgery can cause epithelial injury and inhibit healing, including topical anesthetics, antibiotics, and steroids. If the epithelial insult is extensive or chronic, the patient may develop a persistent epithelial defect or recurrent erosion syndrome. Pre-existing dry eye syndrome may complicate the postoperative course.

Epithelial ingrowth is a rare cause of corneal edema after cataract surgery. It is thought that epithelial cells gain access to the anterior chamber through a defect in the surgical wound. A sheet of epithelial cells may be seen on the posterior corneal surface, or cells may proliferate and extend over the iris and trabecular meshwork (Plates 24.8 and 24.9). Pressure may initially be low to normal but can increase to very high levels if the trabecular meshwork is involved. A conjunctival bleb may be seen, as well as flattening of the iris architecture in the area of involvement. Treatment is difficult and a combined approach with surgical resection, cryotherapy, and photocoagulation may be needed, but results are frequently disappointing [53]. Meticulous wound closure will minimize the incidence of this disastrous complication.

A flat anterior chamber due to a wound leak can cause serious endothelial cell damage, particularly if there is contact between the endothelium and the lens implant. If a wound leak is noted postoperatively, the depth and integrity of the anterior chamber should be restored without delay.

Intraocular pressure

Short- and long-term elevations of intraocular pressure are possible following cataract surgery. As discussed earlier, the cornea is particularly susceptible to pressure increases in the postoperative period when endothelial function is likely to be compromised. A patient with poorly controlled glaucoma may benefit from a filtering procedure combined with cataract surgery to protect the eye from endothelial damage in the postoperative period. Pressure elevations may be associated with inflammatory debris, vitreous, or other material clogging the trabecular meshwork. Persistent inflammation may lead to the formation of peripheral anterior synechia compromising trabecular function, and pseudophakic pupillary block has been reported. Prolonged use of topical steroids is associated with intraocular

pressure elevation in sensitive individuals. Increased intraocular pressure postoperatively has been well documented with the use of viscoelastics for endothelial protection, particularly if the material is left in the eye at the conclusion of surgery. Use of Healon [54,55] has been associated with increased intraocular pressure on the first postoperative day, and Alpar et al. [55] noted intraocular pressure more than 25 mmHg in 65% of patients 24 h after surgery when Viscoat was not removed at the end of surgery. If aspiration of any viscoelastic agent is not possible at the conclusion of surgery, prophylactic use of acetazolamide is recommended. Long-term control of intraocular pressure by medical and/or surgical means should be vigorously pursued to maximize visual function after surgery.

Inflammation

The degree of postoperative inflammation is dependent on many factors: pre-existing conditions, surgical technique, fluids and instrumentation, lens factors, and medications. As previously discussed, inflammation can be associated with short-term endothelial dysfunction and long-term cell loss. Control of inflammation postoperatively begins with intraoperative steps to minimize it. The use of corticosteroids postoperatively should be tailored to the degree of inflammation present. The use of antibiotic/steroid combination products is undoubtedly more convenient for patients, but their use should include consideration of the actual need for the individual components. It should also be noted that in some combination products the steroid concentration is less than the concentration found in individual products.

IOL problems

Problems related to IOL design have been discussed previously. It should also be noted that problems may be related to displaced IOLs if contact occurs between the lens and the endothelium (Plates 24.10 to 24.12). Displaced IOLs are sometimes associated with vitreous problems that may contribute to persistent inflam-

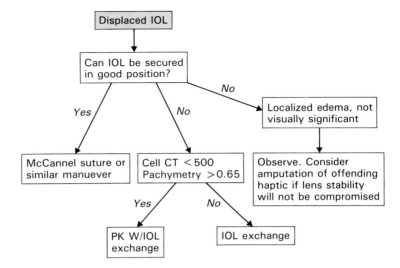

Fig. 24.9 Mangement of displaced intraocular lens (IOL).

mation and corneal decompensation through vitreous touch syndrome. The management of a displaced lens depends on the status of the cornea and the likelihood of surgically securing the lens in good anatomic position (Fig. 24.9). McCannal [56] described a technique for repositioning an IOL using one or two paracentesis sites. When the lens has been repositioned, it is secured to the iris with 10/0 prolene sutures passed through the peripheral cornea (Plate 24.13). Use of McCannal sutures must be weighed against the risks of explantation or exchange of the IOL.

IOL defects or contamination can lead to persistent inflammation requiring explantation in some cases. A "toxic IOL" syndrome has been described where persistent inflammation is felt to be a toxic response to IOL material, but other reports suggest these cases may actually represent smoldering endophthalmitis secondary to an organism of low virulence such as *Propionobacterium acnes*.

Vitreous problems

If the anterior hyaloid face is intact and vitreous prolapse brings it into contact with the corneal endothelium, irreversible corneal edema can follow (Plate 24.14). Vitreous adheres more easily to damaged endothelium and patients with pre-existing endothelial dystrophy are more susceptible, as are patients with compro-

mised endothelium in the early postoperative period. Vitreocorneal touch may be well tolerated if the area of contact is small and peripherally located.

Medical management

The first step in the management of any problem is, of course, establishing the correct diagnosis. The goals of medical (and surgical) management of corneal edema are simply stated as: (a) maximizing visual function; and (b) minimizing patient discomfort. Many patients with early corneal edema note that vision is worse in the early waking hours with improvement as evaporation results in corneal dehydration. This process may be hastened in some patients with the use of hand-held portable hair dryers. A stream of warm air is directed at the ocular surface with the dryer held at arms length, greatly increasing the speed of evaporation and dehydration. This method may not be appropriate for some patients, or effective when early dysfunction progresses. Numerous medical agents are available for the management of corneal edema without surgical intervention.

Hypertonics

The use of topically applied hypertonic agents is one of the mainstays of medical management of corneal edema. The concept is simple: these hypertonic agents applied to the tear film create an osmotic gradient that draws water from the epithelium. It is felt that these agents have little effect on stromal edema as they are soon rendered isotonic by the fluid drawn from the epithelium. Because the primary cause of stromal edema is endothelial dysfunction, and fluid drawn from the stroma is quickly replaced with leakage through the dysfunctional endothelium.

The most commonly used agents are solutions of sodium chloride in 2% and 5% concentrations used 4–6 times a day (ointments are also available and are usually used at bedtime because of their effect on vision). Glycerin is also available for corneal dehydration but is more painful for patients to apply than salt solutions. The use of hypertonics will allow many individuals with marginal corneal edema a significant period of reasonably good acuity and comfort. This can be particularly important if the status of the fellow eye has to be addressed before undertaking penetrating keratoplasty with its lengthy period of visual rehabilitation, or if the patient's age or general medical condition make the delay of surgery desirable. Failing corneas will not, however, be saved by these methods.

Control of inflammation

Because persistent inflammation can have a detrimental effect on both the pump mechanism of the endothelium and its barrier function, it is essential to control inflammation as quickly as possible when it is noted. Topical corticosteroids are applied with sufficient frequency to control inflammation or establish the necessity of another approach. Steroids may also be given orally or by sub-Tenon's injection. The control of inflammation may require lens explantation or exchange, combined with vitrectomy or penetrating keratoplasty in some cases.

Control of intraocular pressure

As noted earlier, elevated or normal intraocular pressure can overwhelm a marginally functioning cornea and decompensation with painful

bullous keratopathy may ensue. It should be remembered that the SP of the stroma decreases sharply as the thickness of the stroma increases and the difference between the stromal SP and the intraocular pressure is the IP of the cornea. When the intraocular pressure exceeds the SP, fluid moves into the cornea and eventually collects beneath the epithelium and bullae are formed. Postoperative pressure elevations are very common. The use of viscoelastic substances for the protection of the endothelium are associated with increased intraocular pressure if they are incompletely removed. In addition, phacoemulsification may be associated with a higher incidence of postoperative pressure spikes. The growing popularity of this procedure requires additional attention to the intraocular pressure in the early postoperative period.

Contact lens

The use of therapeutic hydrogel lenses in aphakic and pseudophakic corneal edema has been of great benefit in patients for whom the visual prognosis is poor or the delay of surgery is desirable for any reason. These lenses, available since the early 1970s, may improve visual acuity in rare cases, but their main use is pain management. They provide relief in approximately 75% of patients with pseudophakic bullous keratopathy [56]. Our approach is to use a high water content lens if there is mild to moderate inflammation. If the inflammation is minimal or the patient has dry eye syndrome, the authors favor the use of a thin membrane lens. These lenses may be used in conjunction with hypertonics and other eye medications.

Surgical intervention

The failure of medical management in pseudophakic bullous keratopathy requires surgical intervention. The surgical approach must be tailored to the specific requirements of the patient, and many factors must be considered including the status of the fellow eye, IOL design and stability, associated anterior or posterior segment abnormalities, and the status of the posterior capsule and vitreous. Management of the IOL at the time of surgery remains an area of debate, but the situation is becoming clearer as our understanding of the pathophysiology of pseudophakic bullous keratopathy increases.

Vitrectomy/laser lysis of vitreous strands

If vitreous touch is noted in the early postoperative period with evidence of corneal decompensation, most authors believe vitrectomy should be undertaken. Anterior vitrectomy with retention of the IOL is possible in some cases if the lens design and placement are not likely to cause further endothelial damage. Both pars plana and anterior approaches have been used. In recent years some clinicians have used the YAG laser to cut vitreous adhesions if endothelial contact is limited to a few vitreous strands.

IOL removal/exchange

The removal of an IOL in an eye with a clear cornea is indicated if there is evidence of ongoing endothelial damage with sufficient endothelial reserve to withstand another intraocular procedure. A lens should not be removed from a quiet, stable eye with good acuity even if it is known to be associated with a high incidence of endothelial injury. Indications for IOL removal include:

1 persistent pain;
2 inflammation;
3 cystoid macular edema;
4 increased intraocular pressure refractory to treatment;
5 progressive endothelial cell loss;
6 IOL instability;
7 intermittent corneal touch; and
8 UGH syndrome.

In these patients lens removal or replacement with a lens of better design may prevent decompensation requiring penetrating keratoplasty in the future. Serial pachymetry or endothelial cell counts in eyes suspected of ongoing IOL-related endothelial damage may help clarify both the necessity and timing of surgery. As indicated earlier, the absolute endothelial cell count required for corneal clarity is not known and may vary between individuals. Corneas with cell counts less than 500 cells/mm^2 or pachymetry readings greater than 0.65 mm are unlikely to withstand the stress of additional surgery and consideration should be given to combining lens exchange with penetrating keratoplasty. In eyes with marginal cell counts or pachymetry, the importance of informed consent is stressed. Eyes with localized edema outside the visual axis which does not progress on serial observations may not require explantation. If segmental corneal edema overlying an area of lens touch is present and progresses, a lens exchange should be considered. Amputation of the haptic may suffice if lens stability will not be compromised.

Penetrating keratoplasty with IOL removal/exchange

If corneal decompensation cannot be managed by conservative measures, penetrating keratoplasty may restore both vision and comfort. Pseudophakic corneal edema is now the most common indication for penetrating keratoplasty in the USA [57]. Although clear grafts are reported in 85–90% of patients undergoing penetrating keratoplasty for pseudophakic corneal edema, reports of visual acuity of 20/40 or better vary from 16% to 87% [58–65]. The wide range reported underscores the fact that this a heterogeneous group with variable length of follow up, and several different surgical procedures are being compared. The most common reason for poor postoperative visual acuity is chronic cystoid macular edema. The patients with the best prognosis are patients with pseudophakic corneal edema associated with posterior chamber IOLs and intact posterior capsules [60]. This group in general experiences the onset of symptoms sooner after surgery and it is felt that the decompensation is due to unusual surgical trauma or an unrecognized pre-existing endothelial dystrophy. The group with the worst prognosis is patients with closed loop anterior chamber lenses retained at the time of keratoplasty. Patient selection is important and a potential acuity measurement may be helpful, although this test is difficult and unreliable in pseudophakic corneal edema patients. The visual acuity of the eye prior to the onset of corneal edema may be a more reliable indicator of the eye's visual potential. The status of the fellow eye must be considered in the timing of keratoplasty with its lengthy period of visual rehabilitation.

Management of the IOL at the time of penetrating keratoplasty entails the same considerations outlined previously. The authors' approach has been to remove iris-fixated lenses in all cases involving: (a) lenses with metal haptens; (b) marked iridodonesis or excessive lens movement; (c) sputnik lenses and patients with a history of chronic inflammation in an uncomplicated insertion; and (d) if intermittent corneal touch is suspected. All closed loop anterior chamber lenses should be removed. In general, if the lens if felt not to be an acceptable style for implantation, it should probably be removed or exchanged. Careful attention to the vitreous is essential in lens explantation and anterior vitrectomy should be performed to ensure that the iris surface and pupillary plane are free of vitreous strands.

Waring [65] advocates reconstruction of the anterior chamber at the time of penetrating keratoplasty, with restoration of normal architecture to the extent possible using lens removal, vitrectomy, lysis of peripheral anterior synechiae (PAS), and closure of large iridectomies with prolene or nylon. He feels that although this approach requires more extensive surgery, the restoration of the anterior segment results in less chronic inflammation, less cystoid macular edema, and better visual results. If the IOL is to be removed, anterior vitrectomy to reduce traction on the vitreous is recommended. Careful inspection of the angle by direct visualization or use of a dental mirror will reveal the extent of PAS and the condition and position of the IOL haptics. Fibrous adhesions may surround the haptics, necessitating blunt or sharp dissection. Amputation of a closed loop haptic followed by careful rotation of the fragment to free it from the angle adhesions may cause less damage to angle structures. Lysis of peripheral anterior synechiae to the extent possible may help to prevent progressive iridocorneal adhesions and severe glaucoma but it is unlikely that trabecular function is restored in these areas of scarring. Control of bleeding that may occur with angle manipulation is essential, and the use of an underwater diathermy tip or fine tip bipolar cautery is recommended.

When the IOL is to be exchanged, the choice between replacement with an anterior chamber lens or a posterior chamber lens must be made. The anterior chamber lenses recommended are open loop designs with enough flexibility to avoid undue stress on the trabecular meshwork and ciliary body, but sufficient anterior–posterior stability to avoid intermittent corneal touch postoperatively. The Feaster Model 120, and Kelman Multiflex designs are examples of lenses that meet these criteria [47]. There have been recent changes in the status of some of these lenses regarding their approval by the Food and Drug Administration (FDA) and may affect availability of these lenses.

Several methods have been developed which allow the placement of a posterior chamber lens in the absence of capsular support. A posterior chamber lens may be sutured to the iris with prolene sutures placed through holes in the optic or haptic, or sutures may be looped around the haptic, passed through the iris, and tied. In recent years, various authors have described methods of transscleral suture fixation of posterior chamber lenses in the absence of capsular support [66–68] (Fig. 24.10). The advantages of these methods are chiefly related to avoiding complications associated with anterior chamber lenses, including endothelial injury, secondary glaucoma, uveitis, and cystoid macular edema. The procedure is technically more difficult than anterior chamber lens placement and potential complications include damage to the ciliary body or the major arterial circle of the iris, suture irritation, and endophthalmitis. Based on their anatomic studies, Duffey et al. [69] suggest use of a one-piece PMMA lens with a single suture tied to each haptic at the greatest diameter of haptic spread. The needle should be passed through the ciliary sulcus, exiting 1 mm posterior to the posterior surgical limbus in an oblique meridian. They feel this method

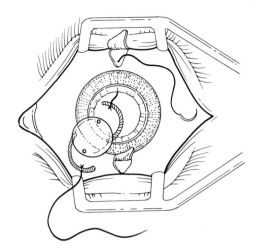

Fig. 24.10 Penetrating keratoplasty with removal of anterior chamber lens and transscleral fixation of a posterior chamber lens. The prolene suture is covered with partial thickness scleral flaps to prevent it from eroding through the conjunctiva, increasing patient comfort and decreasing the chances of endophthalmitis.

gives maximum lens stability with minimal risk to vascular structures [69]. There is as yet no convincing evidence that patients who undergo this procedure have any better visual result or prognosis than patients who receive one of the anterior chamber lenses of the designs listed above. As the length of follow up and patient numbers increase the value of this procedure will become clearer.

Conjunctival flap

The use of conjunctival flaps in the management of bullous keratopathy has significantly decreased in recent years with the advances in microsurgical techniques and the use of bandage contact lenses. This procedure may be a useful measure in the patient with good vision in the fellow eye and poor prognosis secondary to retinal problems in the affected eye. It may also have a place in the management of the patient with poor visual prognosis who cannot manage a therapeutic bandage lens.

The surgical technique most commonly used today was described by Gundersen [70]. Like all ocular surgical procedures, the completion of a successful Gundersen flap requires atten-

tion to detail and can be a difficult procedure [70] (Plate 24.15). A conjunctival flap is considered a reversible procedure and may be used to temporize if delay of definitive surgery is desirable for any reason.

Corneal cautery/diathermy

This procedure is also useful in patients with painful bullous keratopathy, poor visual prognosis due to retinal or optic nerve pathology, and good vision in the fellow eye. Cautery may also be useful for those patients who cannot manage a contact lens or find the appearance of a conjunctival flap unacceptable. The procedure can be performed with topical anesthesia, but retrobulbar injection is preferred. Loose epithelium is removed with a blade or weck sponge. Diathermy is then applied with increasing power until a small stellate contraction of Bowman's layer is noted. Diathermy is then applied in circular fashion starting in the periphery and working centrally for a total of 400–500 applications. A bandage lens is applied at the end of the procedure and the patient is placed on a topical antibiotic steroid combination. It is important to monitor intraocular pressure immediately after the procedure as thermal shrinkage of the cornea may cause pressure elevation. The cornea re-epithelializes over several weeks and the subepithelial scarring establishes a barrier to fluid movement. Farria *et al.* [71] report partial or complete pain relief in 98% of their patients treated with this technique.

Summary

Pseudophakic corneal edema is an entity in constant evolution as changes occur in both pathogenesis and management. Individual approaches to medical and surgical management of postoperative corneal edema in the cataract patient depend on many factors. Each surgeon will develop his or her own guidelines based on clinical experience, surgical techniques, and changes in IOL design and instrumentation. The guidelines we have developed are summarized in Fig. 24.11. Changing trends in surgical procedures are reflected in the speci-

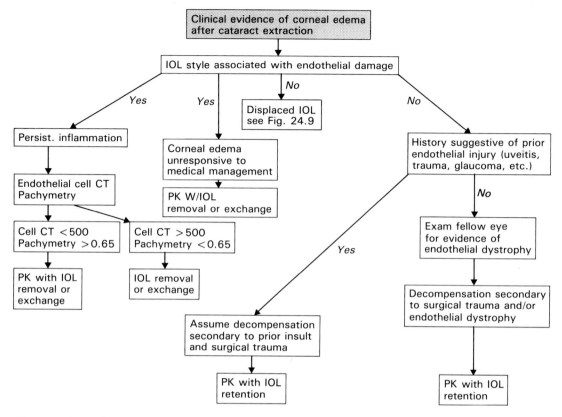

Fig. 24.11 Surgical management of corneal edema following cataract extraction.

fic associations reported in the literature, however, it must be remembered that a significant delay sometimes exists in the identification of these associations. Long-term evaluation of any change in instrumentation and technique is essential in minimizing the incidence of corneal edema after cataract surgery. Careful attention to details and the current literature is essential in providing the best medical and surgical management when it does occur.

References

1 Zucker BB. Hydration and transparency of the corneal stroma. *Arch Ophthalmol* 1966; **75**: 228–31.

2 Hart RW, Farrell RA. Light scattering in the cornea. *J Opt Soc Am* 1969; **59**: 766–74.

3 Dohlman C. Physiology of the cornea: corneal edema. In: Smolin G, Thoft RA, eds. *The Cornea*. 2nd edn. Boston: Little, Brown and Co., 1987: 3–16.

4 Klyce SD, Beuerman RW. Structure and function of the cornea. In: Kaufmann HE, McDonald MB, Barron BA, Waltman SR, eds. *The Cornea*. New York: Churchill Livingstone, 1988: 3–54.

5 Dohlman CH, Hedbys BO, Mishima S. The swelling pressure of the corneal stroma. *Invest Ophthalmol* 1962; **1**: 158–62.

6 Abbott RL, Beebe WE. Corneal edema. In: Abbott RL, ed. *Surgical intervention in Cornea and External Diseases*. Orlando: Grune & Stratton, 1987: 69–85.

7 Hoffer KJ, Kraft MC. Normal endothelial cell count range. *Ophthalmology* 1980; **87**: 861–5.

8 Rao GN, Aquavella JV, Goldberg SH *et al*. Pseudophakic bullous keratopathy: relationship to preoperative corneal endothelial status. *Ophthalmology* 1984; **91**: 1135–40.

9 Ytteborg J, Dohlman CH. Corneal edema and intraocular pressure. II. Clinical results. *Arch Ophthalmol* 1965; **74**: 477–84.

10 Rolando M, Reforo M. Tear evaporimeter for measuring water evaporation rate from the tear film under controlled conditions in humans. *Exp Eye Res* 1983; **36**: 25–33.

11 Bourne WM, McCarey BE, Kaufman HE. Clinical specular microscopy. *Trans Am Acad Ophthal Otolaryngol* 1976; **81**: 743–53.

12 Laibson P. Inferior bullous keratopathy. *Arch Ophthalmol* 1965; **74**: 191–7.

13 Wilson SE, Bourne WM. Fuchs' dystrophy. *Cornea* 1988; **7**: 2–18.

14 Lugo M, Cohen EJ, Eagle RC Jr et al. The incidence of preoperative endothelial dystrophy in pseudophakic bullous keratopathy. *Ophthal Surg* 1988; **19**: 16–19.

15 Burns RR, Bourne WM, Brubaker RF. Endothelial function in patients with corneal guttata. *Invest Ophthalmol Vis Sci* 1981; **20**: 77–85.

16 Wilson SE, Bourne WM, O'Brien et al. Endothelial function and aqueous humor flow rate in patients with Fuchs' dystrophy. *Am J Ophthalmol* 1988; **106**: 270–8.

17 Spencer WH, Fergeson WJ, Shaffer RN, Fine M. Late degenerative changes in the cornea following breaks in Descemet's membrane. *Trans Am Acad Ophthal Otolaryngol* 1966; **70**: 973–83.

18 Olson T. The endothelial cell damage in acute glaucoma on the corneal thickness response to intraocular pressure. *Acta Ophthalmol* 1980; **58**: 257–66.

19 Bigar F. Specular microscopy of the corneal endothelium: optical solutions and clinical results. *Dev Ophthalmol* 1982; **6**: 1–94.

20 Hong C, Itazawa Y, Tanishima T. Influence of argon laser treatment of glaucoma on corneal endothelium. *Japan J Ophthalmol* 1983; **27**: 567–74.

21 Pfister RR, Burstein N. The effects of ophthalmic drugs, vehicles and preservatives on the corneal epithelium. *Invest Ophthalmol Vis Sci* 1976; **15**: 246–59.

22 Gasset AR, Ishii Y, Bach F et al. Cytotoxicity of ophthalmic preservatives. *Am J Ophthalmol* 1974; **78**: 98–105.

23 Lemp MA, Zimmerman LE. Toxic degeneration in ocular surface diseases treated with topical medications containing benzalkonium chloride. *Am J Ophthalmol* 1988; **105**: 670–3.

24 Stocker EG, Schoessler JP. Corneal endothelial polymegathism induced by PMMA contact lens wear. *Invest Ophthalmol Vis Sci* 1985; **26**: 857–63.

25 Lass JH, Dutt RM, Spurney RV et al. Morphologic and fluorophotometric analysis of the corneal endothelium in long-term hard and soft contact lens wearers. *CLAOJ* 1988; **14**: 105–9.

26 Sweeny DF, Holden BA, Vannas A. The clinical significance of corneal endothelial polymegathism. *Invest Ophthalmol Vis Sci* 1985; **26** (suppl): 53.

27 Hoffer KJ. Preoperative cataract evaluation: endothelial cell evaluation. *Int Ophthalmol Clinics* 1982; **22**: 15–35.

28 Hansen FK. A clinical study of the normal human central corneal thickness. *Acta Opthalmol* (Copenh) 1971; **49**: 82–9.

29 MacRae SM, Brown B, Edelhauser HF. The corneal toxicity of presurgical skin antiseptics. *Am J Ophthalmol* 1984; **97**: 221–32.

30 Carr M. Cataract, intraocular lens, and refractive surgery in 1987 with a forecast to 1995. *J Cataract Refract Surg* 1988; **14**: 664–7.

31 Sugar J, Mitchelson J, Kraft M. The effect of phacoemulsification on corneal endothelial cell density. *Arch Ophthalmol* 1978; **96**: 446–8.

32 Abbott RL, Forster RK. Clinical specular microscopy and intraocular surgery. *Ophthalmol* 1979; **97**: 1476–9.

33 Yang HK, Kline OR Jr. Specular microscopy and intraocular lens implantation. *Am Intraocul Implant Soc J* 1981; **7**: 31–5.

34 Colvard DM, Mazzocco TR, Kratz RP et al. Endothelial cell loss following phaco-emulsification in the pupillary plane. *Am Intraocul Implant Soc J* 1981; **7**: 334–6.

35 Kraff MC, Sanders DR. Planned extracapsular extraction versus phacoemulsification with IOL implantation: A comparison of concurrent series. *Am Intraocul Implant Soc J* 1982; **8**: 38–41.

36 Kraff MC, Sanders DR, Lieberman HL. Specular microscopy in cataract and intraocular lens patients: A report of 564 cases. *Arch Ophthalmol* 1980; **98**: 1782–4.

37 Davison JA. Endothelial cell loss during the transition from nucleus expression to posterior chamber-iris plane phacoemulsification. *Am Intraocul Implant Soc J* 1984; **10**: 40–3.

38 Levy JH, Pisacano AM. Endothelial cell loss in four types of intraocular lens implant procedures. *Am Intraocul Implant Soc J* 1985; **11**: 465–8.

39 Oxford Cataract Treatment and Evaluation Team (OCTET). Long-term corneal endothelial cell loss after cataract surgery. *Arch Ophthalmol* 1986; **104**: 1170–5.

40 Rao G, Stevens R, Harris J et al. Long-term changes in corneal endothelium following intraocular lens implantation. *Ophthalmology* 1981; **88**: 386–97.

41 Schultz RO, Glasser DB, Matsuda M et al. Response of the corneal endothelium to cataract surgery. *Arch Ophthalmol* 1986; **104**: 1164–9.

42 Donshik PC. Pseudophakic bullous keratopathy—an overview. *Cataract* 1984; **2**: 30–3.

43 Bourne WM, Kaufman HE. Cataract extraction and the corneal endothelium. *Am J Ophthalmol* 1976; **82**: 44–7.

44 Waltman SR. Corneal changes from intraocular surgery. In: Kaufman HE, McDonald B, Barron BA, Waltman SR, eds. *The Cornea*. New York: Churchill Livingstone, 1988: 911–33.

45 Kraff MC, Sanders DR, Raanan MG. A survey of intraocular lens explantations. *J Cataract Refract Surg* 1986; **12**: 644–50.

46 Smith PW, Wong SK, Stark WJ et al. Complications of semiflexible, closed-loop anterior chamber intraocular lenses. *Arch Ophthalmol* 1987; **105**: 52–7.

47 Apple DJ, Olson RJ. Closed-loop anterior chamber lenses. *Arch Ophthalmol* 1987; **105**: 19–20 (letter).

48 Cohen EJ, Brady SE, Leavitt K et al. Pseudophakic

bullous keratopathy. *Am J Ophthalmol* 1988; **106**: 264–9.

49 Levy JH, Pisacano AM. Clinical endothelial cell loss following phacoemulsification and silicone or polymethylmethacrylate lens implantation. *J Cataract Refract Surg* 1988; **14**: 299–302.

50 Graue EL, Polack FM, Balazs EA. The protective effect of sodium hyaluronate to the corneal endothelium. *Exp Eye Res* 1980; **31**: 119–27.

51 Holmberg AS, Philipson BT. Sodium hyaluronate in cataract surgery II. *Ophthalmology* 1984; **91**: 53–9.

52 Hull DS, Chessotti MT, Edelhauser HF *et al*. Effect of epinephrine on the corneal endothelium. *Am J Ophthalmol* 1975; **79**: 245–50.

53 Maumenee AE, Palton D, Morse PH *et al*. Review of 40 histologically proven cases of epithelial downgrowth following cataract extraction and suggested surgical management. *Am J Ophthalmol* 1970; **69**: 598–603.

54 Barron BA, Busin M, Page C. Comparison of the effects of Viscoat and Healon on postoperative intraocular pressure. *Am J Ophthalmol* 1985; **100**: 377–84.

55 Alpar JJ, Alpar AJ, Baca J. Comparison of Healon and Viscoat in cataract extraction and intraocular lens implantation. *Ophthal Surg* 1988; **19**: 636–42.

56 McCannal MA. A retrievable suture idea for anterior uveal problems. *Ophthal Surg* 1976; **7**: 98–103.

57 Robin JB, Gindi JJ, Schanzlin DJ *et al*. An update of indications for penetrating keratoplasty. *Arch Ophthalmol* 1986; **104**: 87–9.

58 Langston RHS. Prevention and management of corneal decompensation. *Int Ophthal Clin* 1982; **22**: 189–95.

59 Terry AC, Snip RC, Snip RT. Improved vision following penetrating keratoplasty for pseudophakic corneal edema. *Ophthal Surg* 1984; **15**: 752–6.

60 Koenig SB, Schultz RO. Penetrating keratoplasty for pseudophakic bullous keratopathy after extra-

capsular cataract extraction. *Am J Ophthalmol* 1988; **105**: 348–53.

61 Schanzlin DJ, Robin JB, Gomez DS *et al*. Results of penetrating keratoplasty for aphakic and pseudophakic bullous keratopathy. *Am J Ophthalmol* 1984; **98**: 302–12.

62 Speaker MG, Lugo M, Laibson PR, *et al*. Penetrating keratoplasty for pseudophakic bullous keratoplasty; management of the intraocular lens. *Ophthalmology* 1988; **95**: 1260–7.

63 Polack FM. Pseudophakic corneal edema; an 11-year study of its development, incidence, and treatment. *Cornea* 1989; **8**: 306–12.

64 Waring GO III, Stulting RD, Street D. Penetrating keratoplasty for pseudophakic cornea edema with exchange of intraocular lenses. *Arch Ophthalmol* 1987; **105**: 58–62.

65 Waring GO III. Management of pseudophakic corneal edema with reconstruction of the anterior ocular segment. *Arch Ophthalmol* 1987; **105**: 709–15.

66 Stark WJ, Goodman G, Goodman B, Gottsch J. Posterior chamber intraocular lens implantation in the absence of posterior capsular support. *Ophthal Surg* 1988; **19**: 240–3.

67 Cowden JW, Hu BV. A new surgical technique for posterior chamber lens fixation during penetrating keratoplasty in the absence of capsular or zonular support. *Cornea* 1988; **7**: 231–5.

68 Pannu JS. A new suturing technique for ciliary sulcus fixation in the absence of posterior capsule. *Ophthal Surg* 1988; **19**: 751–4.

69 Duffey RJ, Holland EJ, Agapitos PJ, Lindstrom RL. Anatomic study of transscleral sutured intraocular lens implantation. *Am J Ophthalmol* 1989; **108**: 300–9.

70 Gundersen T. Surgical treatment of bullous keratoplasty *Arch Ophthalmol* 1960; **64**: 260–7.

71 Farria RL, Iwamoto T, DevVoe AG. Cautery of Bowman's membrane. *Am J Ophthalmol* 1974; **77**: 548–54.

25: Vision Correction after Cataract Surgery

DAVID D. MICHAELS

Optical correction is the final step in the visual rehabilitation of the cataract patient. Since refraction is an integral part of postsurgical management, it must necessarily be carried out in a setting where adequate instrumentation is available to diagnose and treat any complications which may affect the visual result. This chapter reviews both routine and special postoperative refractive problems.

Useful refractive techniques

Refraction might be attempted one or more weeks after surgery, depending on the status of the eye and the type of surgery. Examination is repeated at weekly intervals until measurements are stable. Temporary lenses can be given if the operated eye is the only one with useful vision. In most cases, the final prescription can be ordered after 6–8 weeks. Periodic refractions are scheduled thereafter because healing is not always predictable, measurements may change from intercurrent disease such as diabetes or capsular opacification, a cataract may progress in the other eye, or lens modifications are dictated by new visual habits.

Since most cataract patients are older and the effort to see with an eye that has not been used is tiring, allow enough time for indecisions and indispositions. Begin with greater targets, closer test distances, brighter lights, maximum contrast, and larger lens change increments.

Aphakic refraction

A certain number of patients from preimplant days as well as some for which implants were contraindicated constitutes a significant, if decreasing, proportion of every surgical practice. Aphakic problems are thus likely to remain with us for some time to come.

Because initial vision is often poor, compounded by glare and photophobia, early acuity is checked with a simple +12 D sphere coupled to a pinhole disc. A smile of recognition provides reassurance to both patient and surgeon. After the first week, keratometry is used to follow wound healing, to identify the degree and axis of astigmatism, and to provide a basis for eventual contact lens fitting. The calibration of the keratometer should be checked periodically against a steel sphere. Comparing the presurgical and postsurgical k-readings, gives a clue to the amount of induced corneal astigmatism. If there is much corneal surface irregularity, k-readings may be misleading because the mires cover only a central 3 mm area. Recall that in aphakia the spectacle cylinder (because it sits in front of the eye) will be less than the keratometric cylinder.

Retinoscopy is the simplest method of objective refraction. It is easy in aphakia because the cornea is the only refracting surface, and the pupil is generally well dilated. Of course, the reflex will be quite dim until one approaches the neutral range. One might therefore begin with a +10 D sphere and move somewhat nearer the eye than the usual working distance.

As with all high refractive errors, subjective refraction is best performed with a trial frame and trial lenses. The advantage is that it maintains a more precise vertex distance. An approximate formula to compute the vertex effectivity is: $F^2/1000$ per mm displacement, where F is the back vertex lens power (i.e. the power engraved on your trial lenses). Thus if a $+12\,D$ lens is displaced 6 mm further from the eye, the new power is 0.14×6 or $0.86\,D$ more plus (or, conversely, a $+11.14\,D$ lens will correct the same refractive error at the new position). An alternative is to have available some $+12\,D$ spheres made up in suitable (i.e. light, more or less round, small eye-sized) frames and overrefract these with a trial clip. This maintains not only the same vertex distance but preserves the proper pantoscopic tilt. If the overrefracting lens (sphere or cylinder) does not exceed $+4\,D$, this value can be added directly to the initial $+12\,D$. Measure the vertex distance by inserting a stenopeic slit in the trial frame and note distance to closed lid with a metal PD ruler (allow 1 mm for lid thickness). Transmit this value (also necessary in contact lens ordering) to the laboratory.

In binocular aphakia, the fusional potential is evaluated by measuring phorias and vergences. Polarized targets may show suppression despite Worth dot fusion. Stereopsis can be measured with any convenient disparate stereograms. Some time may be necessary to re-establish binocular vision especially when the patient has used only one eye for years. In high anisometropia with astigmatism, fusion may only be achieved with bilateral contact lenses hence a trial fitting with overrefraction should be attempted.

Near vision will naturally require either separate reading glasses or a multifocal. Previous near vision correction serves as a guide. Note that the add should be measured with targets suitable to the patient's needs. The aim is to provide useful near vision, not necessarily maximum near acuity. In aphakia particularly, because of intrinsic magnification, the add can often be weaker and thus allow some intermediate distance focusing.

Pseudophakic refraction

Pseudophakic refraction is relatively straightforward and rewarding for both patient and surgeon. Overrefraction with trial lenses is unnecessary and standard methods with a refractor are feasible. A dilated pupil and a dark room facilitates the examination. Eyes with iris-fixated implants (no longer used) should not be dilated. Acuity targets with good contrast are preferred. Do not use contrast sensitivity charts for refraction because (a) lenses only correct high frequency loss; and (b) optical blur affects all frequencies more or less proportionately. In fact, if contrast sensitivity is used in preoperative evaluation of cataract progression, be sure to correct all refractive errors before attaching diagnostic significance to the results.

Keratometry after surgery allows comparison to preoperative k-readings, used to calculate intraocular lens (IOL) power, and indicates induced astigmatism. Sequential readings evaluate wound healing and stabilization. Persistent astigmatism may suggest cutting sutures (usually at about 6–8 weeks). If the retinoscopic cylinder differs significantly from the k-readings, suspect IOL decentration or tilt.

Retinoscopy may be somewhat more difficult because of reflections. In difficult cases, approach to ophthalmoscopic distances to visualize the reflex. Use a darkened room, dilate the pupil, and allow enough time to dark-adapt your own eyes. Automated objective refractors may help but can mislead if the instrument picks up reflections from loops, holes, or pegs, or if fixation is unsteady.

Subjective refraction might begin with the retinoscopic findings. If retinoscopy is unreliable, start with the preoperative spherical equivalent and add the postoperative keratometric cylinder. Proceed with astigmatic dial or cross cylinder refinements. Recall that it is impossible to find the correct cylinder power if the axis is wrong. If the opposite eye (phakic or pseudophakic) has good vision, balance acuities with the minimum anisometropic correction. If vision cannot be equalized, determine the best spherical correction that avoids diplopia.

A major problem in pseudophakic refraction is achieving cooperation with the other eye which is often phakic and has good vision. Every effort should be made to restore binocularity assuming, of course, that the patient had fusion before surgery. Check motility, phorias, vergences, sensory fusion (or suppression), and the amount of prism (horizontal and/or vertical) needed to abolish diplopia at distance and for near vision.

If initial vision is poor, a 2.2× wide angle telescope can be inserted in a trial frame. Refraction is carried out in the usual way by placing trial lenses behind the telescope. The telescope is subsequently removed. Alternatively, acuity targets are moved to half the conventional test distance to provide sufficient magnification for discriminating lens changes.

Near vision needs are determined in the usual way. In younger patients, the add may be unequal for the operated and unoperated eye. A good way to establish useful add power is to measure the range of vision. The add should err on the weak side to provide intermediate focus. Recommend strong reading light which improves the range through depth of focus. Never prescribe an add on the basis of accommodative amplitude and Donders' table (or any other table). Instead obtain specific individual measurements using print size that the patient is likely to use.

Refractive management of aphakia

Following cataract extraction without an implant, the cornea becomes the only major refractive component of the eye. When this refractive hyperopia is corrected by spectacles, the retinal image is around 30% larger, depending on the previous ametropia. When the corrected aphake reaches for an object, it appears closer which translates into a feeling of instability and insecurity [1]. In fact, many aphakic patients never trusted their spectacles sufficiently to resume driving.

In addition, changing magnification across the field of view causes distortion. Objects seem deformed as the gaze shifts; an expanse of floor appears like a saucer, and squares like pin cushions. Magnification further means that a given retinal area is covered by a smaller visible field through the spectacle lens. Thus a circumferential area of the field has no retinal representation. Objects traversing this so-called ring scotoma appear and disappear with the annoyance of a jack-in-the-box [2]. The ring scotoma shifts with eye movements, whereas head movements produce an unpleasant swim. These optical phenomena can be demonstrated and measured by simple office tests [3].

If the unoperated eye is phakic with good vision, it is generally impossible to achieve binocular vision with spectacles. The retinal image size inequality causes insuperable diplopia. And as if the magnification, distortion, swim, and diplopia were not enough, the aphakic patient is now presented with spectacles whose fried egg appearance must be cosmetically discouraging if not dismaying. Fortunately, a variety of modalities and lens designs are available to ameliorate if not eliminate some of these optical complications.

Aphakic spectacles

Spectacle correction is indicated for those aphakic patients who cannot (or will not) tolerate contact lenses or where the condition of the eye precludes a secondary procedure such as implants or epikeratophakia. Spectacle correction seldom kindles clinical enthusiasm, nor does the patient usually regard his or her glasses as an enviable distinction. To solve the unique optical problems of aphakia, lens design objectives either aim to: (a) maintain optimum acuity through eccentric portions of the lens by balancing front and rear curves and by aspheric curves; or (b) improve the field of vision with larger lenses. Naturally, no lens designer thinks that these aims are mutually exclusive. Nevertheless, they lead to different lens construction within the tolerance limits of mass production. For optimum eccentric acuity, corrected curve and asphericity can be better controlled in a smaller lens (generally 40 mm diameter). This is the principle of the lenticular lens which also lowers weight. On the other hand, to enhance the visible field, larger full field lenses are recommended. Being larger, they require flatter base curves to reduce distortion, minimize thickness and improve appearance. Larger lenses tend to have flat rear curves. In all cases, lenses should be plastic to reduce weight. A variety of high index plastics are now available to reduce thickness. High index materials cause more reflections which can be improved by coatings. Lenses should be aspheric and fit as close to the eye as the lashes allow. The smaller the vertex distance, the less the magnification. Minus cylinders are preferred for the same reason. Little can be done about the magnification of the patient's eye as seen through the lens [4].

The ideal bifocal aphakic spectacle design remains controversial. Neither flat top nor round top are aspheric over the segment except in the fused glass lens. Variable focal lenses can be tried if these are available. The style of previously worn bifocals should also be considered. If the patient was happy with separate distance and reading glasses before surgery, there is little reason to force the additional burden of multifocal adaptation to the post-operative adjustment problems.

Ultraviolet (UV) filtration is probably worth-while. The damaging effects of UV rays on the retinas of animals are well documented but not so well in humans. The most damaging rays are presumably in the range of 280–315 nm (UVB); the same rays responsible for sunburn and keratitis. Photosensitizing drugs (e.g. those used in the treatment of psoriasis) may increase the risks. Whether UV causes cystoid macular edema remains a puzzle (where are all the damaged maculas from the days of simple cataract extraction without plastic lenses or filters?). At any rate, UV protection does no harm and may do good. Polycarbonate is in-trinsically the most protective, CR-39 resin next, and glass last. Adding the proper tints can make these materials more or less com-pletely protective. Specially filtered aphakic contact lenses can also be obtained and most implants are UV absorbent.

Temporary tinted wrap-around aphakic spectacles are available to be worn before the final prescription is ordered. They provide useful vision and help protect the eye (e.g. can be worn while sleeping). Bifocals are not needed if the patient is shown that reading vision can be quite good by simply sliding the single vision lenses down the nose.

Care should be taken in bilateral aphakes to center the lenses correctly. By placing the distance optical centers slightly closer than the interpupillary distance, the excessive load on convergence for reading is relieved through the base in effect. Frames should be adjustable, sturdy, of round shape and small eye size.

Contact lenses for aphakia

Aside from their better cosmetic appearance, aphakic contact lenses decrease most if not all of the optical annoyances of spectacles. Because they correct the refractive error at the cornea and not in front of the eye, they reduce mag-nification by 16% or more. Contact lenses improve the field of view, eliminate distortion, and abolish the ring scotoma. Contact lenses can be fitted once the refraction and k-readings have stabilized. Even if the other eye does not have good acuity and binocularity is not a goal, a contact lens will be an advantage because vision more nearly approximates that before surgery.

Handling contact lenses will almost invari-ably present problems for elderly aphakes, especially if the eye to be corrected is the only one with useful vision. A magnifying mirror can help, or a spouse who will assume responsibility for insertion, removal, and clean-ing. Frequently, the solution is an extended wear lens which is cleaned in the office at reasonable intervals. By having several lenses available, the patient can wear one while the other is cleaned. What determines a reasonable interval will depend on the eye's reaction, the amount of deposits, and the reliability of the patient to report untoward reactions. The usual time interval ranges from 1 month to 1 week. Aphakic back-up spectacles should be available.

Hard aphakic contact lenses are naturally thicker and heavier than cosmetic lenses. Lenses may be small single cut or larger lenticular. Single cut lenses are useful for eyes with decentered pupils. Lenticular lenses are easier to fit because they center better. Tear exchange can be confirmed by fluorescein staining. Materials of higher oxygen trans-mission are preferred if available. Overrefrac-tion determines the proper power.

Soft lenses allow extended wear though they do not correct astigmatism greater than 0.75 D or so. Since the aphake will generally need a reading add in any case, the cylindric correction can be incorporated in the bifocal to be worn over the contact. Fitting technique is similar to cosmetic lenses but of larger diameter and a base curve somewhat flatter. High astigmatic corneal curvatures may destabilize the lens and require a back toric design. Liberal use of lubricants is recommended because of the high incidence of dry eyes in this age group.

The variety of complications accompanying soft contact lens wear grows yearly as more data becomes available from larger population samples. Thus the incidence of infectious corneal ulcers is five times more common in aphakic extended wear than daily wear cosmetic lenses. Corneal neovascularization, sterile infiltrates, and giant papillary conjunctivitis may require frequent lens replacement, switching to different materials, or discontinued lens wear.

Unfortunately, because of the reduced demand many manufacturers have discontinued aphakic contact lens production and newer materials of higher oxygen transmission and disposable lenses are not yet available in aphakic power ranges.

Other methods of aphakic correction

For those aphakic patients who cannot tolerate spectacles or contact lenses, there are several other options at the price of greater risk of complications. Secondary implants may be indicated if the condition of the eye permits. Epikeratophakia is less invasive and might be indicated in glaucoma, chronic uveitis, disorganized anterior segment, or monocular patients.

Acuity results with epikeratophakia are lower than with secondary implants and the postoperative course is longer. The incidence of decreased acuity is also higher with epikeratophakia compared to presurgical vision. Older patients tend to lose more vision than younger ones. Moreover, complications are often irreversible.

Therapeutic soft contact lenses may help in bullous keratopathy and can occasionally improve vision. Bandage lenses may also reform a flat anterior chamber. Soft lenses can act as vectors to concentrate selected ophthalmic drugs and prolong contact time providing the drug does not discolor the lens or bind to the lens matrix. Pinhole contact lenses may improve acuity and mask a large iridectomy. In monocular cases, irrespective of refractive error, plastic safety glasses should be worn for protection.

The aphakic problem patient

The ingredients of an aphakic prescription are complex and if improperly concocted will make a hash of the visual result. Here are some common complaints which may have an optical basis:

Poor acuity: incorrect refraction; transposition errors; changes in refraction; contact lens slipped off cornea; frame misalignment; lens surface imperfections.

Magnification: inevitable with spectacles but less so with contact lenses; excessive vertex distance; base curve too bulgy; lenses too thick.

Distortion: lenses too large; lenses not aspheric; over- or undercorrection of astigmatism; excessive oblique astigmatism; improper frame adjustment.

Spectacles too heavy: glass lenses; lenses too large; frames too heavy; frames improperly adjusted.

Diplopia: excessive anisometropia; incorrect lens centration; contact lens lag; inappropriate prism; insufficient prism.

Monocular diplopia: misaligned bifocal segment; contact lens displaced; double vision confused with blurred vision; spectacle lens reflections; high astigmatism.

Near vision problems: add too strong or too weak; add omitted; progressive lens substituted for blended lens; frame misalignment; segment line in field of vision; poor intermediate vision; convergence insufficiency; reading field too small; change in segment style.

Glare: lenses not coated or tinted; dirty lens; displaced contact lens; improper panto tilt.

Contact lens problems: contact lens displaced, dirty, torn, dried out, lost, excessive movement on blink; poor edge design; warped lens.

Cosmetics: lenses too heavy, too bulgy, too large; frame does not hold lenses or hide edges.

Refractive management of pseudophakia

Although the pseudophakic eye is much like a phakic one from an optical standpoint, there are some differences. First, the operated eye often has an altered (either more or less) refractive power and this change is brought about suddenly, not over years like the natural evolution of ametropia. Second, the induced refractive change may or may not be compatible with the fellow eye. Thus, even if zero post-surgical astigmatism has been achieved, adjustment problems can be anticipated if the fellow eye requires a strong cylinder. Third, if the fellow eye is phakic and has, as is likely, a developing cataract, its progression will in itself induce refractive changes which need to be matched sooner or later. Fourth, when the second eye requires surgery, it is desirable to match its optics to the first. Problems arise when the first has an excessive amount of over- or undercorrection. It follows that the optical management of pseudophakia begins before surgery, in planning the refractive goal; during surgery, in avoiding unwanted results; and after surgery, in correcting whatever results have been obtained.

The other eye

If the other eye has already been operated, the problem of matching it is predetermined. This does not necessarily make it simple. Whether the second eye should be made emmetropic or matched to a stable but substantial refractive error will depend on prior adaptation, the potential for achieving binocularity, and a realistic appreciation of the technical feasibility of achieving a match (e.g. unlikely if the prior refractive result was erratic or due to some operative complication). Some surgeons aim for monovision with implant power of one eye set for distance and the other for near. These options should be discussed with the patient.

If the other eye has uncorrectable poor acuity and no surgery is contemplated, the refractive goal should probably be emmetropia or near-emmetropia. Some aim for slight myopia for minimal near vision needs. It is an optical fact that a moderate amount of postoperative myopia (around 2 D) will cause the least change in retinal image size (compared to the pre-surgical size) irrespective of the prior spectacle correction.

If the other eye has a cataract which one plans to remove later, its refraction (particularly astigmatism) must be considered. It is not easy to prevent induced astigmatism but even more difficult to surgically correct a pre-existing astigmatism. Obviously, the degree of opacification and the history of progression in the eye with the advanced cataract will help in timing the intersurgical interval. If the estimated intersurgical interval is long, one must decide whether the first eye should be made emmetropic or matched to the existing refractive error. If the latter objective is chosen, the surgeon must choose between isometropia or iseikonia.

Preoperative planning

Emmetropia would seem to be an ideal postoperative refractive goal, especially if the eye was previously emmetropic or nearly so. Even if there was a significant refractive error prior to surgery, adaptation will probably be uneventful all other factors being equal. Suppose, however, the other phakic eye has no cataract and 5 D of ametropia with some astigmatism besides. To match such an eye one may aim for an equal refractive error or an equal retinal image size. The latter depends not only on the ametropia but also on whether it is axial or refractive. Isometropia might achieve equal acuity at the expense of aniseikonic headaches, distortion, or nausea. Fortunately, because aniseikonia only arises with minimal image size disparity (5% is less) and in patients who have binocular vision, its correction can often be achieved by additional spectacle lenses whose base curve, thickness, and vertex distance are appropriately adjusted [5]. Or one can order selected contact lens–spectacle combinations. This is preferable to leaving the patient with a large anisometropia and diplopia.

A variety of formulas are used to calculate the desired implant power based on preoperative keratometry, axial length measurements, and refractive error. As is well known, most cataracts induce spherical and cylindric refractive changes as they progress. These, usually myopic, deviations should be taken into account in implant calculations. Ideally, one should have the old refractive records, but if these are unobtainable, compare the axial lengths and k-readings of the two eyes.

Intraoperative factors

Since spherical refraction can now be reasonably well controlled by careful preoperative planning of IOL power, intraoperative considerations are directed primarily at preventing astigmatism. The most important factors are pre-existing astigmatism, length of incision, technique of wound closure, and (least predictably) effect of wound healing. For example, the current trend is towards smaller incisions and few sutures. Note that implicit in this is the idea of leaving the eye not without astigmatism but with an unchanged astigmatism. Thus the importance of the pre-existing cylinder. To modify corneal curvature, many surgeons advocate the use of an operative keratometer.

Other factors, of less importance in preventing postoperative astigmatism, are the location of the incision, the type of implant, IOL tilt or decentration, postoperative medications (e.g. steroids), and premature suture removal [6].

Many IOL types are now available, and marketing claims are often unsubstantiated. While the resolution (lines per mm) is generally good, some designs cause more spherical aberration, more image degradation with decentration, and more internal reflections. Optical configuration (e.g. biconvex, planoconvex, etc.) must also be balanced by weight, anterior–posterior dimensions, and mass [7]. The current trend is towards biconvex and planoconvex configurations, and larger optical diameters (6.5–7 mm) [8].

Postoperative correction

Postoperative optical management of pseudophakia is primarily concerned with problems of anisometropia and astigmatism, either planned or unanticipated [9]. Assuming the refractive measurements have stabilized, the goal is to achieve best acuity, rapid adjustment, and binocular cooperation without distortions, discomfort, or disability.

Management of postoperative anisometropia might proceed along the following lines:
1 give the full correction for maximum acuity. This presents no difficulty if the refractive difference is less than 3 D but may also be tried if the difference is greater. Some patients adapt and become happy alternators. After all it happens with monovision prescriptions;
2 balance the correction, modifying power to achieve best if not optimum acuity;
3 correct one eye (or both) with contact lenses. This applies particularly to astigmatic anisometropia;
4 in selected cases a contact lens–spectacle combination may modify retinal image size sufficiently to achieve fusion; and
5 Remove and/or replace the offending implant (the last resort).

The problems of postoperative astigmatism are closely related to those of anisometropia for it is in using both eyes that unequal astigmatic errors usually cause difficulties. Astigmatism is a vector quantity, having both amplitude and direction. Thus the cylinder before and after surgery may be unchanged at 2 D, but the axis may have shifted from 180° to 45°, a likely reason for distortion. Distortion is caused not so much by the altered corneal curvature but by the spectacle lens used to correct it. This is because the lens is fitted some distance from the eye. It follows that any cylinder should be placed as close to the eye as feasible. At the limit, it is fitted at the cornea, hence the advantage of contact lenses. Cylinder power and axis may also be modified on an empiric basis, balancing acuity against distortion. The lens which provides best acuity without tilting the acuity chart can then be placed in a trial frame for a walk about the office. Movement exaggerates untoward effects and further ad-justments are made as needed. Ordering the spherical equivalent is another option, though acuity may be considerably compromised.

Near vision correction

Most implants do not correct near vision though multifocal pseudophakia is on the horizon [10]. This means that some sort of reading prescription will be necessary, either as separate reading glasses or as bifocals. Since most cataract patients are older, chances are they already wear a near correction and the type and style can serve as a guide.

In patients with significant new aniso-metropia, near vision may be compromised by vertical diplopia [11]. Vertical diplopia is generally more annoying than horizontal because of low fusional vergences. The cause of the diplopia is that the eyes look below the optical centers of the distance prescription, rarely because the add is unequal. Vertical diplopia can be corrected by slab off grinding, compensated segments, prism segments, or unequal style bifocal segments. A simpler alternative is separate reading glasses or a high flat top (or straight across) bifocal which keeps the reading point close to (or identical with) the distance optical center. From Prentice's rule, we know that whatever the anisometropia, no prism is induced through the optical centers. The patient must be instructed to lower the head rather than the eyes when reading.

Indications for trifocals depend on inter-mediate vision needs. While every advanced presbyope complains of poor arm's length vision, certain occupations are particularly difficult (e.g. working with computers; reading music). Such tasks will not be seen clearly with bifocals. An alternative is progressive multifocals. They provide a continuous focus-ing sequence and are cosmetically preferable. Many designs are on the market, and each manufacturer claims its lenses cause less dis-tortion, provide a wider field, and allows more rapid adaptation. Unfortunately, comparisons are difficult because of different criteria (dia-gram, vector plots, astigmatic contour plots). Whichever progressive lens one chooses, re-member that each requires its own method of verification (e.g. UV markings, templates). Probably the best way to select a progressive design is by the criterion of patient adjustment.

Bifocal contact lenses are becoming available in an ever increasing variety of design. With careful patient selection, they provide a useful option. Many clinicians still avoid them by adopting the monovision alternative. One eye is fitted for distance and the other for near vision. Whether the compromised binocularity is worth the cosmetic fatuity must be decided on an individual basis.

Multifocal IOLs are based mostly on diffrac-tion optics. The optical principles are similar to multifocal contact lenses but the implant has the advantage of remaining fixed. Problems of excessive aberrations, double vision, and inadequate visual acuity remain to be solved, especially when the implant is improperly centered or pupil diameter is not optimum.

Special management problems

Unanticipated results are inevitable in every surgical practice. They may be related to the preoperative calculations, the operative pro-cedure, or the postoperative course. The con-sequences are special problems which require special management.

High astigmatism

High degrees of astigmatism (say, over 3 D) may result from a variety of causes previously described [12]. If the vertical corneal meridian is steeper than the horizontal, the astigmatism is said to be with the rule; conversely, if the horizontal is steeper, the astigmatism is against the rule (corrected by plus cylinder axis 180). The axis of the plus cylinder identifies the steeper meridian. If the cause of astigmatism is corneal compression (e.g. tight non-absorbable suture), sutures can be cut at about 6–8 weeks. Retinoscopy and keratometry will usually indicate the appropriate axis. Following the same principles, if the axis of a preoperative plus cylinder is at 135, one might tie the sutures more tightly at axis 45.

If the retinoscopic cylinder differs considerably from the keratometric cylinder, implant decentration or tilt might be suspected. Decentration can be evaluated with the slit-lamp and tilt by observing the Purkinje reflections [13]. If the keratometric axis is shifted by the surgical procedure, comparison to preoperative readings requires the use of vectors and calculating the resultant of obliquely crossed cylinders. A graphic or computer method can also be used.

If high astigmatism persists well into the postoperative period, the three management options are: (a) spectacle correction; (b) contact lens correction; and (c) surgical correction. As regards spectacles, many patients can tolerate high cylinders and this simple method is certainly worth a try. If the cylinder is not tolerated, especially in binocular vision, contact lenses are the next alternative. A conventional hard lens may not stabilize on the cornea and a back toric design is needed.

Astigmatism persisting with a spherical contact lens in place represents the uncorrected (residual) corneal astigmatism (rarely, the astigmatism induced by the contact lens through flexure or warping). If the cylinder is more than 3 D, the rear toric surface which was used to improve the fit must be balanced by a front surface toric to correct the residual astigmatism. The third option is surgical correction by keratotomy or resection. These are discussed elsewhere in this text.

Irregular astigmatism

Irregular astigmatism results from variations in corneal curvature within the same meridian. Corneal pathology is generally severe, often accompanied by opacities. Irregular astigmatism is more common after keratoplasty and keratotomy than after cataract extraction unless there is a corneal complication. One source of irregular astigmatism likely to be encountered by the cataract surgeon is corneal molding from poorly fit or warped contact lenses. Contact lens problems are managed by discontinuing lens wear or switching to a different material and better fit.

The diagnosis of irregular astigmatism is made by observing mire distortions on keratometry and with the slit-lamp. Contact lenses provide the only satisfactory treatment for irregular astigmatism. The pinhole disc and stenopeic slit can be used to identify the visual potential and isolate meridians of best acuity. Of course, contact lenses do not correct for complicating corneal opacities. If opacities are extensive, keratoplasty is a surgical alternative.

Diplopia

We have already seen that diplopia is inevitable with simultaneous spectacle correction of a phakic and aphakic eye. Lesser degrees of anisometropia can also result in double vision from the unequally induced prismatic effect of correcting spectacles. Because of its neurologic implications, the work-up of a patient complaining of double vision generally extends beyond refractive tests. A history of childhood strabismus, Grave's disease, and diabetic neuropathy should certainly be considered. Optic neuropathy, as is well known, can result in secondary exotropia. Improper spectacle lens positioning can be evaluated by noting if diplopia persists without the lenses.

Horizontal diplopia due to anisometropia can often be managed by appropriate prisms or lens decentration. Unequal retinal images or a cloudy capsule can cause phoria decompensation hence the fusional capacity might be checked. A trial fitting with Fresnel prisms can be coupled with orthoptics to build up fusional vergences. At the limit, the optical correction can be modified at the expense of reduced acuity. Contact, instead of spectacle, lenses may reduce the fusional load in anisometropic astigmatism.

Vertical diplopia is not uncommon after cataract surgery and usually resolves during the first week. It has been attributed to surgical trauma or tissue swelling acting on the vertical muscles. Persistent, stable vertical tropia has been reported and may require muscle surgery. Vertical prisms can and have been used successfully in the management of some of these problems. Periodic examinations may reveal that the prism strength must later be increased or decreased.

Monocular diplopia

Monocular diplopia is distinguished from true diplopia by closing one eye. During the early postoperative period, common causes are tear film debris, corneal irregularities, vitreous membranes, and floaters. In the later post-operative period, contact lens displacement or an improperly positioned bifocal or trifocal segment is not unusual. With respect to pseudophakia, unwanted optical images may be due to a decentered lens or positioning holes [8]. Reflections from spectacle lens surfaces are an occasional cause.

Evaluation of monocular diplopia might include a simple pinhole to isolate the source of the ghost images. Keratometry identifies irregular astigmatism, slit-lamp examination evaluates a displaced contact lens or IOL centration, fundoscopy locates vitreous floaters (an occasional cause of intermittent monocular diplopia). Refraction will differentiate blurred images from double images, a common patient error.

Management of monocular diplopia depends on the cause: (a) contact lenses for corneal irregularities; (b) constricting the pupil with a mild miotic if the IOL was decentered; (c) repositioning a grossly displaced lens; or (d) coatings for unwanted spectacle reflections. The trend toward larger IOL optics and the omission of positioning holes may help avoid some unwanted images. Laser ridges do not appear to contribute significantly to this problem. Pupil capture with an anterior chamber lens can expose the optic edge, causing monocular diplopia. A pinhole contact lens may solve this.

Glare and photophobia

Photophobia or excessive sensitivity to light is practically universal during the immediate postoperative period. The usual causes are traumatic iritis, keratitis, suture irritation, and a partially dilated pupil. Prolonged photophobia suggests more serious disease (ulcers, foreign body, ophthalmitis, etc.). The treatment of photophobia is directed at interrupting the trigeminal reflex; cycloplegia and a filter to reduce light intensity.

Glare, on the other hand, is discomfort from excessive illumination or dazzling from secondary light sources which alter target contrast. The usual cause is excessive intraocular light scatter. Scattering may be due to corneal edema, irregularities in the implant, in the media, or within the retina. Postoperative glare can result from capsular opacification and a pupil which fails to fully constrict. IOL decentration and edge exposure are also causes of glare [14]. IOL design does not affect glare; neither does UV coating.

Glare symptoms can be confirmed by glare testing instruments or by acuity reduction in ordinary sunlight (e.g. by placing an acuity chart against a well-lit window). Contrast sensitivity measures have also been recommended though the practical results are often disappointing. Subjective complaints generally suggest the severity of glare symptoms. The history will reveal that they are worse at night, especially when driving. Glare can be reduced by light intensity filters on the same principle as stars becoming visible only against the darkening sky. Glare due to corneal irregularities can be reduced by contact lenses. Ideally, the scattering element should be removed.

Reflections from spectacle lenses may produce an annoying glare effect. They are particularly likely in weak powers and can be managed by altering the pantoscopic tilt and by antireflective coatings.

Low vision

For a variety of reasons, acuity may not reach anticipated levels. The surgeon should therefore be prepared to perform a low vision examination and be familiar with the more common low vision aids.

Patients with low vision require different refractive techniques. Use smaller test distances (3 m or less), trial frames and lenses to allow free head and eye movements, avoid ambient glare sources and change lenses in large increments. Target size should be close to the patient's limit of resolution. Responses are gauged not only by optical factors but by the patient's choice of words and quickness of response. Bracket the spheric lens changes; small astigmatic errors will probably go unnoticed. Postoperative cataract patients are especially likely to be affected by the distribution of light. Thus, in measuring near vision with strong reading adds, an adjustable light source is practically mandatory. Discrepancies between distance and near acuity are not uncommon. For example, in macular degeneration, near acuity with magnifiers is likely to be considerably better than distance vision.

The most commonly used postcataract low vision aids are magnifiers for patients with macular disease. Strong spectacle (+6 D and above) reading glasses achieve their effect by allowing the patient to hold the target closer. A target moved from 100 cm to 10 cm is magnified 10 times. The lens simply acts as a strong presbyopic add. Naturally, the light source must be adjustable. Although such magnification may not restore normal reading habits, they provide adequate vision for recognizing price tags, checks, addresses, etc. Telescopic aids are useful for spotting, movies, and watching television.

References

1 Anonymous editorial. The adjustment to aphakia. *Am J Ophthalmol* 1952; **35**: 118–22.

2 Linksz A. Optical complications of aphakia. *Int Ophthal Clin* 1965; **5**: 271–308.

3 Michaels DD. Spectacle correction of aphakia; how aspheric do they have to be? *Ophthalmology* 1978; **85**: 59–72.

4 Boeder P. Review of aphakic correction by lenses, *Int Ophthal Clin* 1978; **18**: 213–22.

5 Michaels DD. *Visual Optics and Refraction*. 3rd edn. St Louis: CV Mosby, 1985.

6 Rowsey JJ, Rubin ML. Refraction problems after refractive surgery. *Surv Ophthalmol* 1988; **32**: 414–20.

7 Holladay JT. Evaluating the intraocular lens optic. *Surv Ophthalmol* 1986; **30**: 385–90.

8 Friedberg HL, Kline OR, Friedberg AH. Comparison of unwanted optical images produced by 6 mm and 7 mm intraocular lenses. *J Cataract Refract Surg* 1989; **15**: 541–4.

9 Holladay JT, Rubin ML. Avoiding refractive problems in cataract surgery. *Surv Ophthalmol* 1988; **32**: 357–60

10 Hansen TE *et al*. New multifocal intraocular lens design. *J Cataract Refract Surg* 1990; **16**: 38–41

11 Burns CL, Seigel LA. Inferior rectus recession for vertical tropia after cataract surgery. *Ophthalmology* 1988; **95**: 1120–4.

12 Swinger CA. Postoperative astigmatism. *Surv Ophthalmol* 1987; **31**: 219–48.

13 Auran JD, Koester CJ, Donn A. *In vivo* measurement of posterior chamber intraocular lens decentration and tilt. *Arch Ophthalmol* 1990; **108**: 75–9.

14 Koch DD *et al*. Glare following posterior chamber intraocular lens implantation. *J Cataract Refract Surg* 1986; **12**: 480–4.

26: Cystoid Macular Edema: Causes, Diagnosis, and Treatment

DAVID D. SAGGAU & LAWRENCE J. SINGERMAN

Introduction

The most common complication leading to decreased vision after intraocular surgery is cystoid macular edema (CME). Since the initial descriptions of CME after cataract extraction [1–9], there have been many advances and improvements in our surgical methods. A subsequent decline in the incidence of CME and other surgical complications has followed the evolution of surgical techniques. However, compared with other significant complications, the relative frequency of CME has increased, and it has become the most common visually limiting complication of modern cataract surgery.

It is estimated that over 90% of patients undergoing modern extracapsular cataract extraction (ECCE) have a final visual outcome of 20/40 or better [10–12]. An unsatisfactory visual outcome after cataract surgery is usually the result of pre-existent ocular disease or surgical complication. Postoperative reduction in vision secondary to a pre-existing ocular condition such as age-related macular degeneration or diabetic retinopathy is usually beyond the control of the surgeon. However, the responsibility for decreased vision secondary to a surgical complication is the surgeon's, and it should be the surgeon's goal to limit the occurrence of each complication. The goal of this chapter is to help the cataract surgeon decrease the frequency of CME and improve the management of it when it occurs.

History and terminology

In a 1953 report, Irvine described a syndrome occurring after uncomplicated intracapsular cataract extraction (ICCE) [1]. The syndrome consisted of spontaneous rupture of the vitreous face with subsequent development of vitreous adhesions to the wound. It was associated with irritability of the eye and reduced vision secondary to "macular degeneration" or vitreous opacities. Nicholls and other authors described post-ICCE macular edema with or without the vitreous changes described by Irvine [2,3,5–7]. In 1966, Gass and Norton described the classic cystoid changes and characteristic fluorescein angiographic findings of CME after cataract extraction [8,9]. Their description included eyes with or without an intact anterior hyaloid face.

Maumenee chose the name Irvine–Gass for the syndrome of CME following ICCE. He stated that the hyaloid face may or may not be ruptured [13]. To many clinicians, the term Irvine–Gass syndrome is synonymous with CME after cataract surgery. Other authors have used the term aphakic cystoid macular edema (ACME). More recently, the term pseudophakic CME (PCME) has been used when an intraocular lens (IOL) is implanted, and ACME is reserved for eyes without an IOL.

CME following cataract extraction is often classified as either subclinical or clinical CME. Subclinical CME is angiographically proven CME that does not cause visual symptoms, or

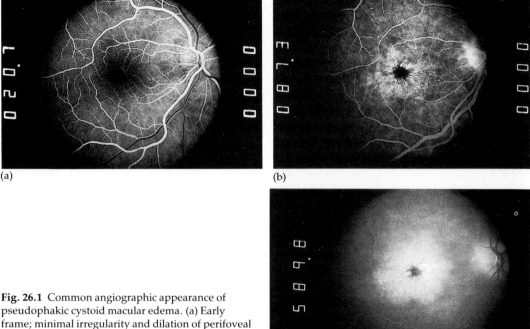

(a)

(b)

(c)

Fig. 26.1 Common angiographic appearance of pseudophakic cystoid macular edema. (a) Early frame; minimal irregularity and dilation of perifoveal capillaries. (b) Gradual leaking spreading centrally and peripherally from normal capillaries. (c) Late frame; typical central hyperfluorescent petalloid figure and leakage from the optic nerve.

at least does not meet the definition of clinical CME. Clinical CME is defined as postoperative visual disturbance or reduced visual acuity secondary to CME. Many authors use a specific level of acuity, most commonly 20/40, to define clinical CME. Fortunately, clinical CME by any definition represents a minority of cases. In our discussion, the term *angiographic CME* implies angiographic findings; it does not imply the presence or absence of symptoms. However, the term *clinical CME* indicates that CME is present and is thought to be the cause of decreased vision. Again, the level of decreased vision used to define clinical CME may vary among clinicians.

Pathology and pathogenesis

The leakage of fluid into the macula in CME is the result of a breakdown in the blood–ocular barrier with leakage from perifoveal retinal capillaries [8]. It is clearly demonstrated by angiography (Fig. 26.1). An animal model of

postoperative CME has shown the blood–ocular barrier at the level of the retinal pigment epithelium (RPE) to be compromised [14]. The contribution of the breakdown in the RPE blood–ocular barrier may be clinically important [15].

Pathologic examination by Martin *et al.* [16] demonstrated an associated retinal phlebitis and other intraocular foci of inflammation in eyes with cystoid edema. This finding supports the concept that a non-specific, generalized, intraocular inflammatory process leads to incompetence of the perifoveal capillaries as a result of a breakdown of the blood–ocular barrier.

The precise mechanism that causes leakage from the perifoveal capillaries is still unclear. One theory is that the detrimental effects of prostaglandins on the vascular endothelium is responsible for breakdown of the tight junctions in the vascular endothelium in the macular area [17]. Prostaglandins are synthesized and released by tissue damaged during initial surgical manipulations and may be continuously released if postoperative anterior segment abnormalities, such as improper IOL fixation or incarcerated tissues, cause persistent inflammation [18]. This may be a cause of prolonged CME following complicated ECCE. Investigation of the treatment of CME with non-steroidal anti-inflammatory agents has supported this theory. These drugs, which have an antiprostaglandin effect, decrease the breakdown of the blood–ocular barrier following cataract surgery [19], decrease the rate of angiographic CME [10,20,21], and may be effective for the treatment of long-standing CME [22].

The effect of ultraviolet (UV) light is also important in the pathogenesis of PCME. Kraff *et al.* [23] found a decreased rate of PCME in eyes with a UV-filtering IOL. They speculated that the increased amount of UVA light reaching the retina after removal of the human lens caused release of free radicals into the eye, with subsequent release of prostaglandins.

Earlier investigators stated that vitreous traction on the macula was probably responsible for the development of CME after cataract surgery [5–7]. Although vitreomacular traction is now a recognized syndrome that can cause macular abnormalities, including cystoid change [24,25], vitreous traction on the macula is usually not observed in the typical case of CME [8,9].

The role of the vitreous is still being investigated. Continued traction on the vitreous base from adhesions to anterior segment structures or incarceration within the wound, is probably important in some cases of persistent CME. Correction of vitreous abnormalities by laser vitreolysis [26–29] or vitrectomy [11,30,31] is effective treatment in some cases of PCME.

The cystoid spaces of CME are intraretinal and are primarily located in the outer plexiform and inner nuclear layers [9,16,32–34]. The outer plexiform layer of Henle is tangentially oriented in the perifoveal region, thereby creating a potential extracellular space. Gass and Norton and other authors have proposed that this potential space can accommodate the fluid leaking from perifoveal capillaries [9,34].

This polycystic pattern of fluid accumulation may account for the typical flower-petal angiographic appearance (Fig. 26.1). Wolter Riemer [33] studied the histopathology of 10 eyes with CME and also concluded that the cystoid spaces were extracellular. Three of the eyes had CME after cataract surgery, and their pathology did not differ from those cases with CME from different causes. He attributed the characteristic fluorescein angiographic appearance to the folding of the inner layers of the retina. Other investigators have found evidence that the edema is intracellular, located in Mueller cells. In their view, extracellular accumulation occurs only if more severe chronic cystoid causes Mueller cell necrosis [35,36]. There is general agreement that the histopathologic and clinical appearance of CME is influenced by the duration and severity of the swelling [9,16,32–36]. Secondary degeneration of the photoreceptors and neuronal elements can occur [32–36]. This can account for the occasional patient who experiences permanent loss of vision following resolution of CME.

Incidence

Various investigators have reported a wide range in the incidence of CME after cataract extraction. This is largely explained by differences in definitions, methods of investigation, and surgical technique. Several studies, especially earlier studies, were not prospective, and angiography was used on a selective basis. These studies were concerned with the rate of clinical CME. Unless angiography is used to evaluate all eyes, the rate of CME will be greatly underestimated. Even prospective studies that obtain either single or serial angiograms do not necessarily detect all cases of CME. The angiogram is usually obtained during the first 4 postoperative months, when most cases of CME occur [37,38]. CME can appear as early as 1 week [39] or as late as several years [9,40–43] after cataract extraction and can resolve after any length of time. Thus, even serial angiogram studies during the first several postoperative months will not detect all cases.

Much of the literature on CME following cataract extraction was written when ICCEs and anterior or iris-support IOLs were popular. It is still necessary [9,40–43] to understand and compare these earlier experiences to gain a comprehensive understanding of ACME and PCME, but because the rate of CME is dependent upon surgical technique, these incidence rates are not applicable to those obtained with modern extracapsular techniques. We will review information from the era of ICCE and then discuss the information on the incidence of PCME that is most useful for today's cataract surgeon: the rate of CME following an ECCE with a posterior chamber (PC) IOL and intact capsule, and the rate after breaking the capsule or losing vitreous.

Cystoid edema of the macula occurs more frequently following intracapsular procedures. If all eyes that have undergone ICCE are examined with careful ophthalmoscopy and angiography at or before the eighth postoperative week, CME is present in 30–60% [37,44–46]. The incidence of angiographic CME is greater than the incidence of clinical CME; how much greater depends to a large extent on the definition of clinical CME used by the investigator and on the type of surgery or IOL.

The reported rate of clinical CME after ICCE, with or without an iris-support lens, at various postoperative times has ranged from 1.4 to 23% [12,47–51]. When compared with no IOL, the presence of an iris-support lens after ICCE may be associated with a greater rate of CME. Taylor et al. [49] reported a 9.9% rate of clinical CME in their patients who had an iris-support IOL and only a 2% rate in patients who did not have an IOL. However, Jaffe et al. [52] and the Miami Study Group [53] found no statistical difference in the incidence of angiographic CME following ICCE with or without an iris-support IOL. Many different designs of iris-support IOLs have been manufactured; the rate of PCME varies according to design [54].

In the early years of ECCE, the iris-support lens was still in popular use. Investigations comparing ICCE/iris-support to ECCE/iris-support lens consistently demonstrated less angiographic and clinical CME with the extracapsular technique [47–49,52,55–59]. This lower incidence was found even though most of the ECCE procedures incorporated a primary capsulotomy, which adversely affects the rate of PCME [60,61]. The reported rate of clinical CME following ECCE with an iris-support IOL ranges from 0 to 4.5% [12,49,56,58,59,62,63].

Jaffe et al. [48] compared eyes undergoing ECCE/Binkhorst iris-support IOL with those undergoing the same procedure, but with a PCIOL. They found no statistical difference in the rates of angiographic CME (4.5% in the iris-support group, 2.9% in the PCIOL group), although a primary posterior capsulotomy was performed in the latter group. No cases of clinical CME occurred in either group.

Two recent articles report incidence rates for CME after uncomplicated ECCE with a PCIOL and intact capsule. A prospective study by Wright et al. [60] found a 16% incidence of angiographic CME 5 weeks after surgery. The prevalence was 4% with a subsequent angiogram performed between 4.6 and 7.3 months after surgery. Kraff et al. [61] reported a comparable incidence of 5.6% when the angiogram was performed between the third and sixth postoperative months (mean 5.2 months). Both of these studies found a low incidence of clinical CME. In the study by Wright et al. only one of 69 patients had clinical CME. Kraff et al. reported that two of 71 patients with angiographic CME had 20/40 vision or worse (one patient had 20/40 vision and the other patient had 20/50 vision).

Other authors [49,62] have reported a 1% incidence of clinical CME following ECCE/PCIOL and an intact posterior capsule. The visual acuity definition of clinical CME in these latter two studies was 20/40 or worse.

The frequency of PCME is greater following a complicated ECCE. Unplanned capsular rupture with or without vitreous loss is experienced by all anterior segment surgeons performing ECCE. The reported rate at which experienced ECCE surgeons encounter vitreous loss ranges between 1.4 and 4.3% [51,64–67]. Intraoperative vitreous loss or rupture of the capsule increases the incidence of CME after ECCE [48,54,62,68,69] and is associated with a poorer prognosis [54,62]. The rate of CME experienced by an individual surgeon depends on the surgical complication rate and the surgeon's management of the complication.

Wright *et al.* [60] and Kraff *et al.* [61] compared eyes after ECCE/PCIOL and an intact posterior capsule with eyes that received a primary planned surgical capsulotomy. They confirmed a lower incidence of CME when the posterior capsule was left intact.

Natural history

The prevalence of CME decreases after the first few postoperative months, with resolution of the CME in a large majority of affected eyes. Permanent visual loss does occasionally occur because of persistent edema or permanent structural change of the macula remaining after resolution. Previous authors have discussed the clinical course of CME following ICCE with or without an IOL [45,68,70,71]. Our discussion will focus on the clinical course of PCME after modern ECCE, both uncomplicated and complicated.

In a prospective study of eyes after ECCE/PCIOL, only one of 69 patients had CME associated with visual acuity less than 20/40 after 6 weeks. Of 49 evaluated at approximately 6 months, there were no patients with CME and visual acuity less than 20/40. The angiographic rate of CME declined during this period from 16 to 4% [60]. No other prospective trials with serial evaluation are available to determine the number of eyes with persistent CME or permanent visual loss secondary to CME after modern uncomplicated ECCE surgery with a PCIOL.

Stark *et al.* [12] reported a 2% incidence of clinically significant CME following ECCE with a PCIOL. Only three of 961 eyes (0.3%) had persistent clinically significant CME. Seventeen patients experienced transient CME, and all eyes except one recovered 20/30 vision or better. Taylor *et al.* [49] had four of 328 eyes (1.27%) with clinical CME after uncomplicated ECCE. Three of the eyes responded to medical treatment. All eyes with CME and visual loss in these two retrospective studies had coexistent macular disease.

In a 1988 article, Bradford *et al.* [72] discussed the outcome of 20 cases of PCME after ECCE/

PCIOL that were referred to their retina practice and had initially presented with 20/30 acuity or less. They mentioned that, in a previous report by Wilkinson [70] on chronic clinical CME associated with iris-support lenses, 54 months were required to collect 93 suitable eyes for investigation, but from the same institution it had taken over 7 years to collect 20 patients with chronic CME associated with a PCIOL.

Resolution of the macular edema was observed in 18 of the 20 eyes. All 18 of the affected eyes had a final vision of 20/40 or better. Edema resolved within 1 year of onset in two-thirds of the eyes and within 2 years of onset in 17 of the 18 eyes. The two eyes with persistent CME had 20/50 vision until corneal problems developed. All eyes received medical treatment, but the management was variable. A primary capsulotomy had been performed in seven of the eyes. One of the eyes with the capsule intact and one with a capsulotomy were treatment failures.

As discussed above, the rate of clinical CME after an uncomplicated modern ECCE may be as high as 3%, but 90% or more of these eyes will recover 20/40 or better vision. The percentage of eyes that experience permanent visual loss of 20/40 or worse secondary to CME after an uncomplicated ECCE with a PCIOL is less than 1%.

Once a complication occurs, the surgical management will determine the visual outcome. When vitreous [68,70], iris, or capsule is left in the wound or entrapped by the IOL, the amount of postoperative inflammation is increased. The severity and duration of the CME and resultant visual loss is also increased after complicated ECCE [48,54,62].

However, relatively good results have been reported after complicated ECCE when a careful vitrectomy and lens implant was performed. Spigelman *et al.* [69] followed 26 patients after ECCE complicated by vitreous loss. A meticulous anterior vitrectomy and placement of a PCIOL (20 patients) or anterior chamber IOL (six patients) lead to 20/50 vision or better in all patients. Nishi [64] reported on 30 eyes that had undergone complicated cataract extraction. Eighteen of these eyes had suffered vitreous loss. A PCIOL was implanted in seven eyes. Only three eyes had clinical CME, and they were all in the group with anterior chamber lenses; one of these eyes had persistent CME.

In our referral retina practice, we reviewed 60 consecutive patients referred for evaluation of PCME. All had undergone cataract extraction; none had had the procedure performed before 1982. Of these cases, only 33% were eyes that had undergone an uncomplicated ECCE with a PCIOL. The remainder were eyes that had suffered a complication at the time of surgery and required an anterior chamber IOL. Assuming that the complication rate of our referring surgeons is similar to that in recently published reports, i.e. 1.4–4.3% rate of vitreous loss or disruption of the posterior capsule [64,66,67], it would seem that our referrals for PCME comprise a disproportionately large number of cases associated with complicated ECCEs.

Clinical presentation and diagnosis

In a clinical trial by Wright *et al.* [60], angiographic CME was identified in 16% of eyes after ECCE with a PCIOL. However, this rate of CME is not seen in the usual practice setting, because only a minority of patients with angiographic PCME will have symptoms. When evaluating a patient with visual loss after cataract extraction, the ophthalmic surgeon must consider all potential causes of visual loss. If CME is discovered, other potential causes of visual loss still need to be excluded because of the large number of eyes with CME that do not have associated visual loss [12]. If all potential causes of visual loss have been excluded and no cystoid edema is seen on biomicroscopy, an angiogram should be obtained, because angiographic CME with minimal biomicroscopic findings can cause visual loss. In addition, the angiogram assists the evaluation of other possible subtle sources of visual loss such as old or small branch vein occlusion or occult choroidal neovascular membranes.

CME after surgery may not be secondary to the cataract extraction. The differential

Table 26.1 Differential diagnosis of cystoid macular edema

Peripheral lesion
  Choroidal melanoma
  Choroidal hemangioma
  Retinal capillary angioma
  Retinal telangiectasis (Coat's disease)
  Retinal detachment
Choroidal neovascular membrane
Epiretinal membrane
Intraocular inflammatory disease
Diabetic retinopathy
Venous occlusive disease
Perifoveal telangiectasis
Vitreomacular traction syndrome
Retinal dystrophies
Medications
  Topical epinephrine
  Oral niacin
Trauma
Intraocular surgery
Many others

diagnosis of CME (Table 26.1) needs to be considered before assuming that the cystoid edema is PCME. When other macular disease, such as diabetic retinopathy, branch vein occlusion, or epiretinal membrane, is present, it may not be possible to determine the cause of the CME. Management of coexistent macular disease will be discussed in the treatment section.

The most common and often only symptom of CME is decreased vision. More specific visual complaints of metamorphopsia or central dimness are occasionally volunteered. CME after uncomplicated ECCE most often occurs between 1 and 3 months after surgery but can occur within a few weeks or after several months [12]. Commonly, the patient recovers relatively good postoperative vision and then experiences a subsequent decrease in vision as the CME manifests. A smaller subgroup of patients, often those who have undergone a complicated extraction, do not experience good immediate postoperative vision.

The severity of visual loss is usually mild with PCME following an uncomplicated ECCE. It is unusual, in the absence of other ocular disease, for significant visual loss to occur. However, following complicated procedures with tissue incarceration and persistent inflammation, the visual loss secondary to PCME can be more severe. Inflammatory symptoms of photophobia, redness, and pain can accompany CME and may occur synchronously with the onset of visual symptoms. Inflammatory symptoms are less common after an uncomplicated ECCE procedure.

The evaluation and management of a patient with PCME begins with the preoperative examination. The anterior segment, vitreous, and retina are evaluated before cataract surgery for evidence of previous ocular disease.

Many causes of decreased postoperative vision fall into the category of ocular surface and refractive disorders. Their diagnosis may prevent unnecessary testing, such as formal visual fields or fluorescein angiography, saving the time and relieving the anxiety of both patient and physician. Thus, the postoperative examination of patients with visual symptoms should begin with best corrected and pinhole visual acuities. Keratometry and retinoscopy are also important adjuncts.

The pupils should be checked for an afferent defect, a finding not caused by PCME. Visual fields are normal by confrontation, but Amsler grid testing can demonstrate central metamorphopsia or relative scotoma when CME is present.

Anterior segment examination should be performed before and after pupil dilation. The presence or absence of intraocular inflammation should be noted. Mild uveitis may accompany typical PCME. The wound should be inspected for possible incarcerated iris, capsule, or vitreous. The undilated iris should be inspected for distortion or peaking (Plate 26.1). The IOL position, stability, and relationship to visual axis and surrounding structures should be evaluated. A malpositioned optic or haptic can lead to increased iris chafing and persistent intraocular inflammation. The vitreous is examined with the slit-lamp for cells, pigment, and debris. After the intraocular pressure is determined, the iris is dilated and slit-lamp examination is again performed with specific attention paid to the iris, IOL position,

remnant lens and capsular fragments, and status of the vitreous.

A peripheral retinal lesion can cause CME of the macula [73]. Indirect ophthalmoscopy must be performed to examine the periphery for retinal breaks or detachment, masses, and retinal exudates or hemorrhages. Shallow or peripheral retinal detachment can mimic or produce CME and can be overlooked unless careful indirect ophthalmoscopy through a well-dilated pupil is performed [74].

The posterior pole and optic nerve are examined with a non-contact or contact lens using stereoscopic biomicroscopy. We prefer the 78- or 90-D lens to the Hruby for non-contact biomicroscopy. It is advisable to use a contact lens after angiography is performed if examination with non-contact lens fails to disclose the cause of the patient's visual disturbance. Subtle biomicroscopic findings of CME and other potential causes of CME, such as a small or old vein occlusion, choroidal neovascular membrane, or epiretinal membrane, are easier to see with a fundus contact lens.

The characteristic retinal appearance of CME has been well described [8,9,75]. Several cysts are usually present within the central macular region. Typically, a single large or several larger central foveal cysts are surrounded by smaller intraretinal cysts. Occasionally, a large thin-walled central cyst can be difficult to differentiate from a macular hole. Macular hole formation has been reported following CME

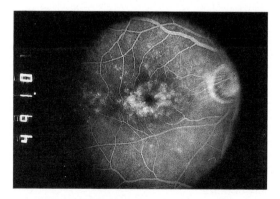

Fig. 26.2 Pseudophakic cystoid macular edema in same eye as Plate 26.1 (20/200).

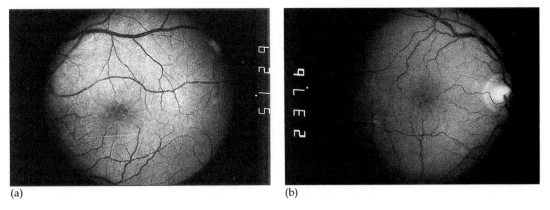

(a)   (b)

Fig. 26.3 (a) Faint outline of central cystoid spaces seen on red-free photo. (b) Cystoid spaces associated with punctate hemorrhage.

[76]. The cysts may be visualized best with the light source directed from the side of the viewing axis. Sometimes they are more easily appreciated if the examiner uses a coaxial thin slit beam and focuses just to the side of the beam on the retroilluminated cysts. Cyst walls are better appreciated with red-free illumination (Fig. 26.2). Retroillumination can also be performed with the beam focused on the fovea as a small spot. Small intraretinal hemorrhages or cysts partially filled with hemorrhage can occur [77]. Their presence necessitates a closer evaluation of other potential retinovascular lesions. If blood is in the subretinal space, an angiogram should be obtained to exclude a choroidal neovascular membrane.

The optic nerve is affected in approximately 20% of PCME cases [45]. Typically there is only mild swelling of the optic nerve, but severe swelling can occasionally occur, sometimes resulting in disc pallor after chronic edema [5,8]. Cells may be present in the posterior vitreous. Optic nerve hyperfluorescence may be seen in the absence of clinical swelling. When optic nerve swelling is identified, the disc of the fellow eye should be examined to rule out papilledema.

The angiogram is the gold standard of diagnosis and is also useful in the management of PCME. The angiographic findings were first detailed by Gass and Norton [8,9]. Early transit frames may appear normal. Dilated or tortuous perifoveal capillaries are often present. Dilated capillaries or vascular malformations need to be closely scrutinized to exclude previous venous occlusive disease. The hyperfluorescence of CME is produced by leaking perifoveal capillaries and may not appear until several minutes have elapsed. Thus, it is necessary when evaluating PCME to perform late frames at least 10 min after injection. The classic petalloid pattern of hyperfluorescence is best appreciated in the late frames. When only a segment of the perifoveal vascular net is leaking, hyperfluorescence will be focal and limited to the leaking segment; the classic petalloid appearance will not be seen (Fig. 26.4). Leaking capillaries may be located well outside the perifoveal region creating atypical patterns of hyperfluorescence (Fig. 26.5). Late frames of the angiogram are also useful to study the optic nerve head. When present, optic nerve leakage can be a useful diagnostic sign of PCME, especially when other retinovascular pathology is present. Fluorescence of the ipsilateral and fellow eye optic nerve should be compared (Fig. 26.6).

The value of fluorescein angiography for routine cases has been questioned [12]. If the retinal examination demonstrates obvious findings of CME, some authors feel that the angiogram is superfluous. The majority of clinical cases resolve within a few months, and angiography can be reserved for those cases that do not resolve as expected. If the CME is persistent or the presentation is atypical or associated with other retinal findings, an angiogram is indicated to rule out other,

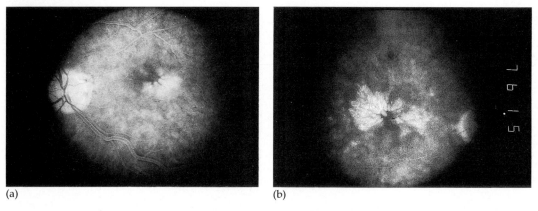

(a)   (b)

Fig. 26.4 (a) Incomplete pattern of perifoveal leakage with intense hyperfluorescence in the temporal and inferior perifoveal ring only. (b) Relative sparing of the vertical perifoveal areas, producing a bow-tie pattern of hyperfluorescence.

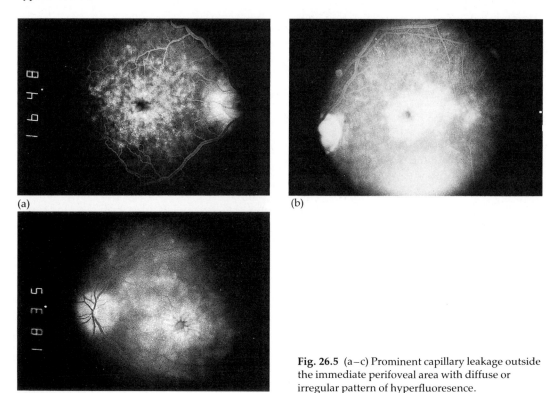

(a)   (b)

(c)

Fig. 26.5 (a–c) Prominent capillary leakage outside the immediate perifoveal area with diffuse or irregular pattern of hyperfluoresence.

potentially treatable causes of the macular edema. Subretinal hemorrhage, subretinal hard exudate, or subretinal fluid are signs of choroidal neovascular membrane and deserve prompt angiographic evaluation.

Use of the indirect ophthalmoscope and appropriate filters to examine the fundus between the transit and late stage of the an-

giogram [78] may detect the macular hyperfluorescence of CME when photographic documentation is precluded by media opacities or miosis. If angioscopy by this method is delayed until after the late stages of the angiogram, the view of the fundus may be limited by fluorescein leakage into the anterior chamber and vitreous.

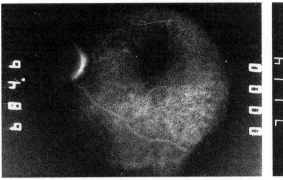
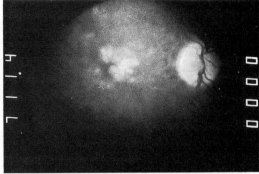

Fig. 26.6 Bilateral comparison of hyperfluorescence from macula and optic nerve demonstrate cystoid macular edema with hyperfluorescent ipsilateral optic nerve.

Prevention and treatment of PCME

The prevention of CME involves preoperative, intraoperative, and postoperative management. Selecting the appropriate timing for an elective cataract extraction is the first step in prevention. Concurrent eye disease should be controlled or stabilized prior to surgery.

Eyes with active inflammation and eyes with retinovascular disease need to be closely evaluated preoperatively. If inflammation is active, eyes with uveitis should not undergo elective cataract extraction [79,80]. CME is more common in these eyes and is usually the determinant of postoperative acuity. The use of aggressive perioperative anti-inflammatory drugs, including oral agents, prevents severe postoperative inflammation and may decrease the incidence of CME [80]. Eyes with background diabetic retinopathy can also have increased macular edema following cataract surgery [81]. When the media permit, clinically significant macular edema [82] should be treated appropriately with retinal photocoagulation and allowed to stabilize before surgery. An angiogram may demonstrate preoperative CME in eyes with concurrent disease such as epiretinal membrane or venous occlusion when the media preclude fundoscopic identification. A baseline preoperative angiogram is useful for the postoperative management of eyes with CME and concurrent disease.

In eyes with concurrent epiretinal membranes and CME following cataract surgery,

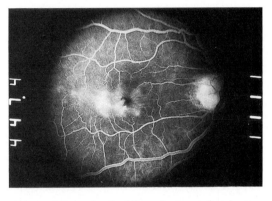

Fig. 26.7 Minimal retinal distortion secondary to an epiretinal membrane, 3 years after cataract extraction (20/50). Mild cystoid macular edema is present. Leakage from the optic nerve head indicates that the edema may be secondary to the pseudophakic state.

the determination of the etiology is difficult. A preoperative angiogram to ascertain the presence or absence of preoperative CME is obviously helpful. If the postoperative angiogram shows optic nerve head fluorescence, then the case should be assumed to be PCME and treated accordingly. A postoperative eye with concurrent epiretinal membrane and CME is demonstrated in Fig. 26.7.

Patients with diabetic retinopathy and CME following cataract surgery are common. When the etiology of the CME is equivocal, they may be treated as PCME for the first few postoperative months. If, thereafter, CME still exists despite medical management, the macular

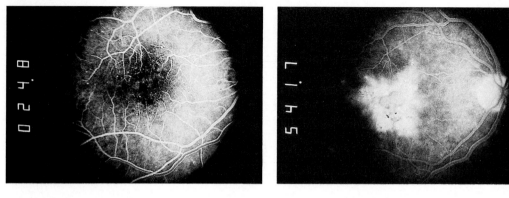

Fig. 26.8 Severe cystoid macular edema with large central cysts associated with diabetic retinopathy in an eye 11 months after cataract surgery (20/60).

edema should be treated according to the recommendations of the ETDRS [82]. If it is clear that significant diabetic macular edema is responsible for a portion of the CME, the individual microaneurysms leaking on fluorescein angiography can be focally treated with laser. Fig. 26.8 shows an eye with background diabetic retinopathy with CME following cataract surgery.

Perioperative topical or oral indomethacin can reduce the incidence of angiographic CME, but it has not been shown to reduce the incidence of clinical CME [10,20,21,83]. Topical indomethacin decreases the breakdown of the blood–ocular barrier in postoperative eyes, especially when it is used together with a topical steroid [19]. In subsets of patients who have an increased rate of CME, such as those with pre-existent retinovascular disease [81], uveitis [80], CME in the fellow eye [8], or previous complicated extraction [48,54,62, 68,69], the use of an antiprostaglandin agent to maintain the blood–ocular barrier may be advantageous.

Good surgical technique is the best method of prevention in all subsets of patients. The surgeon's goal should be to minimize damage to tissues and avoid structural abnormalities that have been shown to increase the breakdown of the blood–ocular barrier. When a complication occurs during surgery, the surgeon should attempt to leave the wound free of incarcerated tissue and the pupil round, small,

and centered. If an IOL is used, it should not distort or capture iris or vitreous. The method of handling vitreous loss or a broken capsule will determine the incidence of CME. As mentioned previously, good results after complicated extractions have been reported [64,69].

In the postoperative period, a YAG laser posterior capsulotomy is frequently necessary. There have been reports in the literature of CME following YAG capsulotomy. In the only well-designed, prospective angiographic study, none of the 136 patients undergoing laser capsulotomy developed CME [84]. The earliest time at which capsulotomy was performed in the study was 4 months. It may be beneficial to delay capsulotomy for at least 4 months, until the initial inflammation has resolved.

PCME can be simply observed, while usual postoperative medications are continued, or it can be treated. The literature is replete with anecdotal accounts of treatment successes using various agents. Reports have found topical and oral steroids to be effective [85–87] and periocular steroids are frequently given by many surgeons, but randomized studies have not been performed. The large majority of PCME cases are self-limited. With a high rate of spontaneous resolution, it is difficult to determine the effects of medical treatment without prospective randomization. The results of a recent double-masked, placebo-controlled, randomized study found ketorolac tromethamine, a non-steroidal anti-inflammatory agent, to be effective treatment for chronic ACME [22]. At this time, any treatment protocol is still largely based on individual experience and preference.

Jampol [88–90] has reviewed the pharmacologic prophylaxis and treatment of CME in several previous articles. He has pointed out the lack of randomized controlled trials of oral, periocular, or topical steroids. The reader is referred to those articles for further information regarding the available literature on the medical management of CME.

Our approach to the management of PCME has developed over many years of treating patients in a referral retinal practice. If CME occurs, we treat with topical steroids. If it persists, we use periocular steroids. A topical steroid is prescribed for use six times a day. Because of the potential theoretic benefits and recent report of effective treatment for chronic CME with ketorolac tromethamine [22], the use of a topical non-steroidal anti-inflammatory agent may be considered. The work presented by Sanders *et al.* [19] found an additive beneficial effect of a topical non-steroidal agent and a topical steroid on the maintenance of the blood–ocular barrier. If there is no subjective or objective improvement after 1 month, and the intraocular pressure has not increased, a peribulbar steroid injection (40 mg of Kenalog) is given, and the patient is rechecked in 1 month. If no treatment effect is seen, the injection is repeated one more time, providing the intraocular pressure is normal. If the patient is improving, we continue the topical medication and begin tapering one agent at a time. Eyes with CME and visible anterior segment inflammation seem to respond to treatment more readily than do eyes without inflammation. Intraocular inflammation should be monitored in eyes with CME and the medical regimen, which may include cycloplegics, should be increased until the inflammation is controlled and tapered slowly with regular observation.

Resolution of chronic CME and improved vision has been related to the administration of 500 mg of acetazolamide (Diamox) each day [15]. Clinical edema returned to pretreatment levels when the Diamox was discontinued. Diamox may be useful in cases of chronic CME when the patients are unresponsive to steroids or if they develop steroid-induced glaucoma.

We do not commonly administer oral steroids or oral non-steroidal anti-inflammatory agents. Because the potential for serious side effects is significant, justification of their use is difficult with the current body of literature. However, an occasional patient with refractory CME is responsive to oral prednisone. CME should be documented with angiography before assuming the risks associated with an oral agent.

We discussed the value of angiography in the previous section. Angiography is necessary for the management of patients with concurrent macular disease, but it is not necessary for all PCME patients. If an excellent view of the macula can be obtained and CME is seen without any other associated findings, then angiography can be withheld unless the CME fails to resolve within the usual time frame. Although abnormalities such as macular branch vein occlusion or choroidal neovascular membranes can be missed without an angiogram, it is uncommon to see CME in one of these entities without associated retinal findings.

If CME is chronic and does not resolve with medical management, attention should be paid to the anterior segment morphology. If there are obvious structural abnormalities, such as vitreous incarceration in the wound, distorted pupil, iris capture, or IOL malposition, CME can be improved by surgical techniques designed to remove these sources of chronic inflammation. YAG vitreolysis, vitrectomy, or anterior segment reconstruction have all been shown to be successful in certain cases.

The ACME collaborative study of aphakic eyes confirmed the effectiveness of vitrectomy for those eyes with CME and vitreous adherent to the wound [11]. The maintenance of the posterior capsule with ECCE techniques and the availability of the YAG laser has decreased the need to perform vitrectomy. YAG vitreolysis has been described by several investigators [26–29]. CME resolved in 40–100% of patients with chronic CME and YAG lysis of vitreous bands to the wound. If there is a large amount of vitreous to the wound or captured by an IOL, YAG vitreolysis is less useful and vitrectomy may be necessary. Vitrectomy for chronic CME with vitreous to the anterior segment IOL or iris without adherence to the wound can also be effective [30,31].

The collaborative ACME vitrectomy study [11] indicated that the benefits of the pars plana approach may be greater than those of vitrectomy through the limbus, but good results with the limbal approach have been reported in aphakic eyes [30,31]. In an eye with an anterior chamber IOL, the pars plana approach allows more complete vitreous removal from the IOL and iris with less trauma to the cornea. We use a typical three-port pars plana approach with two-handed manipulation and vitrectomy through two active ports at 3 and 9 o'clock. It may be beneficial to place the temporal port below horizontal for best access to the superior wound.

Anterior chamber reconstruction has been reported to be successful for eyes with chronic inflammation and PCME associated with corneal edema and structural abnormalities of the anterior chamber [91]. Explantation or exchange of an anterior chamber IOL is also effective in some cases with persistent inflammation and CME [92–94].

Photocoagulation has been reported; however, it is not an accepted modality at this time. Some discussion regarding the use of macular grid laser has begun again because of its effective use in macular edema secondary to background diabetic retinopathy [82] and branch vein occlusion [95]. However, no formal studies are yet organized.

References

1 Irvine SR. A newly defined vitreous syndrome following cataract surgery. *Am J Ophthalmol* 1953; **36**: 599–619.

2 Nicholls JVV. Macular edema in association with cataract extraction. *Am J Ophthalmol* 1985; **37**: 665–72.

3 Nicholls JVV. Concurrence of macular edema with cataract extraction. *Arch Ophthalmol* 1956; **55**: 595–604.

4 Chandler PA. Complications of cataract extraction. *Am J Ophthalmol* 1953; **36**: 599.

5 Welch RB, Cooper JC. Macular edema, papilledema and optic atrophy after cataract extraction. *Arch Ophthalmol* 1958; **59**: 665–75.

6 Tolentino FI, Schepens CL. Edema of posterior pole after cataract extraction. *Arch Ophthalmol* 1965; **74**: 781–6.

7 Algernon BR, Jones IS, Cooper WC. Macular changes secondary to vitreous traction. *Trans Am Ophthalmol Soc* 1966; **64**: 123–34.

8 Gass JDM, Norton EWD. Fluorescein studies of patients with macular edema and papilledema following cataract extraction. *Trans Am Ophthalmol Soc* 1966; **64**: 232–49.

9 Gass JDM, Norton EWD. Cystoid macular edema and papilledema following cataract extraction. *Arch Ophthalmol* 1966; **76**: 646–61.

10 Kraff MC, Sanders DS, Jampol LM, Peyman GA, Lieberman HL. Prophylaxis of pseudophakic cystoid macular edema with topical indomethacin. *Ophthalmology* 1982; **89**: 885–90.

11 Fung WE. Vitrectomy–Aphakic Cystoid Macular Edema Study Group. Vitrectomy for chronic aphakic cystoid macular edema. Results of a national collaborative, prospective, randomized investigation. *Ophthalmology* 1985; **92**: 1102–11.

12 Stark WL, Maumenee AE, Fagadau W *et al.* Cystoid macular edema in pseudophakia. *Surv Ophthalmol* 1984; **28** (suppl): 442–51.

13 Maumenee AE. Further advances in the study of the macula. *Arch Ophthalmol* 1967; **78**: 151–65.

14 Tso MOM. Animal modeling of human cystoid macular edema. *Surv Ophthalmol* 1984; **28** (suppl): 572–9.

15 Cox SN, Hay E, Bird AC. Treatment of chronic macular edema with acetazolamide. *Arch Ophthalmol* 1988; **106**: 1190–5.

16 Martin NF, Green WR, Martin LW. Retinal phlebitis in the Irvine–Gass syndrome. *Am J Ophthalmol* 1977; **83**: 377–86.

17 Sears ML. The pharmacology of ocular trauma. *Surv Ophthalmol* 1984; **27** (suppl): 525–34.

18 Miyake K, Asakara M, Kosayashi H. Effect of intraocular lens fixation on the blood–aqueous barrier. *Am J Ophthalmol* 1984; **98**: 451–5.

19 Sanders DR, Kraff MC, Lederman HL, Peyman LA, Jarabesky S. Breakdown and reestablishment of blood–aqueous barrier with implant surgery. *Arch Ophthalmol* 1982; **100**: 588–90.

20 Miyake K, Sakamura S, Miura H. Long-term follow up study on prevention of aphakic cystoid macular oedema by topical indomethacin. *Br J Ophthalmol* 1980; **64**: 324–8.

21 Yannuzzi LA, Landau AN, Turtz AI. Incidence of aphakic cystoid macular edema with the use of topical indomethacin. *Ophthalmology* 1981; **88**: 947–54.

22 Flach AJ, Dolan BJ, Irvine AR. Effectiveness of ketorolac tromethamine 0.5% ophthalmic solution

for chronic aphakic and pseudophakic cystoid macular edema. *Am J Ophthalmol* 1987; **103**: 479–86.

23 Kraff MC, Sanders DR, Jampol LM, Leberman HZ. Effect of an ultraviolet-filtering intraocular lens on cystoid macular edema. *Ophthalmology* 1985; **92**: 366–9.

24 Gass JDM. *Stereoscopic Atlas of Macular Diseases*. St Louis: CV Mosby, 1987: 676–93.

25 Smiddy WE, Michels RG, Glaser BM, deBustros S. Vitrectomy for macular traction caused by incomplete vitreous separation. *Arch Ophthalmol* 1988; **105**: 624–8.

26 Steinert RF, Watson PJ. Neodynium:YAG laser vitreolysis for Irvine–Gass cystoid macular edema. *J Cataract Refract Surg* 1989; **15**: 304–7.

27 Levy JH, Pisacano AM. Clinical experience with Nd:YAG laser vitreolysis in the anterior segment. *J Cataract Refract Surg* 1987; **13**: 548–50.

28 Katzen LE, Fleischman JA, Trokel S. YAG laser treatment of cystoid macular edema. *Am J Ophthalmol* 1983; **95**: 589–92.

29 Steinert RF, Puliafito CA. *The Nd:YAG Laser in Ophthalmology; Principles and Clinical Applications of Photodisruption*. Philadelphia: WB Saunders, 1985: 115–23.

30 Federman JL, Annesley WH, Sarin LK, Remer P. Vitrectomy and cystoid macular edema. *Ophthalmology* 1980; **87**: 622–8.

31 Robinson D, Landers MB, Hahn DK. An anterior surgical approach to aphakic cystoid macular edema. *Am J Ophthalmol* 1983; **95**: 811–17.

32 Tso MOM. Pathological study of cystoid macular edema. *Trans Ophthalmol Soc UK* 1980; **100**: 408–13.

33 Wolter Riemer J. The histopathology of cystoid macular edema. *Graef Arch Clin Exp Ophthalmol* 1981; **216**: 85–101.

34 Gass JDM, Anderson DR, Davis EG. A clinical fluorescein angiography and electron microscopic correlation of cystoid macular edema. *Am J Ophthalmol* 1985; **100**: 82–6.

35 Fine BS, Brucker AJ. Macular edema and cystoid macular edema. *Am J Ophthalmol* 1981; **92**: 466–81.

36 Yanoff M, Fine BS, Brucker AJ, Eagle RC. Pathology of human cystoid macular edema. *Surv Ophthalmol* 1984; **28** (suppl): 505–11.

37 Irvine AR, Bresley R, Crowder BJ, Forster RF, Hunter DM, Kalvin SM. Macular edema after cataract extraction. *Ann Ophthalmol* 1971; **3**: 1234–40.

38 Sorr EM, Everett WG, Hurite FG. Incidence of fluorescein angiographic subclinical macular edema following phaco-emulsification of senile cataracts. *Ophthalmology* 1979; **86**: 2013–18.

39 Klein RM, Yannuzzi LA. Cystoid macular edema in the first week after cataract extraction. *Am J Ophthalmol* 1976; **81**: 614–15.

40 Epstein DL. Cystoid macular edema occurring 13 years after cataract extraction. *Am J Ophthalmol* 1977; **83**: 501–3.

41 Severin SC. Late cystoid macular edema in pseudophakia. *Am J Ophthalmol* 1980; **90**: 223–5.

42 Weene LE. Delayed onset of aphakic cystoid macular edema. *Ann Ophthalmol* 1984; **16**: 774–5.

43 Mao LK, Holland PM. Very late onset cystoid macular edema. *Ophthal Surg* 1988; **19**: 633–5.

44 Meredith TA, Kenyon KR, Singerman LJ, Fine SL. Perifoveal vascular leakage and macular edema after intracapsular cataract extraction. *Br J Ophthalmol* 1976; **60**: 765–9.

45 Hitchings RA, Chisolm IH. Incidence of aphakic macular oedema. *Br J Ophthalmol* 1975; **59**: 444–50.

46 Hitchings RA, Chisholm IH, Bird AC. Aphakic macular edema: incidence and pathogenesis. *Invest Ophthalmol* 1975; **14**: 68–72.

47 Wetzig PC, Thatcher DB, Christiansen JM. The intracapsular vs. the extracapsular cataract technique in relationship to retinal problems. *Trans Am Ophthalmol Soc* 1979; **77**: 339–45.

48 Jaffe NS, Clayman HM, Jaffe MS. Cystoid macular edema after intracapsular and extracapsular cataract extraction with and without an intraocular lens. *Ophthalmology* 1982; **89**: 24–9.

49 Taylor DM, Sachs SW, Stern AL. Aphakic cystoid macular edema longterm clinical observations. *Surv Ophthalmol* 1984; **28**: 437–41.

50 Stern AL, Taylor DM, Dalburg LA, Consentino RT. Pseudophakic cystoid maculopathy. A study of 50 cases. *Ophthalmology* 1981; **88**: 942–6.

51 Jaffe NS. Results of intraocular lens implant surgery. *Am J Ophthalmol* 1978; **85**: 13–23.

52 Jaffe NS, Eichenbaum DM, Clayman HM, Light DS. A comparison of 500 Binkhorst implants with 500 routine intracapsular cataract extraction. *Am J Ophthalmol* 1978; **85**: 24–7.

53 Miami Study Group. Cystoid macular edema in aphakic and pseudophakic eyes. *Am J Ophthalmol* 1979; **88**: 45–8.

54 Winston RL, Taylor BC, Harris WS. A one-year follow-up of cystoid macular edema following intraocular lens implantation. *Ophthalmology* 1978; **85**: 190–6.

55 Severin TD, Severin SL. Phakic cystoid macular edema. A revised comparison of the incidence with intracapsular and extracapsular cataract extraction. *Ophthal Surg* 1988; **19**: 116–8.

56 Jaffe NS, Luscombe SM, Clayman HM, Gass JDM. A follow-up angiographic study of cystoid macular edema. *Am J Ophthalmol* 1981; **92**: 775–7.

57 Binkhorst CD, Kats A, Tjan TT, Loones LH. Retinal accidents in pseudophakia-intracapsular vs. extracapsular surgery. *Trans Am Acad Ophthal Otolaryngol* 1976; **81**: 120–7.

58 Binkhorst CD. 500 planned extracapsular cataract extraction with indocapsular and iris clip lens implantation in senile cataract. *Ophthal Surg* 1977; **8**: 37–44.

59 Moses L. Cystoid macular edema and retinal detachment following cataract surgery. *Am*

Intraocul Implant Soc J 1979; **5**: 326–9.

60 Wright PL, Wilkinson CP, Balyeat HD, Pophan J, Reinke M. Angiographic cystoid macular edema after posterior chamber lens implantation. *Arch Ophthalmol* 1988; **106**: 740–4.

61 Kraff MC, Sanders DR, Jampol LM, Lieberman HL. Effect of primary capsulotomy with extracapsular surgery on the incidence of phakic cystoid macular edema. *Am J Ophthalmol* 1984; **98**: 166–70.

62 Chambless WS. Phacoemulsification and the retina: cystoid macular edema. *Ophthalmology* 1979; **86**: 2019–22.

63 Sheets JH. Lenses suitable for use after phacoemulsification. *Trans Am Acad Ophthal Otolaryngol* 1979; **86**: 2034–6.

64 Nishi O. Vitreous loss in posterior chamber lens implantation. *J Cataract Refract Surg* 1987; **13**: 424–7.

65 Kratz RP. Teaching phacoemulsification in California and 200 cases of phacoemulsification. In: Emery JM, Paton D, eds. *Current Concepts in Cataract Surgery. Selected Proceedings of the 4th Biennial Cataract Surgical Congress.* St Louis: CV Mosby, 1976: 196–200.

66 O'Donnell FE, Santos B. Posterior capsular–zonular disruption in planned extracapsular surgery. *Arch Ophthalmol* 1985; **103**: 652–5.

67 Pearson PA, Owen DG, Van Meter WS, Smith TSJ. Vitreous loss rates in extracapsular cataract surgery by residents. *Ophthalmology* 1989; **96**: 1225–7.

68 Gass JDM, Maumenee EWD. Follow-up study of cystoid macular edema following cataract extraction. *Trans Am Acad Ophthal Otolaryngol* 1969; **73**: 665–82.

69 Spigelman AV, Lindstrom RL, Nichols BD, Lindquist TD. Visual results following vitreous loss in primary lens implantation. *J Cataract Refract Surg* 1989; **18**: 201–4.

70 Wilkinson CP. A long-term follow-up study of cystoid macular edema in aphakic and pseudophakic eyes. *Trans Am Ophthalmol Soc* 1981; **79**: 810–39.

71 Jacobsen DR, Dellaporte A. Natural history of cystoid macular edema after cataract extraction. *Am J Ophthalmol* 1974; **77**: 445–7.

72 Bradford JD, Wilkinson CP, Bradford RH. Cystoid macular edema following extracapsular cataract extraction and posterior chamber intraocular lens implantation. *Retina* 1988; **8**: 161–4.

73 Brownstein S, Orton R, Jackson B. Cystoid macular edema with equatorial choroidal melanoma. *Arch Ophthalmol* 1978; **96**: 2105–7.

74 Lakanpal V, Schocket SS. Pseudophakia and aphakic retinal detachment mimicking cystoid macular edema. *Ophthalmology* 1987; **94**: 785–91.

75 Gass JDM. *Stereoscopic Atlas of Macular Diseases Diagnosis and Treatment.* St Louis: CV Mosby, 1987: 368–74.

76 Gass JDM. Lamellar macular hole: A complication of cystoid macular edema after cataract extraction: A clinicopathologic case report. *Trans Am Ophthalmol Soc* 1981 1975; **73**: 232–48.

77 Bovino JA, Kelley TJ, Marcus DF. Intraretinal hemorrhages in cystoid macular edema. *Arch Ophthalmol* 1984; **102**: 1151–2.

78 Jampol LM, Goldberg MF. Improved method of fluorescein angioscopy. *Arch Ophthalmol* 1990; **108**: 16 (letter).

79 Diamond JG, Kaplan HJ. Lensectomy and vitrectomy for complicated cataract secondary to uveitis. *Arch Ophthalmol* 1978; **96**: 788–804.

80 Foster CS, Fong LP, Singh G. Cataract surgery and intraocular lens implantation in patients with uveitis. *Ophthalmology* 1989; **96**: 281–8.

81 Jaffe GJ, Burton TC. Progression of nonproliferative diabetic retinopathy following cataract extraction. *Arch Ophthalmol* 1988; **106**: 745–9.

82 ETDRS Group. Treatment techniques and clinical guidelines for photocoagulation of diabetic macular edema. *Ophthalmology* 1987; **94**: 761–74.

83 Klein RM, Katzin HM, Yannuzzi LA. The effect of indomethacin pretreatment on aphakic cystoid macular edema. *Am J Ophthalmol* 1979; **87**: 487–9.

84 Lewis H, Singer TR, Hanscom TA, Straatsma BR. A prospective study of cystoid macular edema after neodymium:YAG laser posterior capsulotomy. *Ophthalmology* 1987; **94**: 478–82.

85 McEntyre JM. A successful treatment for aphakic cystoid macular edema. *Ann Ophthalmol* 1978; **10**: 1219–24.

86 Gehring JR. Macular edema following cataract extraction. *Ann Ophthalmol* 1968; **80**: 626–31.

87 Stern AL, Taylor DM, Oafburg LA, Consentino RT. Pseudophakic cystoid maculopathy: a study of 50 cases. *Ophthalmology* 1981; **88**: 942–6.

88 Jampol LM. Pharmacologic therapy of aphakic cystoid macular edema. *Ophthalmology* 1982; **80**: 891–7.

89 Jampol LM. Pharmacologic therapy of aphakic and pseudophakic cystoid macular edema 1985 update. *Ophthalmology* 1985; **92**: 807–10.

90 Jampol LM. Aphakic cystoid macular edema: A hypothesis. *Arch Ophthalmol* 1985; **103**: 1134–5.

91 Waring GO, Kenyon KR, Gemmill MC. Results of anterior segment reconstruction for aphakic and pseudophakic corneal edema. *Ophthalmology* 1988; **95**: 836–41.

92 Baleut A, Cirerchia L, Mohamadi P. Intraocular lens implant exchange and resolution of cystoid macular edema. *J Cataract Refract Surg* 1986; **12**: 184–5.

93 Smith SG. Intraocular lens removal for chronic cystoid macular edema. *J Cataract Refract Surg* 1989; **15**: 442–5.

94 Beehler CC. Prolapse of a rigid anterior chamber lens through an iridectomy: Report of 10 cases. *J Cataract Refract Surg* 1987; **13**: 436–8.

95 Branch Vein Occlusion Study Group. Argon laser photocoagulation for macular edema in branch vein occlusion. *Am J Ophthalmol* 1984; **98**: 271.

27: The Operation was Successful, but the Patient Cannot See any Better—Where Do We Go From Here?

DONALD C. FLETCHER & AUGUST COLENBRANDER

When a patient has a permanent reduction in vision following cataract surgery, a challenging clinical situation is presented to the ophthalmologist. Through low vision rehabilitation, the ophthalmologist can utilize skills and a position of authority to accomplish worthwhile medical objectives. Just as successful cataract surgery can improve the quality of life, successful rehabilitation of the visually impaired can dramatically improve the quality of life.

Traditional eye care addresses the *causes* of eye conditions, low vision rehabilitation addresses the *consequences*. Traditional eye care approaches the impairment from the point of view of the underlying disease or disorder, which it tries to cure or treat. Low vision rehabilitation deals with the resulting disability; it does not treat the disease, it tries to rehabilitate the individual. The patient needs both services.

Of foremost importance is the realization that low vision is a problem that affects the patient, rather than the eyeball. It may be true that "nothing more can be done" for the macula, but much can and must be done for the patient. We must address the total spectrum of the patient's needs and the reorientation of his or her lifestyle, work, and independence as a result of vision loss.

Functional implications of vision loss

Those with "normal" vision use it in widely varying ways. Likewise for those with decreased vision, the loss can have widely varying functional implications. These are related to the type of loss, the extent of the loss, the type of activities that were previously engaged in, as well as the emotional reaction to the loss.

Central vision loss causes difficulties with detail discrimination as in reading books and traffic signs or doing needlework. Field restrictions are usually associated with orientation and mobility problems. Generally, but not always, the more extensive the vision loss the greater the functional implications are going to be.

The type of activities that the individual has previously made part of his or her life is very significant to the impact of vision loss. A mild reduction in central acuity affects an illiterate warehouse laborer who enjoys participating in wrestling and socializing at the bar very differently than a jeweller who stops at the library every third day to replenish his reading material and plays left field for his baseball team.

The emotional impact of vision loss has a great bearing on the extent of life disruption. It can result in fear and a lack of confidence which can have functional implications far beyond that expected by the level of vision loss alone. For example, individuals with macular degeneration have widely differing abilities to cross streets based primarily on their confidence in doing so. It is not essential to be able to discern the year and model of the large solid object moving down the street toward you to appropriately decide to stay on the curb until all such solid-looking objects have cleared from the intended path. Thus macular patients may stay at home and refuse to travel independently, when they are actually quite capable of doing so. The fear associated with the loss of vision often paralyzes people from appropriately utilizing the visual information they are still receiving.

Types of low vision

Types of low vision are best described by the resulting vision loss, not by the underlying condition. Two types of vision loss are (a) central (reduced visual acuity); and (b) peripheral (reduced field). Central vision loss may be diffuse as in retinal dystrophies, may have a central scotoma as from a disciform scar, or have scattered small scotomata such as with drusen. Peripheral vision loss may be a concentric constriction as in retinitis pigmentosa, may affect a quadrant or hemisphere as in central nervous system (CNS) problems or have segments of the field missing as with Bjerrum scotoma in glaucoma.

Common aggravating problems are decreased night vision as in panretinal photocoagulation treated diabetic retinopathy, slow dark adaptation as in age-related maculopathy, diffuse glare as with cataracts, and slow glare recovery as in age-related maculopathy.

The most prevalent type of low vision is central vision loss; the most common cause is age-related macular degeneration. The most common solution is magnification. But these generalizations should not lead one to equate low vision rehabilitation with magnifiers only.

The low vision history

Whether or not we have the intention of performing any low vision work personally, *all ophthalmologists must be skilled at taking a low vision history*. Dr Eleanor Faye has said that it is not possible to begin rehabilitation "without an understanding of how a person gets through a day, whether doing chores, managing details of a household or job, or taking pleasure in leisure interests."

History taking in low vision rehabilitation is primarily aimed at determining the functional implications of the vision loss. After we are familiar with the visual status we can proceed with an assessment of the impact the loss is having on the individual. A vague question

like: "How are you doing?" may or may not give useful information; a one word answer like "fine" is a frequent response that doesn't mean much. More specific questions are generally needed and they can yield meaningful insights; they also demonstrate a sensitivity that will help to open communication lines further. Some examples of useful questions might include:

1 How are you managing to write checks, pay bills, or balance your accounts?

2 How has your vision loss affected your job?

3 Are you able to read and manage your mail?

4 How has your vision loss affected your leisure time activities?

5 Are you able to do any pleasure reading?

6 How are you managing in the kitchen?

7 Where and how are you traveling independently?

8 How are your family and friends reacting to this?

9 What visual activities do you miss?

10 How has your life changed since your vision loss? and

11 What are your plans for the future?

Once it is decided that a vision loss has functional significance for a patient the next decision is whether to refer for or initiate appropriate rehabilitation efforts.

Vision enhancement

One of the first steps in any low vision evaluation is the determination of visual acuity. A simple, systematic approach can provide an accurate acuity rating and expedite the prescription of appropriate aids.

Visual acuity measurement is traditionally carried out at 6 m (20 ft). For routine eye examinations this measurement is used to determine if the visual system is normal or abnormal and if the refraction can be improved. In low vision work, more accurate measurements in the lower ranges of acuity are necessary to predict function and prescribe aids.

For patients with less than 20/100 acuity the measurement range can be extended by moving the test charts normally used at 6 m (20 ft) to a closer distance. By bringing the chart to a 1 m (3 ft) distance and adopting the metric

Table 27.1 The following table provides metric equivalents for letters designated as 20/xx at 20 ft (6 m)

20/200	20/100	20/80	20/70	20/60	20/50	20/40	20/30	20/25	20/20	20/15	20/12	20/10
60 M	30 M	25 M	21 M	18 M	15 M	12 M	9 M	8 M	6 M	4.5 M	3.5 M	3 M

system many advantages are gained. This extends the measurable range down to 1/50 (20/1000) or 1/60 (20/1200) and makes more letters per line available at each level. One meter is 1 D from optical infinity; thus, a refraction carried out at this distance simply needs 1 D subtracted for distance correction and a 1 D trial lens placed over distance glasses will focus for testing at 1 m (3 ft).

A simple metric Snellen fraction (1/xx) results from testing at 1 m (3 ft). Multiplying the 1/xx Snellen fraction by 20 will give the standard 20/xx score for those accustomed to the traditional notation. Remember: when using the metric system the numerator of the Snellen fraction (indicating the test distance) must be expressed in meters and the denominator (indicating the letter size) in M units. The denominator of this fraction represents the theoretic diopters of add necessary for reading 1 M print (1 M = newsprint). This is known to many as Kestenbaum's rule (dipoters needed = 1/VA). If your chart does not carry metric notation see Table 27.1 for conversions.

After determining the distance and intermediate visual acuity the near acuity must be measured. Since visual acuity is an angular measure, both distance and letter size must be specified. Recording just the "letter size read" (e.g. "J10") without reference to the distance would be meaningless. For a low vision evaluation, the ability to measure at many different distances is crucial, since use of a single "standard" testing distance for all patients is not practical. (By the way, what is "standard": 25 cm, 30 cm, 33.3 cm, 14 in, 40 cm?)

If distance and letter size are properly recorded, the same visual acuity score should be calculated for all distances. The problem is that the most prevalent measures, inches and J-numbers, make visual acuity calculations impossible.

Adopting metric measurements, as we already do in all other parts of our profession, makes calculation far easier. Yet, the traditional notation of the Snellen fraction still leaves us with the need for division of two numbers. It would be easier if we could standardize the numerator to "1" as we did for intermediate acuity. This indeed can be done and actually is rather simple if we remember that the reciprocal of "distance in meters" is known to all of us as the "diopter". If:

$$VA = \frac{\text{test distance}}{\text{letter size}}$$

then:

$$\frac{1}{VA} \text{ (Kestenbaum's value)} = \frac{\text{letter size}}{\text{test distance}}$$

or:

$$\frac{1}{VA} = \frac{\text{size}}{\text{distance}} = \text{size} \times \frac{1}{\text{distance}}$$

$$= \text{size} \times \text{diopters.}$$

Recording the reading distance in diopters may seem unfamiliar at first; yet, it is easily done using the ruler provided with any phoropter. Letter size must, of course, be recorded in M units.

Thus, the procedure is as follows:
1 ask the patient to hold the reading material at whatever distance is in focus with their existing glasses;
2 measure the reading distance in diopters (use a phoropter ruler, or calculate: 100 cm/reading distance in cm);
3 record the letter size in M units and the reading distance in diopters (D);
4 multiply M by D to confirm the consistency of the recorded results. Having determined the starting performance:
5 measure the near acuity with more add (adds do not stop at +3);

Table 27.2 Levels of visual performance and corresponding reading aids

Classification of visual performance			Disability estimates	Visual aids for reading
Near normal vision	Range of normal vision	20/12 20/16 20/20 20/25	Normal performance Normal reading distance	Reading distance 16–30 in Regular bifocals (up to 3 D)
	Near normal vision	20/30 20/40 20/50 20/60	Normal performance, using shorter reading distance	Reading distance 8–12 in Stronger bifocals (4.5 D) Low power magnifier (5 D)
Low vision	Moderate low vision	20/80 20/100 20/125 20/160	Near normal performance with magnifiers, other aids	Reading distance 4–6 in Half-eye glasses (6.1 D) (with prisms for binocularity) Stronger magnifiers (12 D)
	Severe low vision	20/200 20/250 20/300 20/400	Slower than normal, with aids (legal blindness, USA)	Reading distance 2–3 in (cannot be binocular) Hi-power reading lens (12–20 D) Hi-power (stand) magnifiers (20 D)
	Profound low vision	20/500 20/600 20/800 20/1000	Limited reading with aids Orientation Mobility problems	Reading distance 1 in Spectacle mounted magnifier (40 D) Video-magnifier, cane, O + M training
Near blindness	Near blindess	20/1250 20/1600 20/2000 20/2500	Vision unreliable	Video-magnifier Talking books, braille Talking computer, cane, O + M training
	Total blindess	NLP	No vision	Talking devices, cane, O + M training

NLP, no light perception.
O + M, orientation and mobility.

6 adjust the reading distance as the add increases;
7 check the reading distance versus the reading add at each distance;
8 record M and D and check M × D at each distance;
9 continue until 1 M is reached.

Example

Distance acuity: 5/60 or 6/72 (since this is less than 20/200, it would be scored as 20/400 on the usual chart; the actual equivalent is 20/240).
Intermediate acuity: 1/12.
Near acuity:

Size (M)	Distance (meters)	Diopters	Record	Check	Acuity
6	1/2	2	6 M at 2 D	6 × 2 = 12	1/12
4	1/3	3	4 M at 3 D	4 × 3 = 12	1/12
3	1/4	4	3 M at 4 D	3 × 4 = 12	1/12
2	1/6	6	2 M at 6 D	2 × 6 = 12	1/12
1	1/12	12	1 M at 12 D	1 × 12 = 12	1/12

Using the "M unit and diopter" (M & D) notation has several advantages:

1 no need for a prior refraction to correct the patient for your "standard" reading distance;

2 a check on the basic refraction. If the reading add and reading distance (in D) coincide, the basic refraction must be correct;

3 a check on the visual acuity score. Consistent visual acuity scores at each distance reassure us of their reliability. Inconsistencies should not be ignored; they provide additional information that asks for an explanation (see below); and

4 gradually reducing the reading distance encourages the patient with each progressive step, even if 1 M is not achievable. It also eases the patient into the eventual short reading distance which might otherwise be resisted if we jump directly to the highest add based on Kestenbaum's rule.

Discrepancies in the above measurements provide additional information.

A constant difference between reading distance (in D) and reading add indicates an undetected refractive error. This often is an effective way to find lens-induced myopia from nuclear sclerosis in elderly low vision patients and is much less time consuming than a regular subjective refraction at 6 m (20 ft).

An increasing difference between the reading distance (in D) and the reading add may indicate resistance to a close reading distance; in this case the image will not be focused and the visual acuity will not be optimal.

An incorrect reading distance is a common reason for M × D inconsistencies. Fixation problems may also give inconsistent scores indicating the need for eccentric viewing training.

While the patient is reading, note not only the numeric end point, but also the quality of reading for:

1 easy acceptance of a short reading distance and of new modes of reading which allow us to predict easy adaptation;

2 poor fluency, skipping, and guessing indicate that extensive training may be necessary and that our expectations must be tailored not to exceed the patient's ability to perform during the early stages of adjustment;

3 if the patient reads well at one size and poorly at the next, magnification to the first level will restore effective reading;

4 if the patient reads slowly even at the largest sizes, reading will remain difficult even with high magnification; and

5 patients with a small total field or with a small island of high resolution between scotomata, may see small letters more easily than large ones and may actually do better with moderate than with high magnification.

The end point of near acuity testing, as outlined above, is a spectacle correction that allows reading of 1 M print. Knowing the diopters of spectacle add necessary for 1 M can guide the trial of other types of magnifiers. A useful rule of thumb is to start testing magnifiers at the dioptric power where we ended the spectacle testing. This has two reasons:

1 as the lens is moved away from the eye, so is the virtual image, thus requiring more power; and

2 magnifiers are usually held at less than their focal distance; this also reduces their effectiveness.

One of the key factors to remember in recommending low vision devices is that considerable practice is required before they become maximally effective. Reading with a low vision device represents an acquired skill; it is not at all like the quick scanning technique used prior to vision loss. Instruction and practice in their use should be provided prior to discharge from the low vision service. Positive reinforcement that skills will continue to improve through diligent practice will prevent many magnifiers from gathering dust at home on the shelf.

The use of filters is of considerable benefit for many low vision patients. Light yellow filters enhance contrast indoors; this is more noticeable with low contrast items like faces than for high contrast black on white printed material. Dark yellow, orange or amber filters are darker and may provide some contrast enhancement and glare reduction for outdoor settings. The use of a low light transmission filter on a bright sunny day may alleviate glare and be useful in reducing light adaptation time when promptly removed upon entering, say, a dimly lit restaurant.

The use of handheld telescopes for distance spotting tasks such as reading overhead signs at the grocery store or the menu on the wall at a fast food restaurant is often indicated and represents the most common application of telescopic devices. Spectacle-mounted telescopes are sometimes used for theater productions, computer screen viewing, etc.

Special higher technology equipment can provide access to printed or electronically stored material in an ever increasing number of ways. The expense of such equipment is not always prohibitive and it is often of great value. As with all adaptations though, work and practice are required to make them useful and none will magically "restore vision like it used to be."

Addressing other practical problems caused by vision loss

The prescription of low vision devices alone will no more solve all of the difficulties of vision loss than buckling one hole will repairing a retinal detachment caused by multiple breaks. In the low vision history other problem areas that are not directly solved by vision enhancement will have been isolated. These can be addressed by instruction within the low vision service or by referral.

Some of the many suggestions for specific tasks might include:

Writing: felt-tip pens, bold line stationery, large print checks, writing guides, signature/envelop template.

Recognizing people: tell friends and acquaintances about problem; recognize friends by voice, body type, hair style, clothes.

Dialing phone: large-print phone dial, large print phone, memory phone, operator assistance.

Telling time: change watch hands to black ones, low vision watch, talking watch/clock, large print clock.

Mobility: assessment by mobility instructor, instruction if needed, sighted guide technique (spouse). White cane (long: sensing; short: support, identification). Scanning eye movements to reduce blind spots.

Street signs, bus numbers: pocket telescope, ask someone.

Driving: limited license for familiar area.

Shopping: non-busy hours, call ahead to request help, volunteer.

Distinguishing money: serrated and smooth edge, folding different denominations, putting in different wallet compartments.

Housework: counselor/teacher services, adaptation of dials, housekeeper, grid-pattern of cleaning.

Cooking: large-print recipes, adaptation of oven dials, pouring and measuring techniques, timer, counselor/teacher services.

Sewing and handiwork: needle-threader, self-threading needles, dental floss threader, large-print embroidery kits, knitting needles with good contrast. Optical aids for crafts and chores: +6 half-eyes, chest-supported magnifier, illuminated stand magnifier (even if too weak for reading).

Eating: contrasting food/dishes/table cloth, lean over plate a bit, clock method for identification. Feel weight of utensil, resistance, use bread or cracker as a pusher.

Medications: pill-splitter, pill dispenser, shape, color, rubber bands on bottles, friends to fill dispenser, insulin filling guide, talking glucometer.

Games: adapted games, large-print cards.

Television: sit close (12 in screen at 1 ft is larger than 25 in screen at 4 ft).

Music: large-print music, reproduce on enlarging copier, copy-holder that can swing in close to face.

Gardening: pot vs. plot, tactile sense.

For most tasks of daily living, normal vision provides a surplus of information to carry out the task. After functioning with normal vision for many years though, it is not an easy transition to make do with less. Increased attention to more subtle visual clues is necessary; this represents an acquired skill and becomes easier with practice.

For most of life's activities there is a way for the visually impaired to do it. Telling patients how to do it is not as effective as actually giving experience in trying the activity. The biggest obstacle to overcome in adjusting to vision loss is simply gaining the confidence to try. Once patients have felt success at tasks perceived as difficult, they gain confidence to try other activities. (Tasks that may not even require any specific adaptations.) A pressing need today is for more confidence building hands-on experience to be made available for the visually impaired, especially the elderly.

Attitude enhancement

Attitude is one of the key determinants for the outcome of low vision rehabilitation. This was demonstrated in a recent study done by Robbins and McMurray [1]. They surveyed several factors felt to be significant in low vision rehabilitation including personality hardiness, visual acuity, general health, education, income, social network, initial depression, further major life event, etc. Out of all these factors, the personality hardiness (an attitude where the individual maintained a sense of control over life events and viewed the vision loss as a challenge instead of a threat) was the factor most closely correlated with successful outcome of rehabilitation efforts.

Attitude, like residual vision, can be enhanced. Every low vision patient is an individual and has unique coping skills which can be maximized; the ophthalmologist is in a key position to enhance those skills. The most valuable service we can render our patients is to appropriately use our authority to encourage *effort* and give *hope*. Dr William H. Havener has formulated an excellent technique of "reassurance therapy" which appropriately utilizes the placebo effect and stresses the positive aspects of the prognosis. It is outlined in Chapter 4. Reassurance therapy is the cornerstone of low vision rehabilitation.

As Dostoevsky said: "A new philosophy, a way of life, is not given for nothing. It has to be paid for and only acquired with much patience and great effort." All adjustment efforts made by our patients should be copiously praised. Specific techniques can also be used to encourage further effort. A sensitive orientation and mobility specialist, Tim Hindman, asks his clients to tell him about the most difficult thing they have had to do in their past. He gets a variety of answers including accomplishing a college education, surviving divorce, loss of a loved one, etc. He then indicates to them that learning to cope with vision loss will require

at least as much effort as that task. This emphasizes that results come from effort and also points out to people that they have already successfully dealt with major challenges. It starts a focus on what can be done rather than what cannot be done.

To communicate hope to our low vision patients we must first work on our own attitudes and fears about vision loss. If we do not ourselves believe that life can be full, meaningful, and enjoyable despite vision loss nothing we say will have a positive effect. Richard Hoover, MD said: "The ophthalmologist's understanding of the area of visual impairment can be extremely beneficial to his patient. His potential power to encourage the use of rehabilitation services is great and his authority at the time of crisis can contribute significantly to future rehabilitation efforts. The patient senses his attitudes, expressed or unexpressed and responds to them."

There is probably no segment of society that fears vision loss as much as ophthalmologists. When cataract surgery is unsuccessful in restoring vision, the ophthalmologist must not abandon the patient. Visual impairment must be recognized and dealt with in a capable and compassionate manner. The business of saving vision is a noble battle in which vision loss is the enemy. Our most frequent contact with the visually impaired is during the acute stages of vision loss when there is much sadness, discouragement, and fear. We also see those unwilling to accept their diagnosis who are searching for an easy miracle cure. There is far less contact with those who are quietly going on with the work of leading a complete life despite vision loss. Thus our perception of life with a vision impairment is distorted toward the negative side. Gaining positive experiences can be accomplished by seeking contact with visually impaired people who are in control of their lives. If you do not have any other source try a visit to your local school for the blind; there you will see youngsters who are leading happy productive lives despite having no vision. It will be inspiring.

Once you have the confidence that life can be full without vision tell this to your low vision patients. Make it the final communication in your visit. Face them squarely. Talk slowly. Perhaps hold their hand and tell them that you know they can do it. They can.

Reference

1 Robbins HG, McMurray NE. Psychological and visual factors in low vision rehabilitation of patients with age-related maculopathy. *J Vis Rehab* 1988; **2**: 11.

28: Medicolegal Concerns of Cataract Surgeons

SANDER MARC RABIN

The new legal concerns of the cataract surgeon

Today's cataract surgeon is faced not only with the ongoing risk of medical malpractice litigation, but with the added threats of administrative sanctions in the form of expulsion from participation in third-party reimbursement plans, revocation or abridgement of hospital privileges, and limitation or loss of the license to practice. Moreover, competition together with profound changes in the eye care delivery system call for a heightened awareness of legal principles affecting productivity and income creation.

Cataract surgery has become the key focus of legal changes which are converting our profession into a strictly regulated service industry. The two major factors responsible for this conversion are: (a) the widespread prevalence of cataracts, which makes cataract surgery the most frequently performed operation in the USA; and (b) the position of the government of the USA as the largest single purchaser of eye care. Cataract surgery is now being performed under third-party surveillance for cost-containment and quality assurance.

Medical malpractice liability, at one time the major legal concern of cataract surgeons, is now part of a more comprehensive and perhaps more threatening set of legal concerns within which the cataract surgeon must operate. Remaining productive, creative, and fairly paid in this setting is a challenge to twenty-first century ophthalmology.

The legal concerns of cataract surgeons may be now grouped into three categories: (a) con-ventional malpractice liability; (b) surveillance for regulatory compliance; and (c) practice productivity and income creation.

Malpractice liability in cataract surgery

The scope and impact of malpractice liability in cataract surgery

Data collected by the Medical Liability Mutual Insurance Company, a major malpractice carrier in New York State, and the second largest underwriter of malpractice insurance in the USA, revealed that between 1985 and 1988, 525 claims were made against ophthalmologists. Of these, 130 (appproximately 25%), resulted in aggregate payments of $18 678 351, for an average payment of $142 910 per resolved claim.

The Medical Inter-Insurance Exchange of New Jersey, that state's major malpractice carrier, collected data on ophthalmology-related claims between 1977 and 1986. In this period, 348 claims had been reported, of which 62 (18%) arose from cataract surgery; of these, 40 were resolved at the time of the publication of its data in 1987, and 20 resulted in damage awards. The 50% cataract indemnification ratio was higher than the 31% indemnification ratio arising from all eye-related claims in this study.

While the percentage of challenged practices in both states is relatively small when compared to the overall activity of ophthalmology in these states, the personal impact of malpractice litigation on any ophthalmologist can be severe. Moreover, when taken against the annual volume of cataract surgery, the malpractice burden of this form of microsurgery is considerable.

Experience gained in evaluating claims against cataract surgeons has resulted in the formulation of practice guidelines intended to moderate the malpractice risk. These are best appreciated and implemented when taken against the basic principles of the law of medical malpractice and the law of informed consent.

The law of medical malpractice in a nutshell

A claim of medical malpractice is a charge of negligence against a health-care provider. A charge of negligence is a legally cognizable accusation falling within the law of torts, which concerns itself with wrongful departures from civilized rules of conduct. The law of torts is intended to redress legitimately disappointed expectations and to sublimate the urges for vengeance and retribution into the orderly pursuit of monetary recompense.

Generally, the cataract surgeon's duty to the patient arises at the moment the doctor–patient relationship is created, and cataract surgery should be considered as a service which begins with the initial examination of the patient. The cataract surgeon is then obliged to perform the service with a standard of care consistent with that degree of skill and learning ordinarily used under the same or similar circumstances by other competent members of the profession. Expert testimony is required to establish the standard of care and its breach by the defendant.

If the patient can prove that a non-trivial injury was sustained as a result of the departure from the standard of care, and can overcome a defense of causation attributable to an independent intervening incident or the patient's contributory negligence, the malpractice claim will be sustained, subject only to a determination of monetary damages.

Informed consent: untangling the Gordian knot

No medicolegal issue has generated as much controversy as the doctrine of informed con-

sent. Often mistakenly regarded as a special case of medical malpractice, it is actually grounded upon a distinct legal theory. As a failure to give legally sufficient informed consent is itself an independent act of negligence, surgical services performed in the setting of legally insufficient consent need not be proved substandard to support a recovery for an injury. Indeed, totally appropriate performance is no defense in an action grounded upon a lack of informed consent.

From the cataract surgeon's standpoint, the doctrine of informed consent imposes an unrealistic burden—the product of the legal profession's alteration of an accepted ethical obligation into an expansive recitation of possibilities of dubious benefit to patients laboring under duress of illness. Irrationally applied, the doctrine often has the effect of making the cataract surgeon the legal guarantor of a satisfactory outcome. From the attorney's standpoint, the doctrine offers an opportunity to fairly enforce a physician's ethical obligation to provide patients with the information needed to make a decision concerning their most inviolate possession—the body.

The doctrine of informed consent is related to the law of battery. The law of battery creates a claim for the unauthorized touching of another's body. An absolute defense to a charge of battery is proof that the touching followed freely given consent. The practice of eliciting consents for treatments is actually intended to protect physicians from claims of battery by their patients. A cause of action in lack of informed consent actually seeks to invalidate the consent upon which a physician's immunity to a charge of battery is predicated.

Since a battery is legally defined as an *intentional* tort, i.e. a deliberate illegal act *irrespective of any wilfull intention* to cause harm, its commission requires no expert testimony of a breach of an applicable standard of care.

The substantial litigation this cause of action has generated concerns the legal standards of disclosure physicians must satisfy to sustain a defense of a prior consent to "touching." Practically, each case is concerned with retrospectively fashioning a statement of what should have been disclosed, against which a judgment is made of whether the patient would still have submitted to the treatment which occasioned an undesirable outcome. Often, artful persuasion made with the benefit of hindsight play a determinative role in resolving the conflict.

WHAT MUST THE PATIENT BE TOLD?

Generally, consent to cataract surgery is regarded as legally "informed" if the following aspects of the procedure are disclosed by the *operating surgeon*:

1 the diagnosis or nature of the cataract and its relationship to the patient's vision;

2 the nature and purpose of the proposed surgery;

3 the options and risks associated with the various modes of optically rehabilitating aphakia;

4 the likelihood of success;

5 the risks, side effects, and consequences of the surgery;

6 the reasonably available alternatives to the surgery; and

7 the natural history of untreated cataractogenesis and the likely results of foregoing treatment.

There are serveral exceptions to the informed consent requirement, which relieve the cataract surgeon from the duty to disclose fully. These include surgical emergencies, such as phacomorphic glaucoma or anteriorly subluxated lenses; "voluntary waiver," wherein a patient knowingly declines to be fully informed in order to allay anxiety; and, the "therapeutic exception," wherein the cataract surgeon determines that it would be harmful to the patient to make full disclosure. The perils of defenses resting upon a claim of voluntary waiver or the therapeutic exception are obvious.

Preventive guidelines for minimizing malpractice exposure

Treat your patients as if they were guests in your home. Litigation is bred by arrogance, and deterred by clear communication and basic human consideration.

Don't neglect the history. Drug allergies, systemic illnesses and reactions to prior surgery or anesthesia are of obvious importance. If the use of a hyperosmotic agent induced vomiting after a prior cataract operation, its repeated use in cataract surgery on the second eye is difficult to justify. If the second extraction is accompanied by vitreous loss and a retinal detachment, the case may be indefensible. A similar scenario may arise in a case where the surgeon prescribes the liberal use of steroids to a patient with a diagnosis of diabetes, of which the surgeon is unaware.

Obtain consultations in difficult cases. Endorse second opinions and emphasize your patients' free choice in determining the need and source of their care. This practice will engender trust and eliminate any impression of surgical solicitation.

Obtain and document consultations and clearance for the use of general anesthesia; anesthetic complications are the most likely to be catastrophic.

Elicit informed consent personally. Satisfy yourself that the patient understands what you have said.

Maintain impeccable records. Complete, legible records provide an unparalleled defense.

Never discuss your treatment with a patient or another without the chart at your side. Date and annotate telephone conversations regarding requests for medications, refills, inquiries regarding symptoms, and the like. If complications arise, do not use language suggestive of cause and effect such as "secondary to," "possibly or probably arising from," or "associated with." Simply document the occurrence of the complication and your response to it.

Record the non-compliance of difficult or uncooperative patients but do not enter notes suggestive of exasperation or intolerance. Reference to "supratentorial deficits" will not be understood by a jury as they are by your medical colleagues.

Don't discard defective instruments. Claims have arisen involving defective instrumentation.

Whenever any instrument is defective, that finding should be recorded and the defective component should be kept. This practice will help to absolve the cataract surgeon from liability more appropriately borne by the instrument manufacturer or maintenance contractor.

Avoid quarreling with professional associates. Thoughtless remarks may entrap a colleague in litigation, make you an adverse witness, subject you to the risk of a suit in slander, and possibly violate the privacy rights of patients.

Instruct your postoperative patients in writing of signs or symptoms warranting a call to your office.

Err on the side of caution; don't fail to diagnose out of laxity. If your postoperative patient or one for whom you are providing coverage has symptoms suggestive of urgency you must advise of the need for immediate care.

Claims alleging negligent management have, on the average, been more costly per case than those alleging negligent surgery. Patient indemnification is generally higher in claims involving judgmental errors than in those involving technical errors because injuries following judgmental errors tend to be more severe.

Dictate complete operative records. When complications occur, you will have established your own best defense should litigation ensue if you have documented the preventive, diagnostic, and therapeutic measures you employed to anticipate, mitigate, and respond to the complication.

Prescribe medications responsibly. The National Association of Insurance Commissioners has reported that drug-related errors are the source of 10% of claims paid by medical malpractice insurers. Prescribe only within the purview of our specialty. Be vigilant with regard to drug allergies and cross reactions. Consult the Physician's Desk Reference (PDR) liberally. Prescribe legibly, and log prescriptions in the patients' charts.

Delegate responsibly, with discretion and clarity. Remember that your employees are your agents while acting within the scope of their employment. Under the legal principle of respondeat superior, their negligence will be attributed to you. Document job descriptions, responsibilities, and the limits of discretionary action.

What to do if you are sued

The natural tendency is for the emotions to run rampant in response to a lawsuit by one of your patients. You will likely feel anxiety, rage, indignation, and that your best efforts have been repaid by an upsetting and threatening act, or what may be perceived as pure vindictiveness and opportunism.

Do not take the content of the complaint literally or personally. Very few of the allegations will actually contain facts upon which the charge of malpractice is grounded. Do not be distracted by the obvious redundancy of the complaint; your patient's attorney will recast the same set of facts and assertions into multiple, seemingly independent charges of medical malfeasance and neglect. Most of what you will see are standard form recitations from a word processor programmed to print the allegations in every complaint in medical malpractice. These recitations are known as "boilerplate" and should be treated with exactly the concern you would have for a piece of rusted metal in a vacant lot. Above all, do not be outraged by the monetary award requested. Remember that the monetary damages claimed are at best a hope, and will not likely be related to any amount which may ultimately be awarded.

The best attitude to bring to bear is one of respect and detachment. The complaint will serve as a blueprint for preparing your defense. Regard it as something that you will use for that purpose.

In principle, you, your carrier, and your attorney have the same objective—to win the lawsuit or at least to limit the damage. Avoid communicating with your aggrieved patient or the patient's attorney. Leave discussions to your representatives. Be discrete in discussing the case with your professional colleagues, and do not make statements to the media.

Participate in your own defense, but do not let your cooperation be blind. In the current system of malpractice insurance maintaining some skepticism is appropriate; your carrier and its defense attorneys, unlike plaintiffs' attorneys, have no stake in the outcome of a trial. Frivolous defenses may be undertaken while meritorious defenses may be foresaken for expeditious settlements. It is not always clear that the same attorney or firm will be assigned to represent you throughout the course of a claim's resolution. You are as fully entitled to receive explanations and answers from your insurer and attorney as your patients are in receiving informed consent from you. Do not be deterred by the use of the legal vocabulary; insist on clarification until your understanding has been satisfied.

Surveillance: keeping the operating room door open

Living with quality assurance regulation

In the 1980s a process of medical malpractice reform began in several states as an adjunct to the evolving national policy of imposing tighter administrative control over the medical profession, as exemplified by the creation of the National Practitioner Data Bank. The regulation, surveillance, and policing of the medical profession by various third-party private and governmental agencies have created an unprecedented legal practice environment.

In New York's reform legislation, which may serve as an example, hospitals now have a legal duty to monitor the qualifications and performance of their physicians. While credentialing procedures have long been observed, they were never encoded into law. Hospitals must not only scrutinize the performance of physicians seeking to renew or obtain privileges, but must now also investigate physicians' professional histories by obtaining information from prior affiliates. Moreover, each hospital must establish a quality assurance committee to supervise a malpractice prevention program through audits and the reporting of untoward incidents and unexpected outcomes.

Information gathered in the credentialing procedures must include the nature of all pending malpractice actions and professional misconduct proceedings, the number of judgments and settlements of any prior malpractice actions, and facts concerning violations of patients' rights, as suggested by patients' complaints.

The policy of increasing regulation is further reflected in the heightened activities of New York's Offices of Professional Misconduct and Professional Discipline. The activities of peer review organizations, acting under the auspices of Medicare, or performing quality assurance and utilization reviews for hospitals and insurance companies, have also intensified. These agencies may conduct inquests in the form of administrative hearings, governed by non-uniform, vague, or relaxed rules of procedure and evidence, probing allegations ranging from faulty record-keeping, improper billing or overutilization, to professional misconduct or incompetence. Additionally, administrative hearings may not be subject to the same statutes of limitations which delimit the period in which a civil suit may be brought; the threat of their attendant sanctions may have greater longevity.

Administrative hearings: features of concern

In principle, in a civil malpractice action a surgeon will be defended at each procedural step by an attorney. The defense will be heard by an impartial judge, and a jury selected with equal input by the defense attorney and opposing counsel. The jury is presented with facts in accordance with the constitutional standards of procedural due process, elements of which include a hearing, prior knowledge of the charges, time to prepare a defense, representation by counsel, and the right to confront the accusing witnesses.

Moreover, the content and quality of the evidence, its sources, credibility, weight, and legitimate inferences, must meet the requirements of substantive due process. For example, in a criminal trial, guilt must be established "beyond a reasonable doubt"; in a civil trial allegations must be carried by a "preponderance of the evidence." In either forum, the defendant may seek appellate review to challenge non-compliance with both procedural and substantive due process.

In an administrative hearing, by contrast, a surgeon's rights may be compromised. Procedural due process may be undermined by the fact that the accusing party, the hearing officer or panel, and expert or other witnesses may all be related to either the institution in which the hearing is held, or to the accusing party. The administrative standard for meeting the burden of proof may not comply with substantive due process. Moreover, in a judicial review of an administrative proceeding, while available, the court may not have the jurisdiction to review the conclusions of fact reached by the hearing officer from a substantive standpoint; judicial review may be confined only to the adequacy of procedural due process as derived from institutional by-laws.

As administrative hearings in ophthalmology are relatively uncharted waters, questions abound. In charges arising from a review of a surgeon's records, will the records be compared to others of the staff? Will the charged party be allowed access to records for comparative review? Who selects the membership of the hearing panel or appoints the hearing officer? Will the affected surgeon have any participation in selection process? Might not commercial, academic, and political competitors be selected as members? Do the by-laws allow for representation by counsel and may counsel act as an advocate? Do the by-laws grant the right of cross-examination? Will minutes be taken and will they be made available to the accused? What is the substantive standard of proof required to uphold a decision?

Preparing for an administrative hearing

A request for an appearance before an administrative body calls for a carefully considered response. Inevitably, personal principles in possible conflict with realistically available resources and practical consequences will join in the often frustrating formulation of that response. Available options include submission to sanctions without a hearing, compromise, or contested engagement. The following suggestions are helpful for the cataract surgeon in this unenviable position:

1 critically ask whether there is a basis in fact for the decision to conduct an administrative hearing;

2 ask what really underlies the procedure: politics, dislike, competition, incompetence;

3 seek the advice of counsel experienced in representing clients before administrative bodies. Ask for a copy of the institutional by-laws and determine whether they will grant you a hearing consistent with the principles of procedural and substantive due process outlined above. Ask your attorney about available review procedures, and obtain a clear statement of the cost of your representation. Cooperate and involve yourself in your own defense;

4 seek the advice and determine the attitudes of colleagues; marshal the commitment of supportive professional colleagues, if possible. Their willingness to support you or preference for remaining uninvolved must be determined;

5 ask whether a satisfactory informal resolution can be negotiated to head off a formal hearing;

6 consider whether your appearance at the administrative hearing will rock the political boat; is there a risk of professional alienation or a career setback?

7 in evaluating the wisdom of entering a contested proceeding consider the scope, impact and duration of the restriction of privileges; and its effect on your daily professional life and your ability to earn a living;

8 realize that the initial hearing may only set the stage for overturning an unfavorable decision in a higher court, and that the likelihood of compromise diminishes as the hearing progresses. You must be willing to undertake litigation to contest the proceeding, and see the potential conflict and its cost in time and money in this broader context. Assure yourself that your family has the resolve to support you in what may be a formidable undertaking;

9 consider the reporting and dossier-building aspects of the hearing and of allowing an adverse decision to stand;

10 no one can predict what will be at stake in a

given case, but the deeper question of whether you can afford not to fight must be asked in considering the overall cost of your decision; and

11 even if your chances of winning a contested procedure are excellent, don't become a victim of your own pride; assure yourself that your victory will not be pyrrhic.

The National Practitioner Data Bank

The uses and potential abuses of the impending National Practitoner Data Bank will likely become a hotbed of litigation in the near future. Its success as an instrument of malpractice reduction remains to be assessed. Its threat as an instrument for surveillance, misinterpretation, and the erosion of confidentiality arises with its implementation. For better or for worse, medicine is about to become a transparent profession.

Established under the Health Care Quality Improvement Act of 1986, to be operated pursuant to a $15.9 million contract with Unisys, the Data Bank will store and analyze information to be submitted under initial mandatory and voluntary regulations, which are expected to expand.

WHO MUST REPORT AND WHAT MUST BE REPORTED?

1 *Malpractice actions.* Any insurance company or self-insured hospital or practitioner that makes a payment on behalf of a licensed health-care practitioner as a result of a claim or judgment in malpractice must report to the Data Bank and to the appropriate state licensing board(s).

2 *Licensure actions.* State medical boards must report disciplinary actions taken against the license of a health-care practitioner.

3 *Professional review actions.* Hospitals, alternative delivery systems, and certain group practices must report certain adverse actions, e.g. a sanction based on professional incompetence or misconduct taken against clinical privileges lasting more than 30 days.

4 *Society membership actions.* Professional societies must report an adverse action taken against the membership of a practitioner when that action follows from a formal peer review process and the action is based on professional incompetence or misconduct.

WHO MUST QUERY THE DATA BANK?

All hospitals must query the Data Bank every 2 years regarding practitioners on their staff. They must also query the Data Bank when considering an applicant for an appointment or privileges. Hospitals may at other times query as they deem necessary.

WHO MAY QUERY THE DATA BANK?

The law provides that state licensing boards may query the Data Bank. Health-care entities other than hospitals in connection with contemplated employment or affiliation agreements may also query the Data Bank.

An attorney who has filed a medical malpractice action or claim against a hospital may query the Data Bank for information regarding a specific practitioner, but only upon showing that the hospital failed to make a legally required inquiry of the Data Bank with regard to the same practitioner, and provided that the information so obtained is used only with respect to the medical malpractice action or claim against the hospital.

Individual practitioners may query the Data Bank regarding themselves at no cost. Practitioners on whom a report has been made to the Data Bank will routinely receive a copy of that report. Rules and mechanisms for authenticating, challenging, and correcting information have been established.

Aggregate data which do not reveal the identity of any practitioner or institution will be available to interested persons, presumably for statistical and actuarial studies.

Productivity: business law and cataract surgery

As our profession struggles to redefine its functional code of ethics in the new reality of medical practice confronting us, the distinction between service as a profession and service as a business is blurring. Practically speaking you can no longer practice professionally if you do not also function as a person in business.

Being in business demands attention to a myriad of new legal issues in such areas as intellectual property, occupational health and safety, labor law, environmental law, unfair competition and deceptive advertising, contracting with managed care systems, as well as the more traditional issues raised by tax law, partnership agreements, incorporation, and restrictive covenants. These are topics beyond the scope of this chapter.

Anticipating the eye care future will depend on your utilization of the law for productivity, and your keen regard for it in service and accountability.

Further reading

Bettman JW. A review of 412 claims in ophthalmology. *Int Ophthal Clin* 1980; **20**: 131–42.

Byron HM. Intraocular implant surgery. *Int Ophthal Clin* 1980; **20**: 109–19.

Ciaccio P. Data bank to act as repository for adverse action information. *Ocul Surg News* 1990; March 15.

Commonsense ways to reduce your malpractice risk. *Ophthline* 1988; **11**.

Fay MF, Maijer MM, Buchanan J. Regulatory compliance for ophthalmic practices. *Ocul Surg News* 1989; October 15.

Gardinier RH. The nitty-gritty essence of informed consent. *Legal Aspects Med Pract* 1988; **16**.

Goldsmith LS. MDs face greater medico–legal problems than malpractice suits. *Ophthalmol Management* 1989; February: 23–8.

Goldsmith LS. Physicians' hospital privileges may not be forever. *Ophthalmol Management* 1990; April: 17–21.

Kraushar MF, Turner MF. Medical malpractice litigation in cataract surgery. *Arch Ophthalmol* 1987; **105**: 1339–43.

The National Practitioner Data Bank: A Federal Scrutiny. In: *MLMIC Dateline*, the Newsletter of the Medical Liability Mutual Insurance Company. 1990; April.

Medical Liability Mutual Insurance Company Risk Management Department Bulletin. *National Practitioner Data Bank*. 1990; February 2.

Schatz MB. Personal correspondence with accompanying transmittal of data from Medical Mutual Liability Insurance Company. 1989; September 25.

Shemonsky MK, Flannery FT. Medical license— a revocable right. *Legal Aspects Med Pract* 1986; December.

29: Diagnostic Codes and Billing—Dealing with the Changing Socioeconomic Environment

DEBBIE BRANDEL & BARBARA GRENELL

Introduction

Practicing medicine in today's environment requires continued attention to clinical as well as financial matters. Over the past 2 decades, ophthalmologists and other physicians have been faced with cut-backs in reimbursement, third-party intrusion into the clinical process and a significant growth in administrative requirements. One must also be concerned with reimbursement from the patient's stand-point. If forms are not correctly coded or filled out, the patient will not be reimbursed fairly. In this situation, the patient usually will feel that the physician is at fault.

Success, increasingly, will depend on physicians and their office staffs being knowledgeable about reimbursement systems and the complexities of the bureaucratic process. This chapter provides an overview of the current reimbursement and billing system as it pertains to ophthalmologists as well as a summary of the recent changes made in Medicare reimbursement in the 1990 Budget Reconciliation Bill.

Physician reimbursement— an overview

For most ophthalmologists, the payer of primary importance is the Medicare program. Medicare physician reimbursement is generally based on the lesser of:

1 the actual charge;

2 the customary charge, which is the median charge made by the physician for a particular service;

3 the unadjusted prevailing charge, which is equal to the 75th percentile of the customary charges made for a specific service in a particular locality; or

4 the economic adjusted prevailing charge, which is equal to the prevailing charge in 1972 inflated to the current year using an economic index.

Over the past few years, physicians have been subject to a number of other reductions designed to reduce the rate of increase in Medicare expenditures. Some of these reductions apply across the board; others are limited to specific physicians or procedures. Each of the reductions currently in effect are summarized below.

The Deficit Reduction Act of 1984 established a Medicare participating physician program. As part of this program, physicians who elect to participate agree to accept Medicare assignment on all services rendered to beneficiaries during the year. Physicians who do not participate may still accept assignment on individual claims. The advantages and disadvantages of participating are described more fully in a later section, however, the major financial consequences for non-participating physicians are as follows.

1 The prevailing charge calculation for non-participating physicians is 95% of the prevailing charge for participating physicians.

2 Actual charges may not exceed the maximum allowable actual charge (MAAC) on an individual claim. The original MAAC limits were established using the physician's median actual charges during a base period in 1984. In 1990, your MAAC is based on a comparison between the 1989 MAAC and the current prevailing charge for non-participating physicians. If your 1989 MAAC is greater than or equal to 115% of the current prevailing charge, your 1990 MAAC

is 101% of last year's MAAC. If it is less than 115%, your 1990 MAAC is the greater of 101% of 1989's MAAC *or* last year's MAAC plus the difference between last year's MAAC and 115% of the current prevailing charge.

3 In addition to the MAAC, special charge limits also apply to certain procedures, including cataract surgery. The special charge limit is equal to 125% of the prevailing charge. This limit applies only to physicians whose reasonable charge payments were reduced as a result of the prevailing charge reduction.

4 Non-participating physicians who do not take assignment on claims in excess of $500 for elective surgery must inform the patient, in writing, of the charge for the procedure, the Medicare approved charge, and the beneficiaries estimated out-of-pocket expense.

5 If a non-participating physician has two fee schedules, one for Medicare and one for non-Medicare patients, you may not charge a higher fee for a service to Medicare patients than is charged to non-Medicare patients.

6 Due to the Gramm–Rudman law, payments through March 31, 1990 will be further reduced by 2.1%. Beginning April 1, 1990, the reduction will be 1.4%. At the same time, an inflation adjustment of 2% will be provided with three major exceptions:

(a) Primary care services including two ophthalmic office visits (Current Procedural Terminology codes 92002 and 92004) will be increased by the Medicare Economic Index (approximately 4.2%);

(b) Payment for radiology and anesthesiology services will be frozen; and

(c) Certain procedures considered to be overvalued, including 30 ophthalmic procedures, will be reduced (this is discussed in greater detail in the 1990 Budget Reconciliation Act section).

Third-party payer physician reimbursement

Reimbursement by other third-party payers varies depending on the type of contract and the specific payer:

1 Health maintenance organizations (HMOs) and Preferred Provider Organizations (PPOs) often reimburse using a fee schedule that represents anywhere from a 10 to 25% discount. Participating physicians agree to accept the fee schedule as payment in full.

2 Under traditional Blue Cross and Blue Shield insurance contracts, physicians are generally paid at a specified percentile of the usual and customary fee. Patients are responsible for paying the difference between the reimbursed amount and the actual charge.

3 Commercial insurance carriers also offer traditional, PPO, and HMO options. For traditional policies, commercial carriers generally reimburse on the basis of charges.

4 Other government payers, such as Medicaid, reimburse according to a fee schedule which is typically very low. Assignment must be accepted on all Medicaid claims.

Medicare facility reimbursement for cataract surgery

Reimbursement for the facility component in an ambulatory surgery center is based on a prospectively determined rate. All covered ambulatory surgery center procedures are currently classified into four separate payment groups. The payment rates for each group are:

1 group 1—$274;

2 group 2—$326;

3 group 3—$351; and

4 group 4—$399.

The rates are also adjusted for area wage differences. Cataract extractions with the insertion of intraocular lens (IOL) prosthesis (codes 66983 and 66984) are considered to be two separate procedures for payment purposes and are reimbursed at one and one-half times the group 4 rate.

There are several other provisions related to cataract surgery.

1 Currently, payment for IOL implant is made at 80% of the reasonable charge. Beginning July 1, 1988, the reasonable charge may not exceed the actual acquisition cost plus a handling fee which is not to exceed 5% of the acquisition cost. Either the surgery center or the physician may bill for the lens.

2 Medicare will not routinely pay for pre-cataract surgery examinations other than a comprehensive eye examination and an A- or B-scan. Other tests will be reimbursed only if there is a diagnosis in addition to cataracts and the need for the other test is fully documented.

3 The prevailing charge for A-mode ophthalmic ultrasound procedures (codes 76511, 76516, and 76519) may not exceed 5% of the prevailing charge for an extracapsular cataract extraction (ECCE) with lens implant (code 66984).

4 Ophthalmologists involved in a Food and Drug Administration (FDA) monitored study of an IOL are subject to special coverage rules. All eye care related to the study must be provided by the investigating ophthalmologist. Care provided by another practitioner may only be covered if it is under the direction of the investigator and there is an agreement to provide information to the investigator. When billing for these services, all claims should be annotated with the two-digit modifier—LS.

5 Payment may be made under Medicare for cataract glasses and contact lenses furnished to patients. Payment is based on the reasonable charge for the glasses and lenses and a reasonable charge for related services (i.e. prescription and fitting of contact lens, with medical supervision of adaptation). Payment for the frames is based on the cost of a *standard pair of frames only*. If a patient selects a pair of higher priced frames (i.e. deluxe frames) the participating physician may charge the beneficiary for the difference between the standard frames and the deluxe frames.

On August 18, 1989, proposed regulations were published which would result in several changes to the current reimbursement methodology for cataracts and other types of ambulatory surgery. These regulations are still pending and it is unclear when they will be finalized. Once finalized, however, they may be retroactive to as early as July 1, 1988. The implications of a retroactive ruling would certainly be a financial as well as an administrative nightmare. Hopefully the difficulty of implementing this type of retroactive payment will prevent the ruling. The major provisions include.

1 The number of payment groups would be increased from four to six, ranging in price from $250 to $620.

2 Cataract extractions with lens insertions (codes 66983 and 66984) would be moved from group 4 to group 6. Because of this change, reimbursement would no longer be made at one and one-half times the payment rate.

3 Payment for the IOL implant would be added to the facility payment rate for cataract procedures (codes 66983, 66984, and 66985). The add-on payment would be a flat $200 per lens.

1990 Budget Reconciliation Act

The Budget Reconciliation Act was passed by Congress on November 22, 1989. This bill included some of the most significant changes in physician reimbursement since the Medicare program was enacted. These provisions will have far-reaching implications for all physicians, particularly those in specialties such as ophthalmology which are so Medicare dependent. The major provisions which will affect ophthalmology are summarized below.

1 Beginning in 1992 physicians will be paid according to a resource-based relative value scale (RBRVS). The fee schedule will be based on the Hsaio study after incorporating recommendations made by the Physician Payment Review Commission. The relative value units will be reviewed and adjusted at least every 5 years. The fee schedule will be phased in over 5 years from 1992 to 1996 on the following basis:

    (a) in 1992, charges within 85% and 115% of the fee schedule would be paid at the fee schedule rate;

    (b) charges less than 85% or greater than 115% of the fee schedule would be increased or decreased by 15% in 1992;

    (c) the remaining difference will be reduced by 25% each year; and

    (d) in 1996, all payments will be based on the fee schedule.

2 Non-participating physicians will be paid at 95% of the fee schedule amount.

3 The Secretary of the Department of Health and Human Services (HHS) is required to recommend a Medicare voluntary performance standard (MVPS) each year on April 15. The Physician Payment Review Commission will also recommend an MVPS. The MVPS is an estimate of the rate at which part B expenditures should grow during the subsequent fiscal year. It will be based on the growth in beneficiaries, inflation, changes in volume and technology as well as other factors. The MVPS, in comparison to the previous year's actual performance, will be used by Congress to set the annual updates in the conversion factor for the fee schedule.

4 Limits will also be placed on how much physicians may charge beneficiaries on unassigned claims. In 1991, charges will be limited to 125% of the prevailing charge. In 1992 and 1993, the limit will drop to 120% and 115% respectively. In addition, beginning in April 1990, physicians must accept assignment for beneficiaries with incomes low enough to qualify for Medicaid. In September 1990 physicians will also have to submit claims for beneficiaries, whether or not assignment is accepted.

5 Beginning April 1, 1990 and until 1992 when the RBRVS fee schedule is implemented, fees for "overpriced" procedures will be reduced by one-third of the amount determined to be overpriced. Over 500 procedures are affected, including 30 ophthalmic procedures. The annual reductions range from 6% for cataract extractions with an IOL implant to 12% for fluorescein photography.

Peer review organizations

Effective from April 1, 1989 all ophthalmologists are required to obtain prior approval for cataract surgery performed on Medicare patients. The Peer Review Organization (PRO) in each State is responsible for administering the program. The approval criteria varies from State to State but the majority of States require vision of 20/50 or less by Snellen, contrast, or glare measurement as the criteria for surgery. Most PROs use a phone-in process and often an authorization number can be provided immediately. This authorization number must appear on the claim submitted to the Health Care Financing Administration (HCFA). Without this number the claim will not be processed. Approvals are usually good for between 7 and 30 days. Very few procedures

have been denied and most of the administrative problems are generated by missing information. The caller should have the following information on hand:

1 patient name, sex, date of birth, address, and Medicare ID number;
2 surgeon's name, address, telephone number, license number, and facility provider number; and
3 patient history and reason for surgery.

It is important to know the process as well as the criteria used in your State in order to incorporate it into the office routine.

Under a 2-year demonstration project recently initiated by HCFA, PROs will begin reviewing care provided in physician offices. The Wisconsin PRO was selected to head the project with PROs in six other States participating as well. Approximately 120 physicians in each State will be asked to participate in the project on a volunteer basis. The review will focus on 16 common medical conditions, including cataracts. It is expected that the care provided for approximately 1–2% of all beneficiaries in the seven States will be reviewed.

Medical necessity

Medicare coverage is limited to those services which are determined to be "medically necessary." In some instances, the physician may be liable for services rendered to Medicare beneficiaries which are deemed medically unnecessary. In particular non-participating physicians who provide services to beneficiaries on an unassigned basis which are subsequently determined as not reasonable and necessary must refund any amounts collected from the beneficiary. The two circumstances under which the physician would not be required to make a refund are:

1 you did not know, or could not reasonably have expected to know that Medicare would not pay for the service; or
2 the beneficiary was notified that Medicare would not pay for the service prior to it being furnished, and the beneficiary agreed to pay for it.

In the case of a participating physician where

the service is determined to be unnecessary, the fee cannot be collected unless the patient was informed in advance that Medicare may not pay for the service and the patient agrees to pay if payment is denied. In either case, it is extremely important that proper documentation be used to support any claims which might be denied. An example of the type of notices which will satisfy the advance notice requirements and protect you from liability is as follows:

Physician Notice

Medicare will only pay for services that it determines to be 'reasonable and necessary' under section 1862(a)(1) of the Medicare law. If Medicare determines that a particular service, although it would otherwise be covered, is 'not reasonable and necessary' under Medicare program standards, Medicare will deny payment for that service. I believe that, in your case, Medicare is likely to deny payment for (*specify service*) for the following reasons: (*state reasons for your belief*).*

Beneficiary Agreement

I have been notified by my physician that he or she believes that, in my case, Medicare is likely to deny payment for the services identified above, for the reasons stated. If Medicare denies payment, I agree to be personally and fully responsible for payment.

Signed,
(*beneficiary signature*).

Medicare billing

Claim forms/coding

The HCFA 1500 is the insurance claim form used for services rendered to Medicare beneficiaries. Full completion of this form along with proper documentation are the key to

*Source: *Medicare Bulletin*, Empire Blue Cross and Blue Shield, September 1988.

accurate and timely payment. Although many physicians currently submit their claims using a superbill, there have been some discussions about increasing physician use of the 1500. While it is unlikely that HCFA will mandate submission of the 1500, they are beginning to require that superbills contain all the same information fields contained on the 1500. This may render superbills obsolete in the near future.

The coding system used for Medicare is the Health Care Financing Administration Common Procedure Coding System (HCPCS) and it is based on the five digit CPT alpha–numeric codes. In addition to the CPT codes, which comprise 95% of all Medicare Part B coding, there are nationwide codes assigned by HCFA for services not contained in the CPT system. Effective for claims submitted on or after January 1, 1990, all *carrier-assigned local codes* have been eliminated. All physicians should have been notified of this change and received a list of replacement codes.

On April 1, 1989 two other major data requirements became effective. Section 202 of the Medicare Catastrophic Bill required the reporting of diagnostic codes on each request for payment under Part B of Medicare. The coding system to be used is the International Classification of Diseases, Ninth Revision, Clinical Modification (ICD-9-CM). The second requirement is the specific identification of all providers relative to the services billed. This includes the billing, rendering, ordering, or referring provider. Identifying information (name and provider ID number) is required on the ordering and referring physician on any claim in which the provider did not initiate the service being billed. This would include, for example, a clinical lab as the biller and the physician as the ordering provider.

Modifiers

Modifiers are used when there is a specific circumstance which must be identified. The modifier is either a two-digit number placed after the usual procedure code or it may be reported by a separate five-digit code. For example, if multiple procedures are performed at the same operative session, the major procedure is reported as listed. The secondary procedure is identified by adding modifier -51 to the second procedure code or by using code number 09951. An example specific to ophthalmology is when an optometrist performs the postoperative management for a cataract case. In this case the surgeon reports the surgical procedure by adding modifier -54 to the procedure code for cataract surgery while the optometrist adds modifier -55.

Filing requirements

All claims must be filed by the provider no later than the end of the calendar year following the year in which the service was furnished. If, however, the service was furnished in the last 3 months of the year, it can be treated as though the service was furnished in the subsequent year. Currently all claims are held for 14 days before they can be paid. Participating physicians claims are paid within 18 days while nonparticipating claims are paid with 25 days.

General billing issues

Specific issues to be aware of for Medicare billing include.

1 Refractive procedures are not covered. Many ophthalmologists, however, do not separately identify the refraction when billing for a diagnostic examination. The carrier will automatically exclude a portion of the charge unless a separate charge has been identified or the claim indicates that a refraction was not performed. Beginning March 1, 1990 if a refraction was not performed, it must be indicated on the claim.

Guidelines provided to the carriers by HCFA state that in a comprehensive eye examination, the value of the refraction is about 20% of the total charge. In a follow-up examination, the percentage may be as high as 33.3%. Depending on your own fee structure, it may be advantageous to separately identify the charge for the refraction rather than having the carrier calculate it independently.

2 All carriers are required to conduct pre- and postpayment medical review. HCFA has mandated certain medical necessity prepay-

ment screens which are specific to the field of ophthalmology. These include:

(a) screens which identify claims involving replacement of an unusually large number of postcataract external prosthetic contact lenses; and

(b) screens which determine that the A-mode scan was performed in conjunction with cataract surgery.

It is important to maintain clear and detailed documentation for all claims. It is also advantageous for a member of your staff to develop a working relationship with a contact person at the carrier. This will ensure that when a problem arises someone will follow through and assist the practice in resolving it. It will also help the staff identify those issues which the carrier is likely to focus on in reviewing claims.

Payment policies and patient relations

The ophthalmologist's office should have clearly established payment policies which are not only communicated to the office staff but to patients as well. From the office staff's perspective, it is important that billing procedures be delineated for each payer and that one individual be designated as having overall responsibility for the billing process. A list of all managed care plans with which the physician participates should be available to each member of the staff. Computerized billing systems and electronic submissions can be extremely useful in standardizing procedures, reducing errors, and increasing efficiency.

Electronic claims

Over 35% of all Medicare physician claims are currently being submitted electronically. This includes claims submitted directly by the provider to the Medicare carrier via personal computer, diskette or other means as well as those claims submitted through a billing service or other vendor. Many companies will take care of all billing activities, including conversion of paper claims into an electronic format, for a monthly fee.

By ensuring the accuracy and completeness of the claim, electronic submissions can significantly reduce the number of claims rejected by the carrier. Experts within the industry suggest that 30% of paper claims are rejected at the outset compared to a very small percentage of electronic claims. Medicare had also established incentives for electronic submissions by guaranteeing faster turnaround times. This incentive, however, was eliminated when a minimum floor (14 days) was created for the number of days in which a claim could be paid. At some point in the future this incentive may be reinstated. HCFA, in conjunction with the private insurance carriers, is now studying various ways of promoting electronic submissions as well as the best format to be used.

Physicians can save in other ways through electronic submissions by reducing postage costs and freeing up office staff to perform other functions. It is estimated that it costs approximately $1.50–2.00 to submit a claim manually compared to less than $1 for an electronic claim. Electronic claims submission is clearly one option to be considered to reduce costs and increase the efficiency of your office.

Collection policies

Specific payment policies are also needed regarding the collection of copayments and deductibles and the treatment of late/delinquent payments. Certain techniques, for example, are extremely effective in pursuing unpaid bills:
1 telephone calls to the delinquent patient should be made between 5 and 7 p.m. when they are more likely to be home. Male voices are often more effective;
2 letters sent to the patient should indicate that the matter will be referred to a collection agency and that the credit card bureau will be notified if payment is not received;
3 collection agencies can be used for bills above a certain dollar threshold that have been outstanding for more than a specified time period;
4 patients should be notified that they will not be seen except in an emergency within a specified time frame; and
5 careful documentation should be kept including a record of all unanswered calls.

Routine waivers of required coinsurance and deductibles under Medicare is expressly prohibited. If there is evidence that this is occurring, the physician's actual charge will be assumed to be reduced and the customary charge screens will be reduced by 20%. If the physician makes a reasonable collection effort, failure to collect the payment is not considered a reduction in the charge. If the physician advertizes his or her intention to waive the coinsurance, if charges to Medicare beneficiaries are higher than those made to other persons for similar services, or if waivers are made for the majority of Medicare patients, this will be considered evidence that the actual charge has been reduced.

Patients should be given a written statement of all payment policies. This will help inform the patient of what is expected, reduce the possibility of subsequent misunderstandings and reduce the time your office staff will have to spend explaining the policy to patients.

To participate or not participate

The decision on whether to participate in the Medicare program should be made after a careful evaluation of all the factors involved. Participating physicians are given a number of incentives including:
1 higher prevailing charges;
2 faster payment of claims;
3 exempt from financial disclosure requirements for elective procedures over $500;
4 no limits on actual charges which enables you to maintain a single fee schedule for all patients; and
5 automatic forwarding of claims to the patient's supplemental insurer.

In order to make this decision, physicians should identify:
1 the most frequently performed procedures;
2 the number of times the procedure will be provided;
3 the percentage of claims which you are likely to accept assignment on;
4 the 1990 MAAC; and
5 the 1990 participating approved amount for each procedure.
This will enable you to determine how much you are likely to gain or lose by participating. There are several other equally important

issues, however, which should be considered.

1 The percentage of ophthalmologists who participate in the local area. If a high percentage is participating, you may be at a competitive disadvantage if you do not participate.

2 If you are already experiencing difficulty in collecting from Medicare patients, participating in the Medicare program may resolve some of these problems.

3 If you are already accepting assignment on a large proportion of claims, participating may simplify matters for you and your office staff without having a significant financial impact.

4 If you participated in previous years, a decision to stop participating may be viewed negatively by your patients.

Whatever decision is made, patients should be notified of your status and made aware of the billing implications. This is particularly important if you decide not to participate in 1990 when reimbursement for many ophthalmic procedures will be reduced even further.

Conclusion

A physician office's billing system is one of the most critical components in a practice's fiscal health and this is important for the patient as well as the physician. Even the best known clinician and the most effective marketing program cannot guarantee a steady stream of income if the billing process is inefficient. It is,

therefore, extremely important that the practice be knowledgeable about the various payment rules used by third-party payers. In addition to designating one individual who is responsible for all billing functions, the physician should have a basic understanding of the system in order to provide direction to the office staff. One way of reducing errors, speeding up turn-around time, and increasing office efficiency is to submit claims electronically either directly or through a billing service or other vendor. Accurate and full documentation is another key factor to ensure timely payment of claims. It is essential to support your case in the unfortunate event of an audit.

With the constant barrage of cuts and the impending changes in the Medicare reimbursement system, physicians must stay abreast of new developments which regularly come from both Washington and the private sector. Cataract PPO demonstrations, for example, have been widely discussed in the ophthalmology journals and may in fact become a reality before 1991. The demonstrations which are intended to achieve further savings for HCFA will be focused on "the one price cataract" which will include both the professional and facility fees. Being aware of these types of initiatives as well as local market conditions will help you to develop your own policies and strategies to achieve your individual practice goals.

30: AIDS, Cataracts, and the Ophthalmologist

WILLIAM L. HOPPES

As of November 30, 1990, 157 525 cases of the acquired immune deficiency syndrome (AIDS) had been reported in the USA [1]. An estimated 1 million persons are infected with human immunodeficiency virus (HIV) in this country. Persons at increased risk for HIV infection include male homosexuals, intravenous drug abusers, promiscuous heterosexuals, children born to HIV positive mothers, and recipients of multiple units of blood and blood products (including hemophiliacs) prior to April, 1985, when universal HIV testing of all blood products was initiated. Heterosexual cases are now 5% of all AIDS in the USA, with the cases in 1990 showing a 38% increase over the number reported during 1989. This increase is the largest percentage increase of any risk group, and is primarily, but not exclusively, due to heterosexual contact with other risk groups. In larger urban areas, HIV infection is now seen in heterosexuals where neither partner belongs to one of the established risk groups. Asymptomatic HIV-infected individuals often go undetected in the health-care setting, and thus precautions must be taken by all health-care workers with all patients to prevent occupational exposures.

Detailed guidelines for protection of health-care workers against HIV and hepatitis B virus (HBV) have been published [2]. The mode of transmission of HIV is similar to HBV, however, the potential for occupational transmission of HBV is much greater than that of HIV. Although much more is known about transmission of HBV than of HIV, practices known to be effective in prevention of HBV in the workplace should decrease chances of transmission of HIV and other blood-borne pathogens. HBV and HIV may be acquired by percutaneous inoculation or contact of open wounds, non-intact skin (chapped, abraded, weeping, dermatitis), and mucous membranes with blood, or blood-contaminated body fluids or to concentrated virus in a laboratory. Blood is the most important fluid involved in transmission and precautions should be geared to prevention of exposures to blood and any fluid which is visibly contaminated with blood. HBV vaccine is essential in the protection of persons exposed to these substances.

The degree of risk of blood exposure can be estimated by the probability that blood contains either HBV or HIV, the immune status of the person exposed, and the efficiency of transmission of the virus. The probability of blood being HBsAg positive varies from 1 to 3 per 1000 in the general population to 5–15% in high-risk groups including natives of China, south-east Asia, sub-Saharan Africa, most Pacific islands, and the Amazon Basin; residents of institutions for the mentally retarded, intravenous drug abusers, active homosexual males, and household contacts of chronic carriers (both sexual and non-sexual). The risk of transmission of HBV from a single needle stick in a person who has received neither HBV vaccine or postexposure prophylaxis is 6–30%. The risk of one needle-stick exposure to HIV positive blood is approximately 0.5%; the risk of non-intact skin or mucous membrane contact is far less, but there are inadequate data to quantitate that risk [3].

In 1987, the Center for Disease Control (CDC) estimated 300 000 HBV infections in the

USA per year. Of these 25% develop acute hepatitis, and 6–10% become chronic HBV carriers with increased risk for chronic active hepatitis, cirrhosis, and primary liver cancer, and are contagious risks for others. The CDC estimates that of health-care workers whose jobs entail exposure to blood, 12 000 per year become infected with HBV. Of these, 500–600 are hospitalized, 700–1200 become HBV carriers, and 250 will die, 12–15 from fulminant hepatitis, 170–200 from cirrhosis, and 40–50 from liver cancer. Approximately 10–30% of all health-care and dental workers show serologic evidence of past or present HBV infection. HBV vaccine, which should be provided *at no cost* to all health-care workers who are exposed to blood, will provide greater than 90% protection for 7 or more years. If given within 1 week of exposure to HBV, vaccine is 70–88% protective. Addition of hepatitis B immunoglobulin (HBIG) to postexposure prophylaxis increases the protection to 90% [3].

As of September 19, 1988, there were 3182 health-care workers who had been diagnosed with AIDS. Of these, 95% admitted to high risk behavior. In the remaining 5%, or 169 workers, the means of HIV infection is of undetermined source. Twenty-eight workers had incomplete information available (died or refused interview), and 97 cases are still being investigated. Of the 44 workers in whom information is complete, there are nine nursing assistants, eight physicians (four surgeons), eight housekeeping or maintenance workers, six nurses, four laboratory technicians, two respiratory therapists, one dentist, one paramedic, one embalmer, and four who had no patient contact. Eighteen workers had blood exposures, none were to known HIV positive patients, and there were no seroconversions documented by blood samples before and after the contacts [3].

Fear and anxiety out of proportion to documented risk on the part of health-care workers may lead to decreased quality and access to medical care for persons who are HIV positive, and discourage health-care workers from working in areas which they perceive as placing them at greater risk of HIV exposure. The goal of the medical community should be to stress protective guidelines which should make the risk acceptable to most health-care workers. Retrospective reviews of instances of occupational transmission of HIV shed no light on the risk per exposure. Only carefully controlled prospective studies will determine the true risk. Information that should provide more of a sense of security to health-care workers include the facts that the demographics of AIDS cases in the USA and Africa are the same in health-care workers as in non-health-care workers. In the USA, health-care workers make up 5.5% of the work force, and 5.5% of reported cases of AIDS in adults, indicating that careful studies of large numbers of HIV exposures are necessary to discover the apparent small additional risk of working in the health-care field [4].

There are several ongoing prospective studies of the risk of HIV exposures in health-care workers [5–11]. Data from the CDC as of October, 1990 show four documented seroconversions in 1237 injuries with sharp instruments (0.32%), 0/170 mucous membrane exposures, and 0/88 non-intact skin exposures [9]. San Francisco General Hospital has reported only one seroconversion following a "severe needle stick" out of 758 health-care workers tested (0.34%) [12]. There were no delayed seroconversions, and a large number of their workers were tested with the polymerase chain reaction (PCR), a very sensitive method of detection of HIV antigen in clinical specimens [11]. In more than 1300 blood exposures studied by the National Institute of Health (NIH), there were no seroconversions with skin or mucous membrane exposures, and only one (0.31%) following sharp injuries. Many of their subjects were studied with p24 antigen detection and PCR, and the conclusion was that if seronegative latent infection following occupational exposure exists at all, it must be very rare [10]. The known seroconversions that have been reported in the literature have been dramatic needle sticks; milder injuries are probably of less risk.

Several studies have shown that surgeons including ophthalmologists are at higher risk of HBV infection compared to other health-care workers, with trauma and operating rooms having the highest risks [13]. The operating room is also a common site for needle-stick

Table 30.1 Surgical risks of blood exposure [15]

	SP	SMMC/100 SP	SI/100 SP
Cardiothoracic	33	182	9
General	124	63	10
Gynecology	86	91	15
Orthopedic	116	52	3
Trauma	37	158	3

SP: Surgical procedures, SMMC: skin/mucous membrane contacts, SI: sharp injuries.

injuries to nurses [14]. A recent CDC study has further delineated surgical risks of blood exposures [15]. The data is summarized in Table 30.1. This was a four hospital study, one inner-city and one suburban hospital each in a high- and low-incidence AIDS area. There were 334 skin/mucous membrane contacts (SMMC) per 174 surgical procedures (SP), and in 44% of the cases, there was more than one SMMC. There were 33 sharp injuries (SI) per 32 SP, with one case having two SI. Gynecologic surgical procedures had 15% SI, all other procedures combined had only 6%. Out of 33 SI, 22 (67%) were due to suture needles, 16 (48%) were due to sharps held by co-workers, and nine (27%) due to use of fingers to guide the needle or hold tissue. The most common victims of needle sticks were residents and attending surgeons. The most common site was the non-dominant forefinger, and the suture needle was the most likely source of SI. The most obvious protective measure would be a thimble for the non-dominant forefinger. The most promising finding was that no one has ever seroconverted after a non-hollow needle stick injury! Sharp injuries occurred in only 1/40 (2.5%) of exposures to patients who were known to be HIV positive, and in 32/356 (9%) of patients where the HIV status was positive, but unknown at the time of surgery. This would seem to support the findings of others that the identification of high risk or HIV positive patients should be a measure taken in addition to general blood and body fluid precautions (BBFP).

Precautions for ophthalmologists should be the same as for any surgeon. Universal BBFP assumes that all patients' blood and secretions are potentially infectious. Fluids with which precautions are indicated include blood, amniotic fluid, pericardial fluid, peritoneal fluid, pleural fluid, synovial fluid, cerebrospinal fluid, semen, cervicovaginal secretions, and any body fluid visibly contaminated with blood. There have been no documented HIV or HBV transmissions with feces, nasal secretions, sputum, sweat, tears, urine, or vomitus. Saliva is of concern primarily in the dental setting when it is contaminated with blood. HIV transmission has been documented epidemiologically only with blood, semen, and cervicovaginal secretions.

Guidelines incorporated in universal precautions are published by the CDC for health-care worker exposures to blood or blood-stained body fluids [2]. Hands and other skin surfaces should be washed immediately with soap and water or waterless antiseptic hand cleansers. Gloves should be worn when blood exposure is anticipated. Hands should always be washed after gloves are removed, even if the gloves appear to be intact. Protective eyewear and masks to cover the nose and mouth or total face shields should be worn if splash of blood is anticipated. Impervious gowns or aprons should be worn for heavy blood exposures such as childbirth. Blood spills should be cleaned up with Environmental Protection Agency (EPA) approved germicides or a 1:100 solution of household bleach; gloves should always be worn. Visible blood should first be removed with disposable towels, the site decontaminated with the appropriate germicide, and hands washed after gloves are removed. Soiled cleaning equipment should be cleaned and decontaminated or disposed of in plastic bags. Clothing and laundry should be bagged in leak-proof bags and processed by the normal washing cycle.

Rubber gloves do not protect against injuries from sharp instruments. All health-care workers should take precautions against injuries by needles, scalpel blades, and other sharps during procedures, cleaning of used instruments, and disposal of used sharps after procedures. Needles should not be recapped, bent or broken by hand, removed from disposable syringes, or otherwise manipulated.

All sharps should be placed in puncture-proof containers located in patient care areas. Specific operating room recommendations include avoidance of hand-passing of sharp instruments, use of heavy puncture-proof gloves where possible (as in some orthopedic procedures), development of techniques to minimize manipulation of needles by feel, use of thimbles, use of electrocautery instead of sutures when possible, and exclusion of persons in training from certain activities.

When a needle-stick injury occurs, the victim should immediately stop what he or she is doing, squeeze the area involved to cause bleeding, vigorously clean the site, and report the incident to the appropriate supervisor. Policies should be in force, according to local laws, for obtaining consent for HIV and HBV testing of the source of the injury, and for providing for situations where consent cannot be obtained, or is refused. Pre- and post-test counseling of the worker is essential. If the source is HBV positive, and the health-care worker has not been vaccinated against HBV, vaccine should be initiated, and HBIG administered if the injury is not more than 1 week old. If the health-care worker has received HBV vaccine, serological testing for HBsAb should be done, and if less than 10 U by radio-immunoassay (RIA) or a negative enzyme-linked immunoadsorbent assay (ELISA) is found, the worker should receive one booster dose of vaccine and one dose of HBIG. If the source is HIV positive, the worker should be counseled, examined, tested for HIV, advised to report any febrile illness within 12 weeks of the injury (fever, rash, lymphadenopathy), and retested at 6 weeks, 3 months, and 6 months (and at 1 year in the CDC needle-stick study). During the first 6–12 weeks the worker should refrain from donating blood, and should abstain from sex, or engage in safe sex practices. Strict confidentiality should be maintained.

There is considerable controversy as to whether or not people injured via needle-stick should be offered zidovudine (AZT) as post-exposure prophylaxis [15]. Data from animal studies are inadequate to support or reject the use of AZT in this situation. There are insufficient data in humans regarding efficacy or safety, though there are now two reports of failure of postexposure AZT prophylaxis [16,17]. Studies [9,10,12,18] have shown that healthy health-care workers tolerate AZT with only mild and reversible side effects such as nausea, vomiting, and headaches in less than half of the subjects. Mild anemia and granulocytopenia occur in only 5%. On the reverse side, AZT has been associated with vaginal tumors in rats. In the early CDC studies, 20% of physicians took AZT as opposed to 9% of other health-care workers. Presently, 50% of health-care workers in the CDC studies are electing to take AZT [9]. The dose and duration of treatment varies from 400 to 1200 mg per day for 4–6 weeks. Although the option of taking AZT should probably be offered to all health-care workers, they should be informed that diverse opinions exist, and that definite recommendations for or against the use of AZT cannot be made. If post-exposure AZT is offered, policies should be in place to provide the drug within 1 hour of exposure and stop as soon as the source is proven to be HIV negative.

Another controversy in the realm of HIV infection is that of the infected health-care worker, and this has been amplified by the recent report of a dentist who may have transmitted HIV to as many as three patients during invasive dental procedures [19]. The subject has been extensively reviewed in a position paper written by experts in infection control and hospital epidemiology across the USA [20]. A number of salient points in this paper are worth reviewing. Transfer of blood from a patient to a health-care worker is far more common than the reverse situation of the health-care worker's blood being injected into the patient. Oral and gynecology surgeons have been infrequent sources of HBV infection in their patients. In these cases, the health-care workers have been shown to have at least 100 million viral particles per ml of blood, an amount considerably higher than the estimated 1–100 viral particles in 1 ml of blood in an HIV positive patient. The CDC recommends that a surgeon who has been shown to have transmitted HBV through a puncture wound during surgery, from weeping skin lesions, or micro-lacerations should be excluded from further practice involving invasive procedures [2].

In the position paper, the authors felt that, in the case of the dentist and the possible HIV transmission, such a single or rare situation should not become the basis for policy, but should rather be a stimulus for careful studies to determine the true risk. It was stated that some issues cannot be resolved at this time with our present level of knowledge.

The health-care worker cannot ethically or legally deny treatment to an HIV-infected patient. The obligation of a patient to receive care from an HIV-infected health-care worker is less clear. They felt that a health-care worker who is HIV positive should not be "broadly prohibited from practice" [20]. There have been 19 outbreaks world-wide, over the past 20 years, where health-care workers have transmitted HBV to patients during vaginal hysterectomy, oral, major pelvic, or cardiac surgery. The risk is increased in the situation of the chronically infected worker with dermatitis on the hands. The risk is still small, since there are 4000 health-care workers in the USA performing invasive procedures who are HBV positive.

Professional societies need to identify high-risk procedures and encourage development of techniques to minimize manipulation by feel of sharps not directly visualized. Other protective measures would include wire-mesh gloves, exclusion of persons in training from certain activities, avoidance of direct hand-to-hand passage of sharps by use of instrument trays placed closer to the field, and use of cautery instead of sutures.

HBV mortality averages 1–2%. HIV mortality is much higher, but transmission rates are substantially lower. HIV positive health-care workers could voluntarily not perform high-risk procedures known to have transmitted HBV in the past. The alternative would be to receive counseling in order to help lower risk. However, the risk of transmission of HIV is felt to be so small that mandatory proscriptions are not justified, and would decrease the voluntary coming forward for counseling. This might then result in calls for mandatory testing for health-care workers who perform high-risk

procedures, which was felt to be "far out of proportion to the magnitude of risk" [20].

When HIV infected workers become mentally or physically impaired, they must cease practice. Comprehensive programs are needed to evaluate the ability of workers to carry out their duties.

Confidentiality is essential in handling information on HIV positive workers. Their medical records should be kept separate from other medical records, and laboratory results should not be entered in hospital computer systems. This should include evaluation for needle stick protocols and the worker's compensation claims for work-related exposures. Personnel should never discuss the presence, absence, or numbers of HIV infected health-care workers in an institution, because of the possibility of inadvertent breaches of confidentiality.

The risks of exposures to infections in the hospital setting for the HIV infected worker is not great if usual precautions are observed. No health-care worker susceptible to varicella, rubella, or measles should care for patients with these conditions, irrespective of their immune status! If the worker has a chronic cough, he or she should be evaluated for tuberculosis. All other AIDS-associated infections are acquired by breaks in technique (*Salmonella*, cytomegalovirus, herpes simplex virus), or colonized from infancy (*Pneumocystis carinii*), or are not transmitted from person to person (*Toxoplasma, Mycobacterium avium-intracellulare, Cryptococcus*).

The final controversy involves testing and disclosure of a health-care worker's HIV status. With the exception of the situation where a patient is clearly exposed to a worker's blood, the worker should not be required to disclose HIV/HBV status to any patient. The risk to the patient is so low, and the jeopardy to the health-care worker's career is so overwhelming, that routine disclosure is not felt to be justified. Direct questions from patients should be discussed by an experienced individual in the above manner, or answered indirectly, and have further questions referred to administration, who should handle them with strict confidentiality. The health-care worker who is a source of patient exposure is ethically obligated to be tested, and be sanctioned, if they refuse. Patients should be notified of the exposure, but not the name of the source, or exact nature of the incident. They should be informed of the worker's HIV/HBV/HCV status, be counseled, offered effective postexposure prophylaxis, and have long-term medical follow-up arranged.

Baseline testing of the exposed patient should be done after informing them of the importance (in subsequent claims against the institution) of a negative test, and the risks of a positive test. If this is refused, an attempt should be made to get a carefully identified serum for storage and later testing for evidence. If this is also refused, the patient should be asked to sign a formal document attesting to this refusal.

Finally, health-care workers need not be routinely tested nor have mandatory screening for HIV/HBV unless they are the source of a patient's exposure. Policies to cover all contingencies should be drawn up by hospital attorneys and approved by the board.

References

1 *AIDS, Data for Ohio and the United States: US data through November 30, 1990, Ohio data through December 31, 1990.* Ohio: Ohio Department of Health, AIDS Activities Unit.

2 Guidelines for prevention of transmission of human immunodeficiency virus and hepatitis B virus to health-care and public-safety workers. *MMWR* 1989; **38** (RR S–6).

3 Guidelines for prevention of transmission of human immunodeficiency virus and hepatitis B to health-care and public-safety workers. *MMWR* 1989; **38**: 5–7.

4 Stapleton JT. HIV transmission, healthcare workers and media hype. *Infect Control Hosp Epidemiol* 1989; **10**: 503–4.

5 Marcus R, the CDC Cooperative Needlestick Surveillance Group. Surveillance of health care workers exposed to blood from patients infected with the human immunodeficiency virus. *N Engl J Med* 1988; **319**: 1118–23.

6 Henderson DK, Fahey BJ, Saah AJ, Schmitt JM, Lane HC. *Longitudinal assessment of risk for occupational/nosocomial transmission of human immunodeficiency virus, type 1 in health care workers.* Presented at the 1988 ICAAC Conference, New Orleans (Abstract 634).

7 Barnes DM. Health workers and AIDS: questions persist. *Science* 1988; **241**: 161–2.

8 Gerberding JL, Littell CG, Chambers HF et al. *Risk of occupational HIV transmission in intensively exposed health-care workers: follow-up.* Presented at the 1988 ICAAC Conference, New Orleans (Abstract 343).

9 Tokars JI, Marcus RA, Culver DH, McKibben PS, Bell DM. *Zidovudine (AZT) use after occupational exposure to HIV-infected blood.* Presented at the 1990 ICAAC Conference, Atlanta (Abstract 490).

10 Fahey BJ, Beekmann SE, Schmitt J, Fedio J, Henderson DK. *Assessment of risk for occupational HIV-1 infection in health-care workers and safety of zidovudine (AZT) administered as postexposure chemoprophylaxis for occupational exposures.* Presented at the 1990 ICAAC Conference, Atlanta (Abstract 960).

11 Gerberding JL, Littell C, Brown A, Ramiro N. *Cumulative risk of HIV and hepatitis B (HBV) among health care workers: longterm serologic followup and gene amplification for latent HIV infection.* Presented at the 1990 ICAAC Conference, Atlanta (Abstract 959).

12 Gerberding JL, Wugofski L, Berkvan G et al. *Facilitated surveillance and post-exposure AZT prophylaxis for health care workers: The San Francisco General Hospital model.* Presented at the 1990 ICAAC Conference, Atlanta (Abstract 961).

13 Rosenberg JL, Jones DP, Lipitz LR. Viral hepatitis: an occupational hazard to surgeons. *JAMA* 1973; **223**: 395–400.

14 Ruben FL, Norden CW, Rockwell K, Hruska E. Epidemiology of accidental needle-puncture wounds in hospital workers. *Am J Med Sci* 1983; **286**: 26–30.

15 Tokars JI, Marcus RA, Culver DH, Bell DM. *Blood contacts during surgical procedures.* Presented at the 1990 ICAAC Conference, Atlanta (Abstract 958).

16 Lange JMA, Boucher CAB, Hollak CEM et al. Failure of zidovudine prophylaxis after accidental exposure to HIV-1. *N Engl J Med* 1990; **322**: 1375–7.

17 Bernard N, Boulley AM, Perol R, Rouzioux C, Colau JC. Failure of zidovudine prophylaxis after exposure to HIV-1. *N Engl J Med* 1990; **323**: 915–16.

18 Lafon SW, Mooney BD, McMullen JP et al. *A double-blind, placebo-controlled study of the safety and efficacy of Retrovir as a chemoprophylactic agent in health care workers exposed to HIV.* Presented at the 1990 ICAAC Conference, Atlanta (Abstract 489).

19 Update: transmission of HIV infection during an invasive dental procedure in Florida. *MMWR* 1991; **40**: 21–33.

20 The Association for Practitioners in Infection Control; The Society of Hospital Epidemiologists of America. Position paper: the HIV-infected health care worker. *Am J Infect Control* 1990; **18**: 371–82.

Index

353